Official Textbook for the Nutrition Specialist Certification

Nutrition for Professionals

The Ultimate Nutrition Resource Textbook
for Health and Fitness Professionals

by Dr. Jane Pentz
and Michael McElveen
www.aasdn.org
info@aasdn.org

Cover Designed By The Fred Group, LLC

Nutrition for Professionals

Official Textbook for the Nutrition Specialist Certification

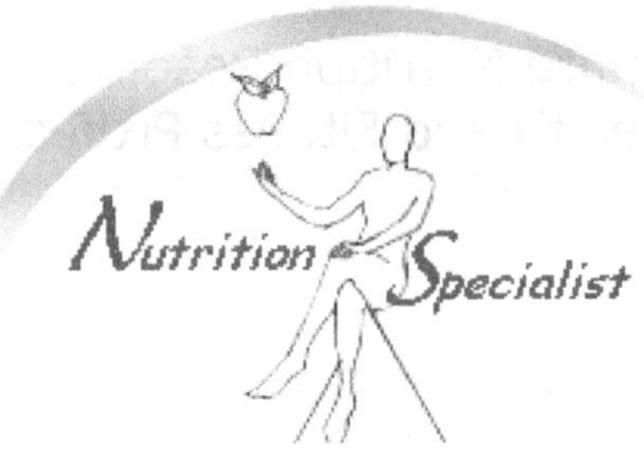

Printed in the United States of America
ISBN: 978-1-892426-22-2
Contact Information:
info@AASDN.org
http://aasdn.org/

Authors

Dr. Jane Pentz, PhD
Michael McElveen, MS, CSCS

Reviewers

Greg Salgueiro, MS, RD, LDN
Lisa Carr, BS, CPT
Erin Franklin, MS Nutrition, ASSA
Joseph F. Reza, RD, CPT, CHC

Speciality Reviewers

Marcy Pugliese, RD, LD, CSR: Chapter 6 – Nutrition and Disease
Lisa Carr, BS CPT – Chapter 11 – Coaching Skills
Carol Ballard, Psy.D – Chapter 11 - Coaching Skills – Counseling Versus Coaching
Greg Salgueiro, MS, RD, LDN: Chapter 13 – Building a Successful Nutrition Business

Biographies

Dr. Jane Pentz

Dr. Jane began her career in nutrition with an undergraduate degree in nutritional biochemistry from Vassar College while simultaneously raising three children. Her education continued at Tufts University where she received her Masters and Ph.D. degrees in Human Nutrition Sciences from the USDA Human Nutrition Research Center on Aging at Tufts University. In addition, Dr. Jane worked with the USDA Human Nutrition Research Center's team that completed ground breaking research on the effects of weight training in 80 and 90 year olds. As the president and CEO of Lifestyle Management Associates, a company dedicated to providing the highest quality nutrition education to professionals, Dr. Jane developed the Nutrition for Professionals course; authored the textbook for the course; and her book, "If You Don't Take Care of Your Body, Where Are You Going to Live!", contains the philosophy of healthy eating along with individualized menu plans. After almost a decade of experience, Dr. Jane along with several colleagues founded the American Academy of Sports Dietitians and Nutritionists (AASDN) has established the Nutrition Specialist Certification. Now, after over 30 years experience in the industry Dr. Pentz has refocused her efforts to educating children. She along with co-author Doug Dwyer have written a children's novel with a purpose! No – *Book one of the 8th Day Mystery Series* deals with the issue of obesity and school lunches. This first novel of the 8th Day series inspires and motivates young readers to make healthy school lunch choices.

Michael McElveen MS, RCRSP, CSCS

Michael McElveen holds a bachelors of science in health science and a master of science in sports medicine. Michael has been instructing the two-day Nutrition for Professionals course with Dr. Jane since July 2011. He began instructing the course after completing the sports nutrition certificate program through AASDN. Michael has experience working in a variety of settings including hospitals, other non-profit organizations and in the private setting. For the last eight years, Michael has worked full time in higher education. He currently serves as the associate director of wellness and recreation programs at Florida Southern College. He is an active member of the NSCA, currently serving on the membership committee, and an active in the NIRSA, currently serving on the editorial board for the *Recreational Sports Journal*, NIRSA's scholarly publication. In addition, Michael works with Florida Area Health Education Centers to facilitate tobacco cessation classes in the central Florida community. Michael's other credentials include: NSCA's certified strength and conditioning specialist, AASDN's nutrition specialist, NASM's performance enhancement specialist, FCB's certified tobacco treatment specialist and is a certified instructor through the American Red Cross.

Greg Salgueiro, MS, RD, LDN

Greg Salgueiro is a Registered and Licensed Dietitian in the State of Rhode Island. Greg began teaching the two-day Nutrition for Professionals course with Dr. Jane in 2008. He also held the position of the Director of Sports Nutrition for Lifestyle Management Associates and currently is the AASDN-BOC Program Director. Greg has experience in corporate, as well as hospital based, fitness and wellness programming. In the past he has been called upon to lecture on Sports Nutrition and Weight Management for the United States Coast Guard Academy. Greg has performed Sports Nutrition workshops for Division I Collegiate athletic teams and works with local high school and college athletes to help them fuel their bodies for optimal athletic performance. Greg is also certified through the Cooper Institute as a Health Promotion Director and through Totally Coached as an Intrinsic Coach. Greg is an ACSM Certified Health Fitness Specialist, an ACSM Certified Advanced Personal Trainer, and possesses a B.S. in Nutritional Sciences from Cornell University. Greg completed his Dietetic Internship at the Bronx VA Medical Center while simultaneously completing his M.S. in Clinical Nutrition at New York University. He also received advanced training at the Human Performance Institute in the Power of Full Engagement and works with clients to optimize human performance through energy management. Greg currently works full-time as the Manager of the Lifestyle Medicine Center and the Women's Medicine Collaborative for Lifespan.

Erin Coates, MS

Erin Coates has a Master's degree in Human Nutrition and is the owner of Body in Balance Wellness Consulting in Vancouver, BC, Canada. She has worked in various health settings, from an endocrinology practice to yoga centers to elementary schools, providing nutrition education to a wide client base. Erin is also a Senior Level Instructor for Lifestyle Management Associates and holds a 200-hour certification as a Registered Yoga Teacher through Yoga Alliance.

Marcy Pugliese, RD, LD, CSR

Marcy Pugliese, RD, LD, CSR is a Board Certified Specialist in Renal Nutrition and an Employee Wellness Consultant for Harbin Clinic, a multispecialty physician's group in Northwest Georgia. As a renal dietitian, she provides medical nutrition therapy, anemia management and mineral bone disease management for people on hemodialysis and peritoneal dialysis. She also initiated a chronic kidney disease medical nutrition therapy class for those with impaired kidney function but not on dialysis. As a member of the corporate wellness program, she writes nutrition blogs and tips, presents seminars on nutrition related topics including reading food labels, portion control, hypertension and hyperlipidemia, and collaborates on Harbin Strong wellness initiatives for her co-workers.
Mrs. Pugliese is an active member of the local and state Academy of Nutrition and

Dietetics having served as a board member for many years. She has taken her passion for nutrition, wellness and disease management home, where she is an avid gardener and food preservationist.

Joseph F. Reza, RD, CPT, CHC

Joseph has been a Medical Nutrition Therapist for 25 years working with patients as a Nutrition support Clinical Dietitian in various hospitals in Southern California. He is currently working as a consultant RD in Long Term Care, Skilled Nursing Facilities and Rehab Centers; he Has 13 years experience as an accomplished healthcare sales and marketing specialist. For over 25 years, Joseph has been coaching various class formats, currently he is Group Exercise Certified, teaching Indoor Cycling and Les Mills Body Pump classes. He has been a sports nutrition presenter since 1989, starting as a corporate gym employee educating over 200 personal trainers with the goal of keeping gym personal trainers current with sports nutrition education. Joseph currently works with clients primarily focusing on the elderly population with some type of medical nutrition therapy need and is a presenter for the Nutrition Specialist Certification program.

Lisa Carr, BS, CPT

Lisa holds a B.S. in Exercise Science from Bridgewater State College. Lisa is an ACE Certified Personal Trainer and Health Coach, as well as an AASDN Nutrition Specialist and Licensed Nutrition Manager Consultant. Lisa began instructing the two-day Nutrition for Professionals course in February 2013 after completing the sports nutrition certificate program through AASDN. Lisa has over 12 years of experience in the health, fitness and wellness industry and has worked in a variety of settings including hospitals and private, public and corporate based fitness facilities. Lisa worked for four years as an exercise physiologist in cardiac and pulmonary rehabilitation; a clinical wellness program that emphasized disease risk factor modification; and an exercise program for patients with Parkinson's disease. She also has six years of experience as a Wellness Director for a corporate fitness company, creating and implementing wellness education programs and directing health promotion initiatives. In 2011 Lisa incorporated and opened her own practice where she currently serves the Rhode Island community offering fitness programs for preschool aged children and adults, as well as nutrition seminars and individual nutrition consultations through AASDN. Lisa combines her nutrition and exercise expertise with health coaching, motivating her clients to tackle common barriers to weight management success. Lisa is passionate about educating, equipping and empowering her clients with knowledge and educational tools to improve their overall health and quality of life.

Questions for Professionals

- ✓ Are your clients not able to lose weight even after exercising an hour a day or five times a week?
- ✓ Are you confused about the role of supplements in fat utilization, muscle hypertrophy, and energy production?
- ✓ Are you unsure of what constitutes adequate protein intake necessary to build muscle?
- ✓ Are you frustrated because you can't seem to help your clients achieve their weight loss or performance goals?
- ✓ Have you been told that nutrition education is beyond your scope of practice?
- ✓ Would you like to incorporate nutrition services into your program while still adhering to all state licensure laws and the Academy of Nutrition and Dietetics guidelines?

The Nutrition for Professionals Textbook has been specifically designed to provide answers to these and many other questions facing fitness and wellness professionals, as well as educators and athletic trainers. This book contains all the details needed to incorporate nutrition services safely and professionally while still adhering to all state licensure laws and the Academy of Nutrition and Dietetics guidelines.

Background

AASDN was founded in 2001 with a mission to disseminate accurate, sound, scientific wellness information by qualified individuals. In 2005 AASDN created the AASDN Credentialing Commission as the credentialing body for the newly acquired Nutrition Specialist Certification. The Nutrition Specialist Certification Program was designed for fitness/wellness professionals who wish to incorporate a nutrition component into their wellness programming. The AASDN Nutrition Specialist Certification is the only non-regulatory nutrition certification program that includes all materials required to implement a nutrition program including documents and scripted programs. The AASDN Nutrition Specialist program is also the only non-regulatory nutrition certification program that includes unlimited sports dietitian support. Hence, The AASDN Nutrition Specialist Certification program standards provide safe, effective and legal programs to the public.

Also created in 2005, the Nutrition Manager Program allows Nutrition Specialists to work with more diversified populations and provide specialized services by working directly with an AASDN Sports Dietitian.

In 2009 AASDN partnered with the USDA Center for Nutrition Policy and Promotion. As a community partner, AASDN is committed to establishing programs that promote physical fitness and the Dietary Guidelines for Americans.

In January 2012, for the first time in 15 years, the USDA issued new guidelines for school meals. These new guidelines double the amounts of fruits and vegetables in school lunches and boost offerings of whole grain-rich foods. During the summer of 2012 AASDN was invited to join the National Alliance for Nutrition and Activity (NANA). NANA, a Center for Science in the Public Interest (www.cspinet.org) advocacy group, advocates federal policies and programs to promote healthy eating and physical activity to help reduce the illnesses, disabilities, premature deaths, and costs caused by diet and inactivity-related diseases, such as heart disease, cancer, high blood pressure, diabetes, and obesity. NANA is made up of more than 300 organizations including steering committee members, national organizations, and state/local organizations. Dr. Jane Pentz of AASDN was appointed to the *NANA School Foods Subcommittee and the NANA Food Marketing Workgroup.*

The combination of the new USDA school lunch guidelines, the publication of Dr. Pentz's children's novel, partnership with USDA Center for Nutrition Policy and Promotion, and appointment to the NANA coalition lead to the creation of the *AASDN National School Lunch Awareness Initiative (NSLAI)*. This initiative is implemented through the *AASDN*

Lunch Placemat™ which incorporates a star-associated food rating system. This simple, colorful, interactive tool provides a simple yet effective tool for educating, inspiring and motivating children to make healthy school lunch choices.

On November 2nd, 2012 almost 3000 children across the country participated in the "Shoot for 20 Stars Day". This first initiative produced data indicating that the participating children consumed more fruits, vegetables and whole grains as a direct response to the AASDN Placemat.

In response to the 2012 NSLAI, AASDN initiated a collaborative research project with The University of South Florida. The purpose of the project is to determine the impact of the AASDN placemat on the fruit and vegetable intake of second grade school age children attending the Villages, FL Charter School.

In 2013 AASDN released it's first educational multi-part series *Strategies for Prevention of Childhood Obesity*. The specific goal of this series is to consolidate the plethora of information concerning childhood obesity and provide solutions and strategies that can be implemented at the family and school level. This series includes determining children's caloric needs and sample menu plans based on these caloric needs. This multi-part educational series is FREE. Continuing education units are also available for professionals wishing to receive contact hours.

As of the date of this publication, AASDN continues to remain the leader in nutrition education for fitness/wellness health professionals, as well as a leader in solution based approaches to reducing childhood obesity.

Foreword

This textbook is dedicated to all professionals involved in the pursuit of total fitness/wellness programming. Our nation is currently facing a major long-term public health crisis. If it is not reversed, the gains in life expectancy and quality of life resulting from medical advances will erode, and more health-related costs will burden our nation even further.

Today, two thirds of adults and nearly one in three children struggle with overweight and obesity (1,2). Twenty years ago, no state had an obesity rate above 15 percent. Today, more than two out of three states, 38 total, have obesity rates over 25 percent (1,2). Obesity contributes to two-thirds of all heart disease, according to the CDC (3,32). Sixty-six percent of American adults with doctor-diagnosed arthritis are overweight or obese (1,3) and over 75 percent of hypertension cases are directly related to obesity (3,32). More than 80 percent of people with type 2 diabetes are overweight (3). In 2010, the nonpartisan Congressional Budget Office reported that nearly 20 percent of the increase in U.S. health care spending (from 1987-2007) was caused by obesity (2,3). The annual health costs related to obesity in the U.S. are as high as $168 billion, and nearly 17 percent of U.S. medical costs can be attributed on obesity (2,3).

Our nation faces real, serious, long-term challenges to its future. Two of the biggest challenges are restoring our global economic competitiveness and reining in the skyrocketing costs of medical care that have become, perhaps, the biggest obstacle to our long-term economic strength. Obesity, and the illnesses along with lost productivity, lies at the center of both of these challenges. The new report by the *Campaign to End Obesity* shows that, for policies designed to prevent or reduce obesity, a 75-year window better captures the full extent of a policy's value (2). This is because efforts to prevent chronic health problems like obesity provide value in the short term, but even more value when looking decades down the road (2).

Getting Involved

In the past health and fitness professionals have been told that nutrition is beyond their scope of practice and that nutrition should be left to dietitians. While dietitians are the "go to" experts, the Surgeon General's office has issued a call to action for all professionals to become involved in reducing obesity rates.

The reality is if current trends in obesity continue, for the first time in history children will have shorter and less healthy lives than their parents (2). The reality is that you - the allied health and fitness professional – can and should play a key role in reducing obesity rates. Dr Pentz experienced this reality when working in a large health club and members would go to the fitness staff for nutrition advice, even though she has a PhD in nutritional biochemistry and is licensed in the state of MA. Dr. Pentz notes that she is not alone in believing that fitness/wellness professionals are the ideal professionals to reduce obesity rates. Margaret Moore, of Wellcoaches, witnessed a pilot program in Seattle, WA. The program was a doctor referred obesity clinic. Each patient was provided a physician, a psychologist, a dietitian, and a personal trainer. Guess which professional brought about the greatest lifestyle changes? You Got It: Personal trainers. According to Margaret, "fitness professionals" often have personalities better suited to coaching than other health professionals. Furthermore, according to AND's Nutrition and You: Trends 2011 survey, the American public is just as likely to seek nutrition information from a personal trainer or health club/gym as they are a registered dietitian (7).

With this in mind, allied health and fitness professionals can and should implement a nutrition component into their programs. As fitness/wellness professionals this is our opportunity to take an active role and take up the cause "to help build a community-based infrastructure that embraces prevention as a priority".

Introduction

The goal of this textbook is to provide allied health professionals with all the tools necessary to incorporate a nutrition component into a wellness program. This book also serves as the textbook for the AASDN Nutrition Specialist Certification.

Part 1

- ✓ Discussion of the biology of cells; digestion, absorption, roles, and utilization of essential nutrients
- ✓ Discussion of energy nutrient needs including requirements, production and utilization of carbohydrates, fats, and proteins
- ✓ Discussion of micronutrients
- ✓ Discussion of nutrition and disease
- ✓ Discussion of alternative medicine
- ✓ Discussion of dietary supplement regulation as it relates to botanicals, vitamins and minerals, ergogenic aids, and weight loss supplements
- ✓ Discussion of bias and conflict of interest in research, and skills required to discern unethical practices in the media and scientific journals

Part 2

- ✓ Discussion of prerequisites to incorporating a nutrition program, including legal considerations, educational considerations, scope of practice and required skills such as coaching
- ✓ Discussion on implementation of nutritional programs including: individual program; group program; child and teen program; older adult program; and a program for athletes and vegetarians
- ✓ Discussion of the obstacles to success such as dieting; ambiguous and deceptive labeling regulations; production of high calorie, high fat commodity foods; eating out; and other sabotaging effects
- ✓ Discussion on the components of building a successful nutrition business including steps to starting a business; how to choose a client base; how to develop a pricing scheme; how to attract business; and how to obtain referrals

Appendix

- ✓ Glossary
- ✓ Equations / Conversions
- ✓ Legal and Responsibility Agreement
- ✓ AASDN Children's Meal Plans
- ✓ AASDN Star-Associated Food Rating Placemats

Table of Contents

Questions for Professionals....vii
Background....viii
Foreword....x
Introduction....xii

PART 1

Chapter 1 – The Basics....1
- Introduction....2
- Biology of Cells....2
- Digestion....4
- Absorption....7
- Transport....7
- Nutrition Basics....9
- Healthcare Crisis....22
- Food Guidance System....23
- Harvard Healthy Eating Plate versus MyPlate....24
- Summary....27
- Chapter 1 Sample Test....29
- References....30

Chapter 2 - Carbohydrates....33
- Introduction....34
- Carbohydrates....34
- Digestion....35
- Absorption....36
- Transport....36
- Glycogen....36
- Glucose Homeostasis....37
- Glycemic Index....41
- Insulin Resistance....44
- Fiber....46
- Alcohol....49
- Sweeteners....51
- Summary....57
- Chapter 2 Sample Test....61

References....62
Chapter 3 - Lipids....67
Introduction....68
Lipids....68
Fatty Acids....70
Steroids....80
Digestion....81
Absorption....82
Transport of Fatty Acids and Cholesterol....82
Summary....84
Chapter 3 Sample Test....88
References....89
Chapter 4 - Proteins....93
Introduction....94
Proteins....94
Amino Acids....96
Nitrogen....99
Digestion....100
Absorption....101
Transport....101
Protein Quality....102
Summary....107
Chapter 4 Sample Test....111
References....112
Chapter 5 - Energy....115
Introduction....116
Energy Production....116
Energy Utilization....119
Energy Intake....127
Meeting Energy Needs....134
Summary....138
Chapter 5 Sample Test....142
References....143
Chapter 6 – Nutrition and Disease....149
Introduction....150

Diabetes....151
Cardiovascular Disease....157
Hypertension....165
Stroke....169
Cancer....172
Gastrointestinal Disorders....175
Chronic Kidney Disease....179
Summary....182
Chapter 6 Sample Test....187
References....188
Chapter 7 - Vitamins....197
Introduction....198
Water Soluble Vitamins....199
Fat Soluble Vitamins....206
Summary....216
Chapter 7 Sample Test....219
References....220
Chapter 8 - Minerals....227
Introduction....228
Water....228
Major Minerals....230
Trace Minerals....238
Summary....250
Chapter 8 Sample Test....254
References....255
Chapter 9 – Complementary and Alternative Medicine....261
Introduction....262
NCCAM....262
Supplements....265
Supplement Categories....270
Verification Programs....283
Points to Consider....285
Position Stands....289
Summary....294
Chapter 9 Sample Test....298

References 299

Chapter 10 – Nutrition Research 307

Introduction 308

Bias 308

Conflicts of Interest 308

Critical Analysis of Current Research 315

Reputable Resources 326

Summary 328

Chapter 10 Sample Test 330

References 331

PART 2

Chapter 11 - Prerequisites 335

Introduction 336

Legal Considerations 336

Coaching Skills 345

Summary 358

Chapter 11 Sample Test 362

References 363

Chapter 12 – Implementing Nutrition Programs 365

Introduction 366

Body Composition Measures 367

Caloric requirements 370

Lifestyle Journal 373

Individual Program 376

Group Program 385

Child and Teen Program 388

Obese Population 396

Aging Population 397

Athletic Population 401

Vegetarian Population 401

Summary 403

Chapter 12 Sample Test 407

Case Studies 408

References 417

Chapter 13 – Promoting Success....421
Introduction....422
Diet – A Four Letter Word....422
Labeling Regulations....431
Food Production Commodities....443
Eating Out....444
Building a Successful Nutrition Business....451
Summary....465
Chapter 13 Sample Test....468
References....469
Appendix....475
Glossary....476
Equations / Conversions....492
Legal and Responsibility Agreement....496
AASDN Children's Meal Plans....498
AASDN Star-Associated Food Rating Placemats....500
Index....502

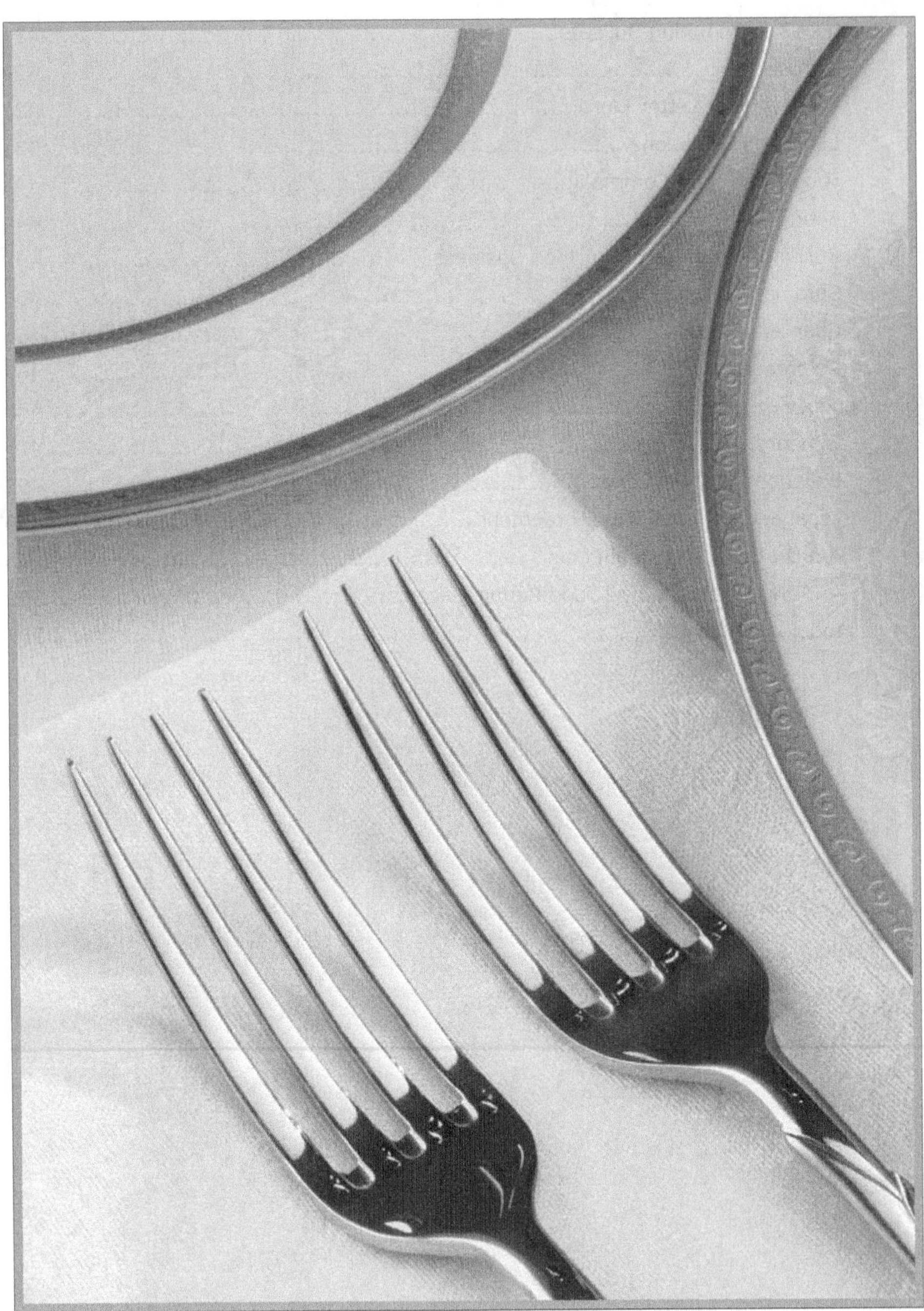

Chapter 1- The Basics

Before we can begin to understand how the body utilizes food for energy, we must first understand some basic principles of cellular biology, physiology, etc.

Objectives:

There are a number of objectives this textbook will attempt to meet. After reading and studying this chapter, you should be able to:

1. Discuss the differences between plant and animal cells, and the differences among muscle cells, fat cells, nerve cells, and red blood cells.
2. Define and recognize the organs involved in digestion and absorption.
3. Be able to recognize the major differences between macromolecules and micromolecules.
4. Define and list the macronutrients and the energy they provide.
5. Discuss Recommended Dietary Allowances in light of the new Dietary Reference Intakes.
6. Discuss the 2010 Dietary Guidelines and their significance.
7. Define homeostasis and provide several examples.

Introduction

Any discussion concerning the basics of nutrition must start with the basic unit of life, the human cell. In all cells oxygen combines with carbohydrate, fat or protein to release the energy required for cell function (8). The body contains about 100 trillion cells (8). While these cells differ markedly from each other, all have basic characteristics that are similar. Each type of cell is adapted to perform one particular function. Cells organize into organs and each organ is an aggregate of many different types of cells held together in supporting structures (8).

Biology of Cells

Cells consist of small membrane bound compartments filled with concentrated aqueous solution (cytosol) (8). Within the cell are smaller membrane bounded compartments known as organelles. Cells can be differentiated by whether or not they contain a nucleus. A cell without a nucleus is called a prokaryotic cell and a cell with a nucleus is called a eukaryotic cell. Bacteria are examples of prokaryotes, while plant cells and animal cells are examples of eukaryotes (8).

The nucleus within a eukaryotic cell contains most of the cell's genetic material, DNA and RNA (8). The nucleus is enclosed by a double lipid layer membrane. The rest of the contents of the cell are suspended in what is known as the cytoplasm. The cytoplasm is a gel-like substance in which most of the cell's metabolic reactions occur (8).

Many of the differences between plants and animals in the areas of nutrition, digestion, growth, reproduction, and defense, can be traced to the differences in cell walls (8). Plant cells have a rigid cell wall composed of tough fibrils of cellulose (fiber) while animal membranes are composed of lipid bilayers.

The plant cell wall is much thicker, stronger, and more rigid than animal cell walls. Rigid plant cell walls prevent the plant cell from movement (8). Plant cells can only receive organic (carbon containing) nutrients through photosynthesis. Photosynthesis is the ability to absorb sunlight and to convert solar energy to chemical energy. The products of photosynthesis can be used directly by the cell for energy or converted to a sugar that can be used by other tissues in the plant (roots). Plant cells also have large vesicles called vacuoles. As plant cells grow, they accumulate water in these vacuoles (8).

Unlike plant cells, animal cells cannot produce energy through photosynthesis. Animal cells receive nutrients through the bloodstream and are bound together by a loose meshwork of large molecules called the extracellular matrix. Animal cell membranes consist of lipid bilayers and are dynamic, fluid structures that allow molecules to move about rapidly and freely in the plane of the membrane. These lipid layers also serve as impermeable barriers to the flow of most water-soluble molecules (8).

Mitochondria are a feature of many eukaryotic cells. Mitochondria are responsible for respiration (the energy released in the aerobic oxidation of food molecules); this process occurs nowhere else in the cell (8). In other words, mitochondria are the energy factories of the cell. Muscle cells contain many mitochondria while fat cells contain very few; muscle cells utilize many more calories than fat cells (8).

There are over 200 types of human cells. These cell types are assembled into a variety of different tissues such as: epithelia, connective, muscle, and nervous tissue (8):

- Epithelial cells are cells on the surface of the skin and mucous membranes.
- Epithelial tissues serve as selective barriers between the body's interior and the environment (cornea, skin, respiratory and digestive tract lining).
- Connective tissue consists of extracellular structural and supportive elements of the body; i.e., tendons, ligaments, cartilage, and the organic matrix of bones.
- Approximately 40 percent of the body is skeletal muscle, and almost another 10 percent is smooth and cardiac muscle. Smooth muscle is found in the eye, gut, bile ducts, uterus, and many blood vessels. Many of the same principles apply to skeletal muscle and smooth muscle; however, the internal physical arrangement of smooth muscle fiber is different. Smooth muscle fibers are composed of smaller fibers in contrast to the skeletal muscle fibers which are made of numerous fibers, and each fiber in turn is made up of successively smaller subunits, myofibrils. Each myofibril contains about 1500 myosin filaments and 3000 actin filaments, which are large protein molecules responsible for muscle contraction. Cardiac muscle is similar to skeletal muscle with the exception that heart muscle maintains cardiac rhythmicity.
- The nervous system is unique in the vast complexity of the control actions that it can perform. The nervous system, along with the endocrine system (hormonal system), provides most of the control functions for the body including the rapid activities of the body and even the rates of secretion of some endocrine glands.

The four types of cells important in metabolism include the fat cell, the muscle cell, the nerve cell, and the red blood cell. Discussion on metabolism with focus on these four types of cells (8):

- A muscle cell has many mitochondria. It is important to remember that mitochondria are the energy producing factories of the body and they regulate caloric expenditure.
- A fat cell has very few mitochondria; hormones are produced, but very few calories are expended by fat cells.
- A nerve cell has no mitochondria and must obtain its energy from simple sugars (in the form of glucose) in the blood stream.
- A red blood cell also has no mitochondria and must rely on glucose in the bloodstream for its energy supply.

The fact that certain cells have no mitochondria is very important in metabolism (8,10). These cells require a constant flow of glucose from the bloodstream; too much or too little glucose in the bloodstream damages cells. Glucose concentrations in the bloodstream are controlled by hormones. If food is unavailable for long periods of time, the body is forced to produce glucose for these cells. Glucose regulation, as well as how the body makes glucose will be discussed in the next chapter.

Digestion

When foods are ingested, such as bread, meat, and vegetables, they are not in a form that the body can use. They must be broken down into smaller molecules or nutrients before they can be absorbed into the bloodstream and carried to cells throughout the body.

Digestion is the process by which food and drink are broken down into their smallest components so the body can absorb them to build and nourish cells and provide energy (12,13). Digestion involves mixing food with digestive juices, moving it through the digestive tract, and breaking down large molecules of food into smaller molecules (12,13). Digestion begins in the mouth, when you chew and swallow, and is completed in the small intestine.

The digestive system is made up of the digestive tract and other organs that help the body break down and absorb food (see figure) (12,13). The digestive track consists of a series of hollow organs joined in a long, twisted tube from the mouth to the anus. Organs that make up the digestive tract are the mouth, esophagus, stomach, small intestine, large intestine (also called the colon), rectum, and anus. Inside these hollow organs is a lining called the mucosa (12,13).

In the mouth, stomach, and small intestine, the mucosa contains tiny glands that produce juices to help digest food. The digestive tract also contains a layer of smooth muscle that helps break down food and move it along the tract (12,13).

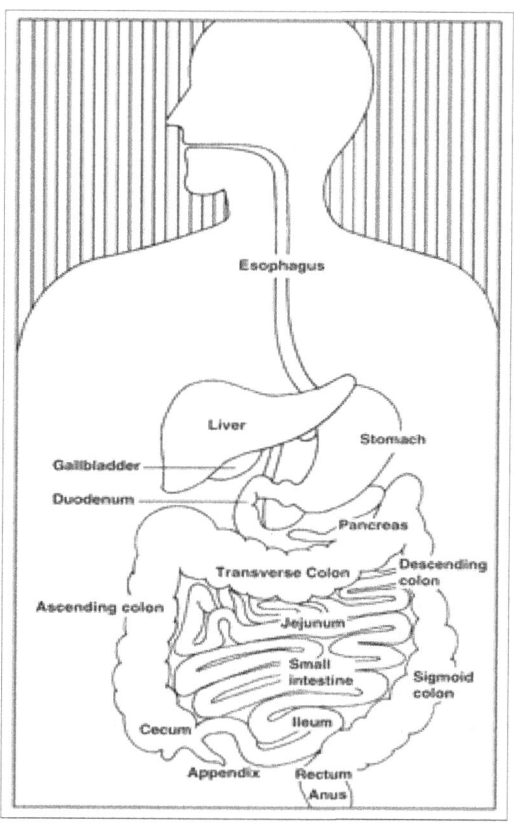

The large, hollow organs of the digestive tract contain a layer of muscle that enables their walls to move (12,13). The movement of organ walls can propel food and liquid through the system and also mix the contents within each organ. Food moves from one organ to the next through this muscle action called peristalsis. Peristalsis looks like an ocean wave traveling through the muscle. The muscle of the organ contracts to create a narrowing and then propels the narrowed portion slowly down the length of the organ. These waves of narrowing push the food and fluid in front of them through each hollow organ (12,13).

The first major muscle movement occurs when food or liquid is swallowed. Although swallowing is by choice, once the swallow begins, it becomes involuntary and proceeds under the control of the nerves.

Swallowed food is pushed into the esophagus, which connects the throat with the stomach. At the junction of the esophagus and stomach, there is a ringlike muscle, called the lower esophageal sphincter, which closes the passage between the two organs (12,13). As food approaches the closed sphincter, the sphincter relaxes and allows the food to pass through to the stomach.

The muscle of the upper part of the stomach relaxes to accept large volumes of swallowed material. Next the food and liquid mix with the digestive juice produced by the stomach. The lower part of the stomach mixes these materials by its muscle action. The final task of the stomach is to empty its contents slowly into the small intestine.

Several factors affect emptying of the stomach, including the kind of food and the degree of muscle action of the stomach and the small intestine (12,13). Carbohydrates, for example, spend the least amount of time in the stomach, while protein stays in the stomach longer, and fats the longest.

The food entering the small intestine dissolves into the juices from the pancreas and liver. The contents are mixed and pushed forward to allow further digestion.

Finally, the digested nutrients are absorbed through the intestinal walls and transported throughout the body (12,134). The waste products of this process (fiber and older cells that have been shed from the mucosa) are pushed into the colon, where they remain until the feces are expelled by a bowel movement.

Production of Digestive Juices

The digestive glands that act first are in the mouth, the salivary glands (12,13). The next set of digestive glands in the stomach lining produce stomach acid and an enzyme that digests protein (12,13). Specific enzymes and their functions will be discussed in subsequent chapters.

A thick mucus layer coats the stomach mucosa and helps keep the acidic digestive juice from dissolving the tissue of the stomach itself (12,13). In most people, the stomach mucosa is able to resist the juice while food and other tissues of the body cannot.

After the stomach empties the food and juice mixture into the small intestine, the juices of two other digestive organs mix with the food (12,13). One of these organs, the pancreas, produces a juice that contains a wide array of enzymes to break down the carbohydrate, fat, and protein in food. Other enzymes that are active in the process come from glands in the wall of the intestine.

The second organ, the liver, produces yet another digestive juice, bile (12,13). Bile is stored between meals in the gallbladder. At mealtime, it is squeezed out of the gallbladder, through the bile ducts, and into the intestine to mix with the fat in food. The bile acids dissolve fat into the watery contents of the intestine, much like detergents that dissolve grease from a frying pan. After fat is dissolved, it is digested by enzymes from the pancreas and the lining of the intestine (12,13).

Absorption

Most digested molecules of food, as well as water and minerals, are absorbed through the small intestine (8,12). Visually, the small intestines look like a tube that has a one inch circumference. This tube extends about twenty feet and contains hundreds of folds. Because of these folds, the area of the small intestines provides a surface comparable to a quarter of a football field (8,12). The mucosa of the small intestine contains many folds that are covered with tiny finger like projections called villi. In turn, the villi are covered with microscopic projections called microvilli (8,12). The microvilli and their membranes contain hundreds of different kinds of pumps and enzymes producing tremendous specialization of absorption of nutrients (8,12). This fact combined with the large surface area allows for quick absorption of nutrients.

The small intestines are divided into three segments: the duodenum, the jejunum and the ileum (8,12). Specialization occurs in these segments of the small intestines (8,12). The nutrients that are ready for absorption early are absorbed near the top of the intestinal tract, those that take longer to be digested are absorbed further down the tract.

Hence, the idea that people should not eat certain foods together because the digestive system cannot handle more than one task at a time is a myth. For example, if only fat is eaten, the protein and carbohydrate carriers for absorption remain idle, while the fat carriers would be working overtime. We will discuss absorption of individual nutrients in future chapters.

Transport

Transport of nutrients throughout the body requires an understanding of the body's circulatory systems - the vascular system and the lymphatic system (9,12).

The vascular system (blood circulatory system) is a closed system of vessels with continuous flow of blood (9,12). The heart serves as a pump, pumping blood to all cells through arteries. Veins are vessels that carry blood to the heart and arteries are vessels that carry blood away from the heart (9,12). Arteries branch into smaller vessels known as capillaries. As the blood circulates through arteries (then capillaries), it picks up and delivers materials to the cells of the body. All cells receive oxygen and nutrients from the blood and all cells deposit carbon dioxide and other wastes into the blood (9,12). Blood entering the digestive system is carried by way of an artery just as with all organs. However, blood leaving the digestive system goes by way of the hepatic portal vein (9,12). The portal vein is unique in that it is a one-way system flowing directly to the liver. Once nutrients leave the intestinal cells they enter the bloodstream via the portal vein and are transported to the liver. The liver is placed in the circulation at this point because it prepares the absorbed nutrients for use by the body (9,12). The liver has many metabolic functions and is truly the body's major metabolic organ. The liver in many ways is an overworked and "heroic" organ.

Functions of the liver include (9,12):

1. Making and storing glycogen
2. Converting all sugars to glucose from amino acids (and glycerin)
3. Converting glycogen to energy when needed
4. Building and breaking down triglycerides, phospholipids, and cholesterol
5. Packaging extra fats into lipoproteins for transport
6. Manufacturing bile which is transported to the gallbladder
7. Making ketones (when needed)
8. Manufacturing dispensable amino acids
9. Removing excess amino acids from the blood and removing the nitrogen
10. Removing ammonia from the blood and converting it to urea (which is then sent to the kidneys)
11. Making DNA and RNA (genetic materials)
12. Making plasma proteins such as clotting factors
13. Detoxifying alcohol, other drugs, wastes and poisons
14. Breaking up old blood cells and recycle the iron
15. Storing some vitamins and minerals
16. Forming lymph

The lymphatic system is also a one-way route. Lymphatic fluid (lymph) circulates between cells of the body and collects into tiny capillary-like vessels (9,12). Lymph is almost identical to blood except that it does not contain red blood cells or platelets. Molecules in the lymphatic system collect in the thoracic duct which terminates in the subclavian vein. Contents are conducted towards the heart where they enter the circulation like other nutrients from the GI tract. One exception, however, is that nutrients entering the blood stream from the lymphatic system bypass the liver (9,12).

Fats are anhydrous (water insoluble) and cannot be transported directly via the bloodstream. Fat products, once inside the intestinal cells, require "packaging" before they can be transported. They are assembled into packaging systems called lipoproteins

(9,12). Some of these lipoproteins - chylomircrons are too large to enter the bloodstream and enter the lymphatic system (12). More details concerning fats are discussed in Chapter 3.

Nutrition Basics

The science of nutrition is the study of the nutrients in foods and how the body utilizes them (including ingestion, absorption, transport, metabolism, interaction, storage, and excretion).

A chemical analysis of the body indicates that it is composed of materials similar to those found in foods (9,10). The molecules found inside cells can be classified as micromolecules or macromolecules. Do not confuse micronutrients (vitamins and minerals) and macronutrients (energy nutrients) with micromolecules (small molecules) and macromolecules (large molecules) (9,10).

Macronutrients are organic (carbon) containing compounds; the word organic means carbon containing. Carbon is unique in the body, in that it alone has the ability to form four bonds with other atoms - hydrogen, nitrogen, oxygen, phosphorous, sulfur - or itself. Because of this unique feature, carbon is central to the biochemistry of life (9,10).

Nearly all of the solid matter in cells is organic and is present in four forms: proteins, polysaccharides, lipids (fats), and nucleic acids (DNA and RNA). Proteins consist of amino acids; polysaccharides consist of simple sugars; lipids (fats) consist of fatty acids (and other components); nucleic acids consists of nucleotides (8,9).

Metabolism is defined as the chemical processes occurring within a living cell or organism that are necessary for the maintenance of life. In metabolism some substances are broken down to yield energy for vital processes (catabolism) while other substances, necessary for life, are synthesized (anabolism). Anabolic reactions are reactions in which small molecules are put together to build larger ones and require energy. Catabolic reactions are reactions in which large molecules are broken down to smaller ones releasing energy (9,10). For example, proteins are broken down into amino acids; polysaccharides are broken down into simple sugars; lipids are broken down into fatty acids; nucleotides are broken down into nucleic acids.

Essential Nutrients

The macronutrient (proteins. fats, carbohydrates) along with vitamins, minerals (micronutrients), and water are the essential nutrients. Water is neither a macronutrient nor a micronutrient, but it is an essential nutrient. Essential nutrients are nutrients a person must obtain from food because the body cannot synthesize them in amounts sufficient to meet physiological needs (9). Eventually, cells will break down and become destroyed if these essential nutrients are not available (9,10).

Categories	Nutrient	Calories/Gram
Macronutrient	Carbohydrate	4
	Fats	9
	Proteins	4
Micronutrient	Vitamins	0
	Minerals	0
Water		0

Calories are the units by which energy released from foods is measured. One kilo-calorie is the amount of heat necessary to raise the temperature of one kilogram of water one degree centigrade. While calories are listed on labels, the measurement is actually kilo-calories (10). One gram of carbohydrate equals 4 Kcal; one gram of protein also equals 4 Kcal; one gram of fat equals 9 Kcal; and one gram of alcohol equals 7 Kcal. One ounce equals 28.35 grams. One half cup of vegetables or juice weighs about 100 grams while one teaspoon of salt weighs about 5 grams.

Another measure of food energy is the kilojoule (kJ), used on nutrition labels in countries outside of the U.S. A joule is the amount of energy expended when one kilogram is moved one meter by a force of one newton. One gram of carbohydrate equals 17 KJ; one gram of protein also equals 17 KJ; one gram of fat equals 37 KJ; and one gram of alcohol equals 29 KJ (10). To convert from Kcal to KJ multiply Kcal by 4.2.

Carbohydrates are the number one energy source for the body. The two categories of carbohydrates include simple and complex.

Simple – One or Two Sugar Units	Complex – Many Sugar Units
Monosaccharide: Glucose, Fructose, Galactose	Starch
Disaccharide: Sucrose, Lactose, Maltose	Glycogen
	Cellulose

Simple carbohydrates, or sugars, consist of one (mono) or two (di) sugar units. Glucose, fructose, and galactose are one unit sugars; while sucrose, lactose, and maltose are two sugar units. Simple carbohydrates are found in fruits, vegetables, table sugar, milk, and malt.

Complex carbohydrates are many sugar units linked together. Complex carbohydrates are found in pasta, potatoes, grains, rice, etc. Carbohydrates from plant foods are called starch. When the plant starches are stored in the body they are called glycogen. Certain parts of plant foods that cannot be digested by enzymes in the body are known as fiber.

Examples of carbohydrate foods are listed in the following table (12).

	Food Amount	**Carbohydrate (g)**	**Calories**
Fruit			
Apple	1 medium	20	80
Orange	1 medium	20	80
Banana	1 medium	25	105
Raisins	¼ cup	30	120
Vegetable			
Corn, canned	½ cup	18	80
Winter squash	½ cup	15	65
Peas	½ cup	10	60
Green Beans	½ cup	7	30
Bread			
Submarine Roll	8" long	60	280
Lender's Bagel	1	30	210
Saltines	5	15	90
Graham Crackers	2 squares	11	60
Grains/Pasta/Starches			
Baked Potato	1 large	55	240
Quinoa	1 cup	39	222
Baked Beans	1 cup	50	330
Lentils, Cooked	1 cup	40	215

We will discuss carbohydrates and fiber in more detail in the next chapter.

Lipids, often referred to as fats, found in foods are triglycerides, phospholipids, and cholesterol (sterol) (12). Triglycerides are the storage form of fat, while phospholipids are part of all cell membranes and are involved in immune system function. The third type of fat found in foods is cholesterol. We obtain cholesterol from our diets, and the human body can also make cholesterol. Fatty acids, structural components of fats, are divided into two broad categories: saturated and unsaturated. Unsaturated fatty acids are either monounsaturated or polyunsaturated. Most foods consist of a combination of both types of fatty acids. The following table provides examples of each (12).

	% Saturated	% Monounsaturated	% Polyunsaturated
Coconut Oil	90	10	
Palm Oil	50	30	20
Butter	65	30	5
Beef Fat	50	45	5
Chicken Fat	30	50	20
Olive Oil	15	75	10
Canola Oil	5	60	35
Peanut Oil	20	50	30
Soybean Oil	23	62	15

When unsaturated fats are turned into solids by hydrogenation, they become trans fatty acids (9,10). Trans fatty acids are similar to saturated fatty acids in that they are considered "unhealthy". Trans fatty acids will be discussed in more detail in chapter 3.

It is very important to have a certain portion of fat in the diet to provide stored energy for sustained activity, to maintain the integrity of cell membranes, for absorption of fat soluble vitamins, and immune system function.

Proteins are a third energy source, in addition to carbohydrates and fats. Amino acids are the basic component of proteins. The table below lists sources of proteins (12).

Item	Serving Size	Protein (g)
Meat, Poultry, Fish	3 oz cooked	21
Milk or Yogurt	8 oz.	8
Cottage Cheese	4 oz.	13
Eggs whites	1 large	4
Beans, Dried Peas, Lentils	½ cup cooked	7

Amino acids contain the element, nitrogen (12). Nitrogen is anabolic (tissue building). The only way our bodies can obtain nitrogen is through amino acid intake. Traditionally amino acids have been distinguished by whether the body can make the amino acid (nonessential) or cannot make the amino acid (essential). Metabolically, however, the distinctions are less clear because a number of essential amino acids can be formed by transamination - a chemical process of transforming one amino acid into another (12). Amino acid essentiality and protein quality will be discussed in detail in Chapter 4.

Protein sources that contain all of the essential amino acids include meats, milk and milk products, eggs, soybeans and wheat germ. Other legumes, grains, and vegetables contain some of the essential amino acids but may be low or missing one or more of the essential amino acids; and for this reason, these foods are considered incomplete protein sources (9,12). Eating these foods in combination or with a complete protein source increases the protein value of the meal (see Chapter 4).

While proteins are a third energy source for the body, they are not a major or direct source of energy. Proteins have many varied roles in the body and the body uses them for energy only when other energy nutrients are not available. The roles of proteins, as well as their digestion and absorption, will be discussed in Chapter 4.

Micronutrients

The micronutrients include vitamins and minerals. Vitamins are a group of organic compounds other than protein, carbohydrates, and fats that cannot be manufactured by the body and are required in small amounts for specific functions of growth (12). The two major categories of vitamins include the water soluble vitamins and the fat soluble vitamins. Water soluble vitamins include the B vitamins and vitamin C. The fat soluble vitamins are vitamins A, D, E, K.

Minerals are inorganic elements essential to life that act as control agents in body reactions and cooperative factors in energy production, body building and maintenance of tissues (12). They retain their identity and cannot be destroyed by heat, air, acid, or mixing (12). The two major categories of minerals include the major minerals (calcium, phosphorus, potassium, sodium, and magnesium) and the trace minerals (iron, zinc, iodine, copper, manganese, chromium, selenium, sulfur) (12).

Vitamins and minerals have many roles in the body. Certain vitamins help "derive" energy from the energy nutrients while not providing energy themselves. These vitamins attach to molecules involved in energy production. Some minerals are also involved in the energy cycle. Other vitamins and minerals have antioxidant properties whose role is to neutralize free radicals that can damage cells (12). These nutrients have many other roles that are pivotal to health and will be discussed in subsequent chapters.

Water

While discussion of water is not a major topic in this textbook, its importance in life and health cannot be minimized. Water constitutes 55 to 60 percent of an adult's body weight (9,10). A person can survive for long periods of time without food but not without water (8,9). Water is inorganic and forms the major part of almost every body tissue (9). Water provides the environment in which nearly all the body's activities occur (9,10). It participates in almost all metabolic reactions and is the medium for transporting molecules in and out of cells. Water lubricates joints and acts as a shock absorber and is the fluid in the eyes as well as in the spinal cord (9,10). The amount of water that must be consumed is enormous relative to other nutrients (18).

Thirst acts to signal the body when water is needed; however, it lags behind the body's optimum need (10). Therefore, responding to thirst will not remedy a water deficiency (10). Because of this, it is important to consistently include adequate amounts of water throughout the day. A general water requirement is difficult to establish since needs are so variable (10).

General water recommendations have been a topic of controversy. The actual research determining water needs does not appear to exist and respected nutrition organizations differ on hydration needs (10). The following calculation, while not proven scientifically, is a good estimate of need. General recommendations under average environmental conditions are as follows: 1.0 to 1.5 ml water per calorie expended (1 ml = .03 ounces) (10). For example, if a person expends 400 calories during exercise, that person should drink 400 to 600 ml, or 12 to 18 ounces. If a person expends 2000 calories per day, he or she should consume 60 to 90 ounces of water per day.

The Dietary Reference Intakes from the Institute of Medicine recommend a total daily beverage intake of 13 cups for men and 9 cups for women (18). This amount is for generally healthy people living in temperate climates. Individual needs vary so some people can be properly hydrated at somewhat higher or lower levels of water intake. Also, keep in mind that water may come from a variety of sources. It includes other beverages, even those containing caffeine, in addition to the water that you drink (18). Also see Chapter 5 for details concerning hydration recommendations before, during and after exercise.

Homeostasis

The human body is endowed with a vast network of feedback mechanisms that control the necessary balances for life. This high level of internal bodily control is called "homeostasis (9,10). In other words, homeostasis is the maintenance of constant internal conditions in body systems; i.e. balance. A homeostatic system is constantly reacting to external forces so as to maintain limits set by the body's needs. Examples include glucose, calcium, alcohol, and cholesterol homeostasis (see individual topics for more information on each).

The human body has a tremendous capacity to return to homeostasis. For example, pH in the bloodstream is regulated within a very narrow range - 7.35 to 7.45. Death occurs at pH levels of 8.0 or greater or pH levels of 6.8 or lower (9,10). Without homeostasis, drinking carbonated beverages would produce large changes in the pH of the bloodstream. However, the body has a tremendous buffering system (chemical reactions) which does not allow the large changes to occur. In other words, homeostasis is the response of the body to maintain a constant pH by utilizing or producing other molecules that will return the internal conditions to "normal". In many instances, this is not simply one chemical reaction, but hundreds, even thousands of reactions. Hence, something so simple as drinking carbonated beverages causes the body to respond through chemical reactions to maintain constant internal conditions.

Controls of Metabolism

To view metabolism as what one eats is simplistic. Metabolism is defined as the complex set of physical and chemical processes occurring within a living cell or organism that are necessary for the maintenance of life (provide energy for maintaining life). There are many factors that control metabolism. Some of these factors are enzymatic, others are hormonal, while still others are controlled at the cellular level through concentration and compartmentalization. The enzymatic controls of metabolism are beyond the realm of this textbook. However, we will examine several hormones as well as several controls at the cellular level including concentration and compartmentalization (10).

<u>Hormonal control</u>

Hormones are chemical messengers secreted in trace amounts by one type of tissue (10). They are carried by the blood to a target tissue and they then stimulate activity in this target tissue (10).

<u>Insulin</u>: Every cell in the body depends on glucose for its fuel to some extent, and certain cells depend primarily on glucose for energy. Insulin moves glucose from the bloodstream into cells. When blood glucose levels rise, special cells of the pancreas secrete insulin into the blood. The circulating insulin binds to receptors on cell membranes which then allow the glucose to enter the cell. Most cells take up only the glucose they need with the

exception of muscle cells and liver cells which can store the glucose as glycogen. Thus, high serum glucose levels are returned to normal.

Glucagon: When blood glucose falls, cells of the pancreas secrete glucagon into the blood. Glucagon counteracts insulin and raises blood glucose by signaling the liver to release its glycogen stores.

Epinephrine: Under stress, epinephrine is released into the bloodstream. This hormone also elicits the release of glucose from the liver cells. Like glucagon, epinephrine works to return glucose to the blood from liver glycogen. This hormone also elicits the breakdown of protein in muscle.

Thyroid hormones: The thyroid hormones control basal metabolic rate (calories expended at rest). High levels of these hormones will produce an increased basal metabolic rate, while low levels will produce a decreased metabolic rate.

Concentration

Concentration of certain nutrients in certain parts of the cell also has an effect on metabolism (10). If too much of a product accumulates in a certain part of the cell, the increased amount of the product signals the cell to stop producing the product or transpose the product into another molecule. For example, when too much glucose enters liver cells, the excess glucose signals the cells to store glycogen.

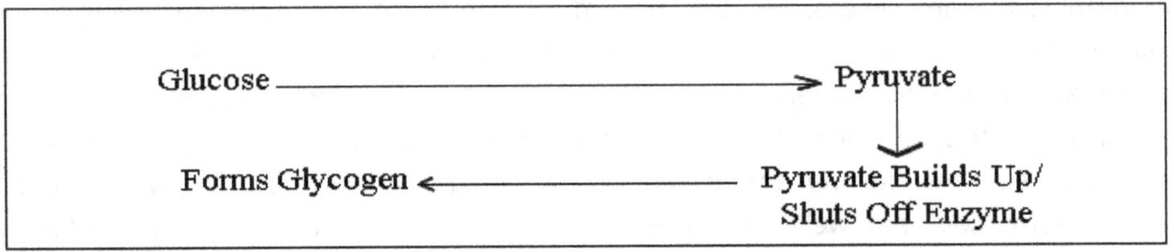

Compartmentalization

Compartmentalization occurs when certain nutrients in different parts of the cell build up, and the increased amounts signal the cell to switch metabolism (10). For example, when fatty acids in the cytosol of the cell build up they become attached to a molecule called carnitine which carries these fatty acids into the mitochondria to be oxidized for energy. If too many fatty acids build up in the mitochondria, the extra fatty acids are then turned into a chemical called citrate. The citrate leaves the mitochondria and goes back into the cytosol where the citrate can be turned back into fatty acids.

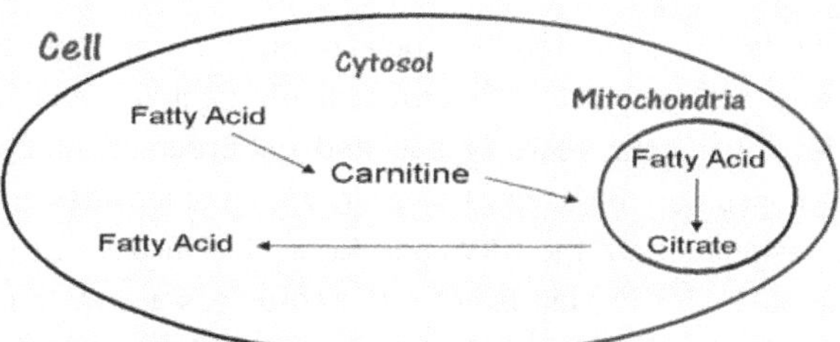

Dietary Reference Intakes

The publication of the first edition of Recommended Dietary Allowances (RDAs) in 1941 was recognized as one of the most authoritative sources of information on recommendations for nutrient intakes for healthy people (24). In 1989, rising awareness of the impact of nutrition on chronic disease dictated an expanded review of uses and misuses of RDAs (24). The new framework for this expanded approach developed by U.S. and Canadian scientists became known as the Dietary Reference Intakes (DRIs). This series of references greatly extends the scope and application of previous nutrient guidelines to include requirements based on how the nutrient may be related to chronic disease or developmental abnormalities (24). This framework also identifies a new reference intake, the Tolerable Upper Intake Level (UL), which if consumed consistently, may result in adverse effects (24).

The DRI's are an average daily dietary intake level sufficient to meet the nutrition requirement of nearly all (97 to 98 percent) healthy individuals in a particular life stage and gender group. They are intended to be used as a guide for daily intake by individuals. RDAs (US standards) depend on Estimated Average Requirements (EAR). If no EAR has been established, then no RDAs are set. If sufficient data is not available to calculate an EAR, then a reference intake - adequate intake (AI) is used instead of an RDA. Less information is available on which to base allowances for certain nutrients (copper, manganese, chromium, molybdenum, and chloride). These nutrients are not included in the RDAs and figures are averages of *Safe and Adequate Intakes* as set by the National Academy of Sciences (20).

Daily Values on Food Labels

There are two sets of reference values for reporting nutrients in nutrition labeling: Daily Reference Values (DRVs) and Reference Daily Intakes (RDIs) (19). These values assist consumers in interpreting information about the amount of a nutrient that is present in a food and in comparing nutritional values of food products. DRVs are established for adults and children four or more years of age, as are RDIs, with the exception of protein (19). DRVs are provided for total fat, saturated fat, cholesterol, total carbohydrate, dietary fiber, sodium, potassium, and protein. RDIs are provided for vitamins and minerals and for protein for children less than four years of age and for pregnant and lactating women (19). In order to limit consumer confusion, however, the label includes a single term (i.e., Daily Value (DV)), to designate both the DRVs and RDIs. Specifically, the label includes the % DV, except that the % DV for protein is not required unless a protein claim is made for the product or if the product is to be used by infants or children under four years of age. The following table lists the Daily values based on a caloric intake of 2,000 calories, for adults and children four or more years of age. Nutrients in the table are in the order in which they are required to appear on a label in accordance with 101.9(c) (19).

Nutrient	Unit of Measure	Daily Values
Total Fat	Grams	65
Saturated Fatty Acids	Grams	20
Cholesterol	Milligrams	300
Sodium	Milligrams	2400
Potassium	Milligrams	3500
Total Carbohydrate	Grams	300
Fiber	Grams	25
Protein	Grams	50
Vitamin A	International Unit	5000
Vitamin C	Milligrams	60
Calcium	Milligrams	1000
Iron	Milligrams	18
Vitamin D	International Unit	400
Vitamin E	International Unit	30
Vitamin K	Micrograms	80
Thiamin	Milligrams	1.5
Riboflavin	Milligrams	1.7
Niacin	Milligrams	20
Vitamin B_6	Milligrams	2
Folate	Micrograms	400
Vitamin B_{12}	Micrograms	6
Biotin	Micrograms	300
Pantothenic Acid	Milligrams	10

Nutrient	Unit of Measure	Daily Values
Phosphorus	Milligrams	1000
Iodine	Micrograms	150
Magnesium	Milligrams	400
Zinc	Milligrams	15
Selenium	Micrograms	70
Copper	Milligrams	2
Manganese	Milligrams	2
Chromium	Micrograms	120
Molybdenum	Micrograms	75
Chloride	Milligrams	3400

Dietary Guidelines

By law (Public Law 101-445, Title III, 7 U.S.C. 5301 et seq.), Dietary Guidelines for Americans is reviewed, updated if necessary, and published every 5 years (18). The U.S. Department of Agriculture (USDA) and the U.S. Department of Health and Human Services (HHS) jointly create each edition (24). The intent of the Dietary Guidelines is to summarize and synthesize knowledge about individual nutrients and food components into an interrelated set of recommendations for healthy eating that can be adopted by the public (21).

In 1980, the U.S. Department of Agriculture (USDA) and the U.S. Department of Health and Human Services (HHS) released the First edition of *Nutrition and Your Health: Dietary Guidelines for Americans* (24). These Dietary Guidelines were different from previous dietary guidance in that they reflected emerging scientific evidence about diet and health and expanded the traditional focus on nutrient adequacy to also address the impact of diet on chronic disease (24).

Dietary Guidelines for Americans, 2010 consists of six chapters (25). This first chapter introduces the document and provides information on background and purpose. The next five chapters correspond to major themes that emerged from the 2010 Dietary Guidelines for Americans review of the evidence. These recommendations are based on a preponderance of the scientific evidence for nutritional factors that are important for promoting health and lowering risk of diet-related chronic disease. Recommendations always refer to individual intake or amount rather than population average intake, unless otherwise noted. Although divided into chapters that focus on particular aspects of eating patterns, Dietary Guidelines for Americans provides integrated recommendations for health. To get the full benefit, individuals should carry out these recommendations in their entirety as part of an overall healthy eating pattern. Taken together, the Dietary Guidelines recommendations encompass two concepts (25):

1. Maintain calorie balance over time to achieve and sustain a healthy weight. People who are most successful at achieving and maintaining a healthy weight do so through continued attention to consuming only enough calories from foods and beverages to meet their needs and by being physically active. To curb the obesity epidemic and improve their health, many Americans must decrease the calories they consume and increase the calories they expend through physical activity.
    - Prevent and/or reduce overweight and obesity through improved eating and physical activity behaviors.
    - Control total calorie intake to manage body weight. For people who are overweight or obese, this will mean consuming fewer calories from foods and beverages.
    - Increase physical activity and reduce time spent in sedentary behaviors.
    - Maintain appropriate calorie balance during each stage of life—childhood, adolescence, adulthood, pregnancy and breastfeeding, and older age.
2. Focus on consuming nutrient-dense foods and beverages. Americans currently consume too much sodium and too many calories from solid fats, added sugars, and refined grains. These replace nutrient-dense foods and beverages and make it difficult for people to achieve recommended nutrient intake while controlling calorie and sodium intake. A healthy eating pattern limits intake of sodium, solid fats, added sugars, and refined grains and emphasizes nutrient-dense foods and beverages—vegetables, fruits, whole grains, fat-free or low-fat milk and milk products, seafood, lean meats and poultry, eggs, beans and peas, and nuts and seeds.
    - Reduce daily sodium intake to less than 2,300 milligrams (mg) and further reduce intake to 1,500 mg among persons who are 51 and older and those of any age who are African American or have hypertension, diabetes, or chronic kidney disease. The 1,500 mg recommendation applies to about half of the U.S. population, including children, and the majority of adults.
    - Consume less than 10 percent of calories from saturated fatty acids by replacing them with monounsaturated and polyunsaturated fatty acids.
    - Consume less than 300 mg per day of dietary cholesterol.
    - Keep trans fatty acid consumption as low as possible by limiting foods that contain synthetic sources of trans fats, such as partially

hydrogenated oils, and by limiting other solid fats.
• Reduce the intake of calories from solid fats and added sugars.
• Limit the consumption of foods that contain refined grains, especially refined grain foods that contain solid fats, added sugars, and sodium.
• If alcohol is consumed, it should be consumed in moderation—up to one drink per day for women and two drinks per day for men—and only by adults of legal drinking age.

A healthy eating pattern should not only promote health and help to decrease the risk of chronic diseases, but should also prevent food-borne illness. Four basic food safety principles (Clean, Separate, Cook, and Chill) work together to reduce the risk of food-borne illnesses. In addition, some foods (such as milks, cheeses, and juices that have not been pasteurized, and undercooked animal foods) pose high risk for food-borne illness and should be avoided.

A basic premise of the Dietary Guidelines is that nutrient needs should be met primarily through consuming foods (23). In certain cases, fortified foods and dietary supplements may be useful in providing one or more nutrients that otherwise might be consumed in less than recommended amounts. Two eating patterns that embody the Dietary Guidelines are the USDA Food Patterns and their vegetarian adaptations and the DASH (Dietary Approaches to Stop Hypertension) Eating Plan (25).

The information in the Dietary Guidelines for Americans is also used in developing educational materials and aiding policy makers in designing and carrying out nutrition-related programs, including Federal food, nutrition education, and information programs (25). In addition, the Dietary Guidelines for Americans has the potential to offer authoritative statements as provided for in the Food and Drug Administration Modernization Act (FDAMA) (25). To obtain a copy of the 2010 Dietary Guidelines visit http://www.cnpp.usda.gov /dietaryguidelines.htm

Dietary Guidelines and Obesity

The recommendations contained in the Dietary Guidelines for Americans traditionally have been intended for healthy Americans ages 2 years and older (25). However, Dietary Guidelines for Americans, 2010 was released at a time of rising concern about the health of the American population. Its recommendations accommodate the reality that a large percentage of Americans are overweight or obese and/or at risk of various chronic diseases. Therefore, the Dietary Guidelines for Americans, 2010 is intended for Americans ages 2 years and older, including those who are at increased risk of chronic disease (25). Poor diet and physical inactivity are the most important factors contributing to an epidemic of overweight and obesity in this country.

Dietary Guidelines and Children

Children are a particularly important focus of the Dietary Guidelines for Americans because of the growing body of evidence documenting the vital role that optimal nutrition plays throughout the lifespan (25). Today, too many children are consuming diets with too many calories and not enough nutrients and are not getting enough physical activity. Approximately 32 percent of children and adolescents ages 2 to 19 years are overweight or obese, with 17 percent of children being obese (25). In addition, risk factors for adult chronic diseases are increasingly found in younger ages. Eating patterns established in childhood often track into later life, making early intervention on adopting healthy nutrition and physical activity behaviors a priority.

Healthcare Crisis

Our nation is currently facing a major long-term public health crisis. How serious is the problem? Obesity has risen a full 34% since 1960 while morbid obesity is up sixfold (26). NPR reports that new research indicates that if people continue to consume food at the rate they do now, a massive 83 percent of men and 72 percent of women will be considered overweight or obese by the year 2020 (27). Reductions in smoking, high blood pressure and high cholesterol have been offset by prediabetes, diabetes and expanding waistbands (27).

More Spending On Healthcare Than Smoking

Our nation spends more on health care than any other country in the world (27). In April of 2012 Reuters reported that obesity in America is now adding an astounding $190 billion to the annual national health care price tag, exceeding smoking as public health enemy number one when it comes to cost (26). Obese men rack up an additional $1,152 a year in medical spending, especially for hospitalizations and prescription drugs (29). Obese women account for an extra $3,613 a year (29).

The high cost of being significantly overweight manifests in a variety of ways, ranging from the increased insurance premiums, to subsidizing the added medical charges, to the surprisingly dramatic impact on energy costs (26). The extra weight carried by vehicles as a result of obese and overweight Americans is responsible for almost *one billion additional gallons* of gasoline being burned each year by automobiles—nearly 1 percent of our total gasoline usage (26). Making the cost impact all the more troubling is the fact that, unlike smokers, obese people tend to live almost as long as those who keep their weight under control (26).

While chronic diseases are among the most common and costly of all health problems, they are also among the most preventable (2). Despite the evidence that prevention works, the focus of our health care system is on disease treatment (26).

Clearly our health care system is not equipped to meet the needs of people with chronic diseases. As stated in the introduction, *health care providers, educators, and all professionals have been called on to work together on implementing the recommendations contained in the Dietary Guidelines for Americans.*

Food Guidance System

In 2005 The Food Guidance System was established to improve the nutrition and well-being of Americans. MyPyramid.gov was developed to carry the messages of the 2005 Dietary Guidelines and to make Americans aware of the vital health benefits of simple and modest improvements in nutrition, physical activity and lifestyle behavior (24). Imagine the monumental task of educating an entire population on lifestyle behaviors required to improve the health of our nation and reduce unmanageable health care costs. The Food Guidance System does a good job of tackling on such an enormous task. There is a plethora of information available on how to make improvements in one's diet (and activity level) for individuals wishing to do so (30).

In 2011 MyPlate was introduced along with updating of the USDA food patterns for the 2010 Dietary Guidelines for Americans (30). The new shape was designed to "grab" consumer attention with a visual cue icon that serves as a reminder for healthy eating. The plate is divided into four quadrants with fruits and vegetables taking up half the plate. Grains take up a bit more than a quarter. The last quadrant, protein, is a term intended to include seafood as well as meat and beans that once made up a section of the old pyramid. There is a separate glass of milk to represent dairy products. Gone completely is any section for sweets and desserts, which once occupied part of the pyramid (30).

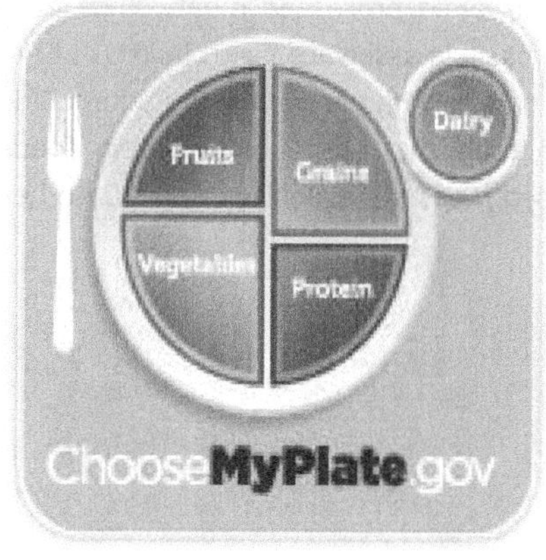

The makeup of the plate was designed to convey the messages in the government's latest

Dietary Guidelines, which recommended consumers eat more fruits, vegetable, substitute sea foods for some meat, and cut back on salt. The new icon is intended to help Americans improve their diets and lose weight. Agriculture Secretary Tom Vilsack, speaking at a news conference said the pyramid that had been used for decades was, "simply to complex to serve as a quick and easy guide for busy American families" (31).

Harvard Healthy Eating Plate Versus MyPlate

The Healthy Eating Plate, created by experts at Harvard School of Public Health and Harvard Medical School, points consumers to the healthiest choices in the major food groups (23) versus the USDA MyPlate icon which does not differentiate between some of the healthier choices. The Healthy Eating Plate is based on the best available science and was not subjected to political and commercial pressures from food industry lobbyists.

The Healthy Eating Plate (23) encourages consumers to choose whole grains and limit refined grains, since whole grains are much better for health. In the body, refined grains act just like sugar. Over time, eating too much of these refined-grain foods can make it harder to control weight and can raise the risk of heart disease and diabetes. MyPlate does not tell consumers that whole grains are better for health (23).

The Healthy Eating Plate encourages consumers to choose fish, poultry, beans or nuts, protein sources that contain other healthful nutrients (23). It encourages them to limit red meat and avoid processed meat, since eating even small quantities of these foods on a regular basis is associated with increased risk of heart disease, diabetes, colon cancer, and weight gain. MyPlate's protein section could be filled by a hamburger or hot dog; it offers no indication that some high-protein foods are healthier than others or that red and processed meat are especially harmful to health (23).

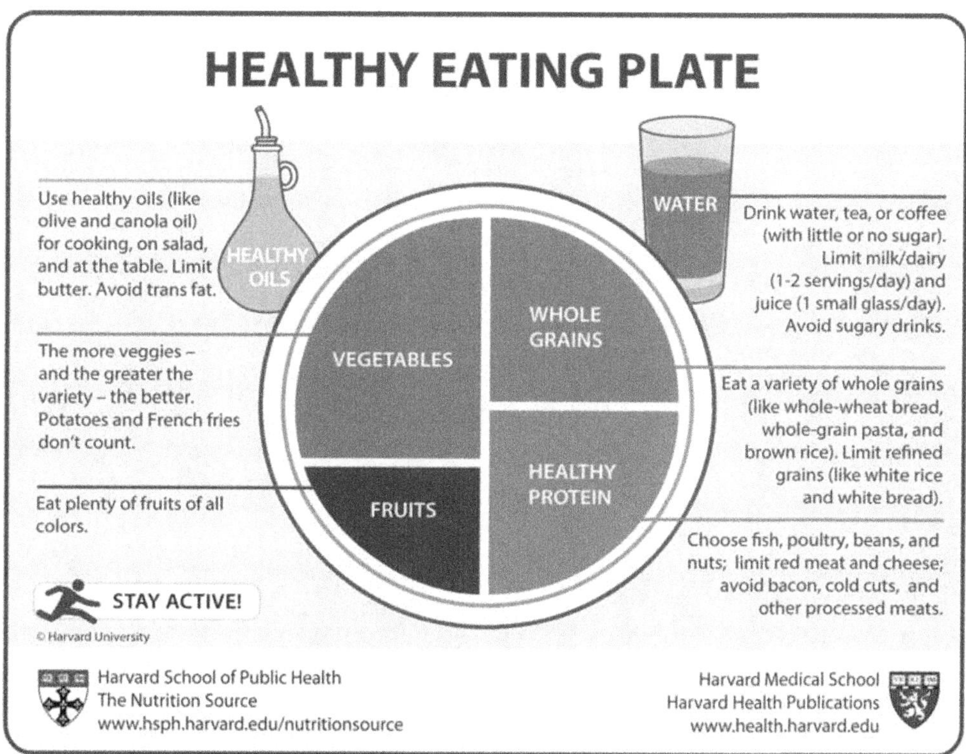

The Healthy Eating Plate encourages an abundant variety of vegetables, since Americans are particularly deficient in their vegetable consumption—except for potatoes and French fries (23). MyPlate does not distinguish between types of vegetables. The Healthy Eating Plate recommends eating a colorful variety of fruits (23).

The Healthy Eating Plate depicts a bottle of healthy oil, and it encourages consumers to use olive, canola, and other plant oils in cooking, on salads, and at the table (23). These healthy fats reduce harmful cholesterol and are good for the heart, and Americans don't consume enough of them each day. It also recommends limiting butter and avoiding trans fat. MyPlate is silent on fat (23).

The Healthy Eating Plate encourages consumers to drink water, since it's naturally calorie free, or to try coffee and tea (with little or no sugar), which are also great calorie-free alternatives (23). It advises consumers to avoid sugary drinks, since these are major contributors to the obesity and diabetes epidemics. It recommends limiting juice, even 100% fruit juice, to just a small glass a day, because juice contains as much sugar and as many calories as sugary soda. MyPlate says nothing about sugary drinks or juice. The figure scampering across the bottom of the Healthy Eating Plate's placemat is a reminder that staying active is half of the secret to weight control. The other half is eating a healthy diet with modest portions that meet your calorie needs. There is no activity message on MyPlate (23).

Summary

Eukaryotic cells have a nucleus which contains most of the cell's genetic material. The nucleus is enclosed by a double lipid layer membrane. The contents of the cell are suspended in what is known as the cytoplasm.

Plant cells have rigid cell walls composed of tough fibrils of cellulose. The plant cells wall is much thicker, stronger, and more rigid than animal cell walls. Rigid plant cell walls prevent the plant cell from moving. Animal cell membranes are composed of lipid bilayers. These cell membranes have dynamic, fluid structures which allow molecules to move about rapidly and freely in the plane of the membrane.

Mitochondria are responsible for respiration and this process occurs nowhere else in the cell. Muscle cells contain many mitochondria, while fat cells contain very few. Cells, such as nerve cells, red blood cells, brain cells, and other cells do not contain mitochondria and can not produce their own energy. These cells rely on glucose in the blood stream for energy.

Digestion is the process by which ingested foods are broken down into smaller segments in preparation for absorption. Absorption is the process by which nutrients enter the small intestinal cells and are absorbed into the body.

Nutrition is the science of how the body breaks down and utilizes the nutrients in foods. The essential nutrients include carbohydrates, fats, proteins, vitamins, minerals and water. The macronutrients - carbohydrates, fats, and proteins provide the body with energy. The micronutrients - vitamins and minerals - do not provide energy, but are just as critical in health. Water provides the environment in which nearly all the body's activities occur. Water participates in almost all metabolic reactions and is the medium for transporting molecules in and out of cells.

Homeostasis is the maintenance of relatively constant internal conditions in body systems by corrective responses to forces that, if left unopposed, would cause unacceptably large changes in those conditions. The human body has a tremendous capacity to return to homeostasis.

The publication of the first edition of Recommended Dietary Allowances (RDAs) in 1941 was recognized as one of the most authoritative sources of information on recommendations for nutrient intakes for healthy people (24). In 1989, rising awareness of the impact of nutrition on chronic disease dictated an expanded review of uses and misuses of RDAs (24). The new framework for this expanded approach developed by U.S. and Canadian scientists became known as the Dietary Reference Intakes (DRIs). This series of references greatly extends the scope and application of previous nutrient guidelines to include requirements based on how the nutrient may be related to chronic disease or developmental abnormalities (24). This framework also identifies a new reference intake, the Tolerable Upper Intake Level (UL), which if consumed consistently, may result in adverse effects (24).

The DRI's are an average daily dietary intake level sufficient to meet the nutrition requirement of nearly all (97 to 98 percent) healthy individuals in a particular life stage and gender group. They are intended to be used as a guide for daily intake by individuals. RDAs (US standards) depend on Estimated Average Requirements (EAR). If no EAR has been established, then no RDAs are set. If sufficient data is not available to calculate an EAR, then a reference intake - adequate intake (AI) is used instead of an RDA. Less information is available on which to base allowances for certain nutrients (copper, manganese, chromium, molybdenum, and chloride). These nutrients are not included in the RDAs and figures are averages of *Safe and Adequate Intakes* as set by the National Academy of Sciences.

The 2010 Dietary Guidelines have been consistent with subsequent editions but they have changed in some significant ways to reflect an evolving body of evidence about nutrition, the food and physical activity environment, and health. The ultimate goal of the Dietary Guidelines for Americans is to improve the health of our nation's current and future generations by facilitating and promoting healthy eating and physical activity choices so that these behaviors become the norm among all individuals.

In 2011 MyPlate was introduced along with updating of the USDA food patterns for the 2010 Dietary Guidelines for Americans. The new shape was designed to "grab" consumer attention with a visual cue icon that serves as a reminder for healthy eating. The plate is divided into four quadrants with fruits and vegetables taking up half the plate. Grains take up a bit more than a quarter. The last quadrant is called "protein," a term intended to include seafood as well as the meat and beans that once made up a section of the old pyramid, officials said. There is a separate glass of milk to represent dairy products.

The Healthy Eating Plate, created by experts at Harvard School of Public Health and Harvard Medical School, points consumers to the healthiest choices in the major food groups. The Healthy Eating Plate is based exclusively on the best available science and was not subjected to political and commercial pressures from food industry lobbyists.

Chapter 1 Sample Test

1. List the energy nutrients and how much energy is derived from each.
2. Explain what constitutes a complete protein (in the traditional sense), and list three sources of complete proteins.
3. What are two major differences between plant cells and animal cells?
4. What are the roles of vitamins and minerals in providing energy?
5. If a man expends 3000 calories per day, what would be his recommended water intake?
6. Define homeostasis and provide several examples.
7. What are the Dietary Reference Intakes? Discuss whether or not they are minimum standard requirements. Also discuss the differences between DRIs and Daily Values.
8. Discuss the Dietary Guidelines and provide details concerning the importance of the guidelines; changes in the guidelines; and the challenges that face our nation as it relates to obesity.
9. Discuss the changes in the "Food Guidance System" with the publication of the latest dietary guidelines.
10. Discuss the Harvard Healthy Eating plate and how it differs from the USDA MyPlate icon.

References

1. Rokholm B. Baker JL. Sorensen TI. (2010), The leveling off of the obesity epidemic since the year 1999—a review of evidence and perspectives. *Obes Rev.* 11: 835–46.
2. Campaign to end obesity. Obesity facts & Resources. (accessed 05/15/2013). http://www.obesitycampaign.org/obesity_facts.asp.
3. Wang Y. McPherson K. Marsh T. Gortmaker S. Brown M. (2011). Health and economic burden of the projected obesity trends in the USA and UK. *Lancet.* 378: 815-25.
4. Wang Y. Beydoun MA. Liang L. Caballero B. Kumanyika SK. (2008). Will all Americans become overweight or obese? Estimating the progression and cost of the US obesity epidemic. Obesity (Silver Spring) 2008; 16: 2323–30.
5. U.S. Department of Health and Human Services. (2013). The Surgeon General's call to action to prevent and decrease overweight and obesity. *Surgeon Generals Report. http://www.surgeongeneral.gov/library/calls/obesity/fact_adolescents.html.*
6. Academy of Nutrition and Dietetics. It's about eating right. How much water do I need each day. (accessed 05/15/2013). http://www.eatright.org/Public/content.aspx?id=6442462188.
7. Gazzaniga-Moloo J. Nutrition and you: trends 2011 webinar. Presented by AND.
8. Alberts B, et al. (2002). Molecular Biology of the Cell, 4th edition. Ny, NY: Garland Publishing.
9. Whitney, E & Rolfes S. (2013). *Understanding Nutrition,13th ed.* Belmont,CA:Wadsworth, Cengage Learning.
10. Lehninger, A. (2013). Principles of Biochemistry, 6th ed NY: W H Freeman and Company. (1-9).
11. Zar, J. (1984). Biostatistical Analysis, 2nd ed. Prentice-Hall Inc: NY.
12. Ross, C (Shils) et al. (2012). *Modern Nutrition in Health & Disease, 11th ed.* Philadelphia PA: Lipincott Wilillians & Wilikins (1115-1116).
13. U.S. Department of Health and Human Services. Your digestive system and how it works. National Digestive Diseases Information Clearinghouse. (accessed 05/15/2013). http://digestive.niddk.nih.gov/ddiseases/pubs/yrdd/index.aspx
14. Recommended Dietary Allowances, 10th ed. Subcommittee on the tenth edition of the RDAs, Food and Nutrition Board Commission on Life Sciences, National Research Council. Washington, DC: National Academy Press, 1989.
15. http://ndb.nal.usda.gov/. USDA National Nutrient Database for Standard Reference. Last modified Dec. 2011.
16. Academy of Nutrition and Dietetics. Nutrition and you: Trends 2011. Public opinion on food and nutrition: 20 years of insights. http://www.eatright.org/media/content.aspx?id=7639
17. Mann D. (2010). Trying to lose weight? Drink more water. (accessed 05/15/2013). http://www.cnn.com/2010/HEALTH/08/23/drink.water.lose.weight/index.html.
18. Dietary Reference Intakes: RDA and AI for Vitamins and Elements http://iom.edu/Activities/Nutrition/SummaryDRIs/~/media/Files/Activity %20Files/Nutrition/DRIs/RDA%20and%20AIs_Vitamin%20and%20Elements.pdf. 2012
19. USDA National Agricultural Library. Dietary Reference Intakes. (accessed 05/15/2013). http://fnic.nal.usda.gov/dietary-guidance/dietary-reference-intakes.
20. USDA National Agricultural Library. USDA Dietary Guidelines. http://fnic.nal.usda.gov/dietary-guidance/dietary-reference-intakes/dri-tables. (accessed 05/15/2013).
21. USDA National Agricultural Livrary. USDA Dietary Guidance. (accessed 05/15/2013). http://fnic.nal.usda.gov/dietary-guidance.
22. U. S. Food and Drug Administration. Guidance for industry: A food labeling guide. Updated 06/24/2013. (accessed 05/15/2013). http://www.fda.gov/Food/GuidanceRegulation

/GuidanceDocumentsRegulatoryInformation/LabelingNutrition/ucm064928.htm.

23. Harvard School of Public Health. Healthy eating plate vs USDA"s MyPlate. 05/15/2013)/ http://www.hsph.harvard.edu/nutritionsource/healthy-eating-plate-vs-usda-myplate/.
24. USDA National Agricultural Library. USDA Dietary Guidelines. A Brief History of the dietary guidelines. (accessed 05/15/2013).http://fnic.nal.usda.gov/dietary-guidance/dietary-guidelines/historical-dietary-guidance.
25. USDA National Agricultural Library. USDA Dietary Guidelines. *Dietary Guidelines for Americans, 2010* (Released 1/31/11) (accessed 05/15/2013). http://www.cnpp.usda .gov/DGAs2010-PolicyDocument.htm.
26. Unger, R. (2012). Obesity now costs Americans more in healthcare spending than smoking. Forbes Magazine. http://www.forbes.com/sites/rickungar/2012/04/30/obesity-now-costs-americans-more-in-healthcare-costs-than-smoking/
27. Kennedy L. Study: 72% of women could be overweight or obese by 2020. (accessed 05/16/2013) http://www.more.com/american-obesity-study.
28. Wang YC, et al. (2011). Health and economic burden of the projected obesity trends in the USA and UK. Lancet. 378: 815-827.
29. Cawley, J. and C. Meyehoefer. (2012). The Medical Care Costs of Obesity: An Instrumental Variables Approach", *Journal of Health Economics.* 31(1): 219:230
30. USDA National Agricultural Library. USDA MyPlate and Food Pyramid Resources (accessed 05/15/2013). http://fnic.nal.usda.gov/dietary-guidance/myplatefood-pyramid-resources/usda-myplate-food-pyramid-resources.
31. Brasher P. (2011). DesMoinesRegister./com. My Plate replaces food pyramid. http://blogs. desmoinesregister.com/dmr/index.php/2011/06/02/my-plate-replaces-food-pyramid/article.
32. Centers for Disease Control and Prevention. (2011). Chronic disease prevention and heath promotion. Health consequences of obesity. (accessed 05/15/2013). http://www.cdc.gov/chronicdisease/resources/publications/aag/obesity.htm.

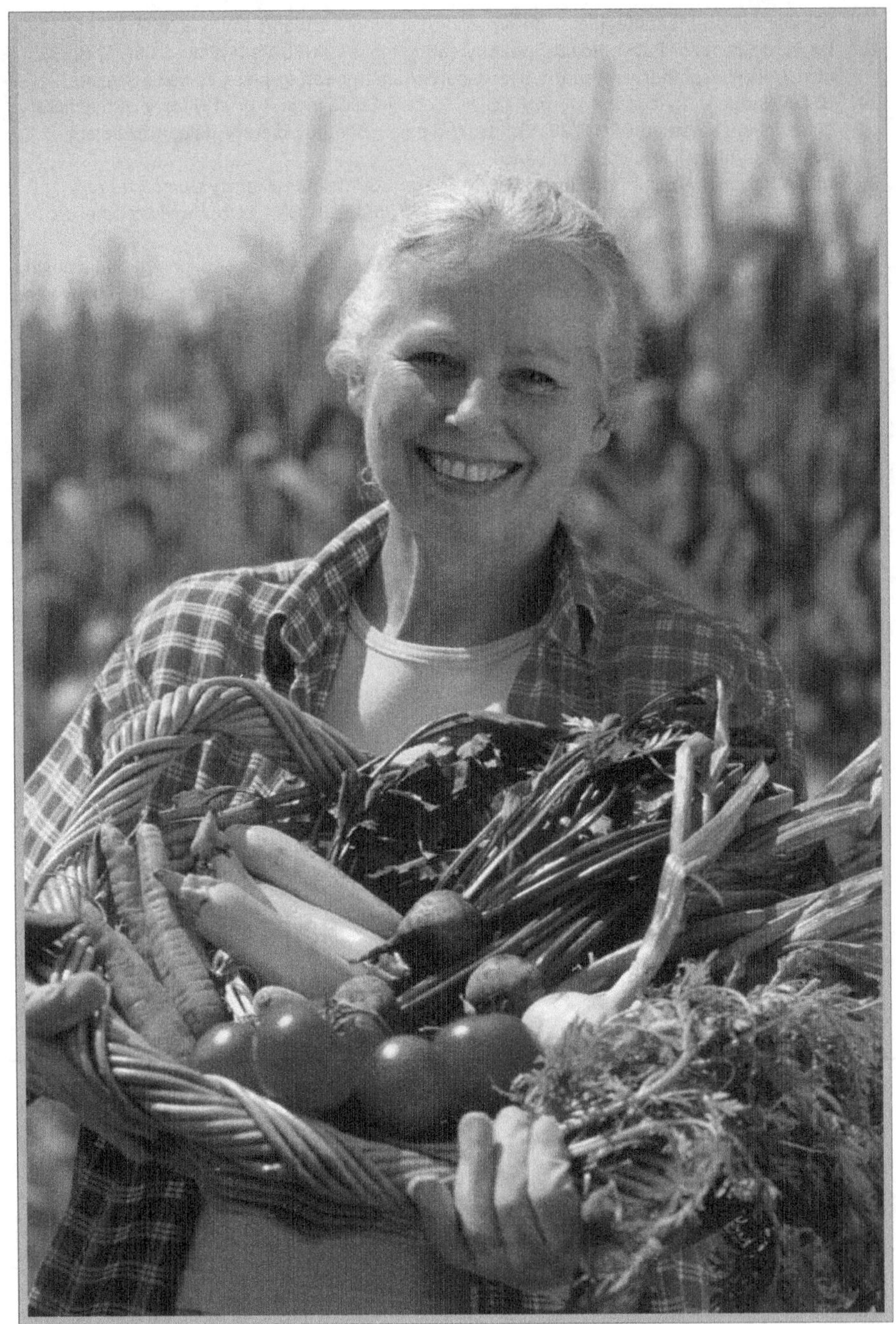

Chapter 2 - Carbohydrates

In the next three chapters we will take a more in-depth look at each of the energy nutrients. Carbohydrates, fats, and proteins provide the body with energy to perform daily activities and sustain life. For optimum health and fitness, these nutrients must be obtained in adequate amounts. In this chapter, we will examine carbohydrates in detail, including digestion, absorption, transport, and their importance in energy production and health.

Objectives

After reading and studying this chapter, you should be able to:

1. List the three classes of carbohydrates and describe each.
2. Describe digestion, absorption, transport, and roles of carbohydrates.
3. Define glycogen and explain its role in metabolism.
4. Discuss fiber and its role in health.
5. Gain an understanding of the positive and negative effects of alcohol.
6. Discuss nonnutritive and nutritive sweeteners.
7. Identify and discuss the controversy over high fructose corn syrup.

Introduction

The body requires larger amounts of carbohydrates than either proteins or fats. According to the Dietary Reference Intakes published by the USDA, 45% - 65% of calories should come from carbohydrate (1). Carbohydrates are the body's main source of fuel. They are needed for the regulation of glucose levels, the central nervous system, the kidneys, the brain, and muscle (including the heart) to function properly (2). Carbohydrates can be stored in the muscles and liver and later used for energy. They are mainly found in starchy foods (like grains and potatoes), fruits, milk, and yogurt. Other foods like vegetables, beans, nuts, seeds and cottage cheese contain carbohydrates, but in lesser amounts (2).

Carbohydrates

The most common and abundant forms of carbohydrates are sugars, fibers, and starches. The basic building block of every carbohydrate is a sugar molecule, a simple union of carbon, hydrogen, and oxygen (2).

There are 3 classes of carbohydrates in foods. Monosaccharides consist of a one sugar molecule, oligosaccharides consist of a few sugar molecules (disaccharide-two sugars), and polysaccharides consist of many sugar molecules (2).

The monosaccharides include glucose, fructose and galactose. Glucose is the simple sugar found in starch and glycogen, and fructose is the simple sugar found in fruit. Galactose is bound to glucose to form the disaccharide, lactose found in milk. The disaccharides are the most common oligosaccharides and include sucrose (fructose and glucose), lactose (galactose and glucose), and maltose (glucose and glucose). Sucrose consists of a fructose and a glucose molecule that forms table sugar. Lactose is the disaccharide found in milk; and maltose occurs when starch is broken down (2).

Monosaccharide	Glucose, fructose, galactose (one sugar link)
Disaccharide	Sucrose, lactose, maltose (two sugar links)
Oligosaccharide	Few sugar links (fructo-oligosaccharide consists of chains of fructose)
Polysaccharide	Starch, glycogen, cellulose (many sugar links)

The polysaccharides include starch, glycogen, and cellulose (2). Starch is a plant polysaccharide composed of glucose and is digestible by humans. Two forms of starch include amylose and amylopectin. Glycogen is the stored form of starch in the body and is composed of glucose molecules. It is manufactured and stored in the liver and muscle. Starch and glycogen consist of many glucose molecules linked together as long branched chains and is more highly branched than starch (2). Cellulose is a complex carbohydrate that is composed of glucose units and forms the main constituent of the cell wall in most plants.

Digestion

Digestion was discussed in general in Chapter 1. We will review digestion of each macronutrient in the next three chapters, beginning with carbohydrates. In review, the goal of carbohydrate digestion is to degrade carbohydrates into their constituent monosaccharides before they can be absorbed and metabolized.

Mouth: Digestion of carbohydrates begins in the mouth (2). Glucose is unique in that small amounts can be absorbed through the lining of the mouth. But for the most part nutrient absorption takes place in the small intestines. An enzyme in saliva, known as salivary amylase, hydrolyzes (breaks) starch into shorter polysaccharides. Because the food is soon swallowed, the job is incomplete (2).

Stomach: The swallowed food mixes with the stomach's secretions (2). The activity of salivary amylase is halted by hydrochloric acid and protein-digesting enzymes. Digestive juices in the stomach contain no enzymes to break down carbohydrates so carbohydrate digestion ceases. Fibers are not digested but they play a role in delaying gastric emptying.

Small Intestines: In the small intestines the major carbohydrate-digesting enzyme, pancreatic amylase, continues breaking down the polysaccharides to shorter glucose chains and disaccharides (2). This enzyme is secreted into the small intestines via the pancreatic duct. The final step takes place on the outer membranes of the intestinal cells where the disaccharides are broken down to monosaccharides (2). Only the indigestible fibers remain in the digestive tract and enter the large intestine. Here, bacterial enzymes digest fiber. Fiber holds water, regulates bowel activity, and also binds cholesterol and some minerals, transporting them out of the body (2).

Large Intestines: Within one to four hours after a meal, all of the available carbohydrates are digested (2). Only the indigestible fibers remain in the large intestines.

Carbohydrate metabolism begins with digestion in the small intestine where monosaccharides are absorbed into the bloodstream and transported to the liver (5).

Absorption

Absorption of carbohydrates occurs when the monosaccharides are absorbed into the small intestinal cells (5). They cross the small intestinal cells and are washed into the bloodstream by a rush of circulating blood which carries them to the liver.

Transport

The monosaccharides are delivered through the bloodstream to the liver where the liver converts them to glucose. There are five possible fates for glucose in the liver:(5)

1. Glucose can be converted into glycogen.
2. Glucose can be used for energy by liver cells.
3. Any amount beyond that which can be stored as carbohydrate will be turned into fatty acids, which in turn can travel to the fat cells and be stored as fat.
4. The liver can add a phosphate group to glucose and store it as glucose-6-phosphate (discussed in more detail in Chapter 5).
5. Glucose can also be made into nucleotides.

Glycogen

After entry into cells, glucose can be used immediately for cellular energy or it can be stored as glycogen. Glycogen is a highly branched polysaccharide consisting of links of glucose molecules. Immediately upon entry into cells, glucose combines with phosphate, a process known as phosphorylation. The phosphorylation of glucose is irreversible in most cells except in liver cells, renal tubular cells, and intestinal epithelial cells. These cells contain the enzyme glucose phosphatase which catalyzes the reverse reaction know as glycogenolysis (the breakdown of glycogen to glucose) (5). In other words, only liver cells, renal tubular cells and intestinal epithelial cells have the ability to catabolize glycogen to glucose. Muscle cells lack the enzyme glucose phosphatase, which is required to release glucose into the blood, so the glycogen stored in muscle is for internal use only and cannot be shared with other cells (5).

Glycogenesis is the process of glycogen formation. Although small amounts of glycogen are synthesized in many cells only liver and skeletal muscle can accumulate large amounts. Liver glycogen is used as a short term energy source by providing a means to store and release glucose in response to blood glucose levels. Liver cells do not use this glucose for their own energy; they prefer fatty acids as an energy supply (5).

Muscle cells can store more glycogen than liver cells. For example, the average 150 pound male can store approximately 1800 calories of carbohydrate, 1400 calories in muscle in the form of glycogen, 320 calories in the liver in the form of glycogen, and approximately 80 calories of glucose in the bloodstream (6).

Glucose Homeostasis

Glucose homeostasis is an example of one of the highest levels of homeostatic control in the human body. A normal fasting blood glucose target range for an individual without diabetes is 70-100 mg/dL. The American Diabetes Association recommends a fasting plasma glucose level of 70–130 mg and after meals less than 180 (7).

Blood glucose homeostasis is regulated primarily by the hormones insulin, glucagon, epinephrine, and norepinephrine. Hormones are chemical messengers secreted by a variety of glands in response to altered conditions in the body. They are secreted from the site of production, through the bloodstream and to other cells throughout the body. Each hormone affects one or more specific target tissues or organs and elicits specific responses to restore normal conditions (2).

Insulin lowers the glucose concentration in the blood, and glucagon raises it (2). Insulin is often called the "hyperglycemic" hormone because of its role in removing excess glucose from the bloodstream. Sugars are absorbed from the intestines into the bloodstream after a meal. Insulin is then secreted by the pancreas in response to this detected increase in blood sugar.

Many cells of the body have insulin receptors which bind the insulin. These types of cells are known as insulin-dependent cells (2). When a cell has insulin attached to its surface, the cell activates other receptors designed to absorb glucose from the bloodstream allowing glucose to enter the cell. Hence, when glucose levels in the bloodstream rise after a meal, insulin promotes glucose absorption by insulin dependent cells. In this manner, glucose levels are restored to normal (2).

Glucagon is the hormone responsible for controlling glucose levels in the bloodstream when levels are low. Glucagon is sometimes referred to as the "hypoglycemic" hormone because of its role in releasing glucose into the bloodstream. Also produced by the pancreas, this hormone signals the liver to convert stored glycogen into glucose which is them released into the bloodstream (2). The action of glucagon is thus opposite to that of insulin.

Epinephrine and norepinephrine produce a similar response as glucagon under stress conditions. During the fight-or-flight (stress) response, the adrenal gland releases epinephrine and norepinephrine into the bloodstream, along with other hormones such as cortisol signaling the liver to release its glycogen (2).

Certain cells of the body do not have insulin receptors and are referred to as non-insulin-dependent cells. Most cells of the body are insulin-dependent cells with the exception of red blood cells, nerve cells, brain cells, and a variety of cells involved in vision. These non-insulin-dependent cells are quite different in that insulin has either little or no effect on glucose utilization or uptake. Another distinguishing factor is that these cells (red blood cells, nerve cells, cells involved in vision, etc.) can only use glucose as an energy source. Therefore, prevention of damage to these cells requires glucose levels to be maintained within the homeostatic range (5).

To review, the role of insulin is to allow glucose to flow from the bloodstream into insulin-dependent cells. This process returns blood glucose levels to normal, thereby protecting non-insulin dependent cells from destruction. When glucose levels are too low, glucagon is released from the pancreas. This event signals the liver to release glucose into the bloodstream, again protecting non-insulin dependent cells from destruction due to insufficient levels of glucose.

Glucose Time Curve

The body has a finite amount of glycogen that can be stored in the liver and muscle. As previously mentioned, the glycogen stored in muscle is not available to supply non-insulin dependent cells with glucose. Therefore, these cells must rely on stored glycogen from the liver when glucose is unavailable (2).

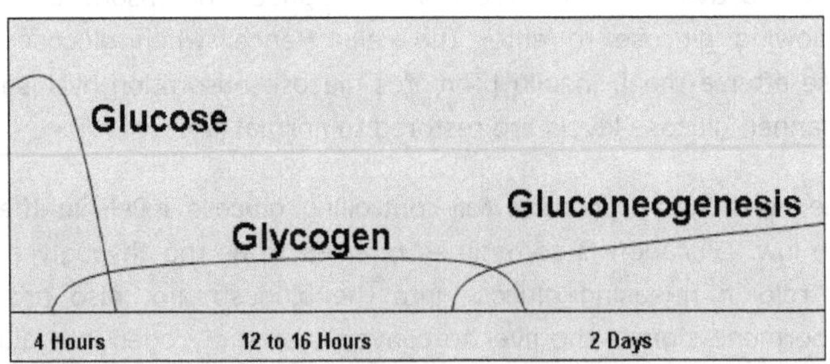

The liver can store enough glycogen to supply non-insulin dependent cells with glucose for about twelve to sixteen hour (2). If liver glycogen stores are depleted and food is not eaten, the body must produce glucose from other sources.

Consider the following example. An individual eats dinner consisting of complex and simple carbohydrates at 6 pm. For the first four hours after this meal, glucose is present in the bloodstream from the meal. At around 10 pm, the individual goes to bed. Even while sleeping, the body utilizes many calories for metabolic reactions (basal metabolic rate). Glycogen stored in the liver is released all night long providing the needed glucose for the glucose requiring reactions. When the individual gets up at 6 am, glycogen in the liver is nearly depleted and by 10 am, is guaranteed to be depleted. Since blood glucose levels must be maintained (homeostasis), if the individual does not eat glucose will be formed through a process known as gluconeogenesis.

Gluconeogenesis

The only way the body can produce glucose after 12 to 16 hours of not eating is through gluconeogenesis, the making of glucose from non-carbohydrate sources (2). The only available source for glucose production in this stage is the breakdown of glucogenic amino acids (amino acids that can synthesize glucose) (2). The body cannot use fat for glucose production because fat cannot synthesize glucose (2). (Glycerol, the alcohol portion of fat can synthesize small amounts of glucose, but the amount is inconsequential.) To obtain these glucogenic (glucose-producing) amino acids the body must catabolize whole proteins from skeletal muscle and eventually other lean organ tissues (2).

In the first few days of a fast, body proteins constitute over 90 percent of the needed glucose. Energy at this point is a homeostatic priority for the body, and since energy from food is unavailable the body must produce energy from gluconeogenesis (2). The only source of energy available is catabolism of proteins which includes both glucogenic and non-glucogenic amino acids (glucose forming and non-glucose forming amino acids). The nitrogen from both glucogenic and non-glucogenic amino acids must be disposed of (this will be also discussed in detail in the section on proteins) which taxes the kidneys and liver.

The process of gluconeogenesis becomes a huge sabotaging effect in weight management and health because muscle is being catabolized for energy. At this point, the scale will go down but is destined to go back up since over half the weight loss can be contributed to muscle loss (see also diets). In other words, the process of energy production from glucogenic amino acids is an "expensive" way to obtain glucose since whole body proteins are catabolized to provide amino acids for glucose production. If the body were to continue to use proteins at the same rate as in the first forty-eight hours, death would ensue within days. Another metabolic process known as ketosis occurs (2).

Ketosis

Ketones, acetoacetate and β-hydroxybutyrate, are small carbon fragments that are the fuel created by the breakdown of fat stores. Ketosis is a metabolic state that occurs when the liver converts fat into fatty acids and ketone bodies.

Biochemically, ketones closely resemble glucose. Some cells (such as muscle cells) can switch to utilization of ketones for energy, while the non-insulin dependent cells previously discussed (brain cells, nerve cells, etc.) cannot. With the use of ketones by muscle cells and other cells, the body can survive weeks and even months (2).

Ketosis is a physiological state associated with chronic starvation (3). Glucose is regarded as the preferred energy source for all cells in the body and ketosis is regarded as a crisis reaction to a lack of carbohydrates in the diet. In the first stage of a low carbohydrate diet ketones build up slowly. After several days, large amounts of ketones are formed.

To reiterate, the liver can store enough glycogen to supply brain cells, nerve cells, and other cells with glucose for about twelve to sixteen hours. A fast longer than 12 to 24 hours produces reduced insulin levels which mobilizes free fatty acids from fat tissue to be converted into ketones and initiates the catabolism of proteins into amino acids (3). The process of ketosis (breakdown of fat into ketones) is always associated with the catabolism of amino acids.

Ketosis is a potentially serious condition if ketone levels rise too high (3). Common short-term side effects include constipation, fatigue, halitosis, headache, thirst, polyuria and nausea (69-73). In pediatric patients, there have been reports of increased rates of dehydration, constipation, kidney stones, hyperlipidemia, impaired neutrophil function, optic neuropathy, osteoporosis, and protein deficiency when following a ketogenic diet (74,76). Ketogenic diets can also affect the central nervous system. In a randomized weight loss study, subjects consuming a ketogenic diet had impairments in higher order mental functions and flexibility (75,76). Death through starvation is the result of loss of muscle tissue, acidosis and other contributing factors. At death, there can still be substantial body fat with very little lean tissue remaining (2). Other effects of low carbohydrates diets and their impact on performance will be discussed in chapter 5.

While the research on ketogenic diets and its efficacy are mixed, the risk of ketosis outweighs any reported benefit in weight loss. In addition, there is an absence of research on the long term health effects of ketogenic diets and their safety (i.e. cancer risk, bone health and kidney health) (5). Moreover, it is important to critically examine the methods of published work on ketogenic diets as there are many variables to consider (i.e. subject size, demographics, caloric intake, specific macronutrients, physical activity level, etc.). How to critically interpret research will be discussed in more detail in chapter 10.

Ketosis should not be confused with ketoacidosis, which is severe ketosis causing the pH of the blood to drop below 7.2 (68). Ketoacidosis is a medical condition usually caused by diabetes and accompanied by dehydration, hyperglycemia, ketonuria, and increased levels of glucagon (68).

Absorption Rate

Absorption rates of carbohydrates differ depending on several factors. Simple sugars in the absence of nutrients such as fiber, fat, and protein are absorbed quickly and enter the bloodstream quickly. As described previously, influx of large amounts of simple sugars into the bloodstream must be removed quickly to prevent damage to non-insulin dependent cells. Triglycerides will be formed from excess sugar and the resulting triglycerides will be stored as body fat. When complex carbohydrates (legumes, breads, etc.) are absorbed in the presence of other nutrients such as fat, protein, or fiber, the absorption rate of the sugar is decreased (slowed). In this circumstance large amounts of simple sugars do not flood the bloodstream and the body is not forced to form triglycerides. For example, calories from an 800 calorie soft drink are absorbed differently than 800 calories from fruit and cottage cheese. While 800 calories may or may not be too many calories (depending on the person and the activity level), much more of the calories from the soft drink will be transformed into triglycerides than the 800 calories from intake of fruit and cottage cheese.

Glycemic Index

The glycemic response refers to how quickly glucose is absorbed after a person eats, how high blood glucose rises, and how quickly it returns to normal. Different foods elicit different glycemic responses, and the glycemic index classifies foods according to this response (2). The glycemic index was designed in Canada by Dr. David Jenkins and his research group at the University of Toronto in the 1980s to assist diabetics with improving carbohydrate food choices (8).

The glycemic index refers to the raising of blood glucose levels by carbohydrate foods (9) and ranks foods and beverages based on how they affect blood sugar levels. Only foods and beverages that contain carbohydrates are ranked, since they have the biggest effect on blood sugar. Foods are scored on a scale of 0 to 100 (12):

- High: 70 and up
- Medium: 56 to 69
- Low: 55 and under

Extensive lists of glycemic index rankings can be found online and in various other resources (11). The following table lists the glycemic index of some popular foods.

Canadian Research		**Glucose Revolution (13)**	
Food	Index	Food	Index
Potato	104	Potato	93
Table Sugar	83	Table Sugar	100
Couscous	93	Couscous	65
Rice Krispies	117	Rice Krispies	55
All Bran	60	All Bran	51
Whole Wheat Bread	100	Whole Wheat Bread	70
White Bread	100	White Bread	70

According to researchers, a high glycemic index is undesirable(12). Foods and beverages with high glycemic index scores are thought to be rapidly digested, which causes a spike in blood sugar, followed by a rapid decline creating wide fluctuations in blood sugar level. In contrast, items with low glycemic index rankings are thought to be digested more slowly, raising blood sugar in a more regulated and gradual way (12).

Researchers debate whether selecting foods based on the glycemic index is practical or offers any health benefits (10). The glycemic index, doesn't rank foods according to how healthy they are. Indeed, some foods with the preferred lower glycemic index ranking may, in fact, be less healthy because they contain large amounts of calories, sugar or saturated fat, especially packaged and processed foods. Whole wheat bread has the same glycemic index as white bread. Carrots have a high glycemic index, and people have eliminated them from their diets. But carrots are a wonderful, healthy food, and a whole bag of carrots contains less than 50 calories. Sweet-tasting watermelon has a very high glycemic index but a slice of watermelon has only a small amount of carbohydrate per serving (as the name suggests, watermelon is made up mostly of water). A Snickers bar has a glycemic index of 41, marking it as a low glycemic index food, but it is certainly not a health food (11).

To make the glycemic index even less useful, each individual has a differing daily glycemic response that can vary 43 percent on any given day (12). Another major concern with the glycemic index is that it ranks foods in isolation. In reality, how the body absorbs and handles carbohydrates depends on many factors, including how much food is eaten; how the food is ripened, processed or prepared; the time of day it's eaten; other foods eaten with it; and health conditions, such as diabetes. See the following table for additional factors (12).

Food Factor (12)	**Examples of Influencing Factors**	**Effect of Glycemic Response and Glycemic Index**
Gross food matrix structure	Grinding	Higher when homogenized
Cell-wall and starch structure	Degree of ripening	Higher when ripened
Granular Starch Structure	Heat treatment	Higher when gelantinized
Amylose and Amylopectin content	Amylopectin is more branched and more rapidly digested than amylose	Lower with higher amylose content
Gelling dietary fiber content	Added gelling fibers	Reduced
Organic acids	Added acids	Reduced
Amylase inhibitor	Added inhibitor	Reduced
Monosaccharide composition	Type of added sugar-glucose fructose ratio	Reduced with increased fructose content
Molecular composition of carbohydrate	Type of monosaccharide bonds in carbohydrate molecule	Reduce with increased number of a1-4 and a1-6
Resistant starch content	Heating-cooling cycles	Indifferent when testing equal amounts of available carbohydrate

So the glycemic index may not give an accurate picture of how one particular food affects blood sugar. Too many factors influence a food's glycemic effect to be an effective tool in choosing healthy carbohydrates.

Glycemic Load

Glycemic load is a related concept that scores a food product based on both carbohydrate content and portion size (14). A food's glycemic load is determined by multiplying its glycemic index by the amount of carbohydrate it contains. In general, a glycemic load of 20 or more is high, 11 to 19 is medium, and 10 or under is low (14).

Food	**Carb**	**X Index**	**= Load**
Baked Potato	34	1.04	35.4
Sugar	4	0.83	3.3
¾ cup Rice Krispies	28	1.17	32.8
Whole Wheat Bread	25	1	25

Food	Carb	X Index	= Load
White Bread	25	1	25

While the glycemic load appears to be a more accurate method than glycemic index, neither of these classification systems are ideal. When it comes to choosing healthy carbohydrates, people should replace highly processed grains, cereals, and sugars with minimally processed whole-grain products.

Insulin Resistance

Insulin resistance, or metabolic syndrome, describes a combination of health problems that have a common link, i.e., an increased risk of diabetes and early heart disease. Described and defined in 1988 by G.M. Reaven, Syndrome X is now referred to as the metabolic syndrome (15).

The cluster of medical conditions that make up insulin resistance (or metabolic syndrome) places a person at risk of developing type 2 diabetes and atherosclerosis (hardening of the arteries) (16). It is estimated that 34% of adult Americans have insulin resistance or metabolic syndrome (17).

Diseases or conditions associated with insulin resistance include the following (18,19,20):

- Obesity
- Type 2 diabetes
- High blood pressure
- Abnormal cholesterol levels
- Heart disease
- Polycystic ovary syndrome

In insulin resistance, the body's cells have a diminished ability to respond to the action of the hormone insulin. To compensate for the insulin resistance, the pancreas secretes more insulin (18).

People with this syndrome have high levels of insulin in the blood as a marker of the disease rather than a cause. Over time people with insulin resistance can develop prediabetes or diabetes as the high insulin levels can no longer compensate for elevated sugars (18).

Signs of Insulin Resistance

The signs of insulin resistance syndrome include (21):

- Impaired fasting blood sugar, impaired **glucose tolerance, or type 2 diabetes** occurs because the pancreas is unable to turn out enough insulin to overcome the insulin resistance. Blood sugar levels rise and prediabetes or diabetes is diagnosed.
- High blood pressure has been associated with insulin resistance. The mechanism is unclear, but studies suggest that the higher the blood pressure, the higher the insulin resistance.
- The typical cholesterol levels of a person with insulin resistance are low HDL, or good cholesterol, and high levels of triglycerides.
- Insulin resistance can result in atherosclerosis (hardening of the arteries) and an increased risk of blood clots.
- A major factor in the development of insulin resistance syndrome is obesity, especially abdominal obesity or belly fat. While obesity promotes insulin resistance, weight loss can improve the body's ability to recognize and use insulin appropriately.
- Protein in the urine, a sign that kidney damage has occurred, is associated with insulin resistance; although not everyone uses this component to define the syndrome.

There is no simple test to diagnose insulin resistance syndrome. Rather, a physician may suspect the syndrome if any three of the following are present (21):

- A waist size of 40 inches or more in men and 35 inches or more in women
- Increased levels of triglycerides (a type of fat in the blood)
- Low HDL, or "good," cholesterol level (Less than 40 mg/dL for men and 50 mg/dL for women)
- High blood pressure of 130/85 or higher, or being treated for high blood pressure
- Fasting blood glucose levels of 100 mg/dL or above, or being treated for diabetes

Note, the current epidemic of obesity in children also puts them at risk for the development of insulin resistance syndrome.

Treatment for Insulin Resistance Syndrome

Getting to and maintaining a healthy weight, as well as increasing physical activity, can help the body respond better to insulin. These lifestyle changes can also reduce the risk for diabetes and heart disease (22).

Insulin Resistance is preventable. Tips to prevent insulin resistance or metabolic syndrome include (22):

- Exercise. Try working up to walking 30 minutes a day for at least five days a week (exercise can be divided into three separate periods of 10 minutes each).
- Get to and maintain a healthy weight.
- Eat right. A healthy balanced diet is recommended.

Fiber

In the 1950's, fiber was described as any nondigestible portion of a plant cell wall (23). In 2002 the Institute of Medicine (IOM) defined total fiber as the sum of dietary fiber and functional fiber (24). Dietary fiber consists of nondigestible carbohydrates and lignin that are intrinsic and intact in plants; functional fiber is defined as isolated, nondigestible carbohydrates that have beneficial physiologic effects in humans (24). Unlike other food components, such as fats, proteins, or carbohydrates, which the body breaks down and absorbs, fiber is not digested. Instead, it passes intact through the stomach, small intestine, and colon and is excreted out of the body (2).

Fiber is commonly classified as soluble (dissolves in water) or insoluble (doesn't dissolve in water) (2). Soluble fiber dissolves in water to form a gel-like material. Soluble fiber is found in oats, peas, beans, apples, citrus fruits, carrots, barley, and psyllium. Insoluble sources of fiber include whole-wheat flour, wheat bran, nuts, beans, and vegetables, such as cauliflower, green beans, and potatoes (2).

Benefits of a High Fiber Diet

Diets rich in fibrous foods, such as whole grains, legumes, vegetables, and fruits, may protect against heart attack and stroke by lowering blood pressure, improving blood lipids, and reducing inflammation (the immune system's response to infection or injury) (25).

High fiber foods also play a key role in managing and preventing diabetes (26). In people with diabetes, fiber, particularly soluble fiber, can slow the absorption of sugar and help improve blood sugar levels.

Another benefit attributed to dietary fiber is prevention of colorectal cancer (27). Fibers may help prevent colon cancer by diluting, binding, and rapidly removing potential cancer-causing agents from the colon (28). Dietary fibers also enhance the health of the large intestine. Large, soft stools ease elimination and reduce pressure in the lower bowel, preventing constipation and making it less likely that hemorrhoids will form (29).

Foods Versus Supplements

Americans should increase their consumption of beans, peas, vegetables, fruits, whole grains, and other foods with naturally occurring fiber. Whole grains vary in fiber content. The Nutrition Facts label can be used to compare whole-grain products and choices that have higher fiber content (30).

Whole foods, rather than fiber supplements, are generally better. Fiber supplements don't provide the variety of fibers, vitamins, minerals, and other beneficial nutrients that foods do. However, some people may still need a fiber supplement if dietary changes aren't sufficient or if they have certain medical conditions, such as constipation, diarrhea, or irritable bowel syndrome. Fiber is also added to some foods; however, it's not yet clear if added fiber provides the same health benefits as naturally occurring sources (30).

Too much fiber eaten too quickly can promote intestinal gas, abdominal bloating and cramping. Increasing fiber gradually over a period of a few weeks helps to eliminate these symptoms by allowing the natural bacteria in the digestive system to adjust to the change. Also, drinking plenty of water is essential. Fiber works best when it absorbs water, making stools soft and bulky. Constipation can occur if insufficient fluid is consumed with a high-fiber diet (2).

Recommended Intake

The recommended intake of fiber includes (34):

	Men	**Women**
Adults under 50 years old	38	25
Adults over 50 years old	30	21

The following table lists fiber content of sample foods (30):

Fiber content of Foods	**Serving Size**	**Total Fiber (Grams)**	**Soluble Fiber (Grams)**	**Insoluble Fiber (Grams)**
Cereals				
All Bran Bran Buds	1/3 cup	13.0	4.0	9.0
All Bran Extra Fiber	1/2 cup	13.0	1.0	12.0
Fiber One	1/2 cup	13.0	1.0	12.0
Quaker Oat Bran	1/2 cup	6.0	3.0	3.0
Raisin Bran	1/2 cup	4.0	0.5	3.5

Fiber content of Foods	Serving Size	Total Fiber (Grams)	Soluble Fiber (Grams)	Insoluble Fiber (Grams)
Cheerios	1 cup	3.0	1.0	2.0
Shredded Wheat	1 1/4 cup	2.9	0.2	2.7
Oatmeal	1/2 cup	2.0	1.2	0.8
Corn Flakes	1 cup	1.0	0.0	1.0
Legumes (cooked)				
Lentils	1/2 cup	9.2	1.5	7.7
Red Kidney Beans	1/2 cup	8.2	3.4	4.9
Split Peas	1/2 cup	8.1	2.5	5.6
Pinto Beans	1/2 cup	7.4	2.7	4.6
Great Northern Beans	1/2 cup	6.2	1.1	5.1
Navy Beans	1/2 cup	5.8	1.7	4.1
Lima Beans	1/2 cup	4.9	1.2	3.8
Breads/Grains/Pasta				
Barley	1/2 cup	6.8	1.4	5.4
Whole Wheat Spaghetti	1/2 cup	3.2	0.4	2.7
Whole Wheat Bread	1 slice	2.2	0.5	1.7
Brown Rice	1/2 cup	1.8	0.2	1.6
Wheat Bread	1 slice	1.6	0.2	1.4
Bagel	1/2 medium	1.3	0.5	0.8
Spaghetti	1/2 cup	1.1	0.5	0.6
White Bread	1 slice	0.6	0.3	0.3
White Rice	1/2 cup	0.6	0.1	0.4
Nuts and Seeds				
Almonds	1/4 cup	3.9	0.4	3.5
Peanut Butter	2 tbsp	2.1	0.6	1.5
Walnuts	1/4 cup	1.4	0.5	0.9
Fresh Fruit				
Apples with Skin	1 large	4.2	1.6	2.6
Pear with Skin	1 medium	4	0.8	3.2
Blackberries	½ cup	3.8	0.9	2.9
Orange	1	3.6	2.1	1.5
Dried Prunes	4	3.1	1.3	1.8
Banana	1	2.8	0.9	1.9

Fiber content of Foods	Serving Size	Total Fiber (Grams)	Soluble Fiber (Grams)	Insoluble Fiber (Grams)
Peach with Skin	1	2.1	0.8	1.3
Grapefruit	½ large	1.8	1.3	0.5
Strawberries	½ cup	1.7	0.6	1.1
Cooked Vegetables				
Corn	½ cup	4.7	0.2	4.4
Green Peas	½ cup	4.4	0.6	3.8
Avocado	½ cup	3.8	1.5	2.2
Brussels Sprouts	½ cup	3.6	1.7	1.9
Sweet Potato (No Skin)	1 medium	3.4	1.7	1.7
Potato (No Skin)	1 large	2.8	0.7	2.1
Broccoli	½ cup	2.3	1	1.3
Carrot Slices	½ cup	2.3	1	1.3
Spinach	½ cup	2.1	0.6	1.4
Green Beans	½ cup	2	0.8	1.2
Cauliflower	½ cup	1.5	0.2	1.3
Raw Vegetables				
Tomato	1 medium	1.3	0.3	1
Celery	½ cup	0.9	0.2	0.7
Green Pepper	½ cup	0.9	0.3	0.6
Romaine Lettuce	1 cup	0.7	0.3	0.4

Alcohol

Alcohols are a class of organic compounds that arise naturally from carbohydrates when certain microorganisms metabolize them in the absence of oxygen (fermentation)(2). Alcohol is not digested like other foods. Once swallowed, it travels down the esophagus into the stomach and the small intestine; it avoids the normal digestive process and goes right into the bloodstream (2).

Alcohols have the ability to dissolve the lipids out of cell membranes allowing the alcohol to penetrate rapidly into cells, destroying cell structures. Ethanol, the type of alcohol we drink, is less toxic and when sufficiently diluted, produces euphoria with low enough risk to be tolerated by the body (2).

Alcohol is a drug (a substance that can modify one or more of the body's functions) and is medically defined as a depressant drug. It is a narcotic that has been used for centuries as an anesthetic (2). People believe alcohol is a stimulant because it seems to relieve inhibitions, but it does so by depressing the activity of the brain (2).

From the moment alcohol enters the body, the tiny molecules need no digestion and are quickly absorbed. About 20 percent of the alcohol molecules are absorbed through the walls of an empty stomach and can reach the brain within a minute. The stomach produces a small amount of an enzyme that breaks down the alcohol (alcohol dehydrogenase) and can thus reduce the amount entering the blood (3). The alcohol that leaves the stomach is absorbed in the intestines and circulates through the bloodstream to the liver. The extra alcohol travels to all parts of the body, circulating until the liver can finally process it. Liver and stomach cells are the only cells that can produce alcohol dehydrogenase (2). The amount of alcohol that the liver can break down is limited to about 1/2 ounce of alcohol per hour; the maximum amount determined by the amount of alcohol dehydrogenase. The amount of this enzyme is genetically determined. Men have more of this enzyme than women(2). Asians, Native Americans, and Inuits secrete less alcohol dehydrogenase than do most Caucasians (2).

The presence of alcohol in the liver disrupts the metabolism of the liver. The liver cells normally prefer fatty acids as fuel and packages excess fatty acids as triglycerides, which is then routed to other tissues of the body. However, when alcohol is present, the liver cells are forced to first metabolize the alcohol, letting the fatty acids accumulate, sometimes in huge amounts. This explains why heavy drinkers tend to develop fatty livers (3). A molecule involved in energy production, known as NADH, is also required for the metabolism of alcohol and is thus not available to produce energy from glucose. The energy cycle is blocked, fatty acids accumulate and hydrogen ions change the pH in the body (2).

The presence of alcohol in the liver can also alter protein metabolism. Synthesis of some proteins important in the immune system function are reduced, weakening the body's defenses against infection. With excessive alcohol consumption, protein deficiency can develop (2).

Alcohol is nonnutritive, contains 7 calories per gram, displaces nutrients from the diet, and can affect every tissue's metabolism of nutrients. Stomach cells begin to over secrete acid and histamine. These changes make the stomach and esophagus linings vulnerable to ulcer formation. Intestinal cells fail to absorb B vitamins, particularly thiamin, folate, and vitamin B12 (2).

Summary of the latest evidence concerning possible benefits of alcohol is that light to moderate consumption may lower mortality from all causes but only in adults 35 and older. No health benefits are evident before middle age and health benefits begin to disappear in older age, as metabolism changes (2).

The following table lists alcohol content of popular beverages

Beverage	Total Calories	Carbohydrate Calories	Alcohol Calories
12 oz. beer	150	50	100
12 oz. lite beer	100	24	76
Brandy (3-4 oz.)	65	0	65
80 proof whiskey (1.5 oz.)	95	0	95
90 proof whiskey (1.5 oz.)	110	0	110
7 oz. red wine	150	20	130
7 oz. white wine	160	30	130
7 oz. dry vermouth	210	10	200

Sweeteners

Sweeteners can be grouped in several ways. The most common approach to classifying sweeteners groups them as nutritive and nonnutritive sweeteners (39). Nutritive sweeteners contain carbohydrate and provide energy; they include sugars, caloric sweeteners, and added sugars. Sugars occur naturally in fruit, vegetables, and dairy products. They are also added to foods in processing or cooking (48). Nonnutritive sweeteners provide little or no calories when ingested (48). They are referred to as high intensity sweeteners since they are many times sweeter than sugar.

The following table lists popular substitutes and how they're commonly categorized (38,39):

Nonnutritive Sweeteners
Acesulfame potassium (Sunett, Sweet One)
Aspartame (Equal, NutraSweet)
Neotame
Saccharin (SugarTwin, Sweet'N Low)
Sucralose (Splenda)
Stevia (Truvia, Purevia, Sun Crystalsl)

Nutritive Sweeteners	
Sugar alcohols	Erythritol, hydrogenated starch, hydrolysate, isomalt, lactitol, maltitol, mannitol, sorbitol, xylitol
Natural Sweeteners	Fruit juice concentrate, honey, maple syrup, molasses

Nonnutritive Sweeteners

Originally termed artificial sweeteners, nonnutritive sweeteners are defined as synthetic sugar substitutes derived from naturally occurring substances, including herbs or sugar itself. They are regulated by the US Food and Drug Administration (FDA) and must be reviewed and approved by the FDA before being made available for sale (44,58,62). The FDA approval process includes establishing the highest no effect level (HNEL) and an acceptable daily intake (ADI) for each artificial sweetener. The HNEL is the threshold of intake at which no adverse effects are seen. The NHEL is divided by 100 and is assigned an ADI. Hence, the ADI is the maximum amount considered safe to consume each day over the course of a lifetime (48).

The approved nonnutritive sweeteners include acesulfame potassium, aspartame, neotame, saccharin, sucralose and stevia. Stevia is considered a nonnutritive sweetener as a Generally Regarded as Safe (GRAS) substance and has not been subjected to the rigorous standards of the other approved sweeteners (43). To be approved as a GRAS substance, generally available data and information about the use of the substance must be known, accepted widely by qualified experts, and a basis to conclude that there is consensus among these experts that the data and information available is sufficient to establish that the substance is safe under the conditions of its intended use. Stevia was given GRAS approval based on scientific data and the fact it has a lengthy history of common use in food (48).

Nonnutritive sweeteners have virtually no calories. In contrast, each gram of regular table sugar contains 4 calories. They are also much sweeter than regular sugar (2) and are widely used in processed foods, including baked goods, soft drinks, powdered drink mixes, candy, puddings, canned foods, jams and jellies, dairy products, and scores of other foods and beverages (2).

One benefit of nonnutritive sweeteners is that they do not contribute to tooth decay and cavities. They may also help with weight control (40). However, some research has suggested that consuming artificial sweeteners may be associated with increased weight, but the cause is not yet known (40).

For diabetics, nonnutritive sweeteners provide an alternative to sugar. Unlike sugar, these sweeteners do not raise blood sugar levels. However, diabetics should always check with their physician about using any sugar substitutes.

Possible Health Concerns

Nonnutritive sweeteners have been the subject of intense scrutiny for decades. In the 1970's saccharin was associated with bladder cancer in laboratory rats (41). Because of this association, saccharin carried a warning label. But according to the National Cancer Institute and other health agencies, there's no sound scientific evidence that any of the artificial sweeteners approved for use in the U.S. cause cancer or other serious health problems. As a result of newer studies, the warning label for saccharin was dropped (34, 41).

Stevia

As previously mentioned, stevia has been approved as a GRAS nonnutritive sweetener. It is about 100 times sweeter than sugar and is obtained from a shrub that is grown in Brazil, Paraguay, southeast Asia, and elsewhere. In the 1990s, the U.S. FDA, Canada, and a European Community scientific panel rejected stevia for use as a food ingredient. High dosages fed to rats reduced sperm production and increased cell proliferation (42).

Two companies developed extracts of stevia that are 95 percent pure rebaudioside and 200 times as sweet as sugar. The companies call their products Truvia (Coca-Cola) and PureVia (Pepsi), respectively, with the nickname of rebiana. In December of 2008, these companies sent a report to the FDA indicating that rebiana should be considered "generally recognized as safe," or GRAS.

UCLA toxicologists and the Center for Science in the Public Interest, however, urged the FDA to reject the GRAS claims for rebiana (49). They indicated that FDA's guidelines call for major new food additives to be tested for two years on both rats and mice, but rebiana had only been tested on rats. The UCLA toxicologists and CSPI said that testing of rebiana in both rats and mice is particularly important because several tests found that rebiana-related substances caused mutations and damaged chromosomes or DNA (50-55). Despite the disagreement about rebiana's safety, in 2009 the FDA approved Stevia as GRAS. The FDA report included a detailed list of international studies, references, and chemical analysis (45). Although the FDA approved highly refined stevia preparations as a novel sweetener (combinations of various types of sweeteners) it has not approved whole-leaf stevia or crude stevia extracts for this use (47).

Nutritive Sweeteners

Sugar and sugar alcohols are each considered nutritive sweeteners because they provide calories when consumed. In the United States, nutritive sweeteners fall under the Generally Recognized as Safe (GRAS) list or as food additives under the 1958 Food Additives Amendment to the Federal Food, Drug, and Cosmetic Act (56,57).

Sugar Alcohols

Contrary to their name, sugar alcohols are neither sugars nor alcohols (sorbitol, mannitol, xylitol, erythritol, isomalt, lactitol, and malitol). They are carbohydrates with structures that only resemble sugar and alcohol. They naturally occur in many fruits and vegetables and are widely consumed in sugar-free and reduced-sugar foods. The sweetness of sugar alcohols varies from 25% to 100% as sweet as table sugar (sucrose). The amount and kind being used is dependent on the food (2).

Sugar alcohols are not as sweet as sugar. As with artificial sweeteners, the FDA regulates the use of sugar alcohols (49).

Uses for Sugar Alcohols

Sorbitol and mannitol are found in hard and soft candies, chewing gum, flavored jam and jelly spreads, frozen food, and baked goods. Xylitol is found in chewing gum, hard candies, and pharmaceutical products. Erythritol is found in chewing gum and some beverages. Isomalt is found in hard and soft candies, ice cream, toffee, fudge, lollipops, wafers, and chewing gum. Lactitol is found in chocolate, cookies, cakes, hard and soft candies, and frozen dairy desserts. Maltitol is found in sugar-free chocolate, hard candies, chewing gum, baked goods, and ice cream (3).

Because sugar alcohols are not completely absorbed, high intakes of foods containing them can lead to abdominal gas and diarrhea. The Academy of Nutrition and Dietetics advises that intakes greater than 50 grams/day of sorbitol or greater than 20 grams/day of mannitol may cause diarrhea (3).

Natural Sweeteners

Natural sweeteners that have GRAS approval include fruit juices, nectars, honey, molasses, and maple syrup (44). Although natural sugar substitutes may seem healthier than processed table sugar, their vitamin and mineral content isn't significantly different from that of sugar; and they are converted by the body into glucose and fructose.

There's no health advantage to consuming added sugar of any type. Consuming too much added sugar, even natural sweeteners, can lead to health problems such as tooth decay, poor nutrition, weight gain, and increased triglycerides. Also, bee honey can contain small amounts of bacterial spores that can produce botulism toxin. For this reason, honey shouldn't be given to children less than 1 year old (49).

High Fructose Corn Syrup

High-fructose corn syrup (HFCS) is any of a group of corn syrups which have undergone enzymatic processing in order to increase their fructose content and are then mixed with pure corn syrup (100% glucose) to reach their final form (59). HFCS is among the sweeteners that have primarily replaced sucrose (table sugar) in the food industry (60).

The process by which HFCS is produced was first developed by Richard O. Marshall and Earl R. Kooi in 1957 and was rapidly introduced into many processed foods and soft drinks (56). Since its introduction, HFCS has replaced sugar in many processed foods in the USA (57). The main reasons for this switch are that HFCS is somewhat cheaper due to the relative abundance of corn and farm subsidies; also sugar import tariffs increase the price for sugar making HFCS more attractive to food processors. HFCS is easier to blend and transport because it is a liquid and usage leads to products with much longer shelf life (61).

HFCS has been classified generally recognized as safe (GRAS) by the U.S. Food and Drug Administration since 1976 (44,58,62).

CSPI Urges FDA to Set Safe Limits

Center for Science in the Public Interest (CSPI) has long been active in seeking to reduce soda consumption, beginning with its landmark 1998 report, Liquid Candy (63). In 2005, CSPI petitioned the Food and Drug Administration to require warning notices on cans and bottles of sugar drinks warning of weight gain and health problems (64,65,66).

In a 54-page regulatory petition filed with the FDA (February 13, 2013), CSPI details the substantial scientific evidence that added sugars, especially in drinks, causes weight gain, obesity, and chronic diseases like diabetes, heart disease, and gout (64,65,66). "If one were trying to ensure high rates of obesity, diabetes, or heart disease in a population, one would feed the population large doses of sugary drinks," said Walter Willett, professor of nutrition and epidemiology at the Harvard School of Public Health (67). "The evidence is so strong that it is essential for the FDA use its authority to make sugary drinks safer" (67). Willett is one of 41 leading scientists and physicians who signed a letter to FDA commissioner Margaret Hamburg in support of the petition (67). CSPI is also petitioning the FDA to determine what level of added sugars would be safe for use in beverages. The petition indicates that several health agencies have identified two-and-a-half teaspoons (10 grams) as a reasonable limit in a healthier drink (67).

Summary

Carbohydrates are the macronutrient that our body needs in the largest amounts. According to the Dietary Reference Intakes published by the USDA, 45% - 65% of calories should come from carbohydrate. Carbohydrates are the body's main source of fuel and regulate blood glucose levels. They are needed for the central nervous system, the kidneys, the brain, and muscle (including the heart) to function properly. Carbohydrates can be stored in the muscles and liver and later used for energy. They are mainly found in starchy foods (like grains and potatoes), fruits, milk, and yogurt. Other foods like vegetables, beans, nuts, seeds and cottage cheese contain carbohydrates, but in lesser amounts.

The most common and abundant forms of carbohydrates are sugars, fibers, and starches. The basic building block of every carbohydrate is a sugar molecule, a simple union of carbon, hydrogen, and oxygen (2). There are 3 classes of carbohydrates in foods. Monosaccharides consist of a one sugar molecule, oligosaccharides consist of a few sugar molecules (disaccharide-two sugars), and polysaccharides consist of many sugar molecules (2).

Every living cell contains carbohydrates, and these nutrients serve vital functions to the human body. Carbohydrates are composed of sugars, which the body digests and converts to glucose, or blood sugar. Glucose is used directly by cells for energy, stored in the liver and muscles as glycogen for later energy use, converted to fat, or used to synthesize amino acids.

Glucose homeostasis is an example of one of the highest levels of homeostatic control in the human body. A normal fasting blood glucose target range for an individual without diabetes is 70-100 mg/dL. The American Diabetes Association recommends a fasting plasma glucose level of 70–130 mg and after meals less than 180.

Blood glucose homeostasis is regulated primarily by the hormones insulin, glucagon, epinephrine, and norepinephrine. Hormones are chemical messengers secreted by a variety of glands in response to altered conditions in the body. They are secreted from the site of production, through the bloodstream and to other cells throughout the body. Each hormone affects one or more specific target tissues or organs and elicits specific responses to restore normal conditions.

Carbohydrates can be stored in muscle and the liver in the form of glycogen. Glycogen storage in muscle is energy for muscle cells only. Glycogen in the liver can be released into the bloodstream and provide glucose for cells that cannot produce their own energy.

The amount of glucose in the bloodstream must be controlled within a very narrow range since these cells are susceptible to damage from excess or insufficient glucose. Homeostasis is the term to describe this fine tuning of the body's glucose environment. If glucose is unavailable, the body must produce it (gluconeogenesis), and in the first few days of a fast, over 90% of glucose production comes from the breakdown of muscle.

To prevent the body from running out of glucose, carbohydrate stores need to be continuously replenished. Absorption rates differ widely depending on the form of the carbohydrate. Large amounts of simple sugars, in the absence of other nutrients known to decrease absorption rate, will force the body to store these rapidly absorbed sugars as fatty acids. Insulin resistance occurs in approximately 25% to 30% of the population. Insulin-resistant individuals need to moderate their carbohydrate intake, not eliminate it.

The glycemic index was designed in Canada by Dr. David Jenkins and his research group at the University of Toronto in the 1980s to assist diabetics with improving carbohydrate food choices. It compares carbohydrates in eaten food on a gram per gram basis. The glycemic index doesn't rank foods according to how healthy they actually are. Indeed, some foods with the preferred lower GI ranking may, in fact, be less healthy because they contain large amounts of calories, sugar, or saturated fat, especially packaged and processed foods. Whole wheat bread has the same glycemic index as white bread. Carrots have a high glycemic index, and people have eliminated them from their diets. But carrots are a wonderful, healthy food, and a whole bag of carrots contains less than 50 calories. Sweet-tasting watermelon has a very high glycemic index, but a slice of watermelon has only a small amount of carbohydrate per serving (as the name suggests, watermelon is made up mostly of water). A Snickers bar has a glycemic index of 41, marking it as a low glycemic index food, but it is certainly not a health food.

Harvard researchers developed a related way to classify foods that takes into account both the amount of carbohydrate in the food and the impact of that carbohydrate on blood sugar levels. This measure is called the glycemic load. A food's glycemic load is determined by multiplying its glycemic index by the amount of carbohydrate it contains. In general, a glycemic load of 20 or more is high, 11 to 19 is medium, and 10 or under is low.

Described and defined in 1988 by G.M. Reaven, Syndrome X became known as the metabolic syndrome or insulin resistance. In insulin resistance, the body's cells have a diminished ability to respond to the action of the insulin hormone. To compensate for the insulin resistance, the pancreas secretes more insulin.

Dietary fiber, also known as roughage or bulk, includes all parts of plant foods that the body can't digest or absorb. Whole foods rather than fiber supplements are generally better. Fiber supplements don't provide the variety of fibers, vitamins, minerals, and other beneficial nutrients that foods do. However, some people may still need a fiber supplement if dietary changes aren't sufficient or if they have certain medical conditions, such as constipation, diarrhea or irritable bowel syndrome. Fiber is also added to some foods. However, it's not yet clear if added fiber provides the same health benefits as naturally occurring sources.

Alcohol is not digested like other foods. Once alcohol is swallowed, it travels down the esophagus into the stomach and the small intestine. It avoids the normal digestive process and goes right into the bloodstream.

From the moment alcohol enters the body, the tiny molecules need no digestion and are quickly absorbed. About 20 percent of the alcohol molecules are absorbed through the walls of an empty stomach and can reach the brain within a minute. The stomach produces a small amount of an enzyme that breaks down the alcohol (alcohol dehydrogenase) and can thus reduce the amount entering the blood (3). The alcohol that leaves the stomach is absorbed in the intestines and circulates through the bloodstream to the liver. The extra alcohol travels to all parts of the body, circulating until the liver can finally process it. Liver and stomach cells are the only cells that can produce alcohol dehydrogenase (2). The amount of alcohol that the liver can break down is limited to about 1/2 ounce of alcohol per hour; the maximum amount determined by the amount of alcohol dehydrogenase. The amount of this enzyme is genetically determined. Men have more of this enzyme than women(2). Asians, Native Americans, and Inuits secrete less alcohol dehydrogenase than do most Caucasians (2).

Originally termed artificial sweeteners, nonnutritive sweeteners are defined as synthetic sugar substitutes derived from naturally occurring substances, including herbs or sugar itself. They are regulated by the US Food and Drug Administration (FDA) and must be reviewed and approved by the FDA before being made available for sale (44,58,62). The FDA approval process includes establishing the highest no effect level (HNEL) and an acceptable daily intake (ADI) for each artificial sweetener. The HNEL is the threshold of intake at which no adverse effects are seen. The NHEL is divided by 100 and is assigned an ADI. Hence, the ADI is the maximum amount considered safe to consume each day over the course of a lifetime (48).

Sugar and sugar alcohols are each considered nutritive sweeteners because they provide calories when consumed. In the United States, nutritive sweeteners fall under the Generally Recognized as Safe (GRAS) list or as food additives under the 1958 Food Additives Amendment to the Federal Food, Drug, and Cosmetic Act (56,57).

High-fructose corn syrup (HFCS) is any of a group of corn syrups which have undergone enzymatic processing in order to increase their fructose content and are then mixed with pure corn syrup (100% glucose) to reach their final form. HFCS is among the sweeteners that have primarily replaced sucrose (table sugar) in the food industry.

Center for Science in the Public Interest (CSPI) has long been active in seeking to reduce soda consumption, beginning with its landmark 1998 report, Liquid Candy. In 2005, CSPI petitioned the Food and Drug Administration to require warning notices on cans and bottles of sugar drinks warning of weight gain and health problems.

Chapter 2 Sample Test

1. List three different food sources of carbohydrates.
2. Discuss the role of carbohydrates in energy.
3. Which cells require glucose for energy?
4. Discuss the value of the glycemic index.
5. Define insulin resistance and the metabolic syndrome.
6. Discuss the types of fiber and importance of fiber in the diet.
7. Discuss sweeteners.
8. Discuss GRAS and the cautions associated with stevia.
9. Discuss the controversy surrounding high fructose corn syrup.
10. Discuss the petition set forth by Center for Science in the Public interest concerning high fructose corn syrup.

References

1. Institute of Medicine, Food and Nutrition Board. Dietary Reference Intakes: Recommended intakes for individuals. http://fnic.nal.usda.gov/dietary-guidance/dietary-reference-intakes/dri-tables.
2. Whitney, E & Rolfes S. (2013). *Understanding Nutrition,* 13th ed. Belmont, CA: Wadsworth, Cengage Learnin (95-121, 213-239).
3. Ross, C, (Shils) et al. (2012). *Modern Nutrition in Health & Disease, 11th ed.* Philadelphia PA: Lipincott Wilillians & Wilikins (59, 37-39, 661-664, 817-818).
4. Lehninger, A. (2013). *Principles of Biochemistry, 6th ed* NY: W H Freeman and Company (37-39).
5. Guyton, A. (2012). *Textbook of Medical Physiology, 11th ed.* Phil: W.B. Saunders Co. (243-243, 744-748, 857-867).
6. Wilmore, JH, Costil DL. (2001). Physical energy: Fuel metabolism, *Nutrition Reviews*, 59:13-16.
7. Klobassa, N, Moreland, P. (2013). Know your blood glucose target range. http://www.mayoclinic.com/health/blood-glucose-target-range/MY00494. Accessed May 23, 2013.
8. Jenkins, D. et al. (1981) Glycemic index of foods. A physiological basis for carbohydrate exchange. *Amer. J. Clin. Nutr.* 34:362-366.
9. Wolever, T. et al. (1991). The glycemic index: methodology and clinical implications. *Amer. J. Clin. Nutr.* 54: 846-854.
10. Sacks, FM, et al. (2009). Comparison of weight-loss diets with different compositions of fat, protein, and carbohydrates. *New England Journal of Medicine*. 859-873.
11. Glycemic index and glycemic load for 100+ foods. http://www.health.harvard.edu/newsweek/Glycemic_index_and_glycemic_load_for_100_foods.htm. Accessed May 23, 2013.
12. Brouns et al. (2005). Glycemic index methodology. *Nutrition Research Reviews* 18:145- 171.
13. Brand-Miller, J. (2003). *The New Glucose Revolution*. Phildelphia, PA: Da Capo Press, Incorporated.
14. Venn BJ, et al. (2007) Glycemic index and glycemic load: Measurement issues and their effect on diet-disease relationships. *European Journal of Clinical Nutrition.* 61(suppl):S122.
15. Reaven, G. (2000) Syndrome X, NY: Simon and Schuster.
16. Puig, J, Angeles, M, Martinez, A. (2008). Hyperuricemia, Gout, and the Metabolic Syndrome. *Curr Opin Rheumatol.* 20:187-191.
17. Ford ES, Giles WH, Dietz WH. (2002). Prevalence of the metabolic syndrome among US adults: findings from the third National Health and Nutrition Examination Survey. *JAMA*; 287:356-359.
18. Lorenzo C, Williams K, Hunt KJ,& Haffner SM. (2007). The National Cholesterol Education Program - Adult Treatment Panel III, International Diabetes Federation, and World Health Organization definitions of the metabolic syndrome as predictors of incident cardiovascular disease and diabetes. *Diabetes Care.* 30:8-13.
19. Kurl S, Laukkanen JA, Niskanen L, et al. (2006). Metabolic syndrome and the risk of stroke in middle-aged men. *Stroke.* 37:806-811.
20. Bataille V, Perret B, Dallongeville J, et al. (2006). Metabolic syndrome and coronary heart disease risk in a population-based study of middle-aged men from France and Northern Ireland: a nested case-control study from the PRIME cohort. *Diabetes Metab.* 32:475-479.
21. Expert Panel on Detection, Evaluation, and Treatment of High Blood Cholesterol in Adults. Executive summary of the third report of the National Cholesterol Education Program (NCEP)

Expert Panel on Detection, Evaluation, and Treatment of High Blood Cholesterol in Adults (Adult Treatment Panel III). (2001). *JAMA.* 285:2486-2497.

22. Mayer-Davis, EJ, D'agostino Jr, Karter AJ, Haffner, SM, Rewers, MJ, Saad, M, Bergman, RN (1998). Intensity and amount of physical activity in relation to insulin sensitivity. *JAMA* 279 (9): 669–674.
23. Hipsley EH, et al. (1953). *Br Med J* 1953:2:420-422.
24. Food and Nutrition Board, Institute of Medicine. Dietary Reference Intakes. Dietary, functional, and total fiber. (2002) *National Academy Press.* Washington, DC.
25. Jacobson, MU. (2010). Intake of carbohydrates compared with intake of saturated fatty acids and risk of myocardial infarction. *Amer J of Clin. Nutr.* 91.
26. Kim, H, et al. (2009) Glucose and insulin responses to whole grain breakfasts varying in soluble fiber. *European Journal of Nutrition.* 48.
27. Dahm, CC, et al. (2010). Dietary fiber and colorectal cancer risk: A nested case-control study using food diaries. *Journal of the National Cancer Institute.*102:614-626.
28. Pan, MH, et al. (2011). Molecular mechanisms for chemoprevention of colorectal cancer by natural dietary compounds. *Molecular Nutrition and Food Research.* 55: 32-45.
29. Tarleton, S, & Dibaise, JK. (2011). Low-residue diet in diverticular disease: Putting an end to a myth. *Nutrition in Clinical Practice.* 26:137-142.
30. Stavin, JL. (1987). Detary Fiber: classification, chemical analysis and food sources. *J of the Amer Dietetic Assoc.* 8:1164-1171, 1987
31. Anderson JW, Baird P, Davis RH et al. (2009). "Health benefits of dietary fiber". Nutr Rev 67 (4): 188–205. doi:10.1111/j.1753-4887.2009.00189.x. PMID19335713.
32. Slavin JL. (2008). Position of the American Dietetic Association: Health implications of dietary fiber. Journal of the American Dietetic Association. 108:1716
33. http://www.cnpp.usda.gov/Publications/DietaryGuidelines/2010/PolicyDoc/Chapter4.pdf
34. http://fnic.nal.usda.gov/dietary-guidance/dietary-reference-intakes/dri-tables.
35. Duyff RL. (2012). *American Dietetic Association Complete Food and Nutrition Guide. 4th ed.* Hoboken, NJ: John Wiley & Sons;:55.
36. Bell, P. (1990). Cholesterol-lowering effects of soluble-fiber cereals as part of a prudent diet for patients with mild to moderate hypercholesterolemia. *Amer J Clin Nutr.* 52: 1020-1026.
37. Ferreira, MP, Willoughby, D. (2008). Alcohol consumption: The good, the bad and the indifferent. *Applied Physiology, Nutrition and Metabolism.* 33:12-20.
38. *American Dietetic Association Complete Food and Nutrition Guide. 4th ed.* (2012). Hoboken, N.J.: John Wiley & Sons. 55.
39. Garner C, et al. (2012). Nonnutritive sweeteners: Current use and health perspectives. A Scientific Statement From the American Heart Association and the American Diabetes Association. *Diabetes Care.* 35:1798-1808.
40. Mattes D, et al. (2009) Nonnutritive sweetener consumption in humans: Effects on appetite and food intake and their putative mechanisms. *American Journal of Clinical Nutrition.* 89:1.
41. Artificial sweeteners and cancer. (2013). National Cancer Institute. http://www.cancer.gov/cancertopics/factsheet/Risk/artificial-sweeteners. Accessed May 23, 2013.
42. Pezzuto JM, et al. (1985)Metabolically activated steviol, the aglycone of stevioside, is mutagenic. *Proc. Natl. Acad. Sci. U.S.A.* 82 (8): 2478–82.
43. Is stevia an FDA-approved sweetener? U.S. Food and Drug Administration. http://www.fda.gov/AboutFDA/Transparency/Basics/ucm214865.htm. Accessed May 20, 2013.
44. Generally recognized as safe. U.S. Food and Drug Administration. http://www.fda.gov/Food/FoodIngredientsPackaging/GenerallyRecognizedasSafeGRAS/ucm2006850.htm.

45. New York Medical College (15 January 2009). "Notice to the U.S. Food and Drug Administration (FDA) that the use of Rebiana (Rebaudioside A) derived from Stevia rebaudiana, as a Food Ingredient is Generally Recognized as Safe (GRAS)" (PDF). p.75.
46. Stevia. Natural Medicines Comprehensive Database. http://www.naturaldatabase.com.
47. What refined stevia preparations have been approved by FDA to be used as a sweetener? U.S. Food and Drug Administration. http://www.fda.gov/AboutFDA/Transparency/Basics/ucm214865.htm. Accessed July 27, 2012.
48. Position of the Academy of Nutrition and Dietetics: Use of nutritive and nonnutritive sweeteners. (2012). *Journal of the Academy of Nutrition and Dietetics*. 112:739.
49. Shapiro, Roger L, Hatheway, C, Swerdflow, DL. (1998). "Botulism in the United States: A Clinical and Epidemiologic Review". *Annals of Internal Medicine*. 129 (3): 221–8.
50. FDA Issues Midnight Go-ahead for Potentially Harmful Stevia Sweetner—Statement of Executive Director Michael F. Jacobson. (December 18, 2008). http://www.cspinet.org/new/200812181.html.
51. Stevia: What's the Rush?—Statement of CSPI Executive Director Michael F. Jacobson. (December 15, 2008) http://www.cspinet.org/new/200812152.html.
52. Lab Tests Point to Problems with Trendy New Sweetener—Press Release. (August 28, 2008). http://www.cspinet.org/new/200808281.html.
53. http://www.cspinet.org/new/pdf/stevia-cspi-cover-letter-8-4-08.pdf. CSPI Letter to the FDA.
54. Stevia: Sweet...but How Safe? (October 2008). *Nutrition Action Healthletter*. http://cspinet.org/new/pdf/stevia_update.pdf.
55. UCLA Toxicologists' Report on Stevia. (August 2008). http://www.cspinet.org/new/pdf/stevia-report_final-8-14-08.pdf.
56. Neltner TG, Kulkarni NR, Alger HM, et al. (2011). Navigating the U.S. food additive regulatoryprogram. *Comp Rev Food Sci Food Safety*. 10(6):342-368.
57. Food and Drug Administration. Determining the regulatory status of a food ingredient. http://www.fda.gov/Food/FoodIngredientsPackaging/FoodAdditives/ucm228269.htm. Updated 2011.
58. Food and Drug Administration. Substances generally recognized as safe, 21 CFR parts 170,184,186. 570.://www.gpo.gov/fdsys/pkg/FR-1997-04-17/pdf/ 97-9706.pdf.
59. Marshall, RO; Kooi, ER, & Moffett, GM. (1957). Enzymatic Conversion of d-Glucose to d-Fructose. *Science* 125 (3249): 648–649. doi:10.1126/science.125.3249.648. PMID1342166.
60. Bray, & U.S. Department of Agriculture, Economic Research Service, Sugar and Sweetener Yearbook series. (2004). Tables 50–52.
61. Food without Thought: How U.S. Farm Policy Contributes to Obesity. (November 2006). *Institute for Agriculture and Trade Policy*. Archived from the original on 2007-09-27.
62. Database of Select Committee on GRAS Substances (SCOGS) Reviews. Accessdata.fda.gov. 2006-10-31. Retrieved 2010-11-06.
63. http://www.cspinet.org/new/pdf/liquid_candy_final_w_new_supplement.pdf. Liquid Candy Report: June 2005.
64. Marriott BP, Olsho L, Hadden L, Conner P. (2010). Intake of added sugars and selected nutrients in the United States, National Health and Nutrition Examination Survey (NHANES) 2003–2006. *Crit Rev Food Sci Nutr* 50(3):228–58.
65. Bowman SA. (1999). Diets of individuals based on energy intakes from added sugars. *Family Economics and Nutrition Review*. 12(2):31–8.
66. Vartanian LR, Schwartz MB, & Brownell KD. (2007). Effects of soft drink consumption on nutrition and health: A systematic review and meta-analysis. *Am J Public Health* 97:667–75.
67. http://www.cspinet.org/new/201302131.html. FDA Urged to Determine Safe Limits on High-Fructose Corn Syrup and Other Sugars in Soft Drinks. February 13, 2013.
68. Eisenbarth GS, Polonsky KS, Buse JB. (2008). Type 1 Diabetes Mellitus. In: Kronenberg HM,

Melmed S, Polonsky KS, Larsen PR. *Kronenberg: Williams Textbook of Endocrinology*. 11th ed. Philadelphia, Pa: Saunders Elsevier. Chap 31.

69. Freeman MR, King J, & Kennedy E. (2001). Popular diets: a scientific review. *Obes Res*. 9: 1S-40S.
70. Yancy WS, et al. (2004). A low-carbohydrate, ketogenic diet versus a low-fat diet to treat obesity and hyperlipidemia. *Ann Int Med.* 140: 769-777.
71. Sondike SB, Copperman N, & Jacobson MS. (2003). Effects of a low carbohydrate diet on weight loss and cardiovascular risk factor in overweight adolescents. *J Pediatr*. 142: 253-258.
72. Westman EC, et al. (2002). Effect of 6 month adherence to a very low carbohydrate program. *Am J Med*. 113: 30-36.
73. Crowe, T. (2005). Safety of low-carbohydrate diets. *Obesity Reviews*. 6(3): 235-245.
74. Tallian K, Nahata M, Tsao CT. Role of ketogenic diet in children with intractable seizures. *Ann Pharmacother*. 32:349–361.
75. Wing RR, Vazquez J, & Ryan C. (1995). Cognitive effects of ketogenic weight reducing diets. *Int J Obes Relat Metab Disord*. 19: 811-816.
76. Denke MA. (2001). Metabolic effects of high protein, low-carbohydrate diets. *Am J of Cardio*. 88: 59-61.

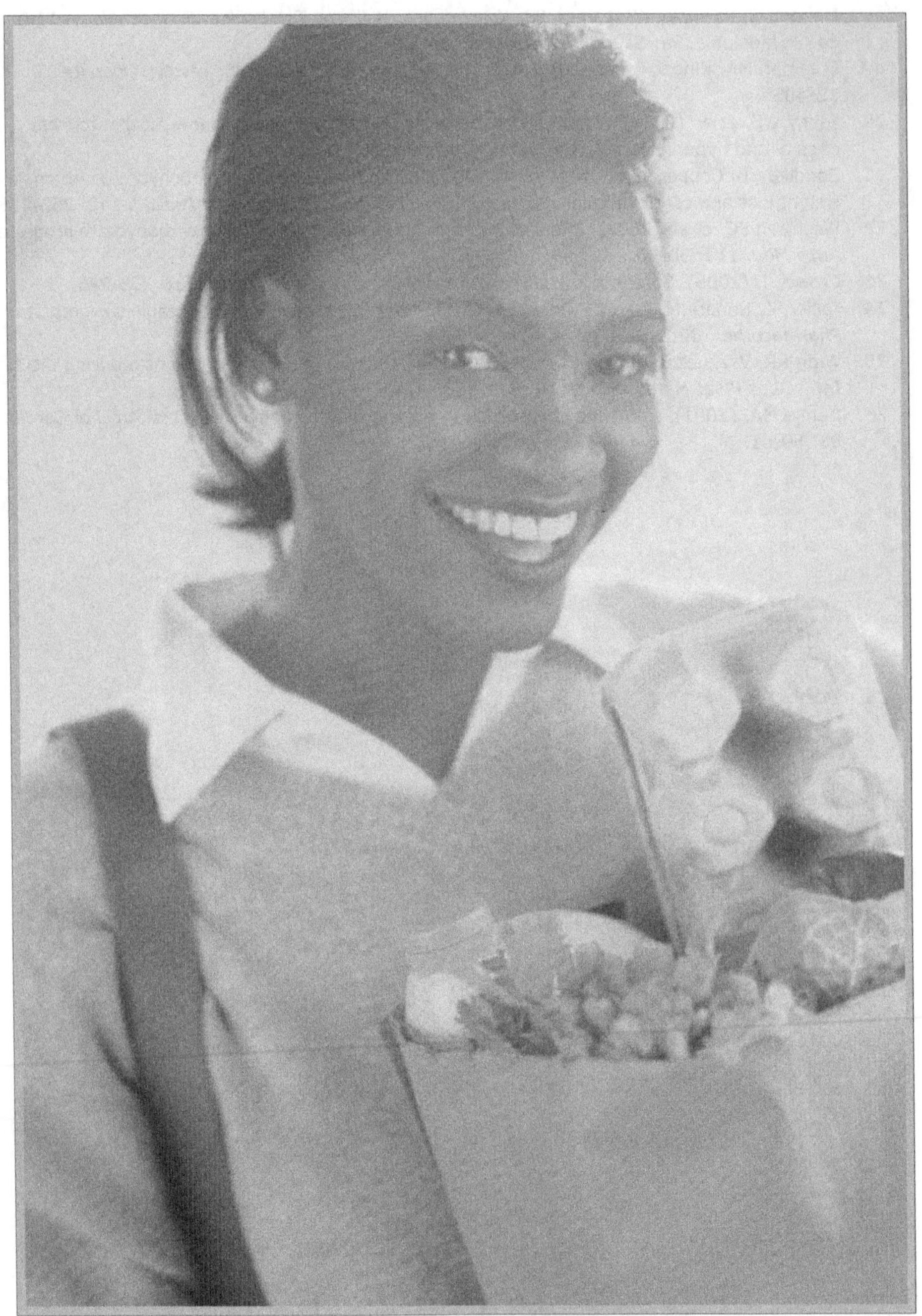

Chapter 3 - Lipids

In this chapter we will take a more in-depth look at the types of fats in the diet and the roles of fats including digestion, absorption, transport, and biochemical roles.

Objectives

After reading and studying this chapter, you should be able to:

1. Define lipids, triglycerides fats, oils, phospholipids, and sterols.
2. Describe digestion, absorption, transport, and roles of lipids.
3. Discuss the different types of fatty acids including trans fatty acids.
4. Discuss essential fatty acids, eicosanoids, prostaglandins and their importance in health.

Introduction

Fats are found in foods from plants and animals and are referred to as dietary fat (3). Dietary fat is one of the three macronutrients, along with protein and carbohydrates that provide the body with energy. In addition to energy, fats are required for absorption of vitamins; necessary for proper growth, and development; and they are an especially important source of calories and nutrients for infants and toddlers (3). The dietary requirements for fats range between 20 to 35% of total caloric intake (1).

Fats refers to a subcategory of nutrients known as lipids. Although the words "oils", "fats", and "lipids" are all used to refer to fats, in reality, fat is a subset of lipid. "Oils" is usually used to refer to lipids that are liquid at normal room temperature, while "fats" is usually used to refer to lipids that are solid at normal room temperature. "Lipids" is used to refer to both liquid and solid fats, along with other related substances. The word "oil" is also used for any substance that does not mix with water and has a greasy feel, such as petroleum (or crude oil), heating oil, and essential oils, regardless of its chemical structure (3).

Lipids

Lipids play a large role in energy storage and in the structure of cells. They are divided into main groups consisting of *triglycerides, phospholipids, and sterols* (subset of steroid hormones)(3).

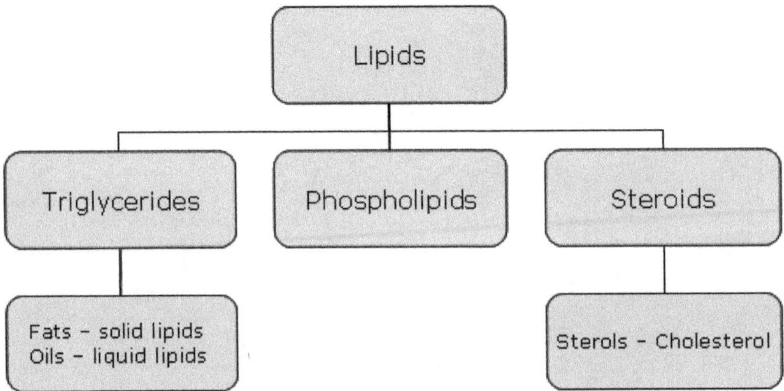

Triglycerides

Most of the stored fat in the body is triglyceride and they are the principal storage forms of energy in the human body. They also form a layer of fat under the skin for insulation and surround organs to protect against shock and injury. Triglycerides consist of a glycerol molecule and three fatty acids (6). Glycerol is an alcohol composed of a three carbon chain that serves as the backbone of the triglyceride molecule (3). In nature, the two outside fatty acids of the triglyceride prefer to hold a saturated fatty acid, whereas the middle position prefers an essential fatty acid (5,6). Fatty acids will be discussed in detail in the following section.

In addition to obtaining triglycerides from the diet, the body can make triglycerides from excess sugars. The body begins by reducing the sugar to a 2-carbon fragment called acetate and synthesizes fatty acids from these excess acetate fragments by hooking them end to end. Glycerol is then added and the resulting triglyceride is stored as body fat. The body can also make triglycerides from alcohol, fats, and proteins (6).

Phospholipids

Phospholipids (also known as phosphatides) are a class of lipids that are a major component of all cell membranes and are involved in immune system function (6).

A phospholipid has a glycerol molecule and two fatty acids. The third fatty acid is replaced by a phosphate group. The phosphate group mixes with water while the fatty acid portion mixes with fat (6).The phosphate group attached to phospholipids is polar and water-soluble, while its fatty acids are oil-soluble. The phospholipids spread out in a thin layer over surfaces of water and form double-layered membranes that surround every living cell of all living organisms (6). They also form membranes around subcellular organelles (mitochondria, nucleus, lysosomes, etc.).

Because of this property, phospholipids are not used as an energy source but are part of all cell membranes. They make up the essential milieu of cellular membranes and act as a barrier for entry of compounds into cells (7). The middle fatty acid of phospholipids is usually an essential fatty acid which, being highly unsaturated, is bent and does not pack tightly. It takes up more space than a straight saturated fatty acid and keeps membranes from hardening. The attached essential fatty acids also perform critical functions within the cell (see section on essential fatty acids) (8). Embedded within the phospholipid structure are proteins, cholesterol, and vitamin E. Fat-soluble toxic substances such as alcohol, barbiturates, drugs, and carcinogens can dissolve in these membranes and can exert their toxic effects (6).

Membranes can contain between 20 and 80% phospholipids, depending on the type of cell or organelle. Red blood cells contain about 45% phospholipids and 55% proteins in their membranes; nerve cell membranes (myelin sheath) contain 80% phospholipids and only 20% proteins. Mitochondrial membranes contain 25% phospholipids, while liver cell membranes contain about 50% phospholipids (6).

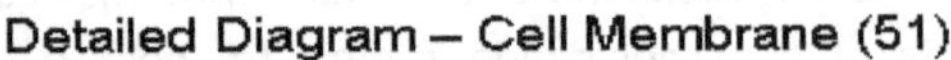

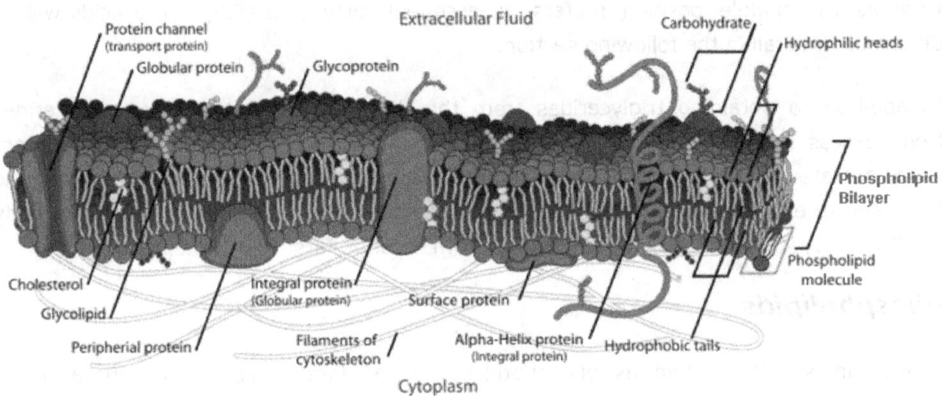

The phosphate groups attached to the phospholipid can have other chemical groups attached, such as choline, inositol, serine ethanolamine. Phosphatidyl choline, or lecithin (a major constituent of cell membranes) is used by food manufacturers to combine ingredients such as water and oil. Lecithin advocates claim that it is necessary to purchase bottles of lecithin in order to receive the daily dose (7). This is false. The digestive enzyme lecithinase in the intestine hydrolyzes most of the lecithin before it enters the body. Also, all the lecithin a person needs for building cell membranes is made in the liver. Therefore, lecithin is not an essential nutrient (3).

Fatty Acids

Fatty acids can be saturated, monounsaturated, or polyunsaturated. They can contain between 4 and 28 carbons (3):

saturated fatty acid: c-c-c-c-c-c-c-

monounsaturated fatty acid: c-c=c-c-c

polyunsaturated fatty acid: c-c=c-c-c=

The single lines between the c's (carbon atom) represent a saturated carbon atom (saturated with hydrogen) bond. A saturated fatty acid has all single lines (bonds).

The double lines (double bond) between the carbons represent an unsaturated carbon atom—not totally saturated with hydrogen. If there is one double bond the fatty acid is a monounsaturated fatty acid; if there are two or more double bonds the fatty acid is a polyunsaturated fatty acid (6).

Saturated Fatty Acids

Saturated fatty acids are the simplest of the fatty acids. They have no double bonds between the carbon atoms of the fatty acid chain; hence, they are fully saturated with hydrogen atoms. The saturated molecule is straight, has no "kinks or bends", contains no double bonds, and is slow to react with other chemicals. Saturated fats are popular with manufacturers of processed foods because they are less vulnerable to rancidity and are generally more solid at room temperature than unsaturated fats (6).

There are several kinds of naturally occurring saturated fatty acids; their only difference being the number of carbon atoms which range from 1 to 24 atoms (4). Some common examples of saturated fatty acids are butyric acid with 4 carbon atoms (contained in butter), lauric acid with 12 carbon atoms (contained in breast milk, coconut oil, palm oil), myristic acid with 14 carbon atoms (contained in cow milk and dairy products), palmitic acid with 16 carbon atoms (contained in palm oil and palm kernel oil), and stearic acid with 18 carbon atoms (contained in meat and cocoa butter) (4).

The body uses saturated fatty acids up to 14 carbons in length for the production of energy. Longer chain saturated fatty acids (14 or more carbons) are not used for energy. They have melting points higher than body temperatures, are insoluble in water, and tend to aggregate or stick together to form droplets or, if hard, plaques (4).

Unsaturated Fatty Acid

An unsaturated fatty acid contains one or more double bonds in the fatty acid chain. A fat molecule is monounsaturated if it contains one double bond and polyunsaturated if it contains more than one double bond. Where double bonds are formed, hydrogen atoms are eliminated (6). Unsaturated fatty acids are less stable than saturated fatty acids, chemically more active, and can react with light, air, and other chemical groups. They melt at lower temperatures than saturated fatty acids that are identical except for the double bond. This makes them vulnerable to destruction from light or air (11).

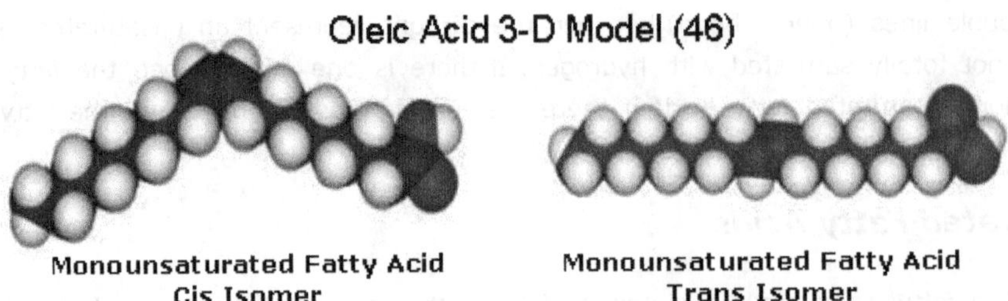

Monounsaturated Fatty Acid Cis Isomer **Monounsaturated Fatty Acid Trans Isomer**

Long chain unsaturated fatty acids are used to build cell membranes as part of phospholipids. Their tendency to disperse balances the tendency of saturated fatty acids to aggregate. In other words, the dispersion ability of long chain unsaturated fatty acids increases membrane fluidity while saturated fatty acids decreases cell membrane fluidity (12).

Double bonds in unsaturated fatty acids may be in either a *cis* or *trans* isomer, depending on the geometry of the double bond. In the *cis* conformation, hydrogens are on the same side of the double bond; whereas in the *trans* conformation, they are on opposite sides (13). Natural sources of fatty acids are rich in the cis isomer; whereas hydrogenated products are rich in the trans isomer.

Again, in the cis configuration, the hydrogen atoms on the carbons involved in the double bond are on the same side of the molecule. The hydrogen atoms repel each other and the fatty acid " kinks or bends". This changes the shape and the properties of the molecule (13). The "kinks" (bends) make it difficult for the fatty acid chains to fit together in cell membranes. They do not aggregate and the membrane remains fluid. It allows molecules within the membrane the freedom to move and fulfill their important chemical and transport functions.

Trans Fatty Acids

In the trans configuration, the hydrogen atoms on the carbons involved in the double bond are on opposite sides of the molecule. This configuration removes the "kink" or bend in the molecule and produces the trans isomer. The molecule now has the same straight configuration of saturated fatty acids, and hence produces many of the same arterial damaging effects as saturated fatty acids. The trans isomer aggregates which decreases cell membrane fluidity. Molecules within the membrane are no longer free to move and fulfill important chemical functions (13). If trans fatty acids are the only fatty acids available, membrane function is compromised.

Trans fatty acids occur from natural sources and are commercially produced. Low quantities of trans fatty acids in food products are derived from ruminant animals, mostly dairy products and meats. Bacteria in animal stomachs hydrogenate the fatty acids from feed (10).

Trans fatty acids are formed when hydrogen is added to unsaturated fats. In the process of hydrogenation, an oil which contains unsaturated fatty acids in the natural cis state is reacted at high temperatures with hydrogen gas in the presence of a metal catalyst for 6 to 8 hours (10). If the process is brought to completion (completely hydrogenated), all of the hydrogen bonds in the oil are saturated with hydrogen (11). The fatty acids that result contain no double bonds, and have no essential fatty acid activity. This fat does not spoil and has a long shelf life. The completely hydrogenated fat can be used for frying, baking, and cooking without being further chemically altered.

When the process of hydrogenation is not brought to completion, partial hydrogenation occurs (the process is stopped when a desired consistency is achieved) (14). The product can contain dozens of intermediate substances. Double bonds may turn from cis to trans, double bonds may shift, and fragments may be produced. Since the hydrogenation occurs at random, it is impossible to predict the outcome. Partial hydrogenation is the process by which margarines, shortenings, and shortening oils are made (14).

Unlike other dietary fats, trans fats are neither required nor beneficial for health. The consumption of trans fats increases one's risk of coronary heart disease by raising levels of "bad" LDL cholesterol and lowering levels of "good" HDL cholesterol (15).

Most trans fats consumed today are industrially created by partially hydrogenating plant oils, a process developed in the early 1900s and first commercialized as Crisco in 1911 (10). The goal of hydrogenation is to add hydrogen atoms to unsaturated fats making them more saturated.

According to several studies, natural trans fats and commercially produced trans fats may have different physiological effects (56-60). The dairy industry published studies in March of 2008 indicating small amounts of "natural" trans fats (0.8% to 1.5% of calories) did not produce the same harmful effects as artificially produced trans fats (56-60). According to a more recent review published by the University of Alberta (Canada), naturally occurring trans fats have a different fatty acid profile than industrial trans fat, which contributes to different physiological effects (61,62). The Alberta, CA Livestock and Meat Agency has awarded a $1 million research grant to the University of Alberta to further investigate health implications of naturally derived trans fats with the goal of changing the way trans fats are listed on food labels in the US and Canada. Presently naturally occurring and industrially produced trans fats are grouped together.

Essential Fatty Acids

Two unsaturated fatty acids are essential; linoleic and linolenic acid. They are deemed essential because the body cannot make them and they are required; hence, they must be obtained from food for life to be sustained. Linoleic acid has two double bonds and is an omega-6 fatty acid, while linolenic has three double bonds and is an omega-3 fatty acid. Omega-3 and omega-6 fatty acids are polyunsaturated fatty acids (PUFA), meaning they contain more than one *cis* double bond (16).

There are the two main types of omega-3 fatty acids (16):

- Long-chain omega-3 fatty acids are EPA (eicosapentaenoic acid) and DHA (docosahexaenoic acid). These are plentiful in fish and shellfish. Algae provides only DHA.
- Short-chain omega-3 fatty acids are ALA (alpha-linolenic acid). These are found in plants, such as flaxseed. Though beneficial, ALA omega-3 fatty acids have less potent health benefits than EPA and DHA. You'd have to eat a lot to gain the same benefits as you do from fish.

Both essential fatty acids have a function in holding oxygen in cell membranes, where they act as a barrier to foreign organisms. These foreign organisms will not thrive in the presence of oxygen (6). As previously mentioned, because of the double bonds, both essential fatty acids are easily destroyed. Linolenic acid is even more sensitive to destruction than linoleic acid because it contains three double bonds.

Essential Fatty Acids Guidelines

The requirements for fats range between 20 to 35% of total caloric intake and include the essential fatty acids (1,17). Adequate intakes have been established for both essential fatty acids. Please note that amounts of linoleic and linolenic acid are not listed on food labels so consumers should be aware of which foods are high in these essential fatty acids. See the following table for essential fatty acid requirements.

	Men 19 - 50	**Men 51+**	**Women 19 - 50**	**Women 51+**
Linoleic Acid	17 grams	14 grams	12 grams	11 grams
Linolenic Acid	1.6 grams	1.6 grams	1.1 grams	1.1 grams

Some foods rich in linoleic acid are listed in the following table.

Some Food Sources of Linoleic Acid (18:2n-6) (50)		
Food	**Serving**	**Linoleic Acid (g)**
Safflower oil	1 tablespoon	10.1
Sunflower seeds, oil roasted	1 oz	9.7
Pine nuts	1 oz	9.4
Sunflower oil	1 tablespoon	8.9
Corn oil	1 tablespoon	7.3
Soybean oil	1 tablespoon	6.9
Pecans, oil roasted	1 oz	6.4
Brazil nuts	1 oz	5.8
Sesame oil	1 tablespoon	5.6

Some foods that are rich in linolenic acid are listed in the following table.

Some Food Sources of Alpha-linolenic Acid (18:3n-3) (50)		
Food	**Serving**	**Alpha-Linolenic acid (g)**
Flaxseed oil	1 tablespoon	7.3
Walnuts, English	1 oz	2.6
Flaxseeds, ground	1 tablespoon	1.6
Walnut oil	1 tablespoon	1.4
Canola oil	1 tablespoon	1.3
Soybean oil	1 tablespoon	0.9
Mustard oil	1 tablespoon	0.8
Tofu, firm	½ cup	0.7
Walnuts, black	1 oz	0.6

The American Heart Association recommends eating fish (particularly fatty fish such as mackerel, lake trout, herring, sardines, albacore tuna, and salmon) at least 2 times a week (17). Major dietary source of EPA and DHA are listed in the following table.

Some Food Sources of EPA (20:5n-3) and DHA (22:6n-3) (17)				
Food	**Serving**	**EPA (g)**	**DHA (g)**	**Amount providing 1 g of EPA + DHA**
Herring, Pacific	3 oz*	1.06	0.75	1.5 oz
Salmon, chinook	3 oz	0.86	0.62	2 oz
Sardines, Pacific	3 oz	0.45	0.74	2.5 oz
Salmon, Atlantic	3 oz	0.28	0.95	2.5 oz

Some Food Sources of EPA (20:5n-3) and DHA (22:6n-3) (17)				
Food	**Serving**	**EPA (g)**	**DHA (g)**	**Amount providing 1 g of EPA + DHA**
Oysters, Pacific	3 oz	0.75	0.43	2.5 oz
Salmon, sockeye	3 oz	0.45	0.60	3 oz
Trout, rainbow	3 oz	0.40	0.44	3.5 oz
Tuna, canned, white	3 oz	0.20	0.54	4 oz
Crab, Dungeness	3 oz	0.24	0.10	9 oz
Tuna, canned, light	3 oz	0.04	0.19	12 oz

*A 3-oz serving of fish is about the size of a deck of cards.

Eicosanoids

Essential fatty acids are precursors to hormone-like substances called eicosanoids (31). The major precursor of these compounds is arachidonic acid (20-carbon polyunsaturated fatty acid), and the pathways leading to the eicosanoids are known collectively as the 'arachidonate cascade' (31). Eicosanoids are not stored and are synthesized in response to immediate cellular need, and include prostaglandins, prostacyclins, the thromboxanes, lipoxins, and the leukotrienes (32,33). The eicosanoids are considered "local hormones." They have specific effects on target cells close to their site of formation.

Eicosanoids exert important effects on the immune system, cardiovascular system, reproductive system and central nervous system. All cells can form eicosanoids, but tissues differ in enzyme profile and hence in the products they can form (32).

Prostaglandins

Prostaglandins are similar to hormones in that they act as chemical messengers, but do not move to other sites and they work within the cells where they are synthesized (33). A diversity of receptors means that prostaglandins act on many types of cells and have a wide variety of effects. A major effect of prostaglandins is control of platelet aggregation. Platelets, along with red cells and plasma, form a major portion of both human and animal blood. Platelets provide the necessary hormones and proteins for coagulation (3).

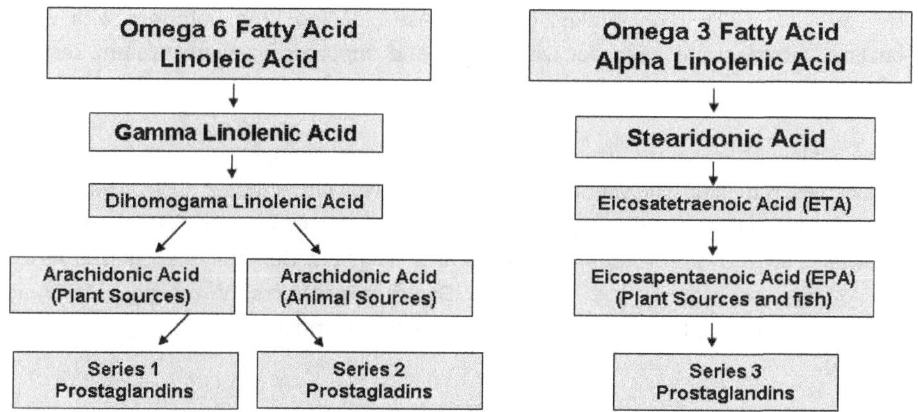

Three major types of prostaglandins active in platelets are (34):

1. *Series 1 prostaglandins.* Omega-6 fatty acids from plant products such as flax, safflower, sunflower, sesame, soybean and walnut go through a series of chemical reactions to form series 1 prostaglandins. These prostaglandins a less inflammatory and anti-aggregating response than series 2 prostaglandins. In other words, these prostaglandins reduce blood clotting.
2. *Series 2 prostaglandins.* The omega-6 fatty acids from animal products go go through a similar series of chemical reactions in which series 2 prostaglandins are formed. These prostaglandins a produce a greater inflammatory and aggregating response than series 1 prostaglandins (increase blood clotting).
3. *Series 3 prostaglandins.* Omega-3 fatty acids go through a different series of chemical reactions which produce series 3 prostaglandins. These prostaglandins produce the least aggregating and inflammatory response and hence, are the "heart healthiest". When choosing fats for optimum health plant products and fish are the healthier choices (12).

Health Effects of Essential Fatty Acids

Research indicates that there are many beneficial effects of omega-3 fatty acids. Regular consumption helps prevent irregular heartbeat and blood clots, improves lipid profile, lowers blood pressure, supports a healthy immune system, and suppresses inflammation (18,19,20,21) .

Increasing omega-3 fatty acid consumption through foods is preferable (22). Because of the potential for side effects and interactions with medications, omega-3 dietary supplements should be taken only under the supervision of a knowledgeable health care provider (22). High intakes may increase bleeding time, interfere with wound healing, increase the need for vitamin E, and suppress immune system response (17,48,49).

Individuals with coronary artery disease may not get enough omega-3 by diet alone. Individuals with high triglycerides may require even larger doses (19). These people may want to talk to their doctor about omega-3 supplements. The FDA has ruled that intakes of up to 3 g/d of marine omega-3 fatty acids are Generally Recognized As Safe (GRAS) for inclusion in the diet (24). Some side effects of omega-3 fatty acid supplementation include fishy after-taste, gastrointestinal disturbances, and nausea (25,26).

Clinical signs of essential fatty acid deficiency include a dry scaly rash, decreased growth in infants and children, increased susceptibility to infection, and poor wound healing (30).

The Mediterranean diet emphasizes foods rich in omega-3 fatty acids, including whole grains, fresh fruits and vegetables, fish, olive oil, and garlic, as well as moderate wine consumption. Research has shown that the traditional Mediterranean diet reduces the risk of heart disease (27,28,29).

Because essential fatty acids are easily destroyed, it's important to be sure that ingested oils be reasonably fresh. If fresh oils are not available, the seeds are the most nutritionally complete way to obtain the essential fatty acids (10). Flax oil spoils when exposed to light, oxygen, or heat, and care needs to be taken in pressing, filling, storing, and shipping of this oil. The oil must be less than 30 days old, stored in a dark, unopened bottle, and once opened, must be discarded after 30 days (10).

<u>Mercury in Fish</u>

Fish and shellfish can be an important part of a healthy diet. They contain high-quality protein, are low in saturated fat, and contain omega-3 fatty acids. A well-balanced diet that includes a variety of fish and shellfish may contribute to heart health.

However, nearly all fish and shellfish contain traces of mercury (57). For most people, the risk from mercury by eating fish and shellfish is not a health concern. The risks from mercury in fish and shellfish depend on the amount of fish and shellfish eaten and the levels of mercury in the fish and shellfish. Farmed fish typically have lower levels of mercury than the wild varieties, hence most consumers of fish in the United States are not in danger of harmful levels (3). Yet, some fish and shellfish contain higher levels of mercury that may harm an unborn baby or a young child's developing nervous system. The Food and Drug Administration (FDA) and the Environmental Protection Agency (EPA) are advising women who may become pregnant, pregnant women, nursing mothers, and young children to avoid some types of fish and eat fish and shellfish that are lower in mercury (see below).

By following the four recommendations listed below for selecting and eating fish or shellfish, consumers can reduce their exposure to the harmful effects of mercury (52).

- Do not eat shark, swordfish, king mackerel, or tilefish because they contain high levels of mercury.
- Eat up to 12 ounces (four 3 ounce servings) a week of a variety of fish and shellfish that are lower in mercury.
- Five of the most commonly eaten fish that are low in mercury are shrimp, canned light tuna, salmon, pollock, and catfish.
- Another commonly eaten fish, albacore ("white") tuna has more mercury than canned light tuna.

PCBs in Fish

Polychlorinated biphenyls (PCBs) are a group of man-made chemicals that exist as oily liquids or solids, are colorless to light yellow in color, and have no smell or taste. They were widely used as coolant fluids in transformers, capacitors, and electric motors. Due to PCBs environmental toxicity and classification as a persistent organic pollutant, PCB production was banned by the United States Congress in 1979 and by the Stockholm Convention on Persistent Organic Pollutants in 2001 (53). Although PCBs are no longer made in the United States, people can still be exposed to them.

How much PCB is allowable? FDA required limits of PCBs include 0.2 parts per million (ppm) in infant and junior foods, 0.3 ppm in eggs, 1.5 ppm in milk and other dairy products (fat basis), 2 ppm in fish and shellfish (edible portions), and 3 ppm in poultry and red meat (fat basis) (54).

Fish consumption appears to be the major pathway of exposure to PCB (54). The Environmental Protection Agency (EPA) regulates commercial fishing to help ensure that fish meet safety standards for mercury, PCBs, and other contaminants.

Should fish be eliminated from the diet? Totally eliminating fish from the diet because of perceived dangers could lead to health consequences that outweigh the alternatives (55). The fact remains that fish is lower in saturated fats than red meat and is an excellent source of omega-3 fatty acids. As with so many other choices in the modern world, a moderate approach to fish consumption is key to reaping the benefits.

Steroids

Steroids are organic compounds derived from 17 carbon atoms composed of four rings. There are hundreds of different types of steroids in plants, animals, and fungi, and they are involved in a variety of physiological processes. Examples of steroids include the dietary fat cholesterol, and the sex hormones estradiol and testosterone (35).

Sterols are special forms of steroids, with a hydroxyl group at position-3 and a skeleton derived from cholestane. Sterols contain a multiple-ring structure and do not contain fatty acids; they are circular molecules made from fatty acids (36).

Cholesterol

Cholesterol, a sterol, is found in animal products; plant products contain larger amounts of phospholipids, smaller amounts of triglycerides, and no cholesterol (6). Cholesterol is a circular molecule that does not contain fatty acids or glycerol (3). It is a hard, waxy substance that melts at 149 degrees centigrade (37). It is made by the body, and is therefore not an essential nutrient. It is manufactured from simple 2-carbon acetate groups which are derived from the breakdown of sugars, fats, and in rare circumstances proteins. The 2-carbon fragments are hooked end to end until 30 of them are chained together. Each step involves enzymes, the chain is cyclized, and 3 carbons are removed to produce the 27 carbon cholesterol molecule (37).

Cholesterol Molecule 3-D (47)

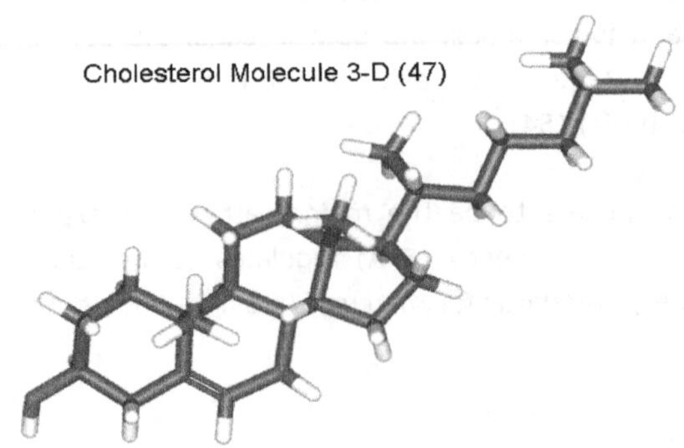

Cholesterol is required to build and maintain membranes; it modulates membrane fluidity over the range of physiological temperatures. The hydroxyl group on cholesterol interacts with the polar head groups of the membrane phospholipids while the bulky steroid and the hydrocarbon chain are embedded in the membrane alongside the nonpolar fatty-acid chain of the other lipids. Through the interaction with the phospholipid fatty-acid chains, cholesterol increases membrane packing, which reduces membrane fluidity (38). In this structural role, cholesterol controls the permeability of the plasma membrane to neutral solutes, protons (positive hydrogen ions), and sodium ions (38).

In addition to its role in modulating membrane fluidity, cholesterol within cells is a precursor molecule in several biochemical pathways (39). In the liver, cholesterol is converted to bile, which is then stored in the gallbladder. Bile contains bile salts, which solubilize fats in the digestive tract and aids in the intestinal absorption of fat molecules as well as fat-soluble vitamins, A, D, E, K. Cholesterol is an important precursor molecule for the synthesis of vitamin D and the steroid hormones, including the adrenal gland hormones cortisol and aldosterone, as well as the sex hormones progesterone, estrogens, and testosterone, and their derivatives (39).

Digestion

Digestion of fat begins in the mouth.

Mouth: The digestion of fats starts slowly in the mouth with some hard fats beginning to melt when they reach body temperature. A digestive enzyme, lingual lipase, found in saliva plays an active role in digestion in infants, but a relatively minor role in adults (3).

Stomach: In the stomach, fat floats as a layer above the other components of swallowed food. As a result, little digestion takes place. Mixing does occur and enzymes that can split fats into their components are present, but they are inactive in stomach acids (3).

Small Intestines: In the small intestines, a hormone, cholecystokinin, signals the gall bladder to release bile which emulsifies the fat. The liver manufactures bile acids from cholesterol, and the gallbladder stores the bile until called for by cholecystokinin. The churning action of the intestines mixes the fat with bile and The fat is emulsified; i.e. broken down to tiny droplets (3). Absorption of fats requires the action of bile acids which surround the fats and makes them water soluble (a requirement for absorption).

During digestion in the small intestines, the fatty acids are separated from the glycerol component by enzymes. Typically the fatty acids are removed and absorbed individually.

However, often the middle fatty acid is not removed and the glycerol is absorbed attached to this fatty acid. Molecules attached to cholesterol are removed and then the cholesterol is absorbed (40).

Absorption

Emulsified fats, not the bile acids, are absorbed into the cells of the small intestine (2). To reiterate, the fatty acid on the middle position of the triglyceride (mono and polyunsaturated fatty acids with lower melting points) is easily absorbed as a monoglyceride even if normally poorly absorbed when present as a free fatty acid. This mechanism assures greater absorption of the essential fatty acids which are preferentially attached to the number two position. Once absorbed, the fats must be reassembled to be transported throughout the body (40).

Transport

Once in the intestinal cell, the fatty acids and glycerol are then reassembled. As previously stated, fats do not mix with water and must be made water soluble to be transported. The packaging systems that transport fats are known as lipoproteins. Lipoproteins are not a type of fat, but are packaging systems that transport fats (36).

The handling of lipoproteins in the body is referred to as lipoprotein metabolism. It is divided into two pathways, exogenous and endogenous, depending in large part on whether the lipoproteins in question are composed chiefly of dietary (exogenous) lipids or whether they originated in the liver (endogenous) (41).

Exogenous Pathway

The exogenous pathway for lipoprotein metabolism begins with dietary lipids (40,41). Epithelial cells lining the small intestines readily absorb lipids from the diet. These lipids, including fatty acids and cholesterol, are assembled into chylomicrons (40,41). These chylomicrons are secreted from the intestinal epithelial cells into the lymphatic circulation because they are too large to enter the bloodstream. They circulate through the lymphatic vessels, bypassing the liver, and drain into the bloodstream (40,41).

In the bloodstream, HDL particles donate proteins to the chylomicron; the chylomicron is now considered mature. An enzyme, lipoprotein lipase (LPL), on endothelial cells lining the blood vessels catalyzes a reaction that ultimately releases glycerol and fatty acids from the chylomicrons (40, 41). Glycerol and fatty acids can be absorbed in tissues, especially adipose and muscle, for energy and storage (40,41).

Endogenous Pathway

The liver is referred to as the endogenous pathway for lipoprotein metabolism. The liver is an important source of lipoproteins, principally very low-density lipoprotein (VLDL) (41). Triglyceride and cholesterol are assembled to form VLDL particles. VLDL particles are released into the bloodstream.

As in chylomicron metabolism, VLDL particles require proteins from HDL to become mature (41). Again like chylomicrons, VLDL particles circulate and encounter LPL on endothelial cells causing hydrolysis of the VLDL particle and the release of glycerol and fatty acids. These products can also be absorbed by peripheral tissues, principally adipose and muscle. The hydrolyzed VLDL particles are now called VLDL remnants or intermediate density lipoproteins (IDL). IDL's are hydrolyzed and become LDL which contain a relatively high cholesterol content (41).

LDL can bind to cells and release its contents into cells. LDL and VLDL circulate through the body depositing triglycerides to all cells (muscle, fat, etc.). These cells also take up cholesterol, fatty acids, and phosphate to build new membranes, make hormones, etc. Most of the triglycerides are taken up by fat cells, although muscle cells can take up and store small amounts (41). The VLDL and LDL remnants are removed by the liver. High levels of LDL and cholesterol damage arteries and increase risk for CVD (36). HDL removes fats that have been released from cells and returns them to the liver for recycling or removal. High levels of HDL are protective and decrease risk for disease (42).

Summary

Fats refer to a class of nutrients known as lipids. Although the words "oils", "fats", and "lipids" are all used to refer to fats, in reality, fat is a subset of lipid. "Oils" is usually used to refer to lipids that are liquid at normal room temperature (70 to 75 degrees Fahrenheit), while "fats" is usually used to refer to lipids that are solid at normal room temperature. "Lipids" is used to refer to both liquid and solid fats, along with other related substances. The word "oil" is also used for any substance that does not mix with water and has a greasy feel, such as petroleum (or crude oil), heating oil, and essential oils, regardless of its chemical structure.

The major lipids found in the foods we eat are triglyceride, phospholipid, and cholesterol (a sterol found only in animal products).

Triglycerides consist of a glycerol molecule and three fatty acids. Glycerol is an alcohol composed of a three carbon chain that serves as the backbone of the triglyceride. In nature, the two outside fatty acids of the triglyceride prefer to hold a saturated fatty acid, whereas the middle position prefers an essential fatty acid. Fatty acids will be discussed in detail in the following section.

In addition to obtaining triglycerides from the diet, the body can make triglycerides from excess sugars. The body begins by reducing the sugar to a 2-carbon fragment called acetate. The body makes saturated fatty acids out of these excess acetate fragments by hooking them end to end. Glycerol is then added and the resulting triglyceride is stored as body fat. The body can also make triglycerides from alcohol, fats and proteins.

Phospholipids (also known as phosphatides) are a second type of fat found in foods. About 5% to 9% of fat in animal products is phospholipid. A phospholipid also has a glycerol molecule, but has only two fatty acids. The third fatty acid is replaced by a phosphate group. The major roles of phospholipids include membrane structure and immune system function. About 1% of the fat in animal products is cholesterol. Cholesterol is a circular molecule that does not contain fatty acids or glycerol.

Fatty acids can be saturated, monounsaturated, or polyunsaturated. Saturated fatty acids are the simplest of the fatty acids. Saturated fatty acids have no double bonds between the carbon atoms of the fatty acid chain; hence, they are fully saturated with hydrogen atoms. An unsaturated fat is a fat or fatty acid in which there are one or more double bonds in the fatty acid chain. A fat molecule is monounsaturated if it contains one double bond, and polyunsaturated if it contains more than one double bond.

Where double bonds are formed, hydrogen atoms are eliminated.

Chemically, trans fats are made of the same building blocks as non-trans fats, but have a different arrangement. In trans fatty acid molecules, the hydrogen atoms bonded to pair(s) of doubly bonded carbon atoms (characteristic of all unsaturated fats) are in the *trans* rather than the *cis* arrangement. Trans fats occur when hydrogen is added to unsaturated fatty acids transforming them from a cis configuration into a trans configuration.

Two fatty acids are essential, linoleic and linolenic. The best sources of essential fatty acids are fish and oils of certain seeds and nuts. Research indicates many beneficial effects of omega-3 fatty acids. Regular consumption helps prevent irregular heartbeat and blood clots, improves lipid profiles, lowers blood pressure, supports a healthy immune system, and suppresses inflammation.

Essential fatty acids are precursors to hormone-like substances called eicosanoids. The major precursor of these compounds is arachidonic acid (20-carbon polyunsaturated fatty acid) and the pathways leading to the eicosanoids are known collectively as the 'arachidonate cascade'. Eicosanoids are not stored and are synthesized in response to immediate cellular need. Eicosanoids include prostaglandins, prostacyclins, the thromboxanes, lipoxins and the leukotrienes. The eicosanoids are considered "local hormones" in that they have specific effects on target cells close to their site of formation.

Eicosanoids exert important effects on the immune system, cardiovascular system, reproductive and central nervous system. All cells can form eicosanoids, but tissues differ in enzyme profile and hence in the products they can form.

Prostaglandins are like hormones in that they act as chemical messengers, but do not move to other sites and work within the cells where they are synthesized. A diversity of receptors means that prostaglandins act on many types of cells and have a wide variety of effects. A major effect of prostaglandins is control of platelet aggregation. Platelets, along with red cells and plasma, form a major portion of both human and animal blood. Platelets provide the necessary hormones and proteins for coagulation.

Three major types of prostaglandins found in platelets are:

- Series 1 prostaglandins: Series 1 prostaglandins are formed when plant products such as flax, safflower, sunflower, sesame, soybean, and walnut are ingested. These prostaglandins are less inflammatory and anti-aggregating. In other words these prostaglandins reduce blood clotting.
- Series 2 prostaglandins: Series 2 prostaglandins are formed from ingestion of

animal products. These prostaglandins are more inflammatory and aggregating. These prostaglandins increase blood clotting.

- Series 3 prostaglandins: Series 3 prostaglandins are formed from ingestion of plant products and fish. These prostaglandins are the least aggregating and inflammatory. They produce the least inflammatory and aggregating response and hence are the "heart healthiest". When choosing fats for optimum health plant products and fish are the healthier choices.

Increasing omega-3 fatty acid consumption through foods is preferable. Because of the potential for side effects and interactions with medications, omega-3 dietary supplements should be taken only under the supervision of a knowledgeable health care provider. High intakes may increase bleeding time, interfere with wound health, increase the need for vitamin E, and suppress immune system response.

Individuals with coronary artery disease, may not get enough omega-3 by diet alone. Individuals with high triglycerides may require even larger doses. These people may want to talk to their doctor about supplements. The FDA has ruled that intakes of up to 3 g/d of marine omega-3 fatty acids are Generally Recognized As Safe (GRAS) for inclusion in the diet (24). Some side effects of omega-3 fatty acid supplementation include fishy after taste, gastrointestinal disturbances and nausea.

Clinical signs of essential fatty acid deficiency include a dry scaly rash, decreased growth in infants and children, increased susceptibility to infection, and poor wound healing.

Cholesterol is found in animal products and is a sterol. It is a hard, waxy substance that melts at 149 degrees centigrade. It is made by the body, and is therefore not an essential nutrient. It is manufactured from simple 2-carbon acetate groups which are derived from the breakdown of sugars, fats, and in rare circumstances proteins. The 2-carbon fragments are hooked end to end until 30 of them are chained together. Each step involves enzymes, the chain is cyclized, and 3 carbons are removed to produce the 27 carbon cholesterol molecule

The digestion of fats starts slowly in the mouth with some hard fats beginning to melt when they reach body temperature. A digestive enzyme, lingual lipase, found in saliva plays an active role in digestion in infants, but a relatively minor role in adults. In the stomach, fat floats as a layer above the other components of swallowed food. As a result, little digestion takes place. Mixing does occur; and enzymes that can split fats into their components are present, but the enzymes are inactive in stomach acids. In the small intestines a hormone, cholecystokinin, signals the gall bladder to release bile

Fats, not the bile acid, are absorbed into the cells of the small intestine. During digestion the fatty acids are separated from the glycerol component by enzymes. Typically the fatty acids are removed and absorbed individually. Attached molecules are removed from cholesterol, and then the cholesterol is absorbed.

The handling of lipoproteins in the body is referred to as lipoprotein metabolism. It is divided into two pathways, exogenous and endogenous, depending in large part on whether the lipoproteins in question are composed chiefly of dietary (exogenous) lipids or whether they originated in the liver (endogenous). The exogenous pathway for lipoprotein metabolism begins with dietary lipids. Epithelial cells lining the small intestines readily absorb lipids from the diet. These lipids, including fatty acids and cholesterol, are assembled into chylomicrons. These chylomicrons are secreted from the intestinal epithelial cells into the lymphatic circulation because they are too large to enter the bloodstream. As they circulate through the lymphatic vessels, they bypass the liver circulation and are drained elsewhere into the bloodstream. The liver is referred to as the endogenous pathway for lipoprotein metabolism. The liver is an important source of lipoproteins, principally very low-density lipoprotein (VLDL). Triglyceride and cholesterol are assembled to form VLDL particles. VLDL particles are released into the bloodstream.

Chapter 3 Sample Test

1. List two other roles for fats in addition to providing energy.
2. Which form of dietary fat is stored in the fat cell, and which form is part of all cell membranes? Explain the roles of each type of fat.
3. What are trans fatty acids?
4. Name the essential fatty acids, and discuss their importance in health.
5. Discuss eicosanoids and prostaglandins and their relative importance in health.
6. Discuss digestion, absorption, and transportation of fats.

References

1. Food and Nutrition Board, Institute of Medicine. (2002). *Dietary Fats: Total Fat and Fatty Acids. Dietary Reference Intakes for Energy, Carbohydrate, Fiber, Fat, Fatty Acids, Cholesterol, Protein, and Amino Acids.* Washington, DC: National Academies Press. 422-541.
2. Maton, Anthea; Jean Hopkins, Charles William McLaughlin, Susan Johnson, Maryanna Quon Warner, David LaHart, Jill D. Wright. (1993). *Human Biology and Health*. Englewood Cliffs, New Jersey, USA: Prentice Hall.
3. Whitney, E & Rolfes S. (2013). *Understanding Nutrition, 13th ed.* Belmont,CA:Wadsworth, Cengage Learnin (128-158).
4. Ross, C (Shils) et al. (2012). *Modern Nutrition in Health & Disease, 11th ed.* Philadelphia PA: Lipincott Wilillians & Wilikins (65-92, 562-564, 584-585, 970-978).
5. Triglyceride molecule. http://smithmeadows.com/farm/not-just-a-by-product/attachment/fat-molecule/.
6. Lehninger, A. (2013).*Principles of Biochemistry, 6th ed.* NY: W H Freeman and Company (368-372, 387-387, 634, 668-672, 857-858, 864-871).
7. Vance, E. Vance, JE. (2008). *Phospholipid biosynthesis in eukaryotes. In: Biochemistry of Lipids, Lipoproteins and Membranes, 5th Ed.* Netherlands: Elsivier Publishing. Chapter 7:214.
8. Dowhan, W, Bogdanov, M, Mileykovskaya, E. (2008). *Functional roles of lipids in membranes.* In: *Biochemistry of Lipids, Lipoproteins and Membranes 5th Ed.* Netherlands: Elsivier Publishing. Chapter 1:7-13.
9. Guyton, A. (2012). Textbook of Medical Physiology, 11th ed. Philadelphia, PA: W.B. Saunders Co. (703, 718-733, 851).
10. Jackson, MA & List, GR. (2007). Giants of the Past: The Battle Over Hydrogenation (1903–1920), Inform 18.
11. Erasmus,U. (1991). Fats and Oils, Canada: Alive Books.
12. Stillwell, W & Wassall, SR. (2003). Docosahexaenoic acid: membrane properties of a unique fatty acid. *Chem Phys Lipids.* 126(1):1-27.
13. Casimir, CA & David, B. ed. (2002). *Food lipids: chemistry, nutrition, and biotechnology*. New York: M. Dekker. 1–2.
14. Freeman, IP. (2005). *Margarines and Shortenings.* Ullmann's Encyclopedia of Industrial Chemistry. Hoboken, NJ: Wiley VCH.
15. Mozaffarian D, et al. (2006). "Trans Fatty Acids and Cardiovascular Disease". *New England Journal of Medicine.* 354 (15): 1601–1613.
16. Miyazaki M. & Ntambi, JM. (2008). *Fatty acid desaturation and chain elongation in mammals. In: Biochemistry of Lipids, Lipoproteins and Membranes 5th Ed.* Netherlands: Elsivier Publishing. Chapter 7:204.
17. Kris-Etherton, PM, et al. (2002). Scientific Statement: Fish Consumption, Fish Oil, Omega-3 Fatty Acids, and Cardiovascular Disease. *Circulation.* 106:2747-2757.
18. Skulas, AC, et al. (2011). Dose response effects on triglycerides, inflammation, and endothelial function in healthy persons with moderate hypertriglyceridemia. *Amer. J. Clin. Nutr.* 93:243-252.
19. Musa-Velosa, K, et al. (2010). Long-chain omega 3 fatty acids does-dependently reduce fasting serum triglycerides. *Nutrition Reviews.* 68:155-167.
20. Bouwens, M, et al. (2009). Fish-oil supplementation induces anti-inflammatory gene expression profiles in human blood mononuclear cells. *Amer. J. Clin. Nutr.* 90:415-424.
21. Duga, K, et al. (2009). Fish oil but not flaxseed oil decreases inflammation and prevents pressure overload-induced cardiac dysfunction. *Cardiovascular Research.* 81:319-327.
22. Kris-Etherton, PM & Hill, A.M. (2008). N-3 fatty acids: Foods or supplements? *J of the Am*

Dietetic Assoc. 108:1125-1130.

23. Department of Health and Human Services, US Food and Drug Administration. (1997). Substances affirmed as generally recognized as safe. Federal Register. Vol. 62, No. 108: 30751-30757. 21 CFR Part 184 [Docket No. 86G-0289].
24. Harris WS, et al. (1997). Safety and efficacy of Omacor in severe hypertriglyceridemia. *J Cardiovasc Risk*. 4:385–391.
25. Sacks FM, Stone PH, Gibson CM, et al. (1995). Controlled trial of fish oil for regression of human coronary atherosclerosis. HARP Research Group. *J Am Coll Cardiol*. 25:1492–1498.
26. Esposito, K, et al. (2010). Prevention and control of type 2 diabetes by Mediterrnean diet: A systemic review. *Diabetes Research and Clinical Practice*. 80:97-102.
27. Buenza, JJ, et al. (2010). Adherence to the Mediterranean diet, long-term weight change and incident overweight or obesity: The Sequimiento Universidad de Navarra cohort. *Amer. J of Clin Nutr*. 92:1484-1493.
28. Sofi F, et al. (2008). Adherence to Mediterranean diet and health status: Meta-analysis. *BMJ*. 337:a1344.
29. Jeppesen PB, Hoy CE, Mortensen PB. (1998). Essential fatty acid deficiency in patients receiving home parenteral nutrition. *Am J Clin Nutr*. 1998;68(1):126-133.
30. Smith, L. Murphy, RC. (2008). *The eicosanoids: cyclooxygenase, lipoxygenase,and epoxygenase pathways. In: Biochemistry of Lipids, Lipoproteins and Membranes* (5th Edition). Chapter 12:332.
31. DeCaterina, R and Basta, G (June 2001). n-3 Fatty acids and the inflammatory response – biological background (PDF). *European Heart Journal Supplements*. 3, Suppl D: D42–D49.
32. Funk, Colin D. (2001). Prostaglandins and Leukotrienes: Advances in Eicosanoid Biology. *Science* 294 (5548):1871–1875.
33. Bagga, D, et al. (2003).Differential effects of prostaglandin derived from ω-6 and ω-3 polyunsaturated fatty acids on COX-2 expression and IL-6 secretion. *PNAS*. 100 (4): 1751-1756.
34. Sadava D, Hillis DM, Heller HC, Berenbaum MR (2011). *Life: The Science of Biology 9th Edition*. San Francisco: Freeman. pp.105–114.
35. G. P. Moss (1989). "Nomenclature of Steroids (Recommendations 1989)". *Pure & Appl. Chem.* 61 (10): 1783–1822.
36. Liscum, L. (2008). *Cholesterol biosynthesis.* In: Biochemistry of Lipids, Lipoproteins and Membranes (5th Edition). Chapter 14:399-402.
37. Yeagle PL. (October 1991). Modulation of membrane function by cholesterol. Biochimie 73 (10): 1303–10.
38. Hanukoglu I. (1992). "Steroidogenic enzymes: structure, function, and role in regulation of steroid hormone biosynthesis.". *J Steroid Biochem Mol Biol*. 43 (8):779–804.
39. Poirier, H, et al. (2009). Intestinal absorption of long-chain fatty acids: evidence and uncertainties review. *Prog Lipid Res*. 48(2):101-15.
40. Fielding, PE & Fielding, CJ. (2008). *Dynamics of lipoprotein transport in the human circulatory system*. In: *Biochemistry of Lipids, Lipoproteins and Membranes 5th Ed*.Netherlands: Elsivier Publishing. Chapter 19:533-553.
41. Brown, V. (2007). High-density lipoprotein and transport of cholesterol and triglyceride in blood. *Journal of Clinical Lipidology*. 1(1).
42. Arsenault BJ, et al. (2009). Beyond low-density lipoprotein cholesterol: Respective contributions of non-high-density lipoprotein cholesterol levels, triglycerides, and the total cholesterol/high-density lipoprotein cholesterol ratio to coronary heart disease risk in apparently healthy men and women. *Journal of the American College of Cardiology*. 55:35.
43. National Cholesterol Education Program National Heart, Lung, and Blood Institute National Institutes of Health. (2002). NIH Publication No. 02-5215
44. ATP III Update 2004: Implications of Recent Clinical Trials for the ATP III Guidelines. (2004).

http://www.nhlbi.nih.gov/guidelines/cholesterol/atp3_rpt.htm.
45. Oleic Acid 3-D Model. http://en.wikipedia.org/wiki/File:Oleic-acid-3D-vdW.png. Accessed 05/25/2013. Permission is granted to copy, distribute and/or modify this document under the terms of the GNU Free Documentation License.
46. Cholesterol 3-D Model. http://en.wikipedia.org/wiki/Cholesterol. Accessed 05/31/2013. Permission is granted to copy, distribute and/or modify this document under the terms of the GNU Free Documentation License.
47. Simopoulos AP. (1999). Essential fatty acids in health and chronic disease. *Am J Clin Nutr.* 70(3 Suppl):560S-569S. Review.
48. Harbige LS. (1970). Fatty acids, the immune response, and autoimmunity: a question of n-6 essentiality and the balance between n-6 and n-3. *Lipids.* 38(4):323-341.
49. Valk EE, Hornstra G. (2002). Relationship between vitamin E requirement and polyunsaturated fatty acid intake in man: a review. *Int J Vitam Nutr Res.*70(2):31-42.
50. U.S. Department of Agriculture, Agricultural Research Service. (2008).USDA National Nutrient Database for Standard Reference, Release 21. 2008. Available at: http://www.nal.usda.gov/fnic/foodcomp/search/.
51. Cell membrane: detailed diagram. http://en.wikipedia.org/wiki/Cholesterol. Accessed 05/31/2013. Permission is granted to copy, distribute and/or modify this document under the terms of the GNU Free Documentation License.
52. What You Need to Know about Mercury in Fish and Shellfish. (2004). EPA: Water: Outreach & Communication. http://water.epa.gov/scitech/swguidance/fishshellfish/outreach/advice_index.cfm.
53. Porta, M, Zumeta, E. (2002). Implementing the Stockholm Treaty on Persistent Organic Pollutants. *Occupational and Environmental Medicine.* 59(10): 651–2.
54. Polychlorinated biphenyls (PCBs). (1997). CASRN 1336-36-3. http://www.epa.gov/iris/subst/0294.htm.
55. Mahaffe, KR, et al. (2011). Balancing the benefits of n-3 polyunsaturate fatty acids and the risks of methylmercury exposure from fish consumption. *Nutr. Reviews.* 69:493-508.
56. Chardigny JM. (2008) Do trans fatty acids from industrially produced sources and from natural sources have the same effect on cardiovascular disease risk factors in healthy subjects? Results of the trans Fatty Acids Collaboration (TRANSFACT) study. *Am J Clin Nutr.* 87:558–66.
57. Mozaffarian D, Katan MB, Ascherio A, et al. (2006).Trans fatty acids and cardiovascular disease. *N Engl J Med.* 354:1601–13.
58. Mensink RP, Zock PL, Kester AD, Katan MB. (2003). Effects of dietary fatty acids and carbohydrates on the ratio of serum total to HDL cholesterol and on serum lipids and apolipoproteins: a meta-analysis of 60 controlled trials. *Am J Clin Nutr.* 77:1146 –55.
59. Aro A., TFA isomers and the missing evidence, *Eur J Lipid Sci Technol.* 106:345-6.
60. Willett WC, Stampfer MJ, Manson JE, et al. (1993). Intake of trans fatty acids and risk of coronary heart disease among women. *Lancet.* 341.
61. Sarah K. Gebauer, Jean-Michel Chardigny, Marianne Uhre Jakobsen, Benoît Lamarche, Adam L. Lock, SD. Proctor, DJ Baer. (2011). Effects of Ruminant trans Fatty Acids on Cardiovascular Disease and Cancer: A Comprehensive Review of Epidemiological, Clinical, and Mechanistic Studies. *Advances in Nutrition.* 2: 332-354
62. University of Alberta (2011, September 7). Expert calls for change in trans fat labeling. Science Daily. Retrieved June 4, 2013, from http://www.sciencedaily.com /releases/2011/09/110907124359.htm.

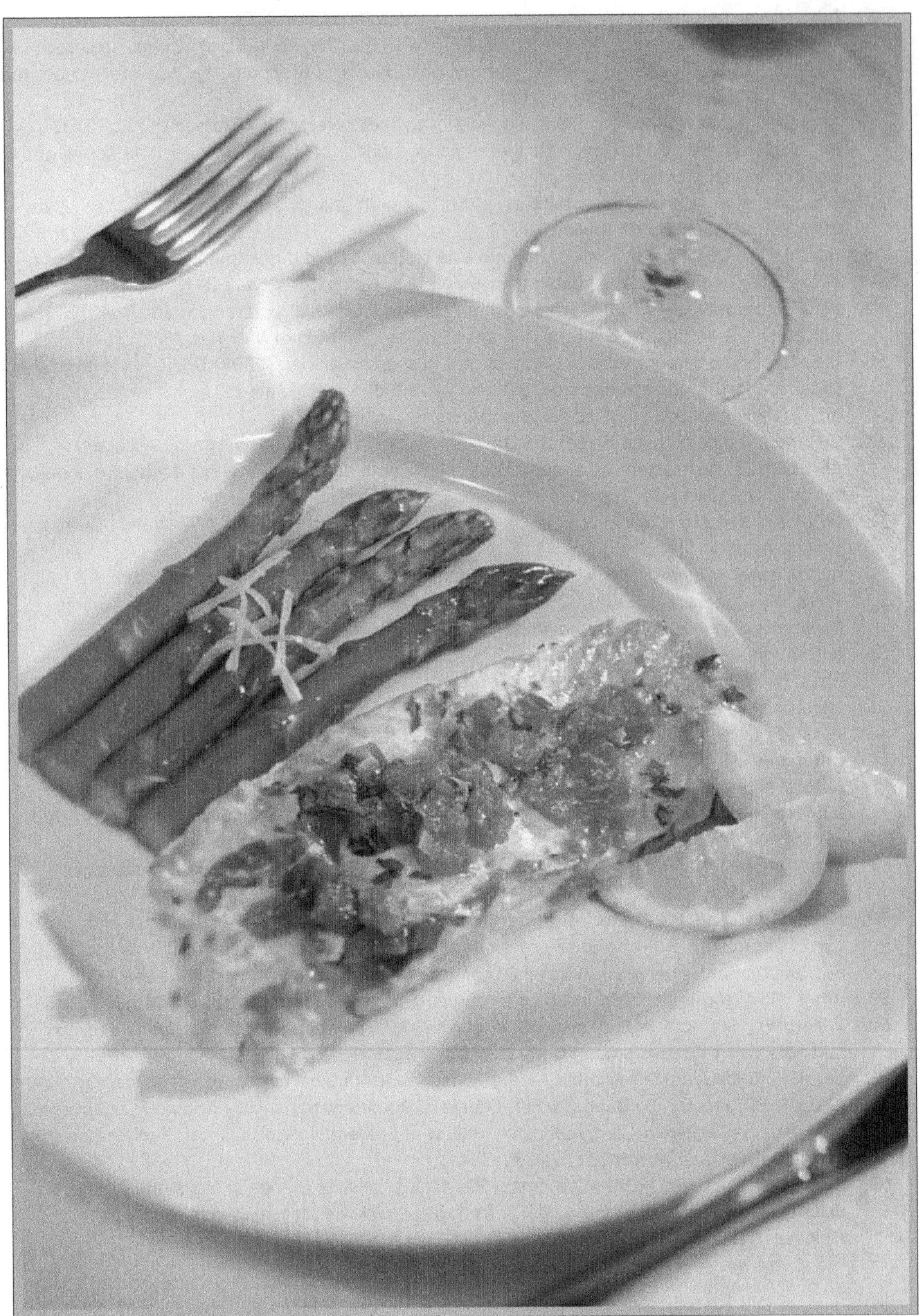

Chapter 4 - Proteins

In this chapter we will take a more in depth look at proteins. Unlike carbohydrates and fats, proteins play a more versatile role in the body. Discussion will center on these roles and roles of amino acids, the building blocks of proteins. We will conclude with a discussion on digestion; absorption and transport of amino acids; and the importance of adequate, high quality protein intake for health.

Objectives

After reading and studying this chapter, you should be able to:

1. Describe digestion, absorption, transport, and roles of proteins.
2. Discuss the types of proteins and metabolic functions.
3. Discuss amino acids and their roles in metabolism; in particular glutamine, alanine and BCAAs.
4. Discuss essential amino acids and their importance in health.
5. Describe nitrogen fixation, biological importance of nitrogen, and the consequences associated with nitrogen toxicity.
6. Discuss transport of amino acids in the bloodstream, including transport through the blood-brain barrier.
7. List the various methods of measuring protein quality and how they differ.

Introduction

Proteins are linear, large organic molecules built from 20 different amino acids. The extraordinary structure of proteins enables them to play more versatile roles in the body than carbohydrates or lipids (6). The dietary requirements for proteins will be discussed in detail in the next chapter on energy.

The words protein, polypeptide, and peptide are a little ambiguous and can overlap in meaning. Protein is generally used to refer to the complete biological molecule in a stable conformation, whereas peptide is generally reserved for a short amino acid chain often lacking a stable 3-dimensional structure (5). However, the boundary between the two is ill-defined and usually lies near 20-30 residues. Polypeptide can refer to any single linear chain of amino acids, usually regardless of length, but often implies an absence of a defined conformation (6).

The table below lists common sources of protein foods (2).

Item	**Serving Size**	**Protein (grams)**
Meat, poultry, fish	3 oz. Cooked	21 grams
Milk	8 oz.	10 grams
Yogurt	8 oz.	8 grams
Cottage cheese	4 oz.	13 grams
Beans, dried peas, lentils	½ cup cooked	7 grams

Proteins

All proteins in all species are built from the same 20 standard amino acids (6). They are assembled from amino acids using information encoded in genes and are defined by their unique sequence of amino acid residues (6). Just as the letters of the alphabet can be combined to form an almost endless variety of words, amino acids can be linked in varying sequences to form a huge variety of proteins.

All amino acids possess common structural features, including a carbon to which an amino group (NH2) is bonded (6). The amino acids in a polypeptide chain are linked by peptide bonds. Once linked in the protein chain, an individual amino acid is called a residue, and the linked series of amino acids is known as the primary structure of the protein (4). The secondary structure of proteins is determined by weak electrical attractions within the polypeptide chain. The tertiary structure forms when long polypeptide chains twist and fold into complex, tangled shapes (6). This extraordinary and unique three-dimensional structure of proteins enables them to perform the various roles in the body. When proteins are subjected to heat, acid, or other conditions that disturb the stability of the structure they uncoil and lose their shape (denaturation) (6). When denaturation occurs the protein loses its activity and no longer functions as a protein.

Proteins are classified according to their structure. Some proteins are large globular compounds and are found in tissue fluids (6). Enzymes, protein hormones, hemoglobin, myoglobin, globulins and albumins of blood are all globular proteins. Other proteins form long chains bound together in a parallel fashion, and are called fibrous proteins (6). These consist of long, folded chains of amino acids and are the proteins of connective tissue and elastic tissue including collagen, elastin, and keratin (6).

The body uses proteins to build and repair all of its tissues. From the moment of conception the body uses proteins to manufacture its cells. Examples include:

- In building bones, cells lay down a matrix of the protein collagen;
- When a tissue is injured, a chain of events leads to the production of fibrin. Fibrin is a stringy insoluble mass of protein fibers that form a clot. A scar forms more slowly to replace the clot and permanently heal the cut (6).
- In skin, new cells are constantly growing from underneath the skin which requires proteins;
- The cells that manufacture hair and fingernails are also constantly synthesizing new protein (4);
- GI tract cells live for only three days and must be replaced; the body constantly deposits protein into new cells that replace the lost ones (4).

Many immune system molecules such as antibodies are proteins and are produced in response to the presence of foreign particles invading the body. A foreign particle may be part of a bacterium, a virus, or a toxin. Once the body has manufactured antibodies against an invader, the body 'remembers' how to produce the antibodies. Hence, the next time the body encounters that same invader, it will produce antibodies even more quickly (6).

Growth hormone, insulin, and glucagon are also proteins, as are many other hormones (4). Various glands in the body secrete hormones in response to changes in the internal environment. The blood carries the hormones to their target tissues, where they elicit the appropriate responses to restore normal conditions. Insulin and glucagon help regulate the concentration of blood glucose. Thyroid hormone, another protein, regulates the body's metabolic rate (4).

Some proteins are transport molecules. These proteins specialize in moving molecules into and out of cells. They reside in cell membranes and work to maintain equilibrium in the surrounding fluids (6). Almost every water-soluble nutrient has its own transport system in cell membranes; in contrast, lipids can cross membranes without the help of proteins. Other transport proteins not attached to membranes move about in fluids carrying nutrients from one organ to another. The protein hemoglobin carries oxygen to all cells. The protein albumin in the bloodstream carries amino acids. The lipoproteins (proteins and lipids) transport lipids throughout the bloodstream. Iron is captured by a protein residing in the cell (ferritin) which will not release the iron unless needed by the body (6).Neurotransmitters

Proteins are involved in the cascade of events in clotting of blood. The light sensitive pigments in the cells of the retina (of the eyes) are also protein molecules called opsin (4).

Proteins are enzymes and are involved in the billions of chemical reactions that take place in the body every millisecond. Enzymes not only break down substances, they also build substances, and transform one substance into another. Each reaction requires its own specific enzyme (6).

Amino Acids

Again, twenty standard amino acids are used by cells in protein biosynthesis, and these are specified by the genetic code. These 20 amino acids are biosynthesized from other molecules, but organisms differ in which ones they can synthesize and which ones must be provided in their diet. The ones that cannot be synthesized by an organism, but required, are called essential amino acids (6).

Besides being the building blocks for proteins, amino acids have other vital roles as well (5). Many amino acids are used to synthesize other molecules, for example:

- Gamma-aminobutyric acid, and glutamate are neurotransmitters.
- Tryptophan is a precursor of the neurotransmitter serotonin and the vitamin niacin.
- Glycine is a neurotransmitter and a precursor of porphyrins such as heme.
- Arginine is a precursor of nitric oxide.
- Carnitine is used in lipid transport within the cell.
- Ornithine and S-adenosylmethionine are precursors of polyamines.
- Homocysteine is an intermediate in S-adenosylmethionine recycling.
- Tyrosine serves as a precursor for norepinephrine and epinephrine. Tyrosine can also make the pigment melanin (4).

- A small group of amino acids comprised of isoleucine, phenylalanine, threonine, tryptophan, and tyrosine give rise to both glucose and fatty acid precursors and are thus characterized as being glucogenic and ketogenic (6).

Transamination is the process in which amino acids are "transformed" into other amino acids. The amino group from the amino acid is transferred to an alpha-ketoacid with the formation of a second alpha-ketoacid and formation of a different amino acid. All amino acids except lysine, threonine, proline and hydroxyproline participate in the transamination process.

Deamination (removal of amino group from an amino acid) occurs in the liver during the metabolism of amino acids. In the liver, the amino acid combines with water; ammonia is formed and is then converted into urea (4). The oxidation pathway starts with the removal of the amino group by a transaminase (enzyme involved in transamination). The amino group then enters the urea cycle. The urea is delivered to the kidneys where it is converted to urine and excreted.

While a cell may need an amino acid to build a vital protein, the need for energy in the form of glucose supersedes these needs. Cells are forced to use amino acids for glucose when glucose is not available. Breakdown of body protein to meet energy and glucose needs can lead to muscle wasting. As discussed in Chapter 2, an adequate intake of carbohydrates spares amino acids from being utilized for energy (4).

Essential/Indispensable Amino Acids

There are nine essential amino acids (also known as indispensable amino acids) that the body cannot synthesize or synthesize in sufficient amounts to meet the needs of the body (4). Traditionally essential and nonessential amino acids have been distinguished on the basis of whether the amino acids can or cannot be synthesized by the body. Metabolically, however, the distinctions are less clear because a number of essential amino acids can be formed by transamination but not in sufficient amounts (4). A third class, known as the conditionally essential amino acids are synthesized from other amino acids (4). For example, the body normally produces tyrosine from phenylalanine. If the diet does not contain enough phenylalanine then tyrosine becomes a conditionally essential amino acid. However, the synthesis of tyrosine from phenylalanine is confined to particular organs and may be limited by certain physiological factors such as age or disease state (4). If phenylalanine is not obtained from food, the body will be forced to break down its proteins (particularly from muscle) to obtain these needed amino acids.

Essential Amino Acids	Nonessential Amino Acids
Histidine	Alanine
Isoleucine	Arginine
Leucine	Asparagine
Lysine	Aspartic acid
Methionine	Cysteine
Phenylalanine	Glutamic acid
Threonine	Glutamine
Tryptophan	Glycine
Valine	Proline
	Serine
	Tyrosine

Glutamine

Glutamine (nonessential amino acid) is the most abundant amino acid in blood and skeletal muscle as well as the body's total free amino acid pool (7,8,10). It is the major transport form of ammonia $(NH4)_2$ in blood. In the liver, glutamine combines with water, and the ammonia formed from nitrogen is converted into urea.

Evidence indicates that glutamine may become a "conditional" amino acid under certain catabolic states such as in illness or surgery. In these cases, glutamine is exported into the blood and tissues such as the gut, kidney; when this occurs immune system cells increase glutamine uptake and metabolism (7). Glutamine supplementation in these conditions appears to be a safe and promising approach to enteral and parenteral nutrition therapy (9).

Alanine

Alanine (a nonessential amino acid) along with glutamine, is an interorgan nitrogen carrier and an energy producing amino acid (5). Alanine plays a key role in the glucose-alanine cycle between tissues and liver. When glucose is unavailable, muscle and other tissues degrade amino acids for fuel, and amino groups are transaminated to form glutamate (10). Glutamate can then transfer its amino group to pyruvate, forming alanine and alpha-ketoglutarate. The alanine formed passes into the blood and is transported to the liver. A reverse of the reaction takes place in the liver in which alanine is transaminated into glutamate forming glucose (through gluconeogenesis) and the glucose formed is released through the circulation system. Glutamate in the liver enters mitochondria and degrades into ammonium which in turn participates in the urea cycle to form urea (10).

BCAA

The branched chain amino acids (BCAA), leucine, isoleucine, and valine, are essential amino acids whose key role is also in the transport of nitrogen. Only muscles have the complete set of enzymes to fully metabolize the BCAA (5)

After a meal, branched chain amino acids are taken up by the muscle and catabolized to branched chain keto acids (5). The branched chain keto acids have several fates; they can be transaminated in the muscle, or they can be transported to the liver. While muscle is made up of 15% BCAA, only 6% is released indicating that much of the BCAAs are transaminated. Alanine and glutamine make up approximately 6% of muscle tissue but are 60% to 70% of amino acids released in fasting (5). As previously discussed, the alanine released by muscle is taken up by the liver where it is converted to glucose. The glucose is released into the bloodstream providing energy for cells.

Larger than physiological levels of BCAA can influence neurotransmitter production. See "Transport of Amino Acids" for details.

Nitrogen

Nitrogen is a chemical element that has the symbol N and atomic number 7 and atomic weight of 14 (13). Elemental nitrogen is a colorless, odorless, tasteless and mostly inert diatomic gas at standard conditions, constituting 78.1% by volume of Earth's atmosphere.

Nitrogen is present in all living organisms in proteins, nucleic acids, and other molecules (14). It is a large component of animal waste, usually in the form of urea, uric acid, ammonium compounds, and derivatives of these nitrogenous products. Molecular nitrogen in the atmosphere cannot be used directly by either plants or animals, and needs to be converted into nitrogen compounds, or "fixed," in order to be used by organisms. Precipitation often contains substantial quantities of ammonium and nitrate, both thought to be a result of nitrogen fixation by lightning and other atmospheric electric phenomena. However, because ammonium is preferentially retained by the forest canopy relative to atmospheric nitrate, most of the fixed nitrogen that reaches the soil under trees is in the form of nitrate. Soil nitrate is preferentially assimilated by tree roots relative to soil ammonium. Some plants are able to assimilate nitrogen directly in the form of nitrates which may be present in soil (15,16). Humans use nitrogen-containing amino acids from plant sources to manufacture proteins and nucleic acids (15,16). Hence, nitrogen cannot be "fixed" (produced) by humans and must be obtained through absorption of amino acids.

Nitrogen is toxic and must be eliminated daily. While amino acids cannot be stored, there does exist a small amino acid pool in the bloodstream and in tissues (4). The concentration of amino acids in these pools is very small compared to the amino acid pool found in skeletal muscle (skeletal muscle makes up 40% of body weight and contains about 75% of whole-body amino acids) (4).

The liver is the major site of nitrogen metabolism in the body. In times of dietary surplus, the potentially toxic nitrogen of amino acids is eliminated via transamination, deamination, and urea formation. The carbon skeletons are generally conserved as carbohydrate, via gluconeogenesis, or as fatty acid via fatty acid synthesis pathways. In this respect amino acids fall into three categories (6): glucogenic, ketogenic, or both glucogenic and ketogenic. Glucogenic amino acids are those that give rise to a net production of pyruvate or energy cycle intermediates, all of which are precursors to glucose via gluconeogenesis. All amino acids except lysine and leucine are at least partly glucogenic. Lysine and leucine are the only amino acids that are solely ketogenic, neither of which can bring about net glucose production (6).

Glucogenic Amino Acids	Ketogenic Amino Acids	Both Glucogenic and Ketogenic Amino Acids
All amino acids except Lysine and Leucine	Lysine and Leucine	Isoleucine, Threonine, Phenylalanine, Tyrosine Tryptophan

Nitrogen balance is the difference between the dietary intake of nitrogen (mainly protein) and its excretion (as urea and other waste products). Healthy adults excrete the same amount as is ingested, and so are in N equilibrium. During growth and tissue repair the body is in positive N balance, i.e. intake is greater than loss and there is an increase in the total body pool of protein. In fevers, fasting, and wasting diseases the loss is greater than the intake and the individual is in negative balance; there is a net loss of nitrogen from the body (4).

Digestion

Through the process of digestion, humans break down ingested protein into free amino acids that are absorbed and enter into metabolic pathways.

Mouth: There is no breakdown of proteins in the mouth.

Stomach: Hydrochloric acid in the stomach begins to denature proteins (uncoils the amino acid chains). Digestive enzymes then break the bonds between amino acids and form peptides (chains of amino acids). Another enzyme (pepsin) breaks peptides into smaller chains. As previously discussed, when denaturation occurs the protein loses its activity and no longer functions as a protein.

Intestines: When these peptides enter the small intestine, pancreatic enzymes break them further into short peptide chains. What remains are free amino acids, dipeptides, and tripeptides. Once in the bloodstream, these amino acids can reach muscles, other cells, and the liver where they can be transaminated (4).

The role of dietary proteins is to provide the body with amino acids that the body can use to synthesize its own proteins (4). A misconception is that proteins in the diet can affect protein synthesis in the body. As previously mentioned, all dietary proteins are digested into amino acids. Once a protein is denatured it no longer functions as a protein but rather is reduced to chains of amino acids. Once absorbed, all amino acids may be used for energy or synthesized into needed compounds, hence proteins in the diet cannot affect protein synthesis in the body. The role of dietary proteins is to provide the body with the necessary building blocks (essential amino acids) needed by the body to synthesize the required proteins. Another misconception is that eating predigested proteins (amino acid supplements) saves the body from having to digest proteins. This is not the case. The digestion system handles whole proteins in a more efficient manner than predigested amino acids because it dismantles and absorbs the amino acids at a rate that is optimal for absorption (4).

Absorption

Free amino acids and dipeptides (sometimes tripeptides) are absorbed into the intestinal cells. In the small intestine, carrier molecules transport these amino acids and small peptides across the intestinal cells, into the bloodstream, and into the body. Once in the bloodstream, amino acids enter cells by transporters. Many different amino acid transport systems exist for different types and groups of amino acids (16,17).

Transport

Amino Acids can enter cells by several mechanisms (16,17). The transport of amino acids into the cytoplasm occurs via biochemically distinct amino acid transport systems. Each system relates to a discrete membrane-bound transporter protein that resides within the cell membrane. This membrane protein functions to transport the amino acid from the extracellular environment into the cytoplasm. Many of these transporters require sodium for maximal activity (17). There are four different classes of transport systems determined by side chains attached to the amino acid (26). The following table lists the four classes of transport systems and the corresponding amino acids involved in each system.

Class	Amino Acid
Non-Polar and Neutral	alanine, glycine, isoleucine, leucine, methionine, phenylalanine, proline, valine
Polar and Neutral	asparagine, glutamine, serine, threonine, tyrosine, cysteine (slightly polar), tryptophan (slightly polar)
Polar and Acidic	aspartic acid, glutamic acid
Polar and Basic	arginine, histidine, lysine

Blood Brain Barrier

The homeostasis of the central nervous system (CNS) environment is maintained by the blood-brain barrier (BBB), which separates the brain from the systemic blood circulation (25). The presence of the BBB has major implications for the passage of molecules into the brain.

The BBB restricts entry of certain molecules into the brain. Essential nutrients are transported into the brain by means of (selective) carrier mechanisms. Several transport systems have been characterized varying from passive transport (such as diffusion) to active and energy requiring processes (25).

The influx of neutral amino acids into the brain is a function of the BBB and plasma amino acid concentrations and does not require specific transport proteins (18). Tyrosine and tryptophan are members of the neutral amino acid category and will compete with phenylalanine, leucine, isoleucine, valine, histidine, and methionine for uptake by the brain. Dietary interventions that influence the relative blood concentrations of tryptophan, tyrosine and the other large neutral amino acids can therefore influence brain neurotransmitter synthesis (18).

To reiterate, the influx of any of the neutral amino acids in larger than physiological amounts, at the exclusion of the other neutral amino acids, can result in changing patterns of neurotransmitter production (18). For this reason, ingesting amino acid supplements is not recommended. Amino acid supplements are discussed in more detail in Chapter 9.

Protein Quality

Protein quality is defined as the measure of the usefulness of a dietary protein for growth and maintenance of tissue. A complete protein contains all of the essential amino acids in relatively the same amounts as the body requires. The protein from animal products is complete, while plant proteins (vegetables, grains, and legumes) tend to be limiting in one or more essential amino acids (4). An essential amino acid supplied in less than the amount needed to support protein synthesis is called a limiting amino acid. Food proteins that offer the body an unbalanced assortment of amino acids in which the body cannot make full use of them are said to be poor quality proteins (4). Vegetarians can receive all the essential amino acids if, over the course of a day, they eat a variety of grains, legumes, seeds, nuts, and vegetables. These foods must also be eaten in sufficient quantities. Some of these foods, such as seeds and nuts, contain large amounts of fat, which could lead to consuming unwanted calories if consumed in large amounts. See Chapter 12 for a list of foods that can be combined to make complete/complimentary proteins.

To be regarded as a high quality protein, a protein must be complete and also digestible. The most complete protein is worthless if it cannot be digested and absorbed. Digestibility depends on the configuration of the protein, other factors in foods eaten with it, and on reactions that influence the release of amino acids. Overcooking (bacon to a crisp) reduces protein bioavailability and the amino acid cysteine is particularly vulnerable to heat destruction (6). Overcooking causes lysine and glutamine residues to bond together hampering digestibility. Overcooking can also cause sugar molecules to cross-link with proteins (Maillard Reaction) and protein digestibility is reduced by this "browning" effect. Excessive heat due to roasting can also reduce protein availability.

In some circumstances, cooking actually improves bioavailability. Cooking improves the absorption of soy protein by inactivating an enzyme inhibitor so that the protein value is improved.

Measuring Protein Quality

In 1985, the Food and Agriculture Organization (FAO), World Health Organization (WHO), and United Nations University (UNU) published a report in which proposed recommendations for total indispensable amino acids (IAAs) as a percentage of protein intake was 43% for infants and 11% for adults (19). Since the FAO/ WHO/UNU report, Young and coworkers presented data that contradicted these findings (20). Young, et al. suggests that the adult requirement for total IAAs be set at 31% of the protein requirement, or about three times the FAO/WHO/UNU estimate. In 1989 Young, et al, derived an amino acid requirement pattern (MIT-AARP) (20,21). In 1999, the Committee on Military Nutrition Research, the Food and Nutrition Board (Institute of Medicine) recommended that amino acid requirements be reexamined but that, in the interim, the MIT-AARP pattern was accepted (22,23).

Amino Acid Score

Amino acid score is the simplest way to evaluate the protein quality of a food. It easily identifies the limiting amino acid and can be used to score mixtures of different proteins (4). Amino acid composition of a protein is determined in a laboratory and its composition compared to that of an ideal reference protein (4). The amino acid pattern for humans aged 2 to 5 years is used as the ideal standard protein. This age group matches or exceeds amino acid requirements of older children and adults. The amino acids in one gram of the dietary protein are expressed as percentages of the amounts of each essential amino acid in one gram of the ideal standard protein. The amino acid showing the lowest percentage is the limiting amino acid, and its percentage determines the chemical score (or amino acid score). For example, the limiting amino acid in cereal protein is lysine (2.4%). The ideal reference protein has 5.5% lysine. The amino acid score is 2.4% divided by 5.5%; the amino acid score for cereal is 44. This measure, however, does not take into account digestibility.

Biological Value

Biological value, another measure of protein quality, attempts to take into account digestibility of the protein. One of the most important complete and digestible proteins available from food is egg protein. Hence, egg protein is a reference protein used as the standard for measuring biological value (4). The biological value (BV) of proteins is the efficiency of a protein in supporting the needs of the body. Protein synthesis stops when an essential amino acid is missing. Because the remaining amino acids cannot be stored they are dismantled, their nitrogen is removed and excreted.

The quality of a given food protein can be tested by feeding it to experimental animals as the sole protein in their diet. Excretion of nitrogen is measured, and the difference is assumed to be retention. The higher the amount of nitrogen retained, the higher the quality of the protein. BV is expressed as a percentage of the nitrogen absorbed that is retained. Egg protein has been given a BV of 100 (by the Food and Agriculture Organization), milk protein 93, beef 75, and fish 75. A BV of 70 or greater can support human growth as long as energy intake is adequate (4). This method has the advantage of being based on experiments in humans and measures actual nitrogen retention; but it is also expensive, cumbersome, and may be based on false assumptions. The retention of the protein in the body does not necessarily mean that it is being well utilized (4). Protein turnover cannot be measured; hence, this method would not detect which tissues are involved.

Net Protein Utilization

Net protein utilization (NPU) like BV, measures nitrogen retention. Instead of retention of absorbed nitrogen, NPU measures retention of food nitrogen (4). The protein efficiency ratio (PER) measures the weight gain of a growing animal and compares that to the animal's protein intake. This method is used more frequently with animals as the test subjects and results offer no help in distinguishing between causes. In other words, there is no way of knowing if the score is due to amino acid composition or poor digestibility (4).

Protein Efficiency Ratio

Protein efficiency ratio (PER) measures the growth of young animals fed a protein source at a standard level and the weight gain per gram of protein eaten provides the PER. Casein has a PER of 2.8 and soy protein 2.4. This means that young animals gained 2.8 grams for every gram of casein eaten, and only 2.4 grams for every gram of soy eaten (4). This method is inexpensive and simple to calculate but the amino acids of animals are not the same as those of human beings and the amino acids necessary for growth are not the same as for maintenance.

PDCAAS

The protein digestibility-corrected amino acid score (PDCAAS) is similar to the amino acid score, but is corrected for digestibility. The amino acid pattern for humans aged 2 to 5 years is used as the basis for determination of PDCAAS. Corrections for digestibility of protein are taken from human data. PDCAA scores range from 1.0 to 0.0, with 1.0 being the upper limit of protein quality able to support growth and health (19). The PDCAA value of casein (milk protein) and egg white is 1.00; soybean has a PDCAA of .99; beef a PDCAA of .92; and whole wheat a PDCAA of .40. Note that 1.00 is the maximum PDCAA a food protein can receive (4).

DIAAS

DIAAS, digestible indispensable amino acid score, has been proposed as the latest measure of protein quality (24). The PDCAAS method has now been in use for some 20 years and limitations have been recognized. In 2011 an FAO Expert Consultation on Protein Quality Evaluation in Human Nutrition was held in Auckland, New Zealand to reevaluate the use of PDCAAS (24). Their report recommends the use of DIAAS to replace PDCAAS. As protein digestibility does not always reflect the digestibility of individual dietary indispensable amino acids, using a score based on individual dietary indispensable amino acid digestibility is preferable. The report also recommends that DIAAS be used to determine protein quality assessment for regulatory purposes. Below is an example of the use of DIAAS for protein quality assessment in the context of making claims (24).

Food	Amount	Protein (g/100g)	DIAAS	Quality	Claim based on quantity	Claim based on quantity and quality
Wheat	100 g	11	40	Low	Yes - high	No, none
Peas	100 g	21	64	Low	Yes - high	No, none
Milk Powder	100 g	28	122	High	Yes - high	Yes, high

Summary

The extraordinary structure of proteins enables them to play more versatile roles in the body than carbohydrates or lipids. The words protein, polypeptide, and peptide are a little ambiguous and can overlap in meaning. Protein is generally used to refer to the complete biological molecule in a stable conformation, whereas peptide is generally reserved for a short amino acid chain often lacking a stable 3-dimensional structure.

Proteins are linear, large organic molecules built from 20 different amino acids. All proteins in all species are built from the same 20 standard amino acids. They are assembled from amino acids using information encoded in genes and are defined by their unique sequence of amino acid residues. This unique sequence is known as the primary structure of the protein. Just as the letters of the alphabet can be combined to form an almost endless variety of words, amino acids can be linked in varying sequences to form a huge variety of proteins. All amino acids possess common structural features, including a carbon to which an amino group (NH2) is bonded. The amino acids in a polypeptide chain are linked by peptide bonds. Once linked in the protein chain, an individual amino acid is called a residue, and the linked series of carbon, nitrogen, and oxygen atoms are known as the main chain or protein backbone.

Proteins are classified according to their structure. Some proteins are large globular compounds and are found in tissue fluids. Enzymes, protein hormones, hemoglobin, myoglobin, globulins and albumins of blood are all globular proteins. Other proteins form long chains bound together in a parallel fashion, and are called fibrous proteins. These consist of long, folded chains of amino acids and are the proteins of connective tissue and elastic tissue including collagen, elastin, and keratin.

Twenty standard amino acids are used by cells in protein biosynthesis, and these are specified by the general genetic code. These 20 amino acids are biosynthesized from other molecules. The amino acids that cannot be synthesized by an organism, but required, are called essential amino acids. Besides being the building blocks for proteins, amino acids have other vital roles as well.

There are nine essential amino acids (also known as indispensable amino acids) that the body cannot synthesize or synthesize in sufficient amounts to meet the needs of the body. Traditionally essential and nonessential amino acids have been distinguished on the basis of whether the amino acids can or cannot be synthesized by the body. Metabolically, however, the distinctions are less clear because a number of essential amino acids can be formed by transamination but not in sufficient amounts. A third class, known as the conditionally essential amino acids are synthesized from other amino acids. For example, the body normally produces tyrosine from phenylalanine. If the diet does not contain enough phenylalanine then tyrosine becomes a conditionally essential amino acid. However, the synthesis of tyrosine from phenylalanine is confined to particular organs and may be limited by certain physiological factors such as age or disease state. If phenylalanine is not obtained from food, the body will be forced to break down its proteins (particularly from muscle) to obtain these needed amino acids.

Nitrogen is present in all living organisms in proteins, nucleic acids, and other molecules. It is a large component of animal waste, usually in the form of urea, uric acid, ammonium compounds, and derivatives of these nitrogenous products. Molecular nitrogen in the atmosphere cannot be used directly by either plants or animals, and needs to be converted into nitrogen compounds, or "fixed," in order to be used by life. Precipitation often contains substantial quantities of ammonium and nitrate, both thought to be a result of nitrogen fixation by lightning and other atmospheric electric phenomena. However, because ammonium is preferentially retained by the forest canopy relative to atmospheric nitrate, most of the fixed nitrogen that reaches the soil surface under trees is in the form of nitrate. Soil nitrate is preferentially assimilated by tree roots relative to soil ammonium. Some plants are able to assimilate nitrogen directly in the form of nitrates which may be present in soil. Humans use nitrogen-containing amino acids from plant sources to manufacture proteins and nucleic acids. Hence, nitrogen cannot be "fixed" (produced) by humans and must be obtained through absorption of amino acids.

Nitrogen balance is the difference between the dietary intake of nitrogen (mainly protein) and its excretion (as urea and other waste products). Healthy adults excrete the same amount as is ingested, and so are in N equilibrium. During growth and tissue repair the body is in positive N balance, i.e. intake is greater than loss and there is an increase in the total body pool of nitrogen.

Through the process of digestion, humans break down ingested protein into free amino acids that are absorbed and enter into metabolic pathways. The role of dietary proteins is to provide the body with amino acids that the body can use to synthesize its own proteins (4). A misconception is that proteins in the diet can affect protein synthesis in the body. As previously mentioned, all dietary proteins are digested into amino acids. Once a protein is denatured it no longer functions as a protein but rather is reduced to chains of amino acids. Once absorbed, all amino acids may be used for energy or synthesized into needed compounds, hence proteins in the diet cannot affect protein synthesis in the body. The role of dietary proteins is to provide the body with the necessary building blocks (essential amino acids) needed by the body to synthesize the required proteins. Another misconception is that eating predigested proteins (amino acid supplements) saves the body from having to digest proteins. This is not the case. The digestion system handles whole proteins in a more efficient manner than predigested amino acids because it dismantles and absorbs the amino acids at a rate that is optimal for absorption (4).

Amino Acids can enter cells by several mechanisms. The transport of amino acids into the cytoplasm occurs via functionally and biochemically distinct amino acid transport systems. Each system relates to a discrete membrane-bound transporter protein that resides within the cell membrane. This membrane protein functions to transport the amino acid from the extracellular environment into the cytoplasm.

Protein quality is defined as the measure of the usefulness of a dietary protein for growth and maintenance of tissue. A complete protein contains all of the essential amino acids in relatively the same amounts as the body requires. The protein from animal products is complete, while plant proteins (vegetables, grains, and legumes) tend to be limiting in one or more essential amino acids. An essential amino acid supplied in less than the amount needed to support protein synthesis is called a limiting amino acid. Food proteins that offer the body an unbalanced assortment of amino acids in which the body cannot make full use of them are said to be poor quality proteins. Vegetarians can receive all the essential amino acids if, over the course of a day, they eat a variety of grains, legumes, seeds, nuts, and vegetables. These foods must also be eaten in sufficient quantities. Some of these foods, such as seeds and nuts, contain large amounts of fat, which could lead to consuming unwanted calories if consumed in large amounts.

To be regarded as a high quality protein, a protein must be complete and also digestible. The most complete protein is worthless if it cannot be digested and absorbed. Digestibility depends on the configuration of the protein, other factors in foods eaten with it, and on reactions that influence the release of amino acids. Overcooking (bacon to a crisp) reduces protein bioavailability. The amino acid cysteine is particularly vulnerable to heat destruction (6). Overcooking causes lysine and glutamine residues to bond together hampering digestibility. Overcooking can also cause sugar molecules to cross-link with proteins (Maillard Reaction) and protein digestibility is reduced by this "browning" effect. Excessive heat due to roasting can also reduce protein availability. The key is not to overcook.

In some circumstances, cooking actually improves bioavailability. Cooking improves the absorption of soy protein by inactivating an enzyme inhibitor so that the protein value is improved.

In 1985, the Food and Agriculture Organization (FAO), World Health Organization (WHO), and United Nations University (UNU) published a report in which proposed recommendations for total indispensable amino acids (IAAs) as a percentage of protein intake was 43% for infants and 11% for adults (19). Since the FAO/ WHO/UNU report, Young and coworkers presented data that contradicting these findings (20). Young, et al. suggests that the adult requirement for total IAAs be set at 31% of the protein requirement, or about three times the FAO/WHO/UNU estimate. In 1989 Young, et al, derived the Massachusetts Institute of Technology Amino Acid Requirement Pattern (MIT-AARP) (20,21). In 1999, the Committee on Military Nutrition Research, the Food and Nutrition Board (Institute of Medicine) recommended that amino acid requirements be reexamined but that, in the interim, the MIT pattern was accepted.

Chapter 4 Sample Test

1. List three different food sources of proteins.
2. List protein classifications and describe several physiological roles for each classification.
3. Describe digestion and absorption of proteins.
4. Define amino acids, and describe their functions in the human body.
5. Define the indispensable amino acids, and discuss the physiological effects of excessive and insufficient amounts in the diet.
6. How is nitrogen obtained in the diet? What is the significance of nitrogen in metabolism? Why is it toxic, and how does the body eliminate it?
7. Discuss the transport of amino acids into cells including transport into the blood-brain barrier.
8. Discuss protein quality as it pertains to digestibility.

References

1. Food and Nutrition Board, Institute of Medicine. (2002) Dietary Fats: Total Fat and Fatty Acids. Dietary Reference Intakes for Energy, Carbohydrate, Fiber, Fat, Fatty Acids, Cholesterol, Protein, and Amino Acids. Washington, DC: *National Academies Press.* 422-541.
2. U.S. Department of Agriculture, Agricultural Research Service. (2008). *USDA National Nutrient Database for Standard Reference*, Release 21. 2008. Available at: http://www.nal.usda.gov/fnic/foodcomp/search/.
3. Maton, Anthea; Jean Hopkins, Charles William McLaughlin, Susan Johnson, Maryanna Quon Warner, David LaHart, Jill D. Wright (1993). *Human Biology and Health*. Englewood Cliffs, New Jersey, USA: Prentice Hall.
4. Whitney, E & Rolfes S. (2013). *Understanding Nutrition,13th ed.* Belmont, CA : Wadsworth, Cengage Learnin (167-188, 341-342).
5. Ross, C (Shils) et al. (2012). *Modern Nutrition in Health & Disease, 11th ed.* Philadelphia PA: Lipincott Wilillians & Wilikins (3-35, 464).
6. Lehninger, A. (2013). *Principles of Biochemistry, 6th ed* NY: W H Freeman and Company (75-190).
7. Lacey, JM. & Wilmore, DW. (1990). *Nutr Rev.* 48:297-309.
8. Ziegler, TR, et al. (1993). *Clin Nutr.* 12 Suppl 1:s82-90.
9. Heyland, DK, et al. (2007). J Parenter Enteral Nutr. 31:109-118.
10. Nelson, DL, Cox, MM. (2005), *Principles of Biochemistry* (4th ed.), New York: W.H. Freeman, pp.684–85.
11. Sakami W, Harrington H. (1963). Amino acid metabolism. *Annu Rev Biochem* 32: 355-98.
12. Brosnan J (2000). "Glutamate, at the interface between amino acid and carbohydrate metabolism". *J Nutr* 130 (4S Suppl): 988S-90S.
13. Lavoisier, AL.(1965). *Elements of chemistry, in a new systematic order: containing all the modern discoveries*. Courier Dover Publications: p15.
14. Emsley, John (2011). *Nature's Building Blocks: An A-Z Guide to the Elements* (New ed.). New York, NY: Oxford University Press.
15. Bothe, Hermann; Ferguson, Stuart John; Newton, William Edward (2007). *Biology of the nitrogen cycle*. Elsevier. p.283.
16. Christensen, HN. (1990). Role of amino acid transport and counter transport in nutrition and metabolism. *Physiol Rev*:43-77.
17. Souba W.W, Pacitti A.J. (1992). How amino acids get into cells: Mechanisms, models, menus, and mediators. *JPEN J Parenter Enteral Nutr.*16:569-578.
18. Friedman, M. (1989). *Absorption and utilization of Amino Acids*. Boca Raton, FL. CRC Press: Vol 3:57.
19. FAO/WHO/UNU (Food and Agriculture Organization of the United Nations/World Health Organization/United Nations University). (1985). *Energy and protein requirements.* Report of a joint expert consultation. World health Organization Technical Report Series no 724. Geneva: World Health Organization.
20. Young, VR. (1987). McCollum Award Lecture: Kinetics of human amino acid metabolism: Nutritional implications and some lessons. *Am. J. Clin Nutr.* 46:709-725.
21. Young, VR et al. (1989). A theoretical basis for increasing current estimates of the amino acid requirements in adult man with experimental support. *Am. J. Clin. Nutr.* 50:80-92.
22. Young, VR. (1994). Adult amino acid requirement: The case for a major revision in current recommendations. *J. Nutr.* 124:1517s-1523s.
23. Institute of Medicine, Food and Nutrition Board, Committee on Military Nutrition Research, Committee on Body Composition, Nutrition and Health. Washington, DC, 1999.

24. Dietary protein quality evaluation in human nutrition: Report of an FAO expert consultation. (2013). *FAO food and nutrition paper 92*. Auckland, New Zealand.
25. Helga E. de Vries, Johan Kuiper, Albertus G. de Boer, Theo J. C. Van Berkel and Douwe D. Breimer (1997). The blood-brain barrier in neuroinflammatory diseases. *Pharmacological Reviews* 49 (2): 143–156
26. Ophardt, CF. (2003). Structure of amino acids. *Virtual Chembook. http://www.elmhurst.edu/~chm/vchembook/561aminostructure.html.* Retrieved 06/02/2013.

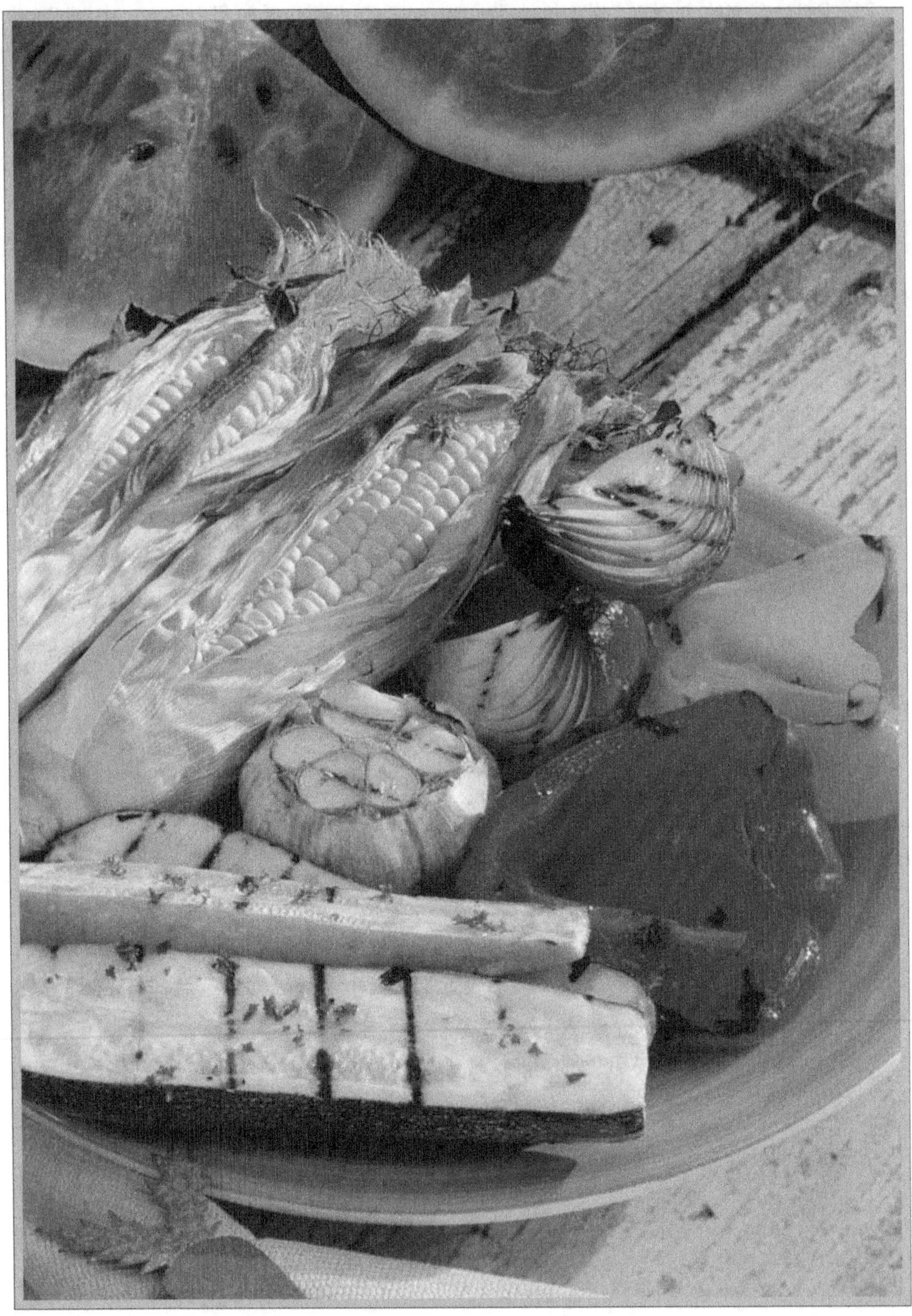

Chapter 5 - Energy

This chapter will focus on energy metabolism including factors involved in energy nutrient utilization, meeting energy nutrient needs through adequate caloric intake, the importance of nutrient timing, and factors involved in energy expenditure.

Objectives

After reading and studying this chapter, you should be able to:

1. Discuss the four phases of energy production.
2. Describe the factors involved in nutrient utilization (diet, rest, exercise intensity, exercise duration, fitness levels, muscle mass).
3. Discuss meeting energy nutrient needs through adequate caloric intake.
4. Describe nutrient timing and the position of the Academy of Nutrition and Dietetics, the American College of Sports Medicine, and the International Olympic Committee.
5. Discuss the position of the Academy of Nutrition and Dietetics, the American College of Sports Medicine, and the International Olympic Committee on adequate fluid intake.
6. Discuss the position of the Academy of Nutrition and Dietetics, the American College of Sports Medicine, and the International Olympic Committee in micronutrient (vitamin and mineral) supplementation.
7. List the three components of energy expenditure (BMR, thermic effect of food, physical activity) and explain each component.

Introduction

Metabolism is defined as the sum of all the chemical reactions in living cells and includes all the reactions by which the body expends energy (production) and obtains energy (consumption from food) (1). Energy is provided in the diet by protein, fat and carbohydrate. With the help of enzymes and coenzymes, cells use these nutrients to build complex compounds (anabolism) or break them down to release energy (catabolism) (2). Our discussion will center on understanding the process of energy metabolism in general terms and will not include the enzymatic reactions involved.

The energy in foods is expressed as a unit of heat, the kilocalorie or kilojoule (see Chapter 1). The potential energy contribution of food is measured in a bomb calorimeter where food is completely combusted to carbon dioxide and water (2). The conversion of food into energy is an inefficient process with approximately 50% lost as heat and approximately 45% available to the body primarily as adenosine triphosphate (ATP) (2).

Before we begin our discussion on energy metabolism it is important to review cellular biology. The human body consists of trillions of cells and the number and type of metabolic activities vary depending on the cell. Liver cells are by far the most versatile and metabolically active cells. A membrane encloses each cell's contents and regulates the passage of molecules in and out of cells (4). The cytoplasm lies inside the cell membrane, and a jelly-like fluid called cytosol fills the space. The breakdown of glucose – glycolysis – occurs in the cytosol of the cell. Mitochondria, often referred to as the power house of the cell, are surrounded by intricately folded membranes that house chemicals required for the tricarboxylic acid (TCA) cycle and electron transport chain (described later in this section) (4). A separate membrane encloses the cell's nucleus.

Energy Production

As discussed in previous chapters during digestion, carbohydrates are broken down to glucose molecules, fats are broken down to glycerol and fatty acids, and proteins are catabolized into amino acids.

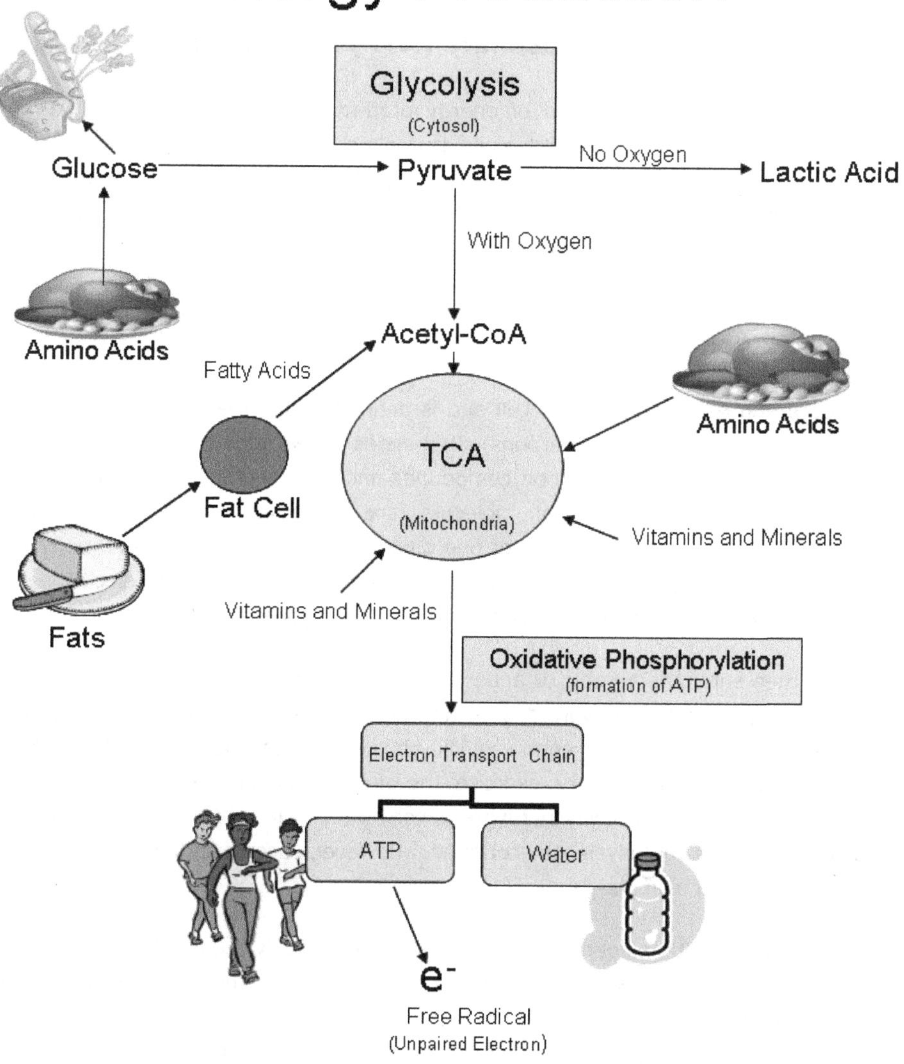
Energy Production
Glycolysis
(Cytosol)
Glucose
Pyruvate
No Oxygen
Lactic Acid
With Oxygen
Amino Acids
Acetyl-CoA
Fatty Acids
Amino Acids
TCA
(Mitochondria)
Fat Cell
Vitamins and Minerals
Fats
Vitamins and Minerals
Oxidative Phosphorylation
(formation of ATP)
Electron Transport Chain
ATP
Water
e-
Free Radical
(Unpaired Electron)

Energy production consists of four phases:

1. ATP-PC
2. Glycolysis
3. Tricarboxylic acid (TCA) cycle
4. Electron transport chain

Anaerobic Adenosine Triphosphate (ATP) Production

The simplest and most rapid method of energy production is the formation of ATP by phosphocreatine (PC) breakdown. Muscle cells can only store a small amount of PC, which limits the amount of ATP that can be produced (80). This combination of ATP and PC is called the ATP-PC system or phosphagen system. It is the energy system that provides energy at the onset of muscular contraction during short, high intensity exercise (i.e. less than five seconds) (80).

Glycolysis -Cytosol

Glycolysis occurs in the cytosol of the cell and is defined as the metabolic breakdown of glucose (6 carbons) to pyruvate (3 carbons). In a series of reactions the 6-carbon glucose molecule is converted to other 6-carbon compounds and then split in half forming two 3-carbon molecules (1). These 3-carbon molecules are converted to pyruvate through a series of reactions; hence, the net yield of one glucose molecule is 2 pyruvate molecules (1). In the process of pyruvate formation, hydrogen atoms with their electrons are released and carried to the electron transport chain (phase 3 of energy production) (1).

Pyruvate can then enter the aerobic or anaerobic pathway (2). In the anaerobic pathway (without oxygen) pyruvate is converted to lactic acid (see Energy Production figure). This pathway yields a small amount of energy quickly but energy can be sustained for only a few minutes. During high intensity exercise the muscles initially rely heavily on the anaerobic pathway. In this pathway pyruvate is converted to lactate, and coenzymes are released which allows glycolysis to continue. However, accumulation of lactate is associated with burning pain and fatigue (1).

The aerobic pathway (with oxygen) produces energy more slowly but can be sustained for long periods of time. When oxygen is available pyruvate enters the mitochondria and is converted to acetyl CoA through a series of reactions. It's important to note that both fatty acids and amino acids can be converted to Acetyl CoA. Acetyl CoA then enters the TCA Cycle (1).

TCA Cycle – Mitochondria

The TCA cycle reactions occur in the inner compartment of the mitochondria (1). The pathway of acetyl CoA is a one way route, and it can not be regenerated (1). When cells need energy, acetyl CoA enters the TCA cycle which begins a series of complicated reactions in which the final compound - oxaloacetate - is also part of the first reaction (circular pathway). Oxaloacetate picks up another acetyl CoA and starts the cycle again. Oxaloacetate is made primarily from pyruvate. Small amounts can be made from amino acids but cannot be made from fat (1). This fact underscores the importance of carbohydrates in the diet.

As compounds in the TCA cycle are catabolized they begin to lose a carbon to carbon dioxide; hydrogens with their electrons are carried off by coenzymes to the electron transport chain. Each turn of the TCA cycle releases a total of 8 electrons (2).

Electron Transport Chain- Mitochondria

The electron transport chain consists of a series of proteins that serve as electron carriers. Electrons enter the transport chain from the TCA cycle, glycolysis and oxidation of fatty acids. As the coenzymes deliver the electrons to the electron transport chain, each carrier receives the electrons and passes them down to the next carrier until the electrons reach oxygen. Oxygen accepts the electrons and combines with hydrogen to form water. As electrons are passed from carrier to carrier, hydrogen atoms are pumped across to the outer compartment of the mitochondria and then back to the inner compartment. This process powers the synthesis of ATP (1).

ATP

ATP leaves the mitochondria and enters the cytosol where it can be used for energy (1). One glucose molecule yields 30 to 32 ATP. One 16-carbon fatty acid chain yields 129 ATP when completely oxidized. Hence, fat is a much more efficient fuel source making it the body's preferred form of energy storage.

Energy Utilization

In this section we will discuss factors involved in energy nutrient utilization under differing circumstances. How much of which fuels are used depends on an interplay among the fuels available from the diet, rest, intensity and duration of exercise, fitness level of the individual, and factors involved in muscle hypertrophy.

Diet

Glycogen storage in muscle and liver depends on foods in the diet. How much carbohydrate is digested and absorbed influences how much glycogen is stored, which in turn influences nutrient utilization (1).

Low-Carbohydrate Diets

While it is difficult to estimate the number of people who have followed low-carbohydrate diets, the number and popularity of articles and books from the lay press advocating their use attest to the interest and demand by the public (5). Numerous professional organizations, including the Academy of Nutrition and Dietetics and the American Heart Association, have cautioned against the use of low-carbohydrate diets (7-10).

A quantitative analysis by Bravada, et al., (107 studies and 94 diets) examined the efficacy and safety of low-carbohydrate diets (5). Their conclusion is that there is insufficient evidence to make recommendations for or against the use of low-carbohydrate diets. In particular, these diets were found to be inadequately evaluated for longer than 90 days, for individuals aged 53 years or older, or for use by participants with hyperlipidemia, hypertension, or diabetes. The lowest-carbohydrate diets (≤20 g/d of carbohydrates) were studied in only 71 participants for whom no data on serum lipid, fasting serum glucose, fasting serum insulin levels, or blood pressure was reported (5). The study also concluded that there is insufficient evidence that low-carbohydrate consumption is independently associated with greater weight loss compared with higher-carbohydrate content (5).

In addition to sacrificing glycogen stores, there are concerns that low-carbohydrate diets lead to abnormal metabolic functioning that may have serious medical consequences, particularly for participants with cardiovascular disease, type 2 diabetes, dyslipidemia, or hypertension (7). Specifically, it has been cautioned that low-carbohydrate diets:

- May cause accumulation of ketones and may result in abnormal metabolism of insulin and impaired liver and kidney function;
- In salt and water depletion, may cause postural hypotension, fatigue, constipation, and nephrolithiasis;
- In excessive consumption of animal proteins and fats, may promote hyperlipidemia;
- In higher dietary protein loads, may impair renal function (7).

Rest

During rest, the body derives slightly more than half of its energy from fatty acids and most of the rest from glucose (2). During a workout, the muscles accumulate microscopic cellular damage. The two factors that expedite convalescence (gradual recovery of health and strength) of the muscles are proper nutrition and rest (11,12). The most important form of rest is sleep, which is essentially just a heightened anabolic state, meaning a time during which larger molecules and tissue are constructed. Sleep also promotes the rejuvenation of the immune, nervous, and muscular systems because protein metabolism occurs at a more proficient rate (11, 12).

Exercise Intensity

ATP is present in small amounts in all body tissues including muscle and is the driving force for contraction. Immediately after the onset of muscle contraction, before muscle ATP pools are depleted, a muscle enzyme begins to break down phosphocreatine. Supplies of ATP and phosphocreatine last for approximately 30 seconds (2). During anaerobic exercise (without oxygen), the body must utilize glucose for energy (since utilization of fat and amino acids requires oxygen), and lactic acid is produced as a by product.

To meet prolonged needs, the body must generate ATP from glucose, fatty acids, and amino acids, and this process requires oxygen (1). During aerobic exercise, the muscles use a combination of energy nutrients for energy. Muscles never use just one single fuel; energy utilization is always a combination of glucose and fat (or fat by-products) and amino acids when caloric needs are not meet.

A popular myth suggests that in order to burn greater amounts of fat, individuals should exercise at a lower intensity. However, at the higher intensity more calories are utilized than at a lower intensity resulting in a greater amount of actual fat being utilized. Dr. Wayne Wescott, Fitness Research Director of the South Shore YMCA, Boston, MA, confirmed the following calculation through research (13,14):

- If a 160 pound male walks for 30 minutes at 3.5 miles/hour he utilizes approximately 240 calories; 40% of those calories would come from fat and 60% from carbohydrates. This results in utilization of 96 calories from fat, or 10.6 grams of fat.
- If the same male runs for 30 minutes at a pace of 6.5 miles/hour, he utilizes approximately 450 calories; 25% of those calories from fat and 75% from carbohydrates. This results in utilization of 112 calories from fat, or 13.5 grams.

Exercise Duration

Exercise duration is also a factor in energy nutrient utilization (1,2). During the first few minutes of exercise, the ATP-PC system, or phosphagen system, and glycolysis provide muscular energy. As exercise continues (10 to 20 minutes), more oxygen becomes available, and aerobic metabolism occurs. When glycogen stores are depleted, activity comes to a near halt (what marathon runners refer to as "hitting the wall") (1,2). See Ketosis in Chapter 2 and Nutrient Timing (later in this chapter) for an in-depth discussion of this process.

Fitness Level

Another critical component in energy nutrient utilization deals with an individuals' fitness level. More oxygen is delivered to muscles cells of aerobically fit individuals. This additional oxygen allows this "fit" individual to utilize more fat in conjunction with glucose, thereby extending glycogen stores. Conditioned muscles also rely less on glycogen and more on fat so that glycogen breakdown occurs more slowly in trained athletes (1,2). Such individuals utilize a greater percentage of fat even at rest.

Muscle Mass

Muscle hypertrophy is a scientific term for the growth and increase of the size of muscle cells. Muscle hypertrophy is dependent on factors such as genetics, gender, age and nutrition (9). Catabolic factors that can lead to muscle catabolism include fasting, starvation, illness, stress, caffeine, alcohol and inadequate amount of rest. We will initially discuss the factors involved in muscle mass and conclude the discussion on factors involved in muscle catabolism.

<u>Muscle Mass - Genetics</u>

While adaptable to training, muscle fiber types are determined genetically and the type of fiber affect skeletal muscle hypertrophy. The force generated by a muscle is dependent on its size and composition of the fiber type. Skeletal muscle fibers are classified into two major categories:

- Slow twitch (type 1) fibers
- Fast twitch (type 2a and type 2b) fibers

The difference between the two fibers can be distinguished by metabolism, contractile velocity, neuromuscular differences, glycogen stores, capillary density of the muscle, and the actual response to hypertrophy (15). Type I fibers are primarily responsible for maintenance of body posture and skeletal support (15). They utilize fats and carbohydrates better because of the increased reliance on oxidative metabolism. Type II fibers require greater amounts of force production for shorter periods of time. These fibers rely on anaerobic metabolism for energy for contraction (15).

<u>Muscle Mass - Gender</u>

Gender differences occur in muscle hypertrophy due to hormones (16,17,18). Testosterone, is present in both males and females, but in greater amounts in males, and has an anabolic effect. Testosterone is an androgen, and the primary physiological role of androgens is to promote the growth and development of male organs and characteristics (16,17,18). Testosterone affects the nervous system, skeletal muscle, bone marrow, skin, hair, and the sex organs. During puberty in males, hypertrophy occurs at an increased rate due to increased testosterone levels; it increases protein synthesis, which induces hypertrophy. This contributes to the gender differences observed in body weight and composition between men and women. (16,17,18).

<u>Muscle Mass - Age</u>

Fast twitch muscles decline with age. However, according to Rosenberg and Evans, a decline in muscle hypertrophy is not inevitable (15). Landmark research has shown that muscle hypertrophy occurs through appropriate resistance training in individuals at any age (15).

<u>Muscle Mass- Nutrition</u>

Nutrition is also a factor in muscle hypertrophy. Without adequate caloric intake, along with adequate protein, fat, carbohydrate and micronutrient intake muscle hypertrophy will not occur. Other nutrition factors include adequate hydration, adequate rest and stress reduction (15,16,17).

Catabolic Factors

Many factors contribute to catabolism of muscle tissue. We will limit our discussion to include the catabolic responses to fasting and starvation, illness, stress, ingestion of caffeine and alcohol, and inadequate rest.

<u>Catabolic Factors – Fasting and Starvation</u>

During fasting, glycogen stores are depleted, and the body must produce glucose from glucogenic amino acids. As discussed in chapter 2, the only way the body can produce glucose after 12 to 16 hours of not eating is through gluconeogenesis, the making of glucose from non-carbohydrate sources (1). The only available source for glucose production in this stage is the breakdown of glucogenic amino acids (amino acids that can synthesize glucose) (1). The body cannot use fat for glucose production because fat cannot synthesize glucose (1). (Glycerol, the alcohol portion of fat can synthesize small amounts of glucose, but the amount is inconsequential.) To obtain these glucogenic (glucose-producing) amino acids the body must catabolize whole proteins from skeletal muscle and eventually other lean organ tissues (1).

Catabolic Factors - Illness

During periods of infection or illness, the immune system must produce immune response proteins quickly. Amino acids from muscle protein catabolism are utilized to form the necessary molecules; hence, muscle tissue is sacrificed (2).

Catabolic Factors - Stress

The body responds to stress with an elaborate series of physiological steps, using the nervous system and hormonal systems to bring about defensive readiness in every body part, i.e. the "fight or flight response" (2). The stress hormone, cortisol is a steroid hormone which is produced in the adrenal cortex of the kidney and is responsible for stimulating gluconeogenesis under stress conditions (2,4). Cortisol also inhibits the use of glucose by most body cells. This process initiates protein catabolism thus freeing amino acids for productions of molecules involved in the stress response (2,4). In terms of muscle, an increase in cortisol is related to an increased rate of protein catabolism and inhibition of skeletal muscle hypertrophy (6). Stress that is chronic will produce a state of constant catabolism - that is, stress can drain the body of its energy reserves and leave it weakened, aged, and vulnerable to disease.

In stress, the heart beats faster, breathing changes, blood pressure increases, serum cholesterol increases, more acid is secreted in the stomach, and muscle proteins are broken down into their constituent amino acids. Some of these amino acids are transported to the liver where glucose is synthesized and released into the bloodstream readying the body to "run or fight". Under chronic psychological stress cells are not able to take up these nutrients in sufficient amounts; these stress products build up in the bloodstream and increase the risk of development of chronic diseases such as diabetes, cardiovascular disease, hypertension, etc. (2).

Catabolic Factors - Caffeine

Early populations found that chewing the seeds, bark, or leaves of certain plants had the effect of easing fatigue, stimulating awareness, and elevating mood (20). It was also found to act as a natural pesticide that paralyzes and kills certain insects feeding on plants (24). Only much later was it found that the effect of caffeine was increased by steeping such plants in hot water.

Caffeine, a stimulant drug, is a xanthine alkaloid compound that acts as a psychoactive stimulant (21,22). It is the world's most widely consumed psychoactive substance, but unlike most other psychoactive substances, it is legal and unregulated in nearly all countries. In North America, 90% of adults consume caffeine daily (21,22).

Caffeine is primarily an antagonist of the central nervous system receptors for the neurotransmitter adenosine. Individuals who regularly consume caffeine adapt to the continual presence of the drug by substantially increasing the number of adenosine receptors in the central nervous system (21,22). This increase in the number of the adenosine receptors makes the body much more sensitive to adenosine in two ways. First, the stimulatory effects of caffeine are substantially reduced, a phenomenon known as a tolerance adaptation. Second, because these adaptive responses to caffeine make individuals much more sensitive to adenosine, a reduction in caffeine intake will effectively increase the normal physiological effects resulting in unwelcome withdrawal symptoms (27,28).

Caffeine content in coffee varies widely depending on the type of coffee bean and the method of preparation used (25,26). Tea is another common source of caffeine but usually contains about half as much caffeine per serving as coffee, depending on the strength of the brew. Certain types of tea, such as black and oolong, contain somewhat more caffeine than most other teas. Tea contains small amounts of theobromine and slightly higher levels of theophylline than coffee (25,26). These chemicals have a similar, but lesser, effect than caffeine (25,26).

Caffeine is also a common ingredient in soft drinks such as cola, originally prepared from kola nuts. Guarana, a prime ingredient in energy drinks, contains large amounts of caffeine with small amounts of theobromine and theophylline (29). Chocolate derived from cocoa contains a small amount of caffeine. The weak stimulant effect of chocolate may be due to a combination of theobromine and theophylline as well as caffeine (27). Chocolate contains too little of these compounds for a reasonable serving to create effects in humans that are on par with coffee (27). A typical 28-gram serving of a milk chocolate bar has about as much caffeine as a cup of *decaffeinated* coffee (25,26).

The precise amount of caffeine necessary to produce effects varies from person to person depending on body size and degree of tolerance to caffeine (30). It takes less than an hour for caffeine to begin affecting the body and a mild dose wears off in three to four hours.

An acute overdose of caffeine, usually in excess of 400 milligrams (more than 3-4 cups of brewed coffee), can result in a state of central nervous system over stimulation called caffeine intoxication (31). The symptoms of caffeine intoxication are not unlike overdoses of other stimulants and may include restlessness, nervousness, excitement, insomnia, flushing of the face, increased urination, gastrointestinal disturbance, muscle twitching, a rambling flow of thought and speech, irritability, irregular or rapid heart beat, and psychomotor agitation. In cases of much larger overdoses mania, depression, lapses in judgment, disorientation, loss of social inhibition, delusions, hallucinations, rhabdomyolysis (the destruction or degeneration of muscle tissue), and death may occur (31).

Beaven and colleagues reported that an 800 mg dose of caffeine was associated with a small improvement in sprint performance, but also attributed to a 52% increase in cortisol during exercise and recovery (82). While the benefits of caffeine as an ergogenic aid have been widely reported, the catabolic effects of increasing cortisol and a decline in testosterone/cortisol ratio when consuming large quantities of caffeine should be considered (82).

The U.S. Food and Drug Administration lists caffeine as a "Multiple Purpose Generally Recognized as Safe Food Substance" (23). However, recently the FDA announced that it will begin to investigate "any and all products with added caffeine." FDA officials indicated they were spurred to take action after the recent introduction of Alert Energy Gum, a new caffeinated gum made by Wrigley (75).

Several studies have confirmed the dangers of caffeine in pregnancy (32). Caffeine crosses the placenta and is poorly metabolized by the fetus which may influence cell development and decrease placental blood flow. Pregnant women who drank the equivalent of at least two cups of coffee daily, or five cans of a soft drink with caffeine, were twice as likely to miscarry as women who consumed no caffeine. Other studies have also reported increased risk of miscarriage with caffeine (32). According to Morgan and colleagues, data suggests that there is not an increased risk of adverse pregnancy, fertility or neurodevelopment outcomes with caffeine consumption of 300 mg/d or less (83). While there is conflicting data on the safety of caffeine consumption during pregnancy, it seems prudent to limit consumption to 300 mg or less a day (83).

<u>Catabolic Factors – Alcohol</u>

Skeletal muscle atrophy is a common feature in alcoholism that affects up to two-thirds of alcohol abusers, and women appear to be particularly susceptible. There is also some evidence to suggest that malnutrition exacerbates the effects of alcohol on muscle (33).

Excessive exposure to alcohol causes damage to skeletal muscle, leading to the development of a specific disease called alcoholic myopathy (33). Predominant features of alcoholic myopathy include difficulties in gait, cramps, impaired muscle strength, and reduced whole body lean tissue mass (33). These pathologies are also accompanied by reductions in amounts of contractile proteins in the muscle, such as myosin, desmin, actin, and troponin (34).

Excessive alcohol ingestion alters the metabolism of most nutrients and includes disorders such as severe hypoglycemia and glucose intolerance, probably due to a inhibition of glucose-stimulated insulin secretion (2).

Excessive alcohol intake also leads to negative nitrogen balance and an increase in protein turnover. It also alters lipid metabolism causing a profound inhibition of lipolysis (34).

Catabolic Factors – Inadequate Rest

Without adequate rest and sleep, muscles do not have an opportunity to recover. Although muscle stimulation occurs during resistance training, muscle hypertrophy occurs afterward during rest (35,36,37). Training at a high intensity too frequently stimulates the central nervous system (CNS) and can result in a hyper-adrenergic state that interferes with sleep patterns (36). To avoid over training, intense frequent training must be met with at least an equal amount of purposeful recovery (35,36,37).

Energy Intake

The first component to meeting nutrient needs is to ensure adequate consumption of calories to offset energy expenditure (47,48,49). An equally important component deals with the timing of nutrients to optimize muscle hypertrophy and fat utilization.

Nutrients

In this section our discussion will concentrate on required intake of each nutrient to meet energy needs of sedentary adults, active adults, and athletes. We will limit our discussion to the Dietary Reference Intakes, the recommendations by the Academy of Nutrition and Dietetics (AND), the International Olympic Committee (IOC) and the American College of Sports Medicine (ACSM). The information presented by AND and ACSM is taken from a joint position statement, authored by AND, Dietitians of Canada (DC), and ACSM (51). Case studies, including calculations of nutrient needs, will be discussed in Chapter 12.

Recommendations (40,41)	Grams/Day	Percentage of Daily Calories
Carbohydrates	130 grams for men and women	45% to 65%
Sugar	NA	Less than or equal to 10%
Total Fats	NA	20 % to 35%
Saturated and Trans Fat	NA	Keep as low as possible
Proteins	.8 grams to 1.8 grams	15 to 20%

Carbohydrates

Adults should get 45 percent to 65 percent of their calories from carbohydrates (40,41). Acceptable ranges for children are similar. The Recommended Dietary Allowances express recommendations in terms of grams per day which includes 130 grams per day for both men and women ages 9 years to 70 years old.

Consensus in the field of sports nutrition has departed from calculating carbohydrate requirements as a percentage to expressing requirements as grams per kilogram (g/kg) body weight per day (BW/day) (52). The g/kg/BW/day requirement ensures that adequate macronutrients are provided in respect to total energy intake (59). Athletes require more energy and macronutrients in proportion to their body weight compared to sedentary individuals. Therefore, according to the ACSM and AND, "expressing energy and macronutrient needs in terms of grams per kilogram body weight is a practical method to document these needs" (51).

Several organizations have determined carbohydrate needs based on grams per kilogram body weight (g/kg/BW/day). The AND and ACSM provide a general recommendation while the IOC provides detailed recommendations (51,52). See the following table for the AND, ACSM and IOC recommendations.

AND, ACSM Carbohydrate Recommendations (51)	IOC Carbohydrate Recommendations (52)
6 to 10 g/kg/BW/day.	3 to 5 g/kg/BW/day, low intensity/skill-based activities;
	5 to 7 g/kg/BW/day, moderate/high intensity (1 hour/day)
	6 to 10 g/kg/BW/day, moderate/high intensity (1 to 3 hours per day)
	4 to 7 g/kg/BW/day for strength athletes
	8 to 12 g/kg/BW/day, extreme commitment (4 to 5 hours per day)

Adequate intake of dietary fiber was discussed in chapter 2. The table below reiterates the recommended dietary intake for fiber (40).

	Men (g/day)	Women (g/day)
Adults under 50 years old	38	25
Adults over 50 years old	30	21

The timing of carbohydrate intake in relation to exercise is also extremely important and will be discussed in the section on Nutrient Timing.

There is controversy about the use of the glycemic index in sports nutrition. Currently, there are no clear recommendations. It has been reported that there is improved metabolism and substrate utilization during exercise when low glycemic index carbohydrate-containing food is ingested with the pre-exercise meal (59). However, these studies have not shown improved exercise performance. Currently, the most important aspects of carbohydrate intake are obtaining daily carbohydrate requirements and ensuring gastrointestinal comfort (50).

<u>Fats</u>

The acceptable macronutrient range for fat intake is 20 to 35% of energy (40). The fat requirements for sedentary individuals and athletes are similar, but slightly higher for athletes. Consuming adequate amounts of fat is required for optimal health, maintenance of energy balance, optimal intake of essential fatty acids and fat-soluble vitamins, as well as replenishing intramuscular triglyceride stores (49,50,51,60). The AND and ACSM recommend that daily fat intake for athletes remains in the range of 20-35% of total energy intake. Intake should not decrease below 20% of total energy intake, as the intake of fat is important for the ingestion of fat-soluble vitamins and essential fatty acids (51). The IOC recommends following a diet that does not contain less than 15-20% of total energy from fat (65).

High-fat diets for athletes are not recommended (51). It is suggested that athletes be cautious of high-fat diets greater than 30% of total energy intake. The recommendation from the AND and ACSM regarding fat intake should suffice for any athlete (51). A high-fat intake can be at the expense of carbohydrate intake and may have negative effects on training and performance.

<u>Proteins</u>

According to the recommended dietary allowance (RDA), the general protein requirement for a sedentary person is 0.8 g/kg BW/day (51,61,63). This requirement appears to suffice for general fitness and can be slightly elevated to 1.0 g/kg BW/day (61).

Dietary protein requirements are elevated with strength, speed, or endurance training because protein supports muscle protein synthesis, reduces muscle protein breakdown, and repairs muscle damage (60,61). Endurance exercise increases leucine oxidation. Therefore, endurance athletes may have slightly higher protein requirements than their sedentary counterparts (61). The AND and ACSM recommend daily protein requirements for strength and endurance athletes of 1.2-1.7 g/kg BW/day.

The IOC protein guidelines for athletes are 1.3-1.8 g/kg BW/day and 1.6-1.7 g/kg BW/day for strength-training athletes (64). Because of the high energy intake of these athletes, these requirements are typically met through diet (64). According to the IOC, protein intake above these guidelines does not have any additional benefit and can promote amino-acid catabolism and protein oxidation (64).

It is recommended by all three organizations that these requirements are reached through diet alone. Additional supplementation is not necessary, especially when the energy intake is optimal (51).

Dietary protein intake should consist of high quality protein. See discussion in Chapter 4 concerning protein quality.

Current research indicates that milk protein, compared to isolated soy protein (with equivalent protein and macronutrient energy) may increase muscle protein synthesis after resistance exercise and may lead to greater muscle hypertrophy (61).

The term "high protein diet" is commonly used to describe a diet with a higher energy intake from protein (84). An issue in discussing the positive and negative effects of a high protein diet is that there is not a standard definition of what constitutes a "high protein diet" (84). In randomized controlled trials reviewed in a meta-analysis by Santesso and colleagues, the percentage of total daily protein intake in high protein diets ranged from 16 - 45 %, with a median of 27% (84). Based on this research, consuming 1.7 grams of protein per body weight (inside ACSM's recommendation) would be considered high especially considering the RDA of 0.8 g/kg BW.

More important than the subjective definition of "high protein" is consuming adequate amounts and types of proteins without sacrificing adequate consumption of carbohydrates and fats. Adverse effects from high protein consumption (higher than recommended) included gastrointestinal problems (constipation, halitosis, and diarrhea), general weakness, headaches, muscle cramps, and rash (84-85). The increase in glomerular filtration rate (a test used to determine how well the kidneys are working) that has been linked to high consumption is likely explained by the increase in renal capillary permeability (86-88). However, this homeostatic response is insufficient in clearing protein by-products, and urea nitrogen levels increase, along with a significant decrease in urinary pH (86,87,89).

Fluids

The Dietary Reference Intake (DRI) for water for males is 3.7 liters (125.1 ounces) per day and 2.7 liters (91.3 ounces) per day for females. Sources include all beverages including water and moisture in foods. High moisture foods include most fruits, and soups.

Micronutrients

The position stand of the AND and ACSM indicate that no vitamin or mineral supplements are necessary for individuals consuming a variety of foods to maintain body weight (51). Supplementation unrelated to exercise include folic acid for women of childbearing age; a multivitamin for dieting individuals; and single-nutrient supplements may be appropriate for specific medical conditions (51). Dietary supplements and the roll of fitness/wellness professionals in regards to supplementation will be discussed in detail in Chapter 9.

Nutrient Timing

In this section, we will discuss the benefits of nutrient timing as it relates to athletic performance, optimizing muscle hypertrophy, and body fat utilization. Again, we will limit our discussion to the recommendations by the Academy of Nutrition and Dietetics (AND), the International Olympic Committee (IOC) and the American College of Sports Medicine (ACSM). The information presented by AND and ACSM is taken from a joint position statement, authored by AND, Dietitians of Canada (DC), and ACSM (51).

Carbohydrates

Carbohydrate recommendations by the ACSM and the IOC are listed in the following table (51,59,69). Recommendations include carbohydrate loading before an event, pre-event requirements, during event requirements and post-event requirements.

	ACSM Carb. Recommendations (51)	**IOC Carb. Recommendations (52)**
Carbohydrate Loading	8 to 10 g/kg/BW/day 1 to 3 days prior to the event	36 to 48 hours of 10 to 12 g/kg/BW per 24 hours
Pre-Event	200 to 300 grams three to four hours prior to event	1 to 4 g/kg/BW consumed one to four hours prior to event (for exercise > 60 minutes.
During Event <45 Minutes		None needed

	ACSM Carb. Recommendations (51)	IOC Carb. Recommendations (52)
During Event – 45 to 75 minutes	.7 grams/kg/BW per hour or 30 to 60 grams for event greater than 60 minutes	Small amounts needed
During Event – one to 2.5 hours		30 to 60 grams per hour
During Event – greater than 2.5 to 3 hours		Up to 90 grams per hour
After Event	1.0 to 1.5 g/kg/BW during first 30 minutes and again every 2 hours for 4 to 6 hours after the event	1.0 to 1.2 g/kg/BW per hour for first 4 hours, then resume daily fuel needs.

Proteins

The AND and ACSM recommend that a moderate amount of protein is added to the pre-event meal. No specific guideline on ingestion of protein before exercise is included in the consensus document (51). The IOC states that although preliminary evidence appears to support increased muscle protein synthesis in response to resistance training when protein is given before exercise, follow-up studies have failed to confirm this finding. Therefore, the current opinion of the IOC is that protein should be ingested after exercise when optimal muscle protein synthesis occurs (64,69).

The AND and ACSM state that evidence of any benefit of additional protein to carbohydrate solutions during exercise is inconclusive. No recommendations are made in this regard in the consensus document (51). The IOC refers to evidence suggesting that ingestion of carbohydrates and essential amino acids is beneficial before and during resistance exercise as it increases substrate availability, exercise performance, stimulates muscle protein synthesis, and decreases muscle damage or tenderness (64,69). However, the IOC agrees with the AND and ACSM and do not provide any recommendations for protein intake before or during a workout (64,69).

There is consensus from the AND, ACSM, and IOC on the beneficial effect of the ingestion of ~20 grams of protein with carbohydrates within 30 minutes post exercise (51,64,69) and this recovery strategy should be achieved through dietary sources. Additional supplementation is not warranted.

After exercise, the AND and ACSM indicate that the primary goals of recovery should be to provide sufficient fluid, electrolytes, energy, and carbohydrates to replace muscle glycogen stores and facilitate recovery (51). The addition of proteins can provide amino acids for the maintenance and repair of muscle protein, but no specific guideline has been provided by the ACSM (51). Current IOC guidelines also advocate the ingestion of protein after exercise, as this is when maximal stimulation of muscle protein synthesis is required (64,69). The IOC recommends that 20-25 grams of high quality protein be included after resistance exercise (61,69). The combination of carbohydrates and protein post exercise is important to restore muscle glycogen and promote protein synthesis (64,69). Protein intake that exceeds this recommended amount does not promote muscle protein synthesis, but can lead to protein oxidation (64). From recent research, the dietary protein form of choice appears to be flavored low fat milk (61,62).

Fluid

Dehydration (water deficit in excess of 2-3% body mass) decreases exercise performance; thus, adequate fluid intake before, during, and after exercise is important for health and optimal performance (51). The goal of drinking is to prevent dehydration from occurring during exercise. After exercise, approximately 16-24 oz (450-675 ml) of fluid should be consumed for every pound (0.5 kg) of body weight lost during exercise (51). The AND and ACSM guidelines for hydration before an event should be initiated several hours before exercise to ensure fluid absorption and normal urine output. Beverages and sodium-containing salted snacks can increase the sensation of thirst and retain fluids. Fluid programs during an event should be customized for each individual, based on body weight measurements before and after exercise. Athletes should aim to prevent greater than 2% body weight loss during exercise. Fluids should contain carbohydrates and electrolytes to maintain fluid balance and exercise performance. After exercise, the ACSM recommends normal meals and beverages. If more rapid recovery is required, 1.5 liters of fluid per kg body weight loss during exercise should be ingested. Beverages and snacks should contain sodium to help with rapid recovery (51,69).

Micronutrients

The AND and ACSM recommend no additional vitamin and mineral supplementation if an athlete obtains sufficient energy from a wide variety of foods (51). Supplementation may be individually prescribed by the attending healthcare professional for certain athletes, such as those restricting energy intake, vegetarians, people who are ill, recovering from injury, or with specific medical conditions (51). Vegetarians may require vitamin B12, iron, calcium, vitamin D, riboflavin, and zinc supplementation (51). Research has indicated that possible supplementation with antioxidants might be warranted. The IOC position supports the AND and ACSM conclusion that energy requirements be met through dietary means, and additional supplementation is not warranted. Toxic levels may impair muscle functioning and reduce training adaptations to exercise (71). The IOC also cautions against the use of single-nutrient, high-dose antioxidant supplements (71).

Meeting Energy Needs

The sum of energy expenditure consists of three components (1):

- Basal Metabolic Rate (BMR)
- Thermic Effect of Food (TEF)
- Physical Activity.

In this section, we will discuss the theory of each of these components. Examples of case studies utilizing these calculations will be discussed in Chapter 12.

Basal Metabolic Rate (BMR)

BMR measurements are typically taken in a darkened room upon waking after 8 hours of sleep, 12 hours of fasting to ensure that the digestive system is inactive, and with the subject resting in a reclined position. Resting Metabolic Rate (RMR) measurements are typically taken under less restricted conditions than BMR and do not require that the subject spend the night sleeping in the test facility prior to testing.

About two-thirds of the energy the average person expends in a day supports the body's basal metabolism. BMR is the rate at which the body expends energy for these activities. Other factors that influence BMR include growth, gender, age, physical activity, body composition and size. BMR is high in people that are still growing (infants, children, adolescents, pregnant and lactating women). Women typically have a lower BMR than men; and BMR decreases with age. The decline in BMR in aging can be attenuated by maintaining muscle mass through resistance training (15). BMR is high in people who are tall and have a large surface area. Similarly the more a person weighs the higher the BMR (1).

Several formulas exist for determining BMR. Fat free mass is a large predictor of BMR and should be included in total energy expenditure calculations.

The Harris-Benedict formula was created in 1919 (43) and due to changing lifestyles tends to overstate calorie needs by 5% (45). This formula tends to be skewed towards both obese and young people (45). Another formula known as the Mifflin-St Jeor equation (44) has been shown to be more accurate than the Harris Benedict equation (45).

Another equation known as the Cunningham equation takes into account lean body mass (39). Fat free mass, i.e., lean body mass, contains the metabolically active compartments of the body and has been shown to be a major predictor of basal metabolism (39). A variation on the basic Mifflin-St Jeor formula developed by Katch-McCardle also takes into account fat free mass or lean body mass.

The Academy of Nutrition and Dietetics (AND) published a comparison of various equations (67). The Mifflin-St Jeor equation is more likely than the other equations to accurately estimate BMR and was the most reliable within 10% of measured in nonobese and obese individuals with the narrowest margin of error. According to AND, older adults and US ethnic minorities were underrepresented; hence, a high level of suspicion exists regarding accuracy (67) for these populations. The table below describes each of the discussed equations.

Mifflin-St Jeor (44)	Katch McCardle (68)	Cunningham (39)
Men 10 x weight (kg) + 6.25 x height (cm) - 5 x age (y) + 5 **Women** 10 x weight (kg) + 6.25 x height (cm) - 5 x age (y) - 161	**Men & Women** 21.6 * Fat Free Mass + 370 Where Fat Free Mass = Weight - (Body Fat Percentage * Weight)	**Men & Women** 500 + 22 (LBM)

Thermic Effect of Food

The second component in total energy expenditure is thermic effect of food. Thermic effect of food is the number of calories the body expends in digesting foods. This amount is dependent on the composition of the diet. If the diet is high in fat (40%) then the estimate is 5% of the BMR; if the diet is higher in carbohydrates or proteins, then the estimate is 10% of the BMR (2).

Physical Activity

The third factor in determining daily energy requirements is physical activity. The amount of energy needed for any activity depends on muscle mass, body weight, and activity. The activity's duration, frequency, and intensity also influence caloric expenditure.

Physical activity is typically estimated by multiplying BMR or RMR by an appropriate activity factor representing light to moderate and very heavy physical activity levels (see below) (54,55).

Estimated Energy Requirements (EER)

The Dietary Reference Intakes (DRI) (40) and the Dietary Guidelines (57) provide energy recommendations for men and women who are slightly active to very active. The Dietary Reference Intakes (DRIs) define the daily requirement for energy as the Estimated Energy Requirement (EER). Estimated Energy Requirement (EER) is the average dietary energy intake that is predicted to maintain energy balance in healthy, normal weight individuals of a defined age, gender, weight, height, and level of physical activity consistent with good health. In children and pregnant and lactating women, the EER includes the needs associated with growth or secretion of milk at rates consistent with good health (54,58). The following table defines the EER equation for men and women (weight is in kilograms and height is in meters).

Men 19 Years and Older
EER = [662 - (9.53 x Age)] + PA X [(15.91 x Weight) + (539.6 x Height)]
Women 19 Years and Older
EER = [354 - (6.91 x Age)] + PA X [(9.36 x Weight) + (726 x Height)]

The EER approach differs from the more commonly used equations previously discussed (i.e. the Harris–Benedict equation) in estimating basal metabolic rate or total energy expenditure (TEE). EER reflects BMR, thermal effect of food and physical activity which includes two important distinguishing components. The EER equation distinguishes between the 'Physical Activity Coefficients (PA)' and the 'Physical Activity Levels (PAL)'. The physical activity coefficients are used in the EER equations to estimate energy requirements and are based on ranges of physical activity levels. The Physical Activity Level is the ratio of total energy expenditure to basal energy expenditure. The Physical Activity Level categories are defined as sedentary (PAL 1.0-1.39), low active (PAL 1.4-1.59), active (PAL 1.6-1.89), and very active (PAL 1.9-2.5). The Physical Activity Coefficients below are used with the EER equations to calculate the amount of calories needed each day (58).

Men > 19 Years (1)	**Women > 19 Years**	**Physical Activity**
Sedentary: 1.0	Sedentary: 1.0	Daily living activities
Low Active: 1.11	Low Active: 1.12	Plus 30-60 min. moderate activity
Active: 1.25	Active: 1.27	Plus >60 min. moderate activity
Very Active: 1.48	Very Active: 1.45	Plus >60 min. moderate activity and 60 min. vigorous activity or 120 min. moderate activity

The EER predictive equation has been shown to be an accurate and applicable method for determining total energy requirements for children; men and women 19 years and older; and pregnant and lactating women (54,57).

In working with children (up to 16 years of age), the EER tends to over estimate total caloric needs for children. Another method from the Institute of Medicine (IOM) utilizes information taken from the IOM Dietary Reference Intakes report, 2002, which utilizes "Reference size," as determined by IOM. Reference size is based on median height and weight for children ages up to age 18 years of age (following table).

Gender	Age (years)	Sedentary [b]	Moderately Active [c]	Active [d]
Child	2-3	1,000	1,000-1,400	1,000-1,400
Female	4-8 9-13 14-18	1,200 1,600 1,800	1,400-1,600 1,600-2,000 2,000	1,400-1,800 1,800-2,200 2,400
Male	4-8 9-13 14-18	1,400 1,800 2,200	1,400-1,600 1,800-2,200 2,400-2,800	1,600-2,000 2,000-2,600 2,800-3,200

In this textbook we will be applying the EER to estimate caloric needs for adults and the IOM Dietary Reference Intakes (based on median height and weight) for determining caloric needs for children.

Body Fat Adjustment

The BMR component of EER does not take into account body composition, which includes the percentages of lean body mass and fat in the body. Muscle burns many more calories than fat. Leaner bodies need more calories than bodies that are less lean. Hence, a person with an above average amount of muscle will have a higher BMR than calculated and therefore a higher EER; and a person with a below average amount of muscle will have a lower BMR than calculated and therefore a lower EER (54,57). The "ideal" lean body mass is based on the ideal body fat percentage of 15% for men and 22% for women. These "factors" will be included in the final EER calculations for adults in Chapter 12.

Summary

Metabolism is defined as 'the sum of all the chemical reactions that go on in living cells'. Chemical energy is stored in food and is the only form of energy humans can use to maintain life. Energy metabolism includes all the reactions by which the body obtains and expends energy from food. Energy is provided in the diet by protein, fat and carbohydrate. With the help of enzymes and coenzymes cells use these nutrients to build complex compounds (anabolism) or break them down to release energy (catabolism). Note: Alcohol contributes calories but is not a nutrient.

The energy in foods is expressed as a unit of heat - the kilocalorie or kilojoule. See Chapter 1 for details concerning the definition of calorie and kilojoule. The potential energy contribution of food is measured in a bomb calorimeter where food is completely combusted to carbon dioxide and water. The conversion of food into energy is an inefficient process with approximately 50% lost as heat and approximately 45% available to the body primarily as adenosine triphosphate (ATP).

Energy production consists of 4 phases: ATP-PC, Glycolysis, TCA cycle, and electron transport chain. Glycolysis occurs in the cytosol of the cell and is defined as the metabolic breakdown of glucose (6 carbons) to pyruvate (3 carbons). In a series of reactions, the 6-carbon glucose is converted to other 6-carbon compounds and then split in half forming two 3-carbon molecules. These 3-carbon molecules are converted to pyruvate through a series of reactions. Hence, the net yield of one glucose molecule is 2 pyruvate molecules. In the process of pyruvate formation, hydrogen atoms with their electrons are released and carried to the electron transport chain. The TCA cycle reactions occur in the inner compartment of the mitochondria. The pathway of acetyl CoA is a one way route, and it cannot be regenerated. When cells need energy, acetyl CoA enters the TCA cycle which begins a series of complicated reactions in which the final compound, oxaloacetate, is also part of the first reaction (circular pathway). Oxaloacetate picks up another acetyl CoA and starts the cycle again. Oxaloacetate is made primarily from pyruvate. Small amounts can be made from amino acids but cannot be made from fat. This fact underscores the importance of carbohydrates in the diet. The electron transport chain consists of a series of proteins that serve as electron carriers. Electrons enter the transport chain from the TCA cycle, glycolysis, and oxidation of fatty acids. As the coenzymes deliver the electrons to the electron transport chain, each carrier receives the electrons and passes them down to the next carrier until the electrons reach oxygen. Oxygen accepts the electrons and combines with hydrogen to form water. As electrons are passed from carrier to carrier, hydrogen atoms are pumped across the outer compartment of the mitochondria and then back to the inner compartment. This process powers the synthesis of ATP.

How much of which fuels are used depends on an interplay among the fuels available from the diet, the intensity of exercise, duration of the exercise and the fitness level of the individual. A quantitative analysis by Bravada, et al.(107 studies and 94 diets) examined the efficacy and safety of low-carbohydrate diets. Their conclusion is that there is insufficient evidence to make recommendations for or against the use of low-carbohydrate diets.

The most important form of rest is sleep, which is essentially just a heightened anabolic state, meaning a time during which larger molecules and tissue are constructed. It is complicit in the rejuvenation of the immune, nervous and muscular systems because protein metabolism occurs at a more proficient rate.

When muscles contract, they respond immediately without metabolizing fat or carbohydrate for energy. In the first fraction of a second, muscles use ATP and Phosphocreatine (PC). Immediately after the onset of muscle contraction, before muscle ATP pools are depleted, a muscle enzyme begins to break down PC (phosphocreatine). Supplies of ATP and PC last for approximately 30 seconds. To meet prolonged needs, the body must generate ATP from glucose, fatty acids, and amino acids (aerobic metabolism), and this process requires oxygen. During aerobic exercise the muscles use a combination of energy nutrients for energy. During anaerobic exercise (without oxygen), the body must utilize glucose for energy (since utilization of fat requires oxygen) and lactic acid is produced as a byproduct. Muscles never use just one single fuel. Energy utilization is always a combination of glucose and fat (or fat by-products). How long glycogen stores last depends on the duration of the exercise. During the first few minutes of exercise the major source of fuel is glycogen since oxygen is not yet available to the muscle cells. As exercise continues (10 to 20 minutes), more oxygen becomes available and greater fat utilization occurs.

Another critical component to extending glycogen stores is an individual's fitness level. More oxygen is delivered to muscles cells of aerobically fit individuals. This additional oxygen allows this "fit" individual to utilize more fat in conjunction with glucose, thereby extending glycogen stores. Conditioned muscles also rely less on glycogen and more on fat so that glycogen breakdown occurs more slowly in these trained athletes. These individuals utilize a greater percentage of fat even at rest.

Muscle mass plays a role in energy nutrient utilization. Muscle hypertrophy is a scientific term for the growth and increase of the size of muscle cells. Muscle hypertrophy is dependent on several factors such as genetics, gender, age and nutrition. Catabolic factors that can lead to muscle catabolism include fasting, starvation, illness, stress, caffeine, alcohol, and inadequate amount of rest.

The AND and ACSM recommend that "athletes need to consume adequate energy during periods of high intensity and/or long duration training to maintain body weight and health and to maximize training effects". The AND and ACSM recommend that energy requirements are calculated using either the Dietary Reference Intakes (DRIs) or prediction equations, such as the Cunningham or Harris-Benedict equations, where the basal or resting metabolic rate is calculated using a physical activity factor of 1.8 to 2.3 depending on the type, duration, and intensity of exercise.

The field of sport nutrition has departed from calculating carbohydrate requirements as a percentage of the total energy requirement to instead focus on determining requirements expressed as grams per kilogram (g/kg) body weight (BW).

There is controversy about the use of the glycemic index in sport nutrition. Currently, there are no clear recommendations for athletes. It has been reported that there is improved metabolism and substrate utilization during exercise when low glycemic index carbohydrate-containing food is ingested with the pre-exercise meal. However, these studies have not shown improved exercise performance.

The fat requirements of athletes are slightly higher than those in non-athletes. It is important to consume adequate amounts of fat to ensure optimal health, maintenance of energy balance, optimal intake of essential fatty acids and fat-soluble vitamins, as well as to replenish intramuscular triglyceride stores.

Dietary protein requirements are elevated with strength, speed or endurance training. Energy intake, exercise intensity and duration, ambient temperature, gender, and age also influence protein requirements. There are increased requirements in the case of strength or resistance training because protein supports muscle protein synthesis, reduces muscle protein breakdown and repairs muscle damage. Endurance exercise increases leucine oxidation. Therefore, endurance athletes may have slightly higher protein requirements than their sedentary counterpart. The AND and ACSM recommend daily protein requirements for strength and endurance athletes of 1.2-1.7 g/kg BW/day. IOC general protein guidelines for athletes are 1.3-1.8 g/kg BW/day and 1.6-1.7 g/kg BW/day for strength-training athletes. Dietary protein intake should consist of high quality protein. Protein quality can be measured by the Protein Digestibility-Corrected Amino Acid Score (PDCAAS) where a score of close or equal to 1 indicates protein of high quality. Dietary protein sources with a similar score include, but are not limited to, milk (casein and whey), egg and meat products. Milk protein, compared to isolated soy protein (with equivalent protein and macronutrient energy) has been shown to increase muscle protein synthesis after resistance exercise and leads to greater muscle hypertrophy.

The AND and ACSM indicate that no additional vitamin and mineral supplementation is needed if an athlete obtains sufficient energy from a wide variety of foods (51). The AND and ACSM allow for micronutrient supplementation that is unrelated to exercise performance, such as folic acid supplementation during pregnancy (51). Supplementation may be individually prescribed by the attending healthcare professional for certain athletes, such as those restricting energy intake, vegetarians, people who are ill, recovering from injury, or with specific medical conditions (51). Vegetarians may require vitamin B12, iron, calcium, vitamin D, riboflavin, and zinc supplementation (51). Research has indicated that possible supplementation with antioxidants might be warranted. However, the IOC position stand supports the AND and ACSM conclusion that energy requirements be met through dietary means, and additional supplementation should not be warranted. Also, toxic levels may impair muscle functioning and reduce training adaptations to exercise (71). IOC also cautions against the use of single-nutrient, high-dose antioxidant supplements (71).

The sum of energy expenditure consists of three components: Basal metabolic rate (BMR), thermic effect of food; and physical activity. About two-thirds of the energy the average person expends in a day supports the body's basal metabolism. BMR is the rate at which the body expends energy for these activities. Other factors include growth, gender, age, physical activity, and body composition and size. The second component in total energy expenditure is thermic effect of food. Thermic effect of food is the number of calories the body expends in digesting foods. This amount is dependent on the composition of the diet. If the diet is high in fat (40%), then the estimate is 5% of the BMR; if the diet is higher in carbohydrates or proteins, then the estimate is 10% of the BMR. The third factor in determining daily energy requirements is physical activity. The amount of energy needed for any activity depends on muscle mass, body weight, and activity. The activity's duration, frequency, and intensity also influence caloric expenditure. The BMR component of EER does not take into account body composition, which includes the percentages of muscle and fat in the body. Muscle burns calories, while fat does not. Leaner bodies need more calories than bodies that are less lean. Hence, a person with an above average amount of muscle will have a higher BMR than calculated and therefore a higher EER; and a person with a below average amount of muscle will have a lower BMR than calculated and therefore a lower EER (54,57). The "ideal" lean body mass is based on the ideal body fat percentage of 15% for men and 22% for women.

Chapter 5 Sample Test

1. What are the four phases of energy production? Provide details concerning each phase.
2. What are the factors involved in nutrient utilization?
3. Discuss how to meet energy nutrient needs through adequate caloric intake.
4. What is the position of the AND, ACSM, and the IOC on nutrient timing before an event, pre-event, during the event and post-event?
5. What is the position of the AND, ACSM, and the IOC on adequate fluid intake?
6. What is the position of the AND, ACSM, and the IOC in micronutrient (vitamin and mineral) supplementation?
7. Define the three components of energy expenditure, and provide details of each component.

References

1. Whitney, E & Rolfes S. (2013). *Understanding Nutrition,*13th ed. Belmont, C A : Wadsworth, Cengage Learnin (198-251).
2. Ross, C, (Shils) et al. (2012). *Modern Nutrition in Health & Disease, 11th ed.* Philadelphia PA: Lipincott Wilillians & Wilikins (88-101, 1540-1562).
3. Lehninger, A. (2013). *Principles of Biochemistry, 6th ed* NY: W H Freeman and Company (587-627).
4. Guyton, A. (2012). *Textbook of Medical Physiology, 11th ed.* Phil: W.B. Saunders Co. (9-22).
5. Bravata, DM. Sanders L., et al. (2003). Efficacy and safety of low-carbohydrate diets: A systematic review. *JAMA.* 289(14):1837-1850. doi:10.1001/jama.289.14.1837.
6. Hernandez RJ. Kravitz L. The mystery of skeletal muscle hypertrophy. http://www.unm.edu/~lkravitz/Article%20folder/hypertrophy.html (accessed 06/09/2013).
7. Stein K. (2000). High-protein, low-carbohydrate diets: do they work? *J Am Diet Assoc.*2000;100:760-761.
8. St Jeor ST, Howard BV, et al. (2001). Dietary protein and weight reduction: a statement for Healthcare Professionals from the Nutrition Committee of the Council on Nutrition, Physical Activity, and Metabolism of the American Heart Association. *Circulation.*104:1869-1874.
9. American Heart Association Statement on High-Protein, Low-Carbohydrate Diet Study. (2002). Presented at: Scientific Sessions for the American Heart Association; November 19, 2002; Chicago, Ill. Available at: *http://www.americanheart.org/presenter.jhtml?identifier=3006728.*
10. American Heart Association. (2003). High-protein diets: AHA recommendation. Available at: *http://www.americanheart.org/presenter.jhtml?identifier=11234.*
11. Takahashi T. Kippid DM. Daughaday WH. (1968). Growth hormone secretion during sleep. J *Clin Invest.* 2079–2090.
12. Cauter V. EKerkhofs M. Caufriez A. Van Onderbergen A. Thorner MO. Copinschi G. (1992). *J Clin Endocrinol Metab.* Jun; 74(6):1441-50.
13. Swain D. (2006). Moderate- or Vigorous-Intensity Exercise: What Should We Prescribe? *ACSM'S Health & Fitness Journal.* Volume 10 - Issue 5 -7-11 doi: 10.1249/01.FIT.0000244891.55243.
14. Westcott WL, Winett RA, Annessi JJ, et al. (2009). Prescribing physical activity: Applying the ACSM protocols for exercise type, intensity, and duration across 3 training frequencies. *Phys Sports Med.* 2: 51–8.
15. Evans, W, IH Rosenberg. (1991). *Biomarkers.* NY: Simon & Schuster.
16. Williams MH. (1983). *Ergogenic Aids in Sports.* Champaign Il: Human Kinetics Publishers.
17. Nieman D. (1991). *Fitness and Sports Medicine.* Palo Alto: Bull Publishing Co.
18. Miller AE. MacDougall JD. Tarnopolsky MA. (1993). Gender differences in strength and muscle fiber characteristics. Eur J *Appl Physiol Occup Physiol.* 1993;66(3):254-62.
19. Fredholm B.B. (1995). Adenosine, adenosine receptors and the actions of caffeine. *Pharmacol. Toxicol.* 76:93–101. [PubMed]
20. Fredholm B.B, et al. (1999).Actions of caffeine in the brain with special reference to factors that contribute to its widespread use. *Pharmacol.* 51:83–133. [PubMed]
21. Griffith R.R. Woodson P.P. (1988). Reinforcing effects of caffeine in humans. *J. Pharmacol. Exp. Ther.* 246:21–29. [PubMed]
22. Fredholm BB, et al. (1999). Actions of caffeine in the brain with special reference to factors that contribute to its widespread use. *Pharmacol Rev.* Mar;51(1):83-133.
23. Database of Select Committee on GRAS Substances (SCOGS) Reviews. U.S. Food and Drug Administration. (1978). Report: 89:58-08-02. http://www.accessdata.fda.gov/scripts/fcn/fcnDetailNavigation.cfm?rpt=scogslisting&id=42.

24. G. Hollingsworth. (2002). Hawaii Department of Agriculture (HDOA) pesticide label (and attachments) for application of caffeine to control Caribbean frogs (Eleutherodactylus coqui and Eleutherodactylus planirostris) in the State of Hawaii. *Nature*. Vol 417:915.
25. Caffeine Content of Food & Drugs. (2012). Center for Science in the Public Interest. http://www.cspinet.org/new/cafchart.htm.
26. Juliano LM. & Griffiths R.R. (2005). "Caffeine." In Lowinson, J.H., Ruiz, P., Millman, R.B., Langrod, J.G. (Eds.). Substance Abuse: A Comprehensive Textbook, Fourth Edition. (pp 403-421). Baltimore: Lippincott, Williams, & Wilkins.
27. Rhoads DE. Huggler Al. Rhoads LJ. (2011). Acute and adaptive motor responses to caffeine in adolescent and adult rats. *Pharmacol Biochem Behav.* 99(1):81-6. doi: 10.1016/ j.pbb.2011.04.001.REVIEW.
28. Yang A. Palmer AA. De Wit. H. (2010). Genetics of caffeine consumption and responses to caffeine. *Psychopharmacology.* 211:245.
29. Bempong DK. Houghton PJ. Steadman K (1993). The xanthine content of guarana and its preparations. *Int. J. Pharmacog.* 31 (3): 175–81.
30. Smith, A (2002). "Effects of caffeine on human behavior". *Food and Chemical Toxicology.* 40 (9): 1243–55.
31. Caffeine Intoxication: Diagnostic criteria for 305.90 Caffeine Intoxication. Psychiatry Online. DSM-IV-TR. *Diagnostic and Statistical Manual of Mental Disorders.* http://dsm.psychiatryonline.org/content.aspx?bookid=22§ionid=1889660.
32. Weng X, et al. (2008). "Maternal caffeine consumption during pregnancy and the risk of miscarriage: a prospective cohort study" *Am J Obstet Gynecol.* DOI: 10.1016/ j.ajog.2007.10.803.
33. Pacy PJ, et al. (1991). The Effect of Chronic Alcohol Ingestion on Whole Body and Muscle Protein Synthesis: A stable Isotope Study. *Alcohol and Alcoholism. Vol 26, Issue 5-6.*505-513.
34. Pruznak AM, et al. (2013). Direct Central Nervous System Effect of Alcohol Alters Synthesis and Degradation of Skeletal Muscle Protein *Alcohol and Alcoholism. 48(2): 138-145 first published online October 18, 201.*
35. Driver HS, et al. (1988). Submaximal exercise effects on sleep patters in young women. before and after aerobic training program. *Acta Physiologica Scandinavica.* 133:8-13.
36. Driver, HS, et al. (1994). Prolonged endurance exercise and sleep disruption. *Medicine and Science in Sports and Exercise.* 26:903-907.
37. Takahashi Y. et al. (1968). Growth hormone secretion during sleep. *J Clin Invest.* 47(9): 2079–2090. doi: 10.1172/JCI105893 PMCID: PMC297368
38. Donahoo W. Levine J. Melanson E. (2004). Variability in energy expenditure and its components. *Curr Opin Clin Nutr Metab.* 7:599-605.
39. Cunningham JJ. (1980). A reanalysis of the factors influencing basal metabolic rate in normal adults. *Am J Clin Nutr.* 33:2372-4.
40. Otten J. Hellwig J. Meyers L, ed. (2006). *Dietary Reference Intakes: The Essential Guide to Nutrient Requirements.* Washington (DC): The National Academies Press.
41. Institute of Medicine. (2005). *Dietary Reference Intakes for Energy, Carbohydrate, Fiber, Fat, Fatty Acids, Cholesterol, Protein, and Amino Acids.* Washington (DC): The National Academies Press.
42. United States Department of Health and Human Services and United States Department of Agriculture. (2005). *Dietary Guidelines for Americans.* Washington (DC): US Government Printing Office. (http://www.health.gov/dietaryguidelines/dga2005/report/HTML/D3_Disccalories.htm)
43. Harris J. Benedict F. (1919). *A Biometric Study of Basal Metabolism in Man.* Philadelphia (PA): F.B. Lippincott Co.
44. Mifflin, MD. St Jeor ST, et al. (2005). A new predictive equation for resting energy

expenditure in healthy individuals. *J Am Diet Assoc.* 51:241-247.

45. Frankenfield DC, et al. (1998). The Harris-Benedict studies of human basal metabolism: history and limitations. *J Am Diet Assoc.* 1998;98:439-445
46. Schuit AJ. Schouten EG, Klaas R. Westerterp W. Saris HM. (1997). Validity of the physical activity scale for the elderly (PASE): According to energy expenditure assessed by the doubly labeled water method. *Journal of Clinical Epidemiology.* Volume 50, Issue 5, Pages 541-546.
47. Leutholtz B. Kreider R. Exercise and Sport Nutrition. In *Nutritional Health.* Edited by Wilson T, Temple N. Totowa, NJ: Humana Press; 2001:207-39.
48. Sherman WM, Jacobs KA. Leenders N. (1998). Carbohydrate metabolism during endurance exercise. In *Overtraining in Sport.* Edited by Kreider RB, Fry AC, O'Toole ML. Champaign: Human Kinetics Publishers; 289-308.
49. Kreider RB, Fry AC, O'Toole ML (1998). *Overtraining in Sport.* Champaign: Human Kinetics Publishers.
50. Kreider RB. (1991). Physiological considerations of ultraendurance performance. *Int J Sport Nutr.* 1(1):3-27. PubMed Abstract.
51. Rodriquez NR. DiMarco NM. Langley S. (2009). Position of the American Dietetic Association, Dietitians of Canada, and the American College of Sports Medicine: Nutrition and athletic performance. *J Am Diet Assoc.* 109(3):509-527 [homepage on the Internet]. c2012. Available from: http://journals.lww.com/acsm-msse/Fulltext/2009/03000/ Nutrition_and_Athletic_Performance.27.aspxPrev Chronic Dis. 2006 October; 3(4): A129. Published online 2006 September 15. PMCID: PMC1784117.
52. International Olympic Committee (IOC) consensus statement on sports nutrition 2010. J Sports Sci. 2011;29(SI):S3-S4.
53. Potgieter S. (2013). Sport nutrition: A review of the latest guidelines for exercise and sport nutrition from the American College of Sport Nutrition, the International Olympic Committee and theInternational Society for Sports Nutrition. *S Afr J Clin Nutr.* 26(1):6-16
54. Gerrior S. WenYen J. Basiotis P. (2006). An Easy Approach to Calculating Estimated Energy Requirements. Prev Chronic Dis. 2006 October; 3(4): A129. http://www.ncbi.nlm.nih.gov/pmc/articles/PMC1784117/
55. Gabel KA. (2006). Special nutritional concerns for the female athlete. *Curr Sports Med Rep.* 5:187-91
56. Interactive DRI for Healthcare Professionals. USDA National Agricultural Library. EER online calculator: http://fnic.nal.usda.gov/fnic/interactiveDRI/. (Accessed 06/08/2013).
57. GlobalRPH. Insittute of Medicine - EER Requirements. EER online calculators: http://www.globalrph.com/estimated_energy_requirement.htm. (Accessed 06/08/2013).
58. Dietary Reference Intakes For Energy, Carbohydrate, Fiber, Fat, Fatty Acids,Cholesterol, Protein,and Amino Acids, Institute of Medicine of the National Academies, 2002 and 2005, THE NATIONAL ACADEMIES PRESS 500 Fifth Street, N.W. Washington, DC 20001.
59. Burke LM. Hawley JA. Wong SH, et al. (2011). Carbohydrates for training and competition. *J Sports Sci.* 29(S1):S17-S27.
60. Kreider RB. Wilborn CD. Taylor L, et al. (2010). ISSN exercise and sport nutrition review: research and recommendations. *Int J Soc Sports Nutr.* 7:7 [homepage on the Internet]. c2012. Available from: http://www.biomedcentral.com/content/pdf/1550-2783-7-7.pdf.
61. Phillips SM. Van Loon LJC. (2011). Dietary protein for athletes: from requirements to optimum adaptation. *J Sport Sci.* 29 Suppl 1):S29-S38.
62. Wilkinson SB, Tarnopolsky MA, Macdonald MJ, Macdonald JR, Armstrong D, Phillips SM. (2007). Consumption of fluid skim milk promotes greater muscle protein accretion after resistance exercise than does consumption of isonitrogenous and isoenergetic soy-protein beverage. *Am J Clin Nutr.* 85 (4): 1031–40.
63. Nutrition Information Centre, Stellenbosch University.(2003). Dietary reference intakes. Washington: The National Academies Press; 2003.

64. Slater G. Phillips SM. (2011). Nutrition guidelines for strength sports: sprinting, weightlifting, throwing events, and bodybuilding. *J Sports Sci.* 29(S1):S67-S77.
65. Sundgot-Borgen J. Garthe I. (2011). Elite athletes in aesthetic and Olympic weight-class sports and the challenge of body weight and body composition. *J Sports Sci.* 29(S1):S101-S114.
66. Kerksick C. Harvey T. Stout J, et al. (2008). International Society of Sports Nutrition position stand: nutrient timing. Int J Soc Sports Nutr. 5:17 [homepage on the Internet]. c2012. Available from: http://www.jissn.com/content/pdf/1550-2783-5-17.pdf.
67. Frankenfield D. et al. (2005). Comparison of predictive equations for resting metabolic rate in healthy nonobese and obese adults: a systematic review. *J Am Diet Assoc.* 105(5):775-89.
68. McArdle, WD. Katch. Katch VL. (2006) Essentials of Exercise Physiology 3rd ed. Baltimore: Lippincott Williams & Wilkins.
69. Sawka M, Burke L, Eicher R, et al. (2007). Exercise and fluid replacement. *Med Sci Sports Exerc.* 39(2):377-390.[homepage on the Internet]. c2012. Available from: http://www.acsm-msse.org.
70. Shirreffs SM, Sawka MN. (2011). Fluid and electrolyte needs for training, competition, and recovery. *J Sports Sci.* 29(S1):S39-S46.
71. Powers S, Nelson WB, Larson-Meyer E. (2011). Antioxidant and Vitamin D supplements for athletes: sense or nonsense? *J Sports Sci.* 29(S1):S47-S55.
72. Jackson, AS; Stanforth, PR; Gagnon, J; Rankinen, T; Leon, AS; Rao, DC; Skinner, JS; Bouchard, C et al. (2002). "True". *International Journal of Obesity* 26 (6): 789–96.
73. ACE (2009) What are the guidelines for percentage of body fat loss? American Council on Exercise (ACE). Ask the Expert Blog. December 2, 2009.
74. Friedl, KE. Moore RJ. Martinez-Lopez LE. Vogel JA. Askew EW. Marchitelli LJ. Hoyt RW. Gordon CC (1994). "Lower limit of body fat in healthy active men.". *J Appl Physiol.* 77(2):933-40.
75. FDA to Investigate Added Caffeine. U.S. Food and Drug Administration. (May 3, 2013). http://www.fda.gov/ForConsumers/ConsumerUpdates/ucm350570.htm.
76. Ciclitiria P.J.(2003).Recent advances in coeliac disease". *Clinical Medicine.* 3(2)166-169.
77. DASH Diet: www.nhlbi.nih.gov/hbp/consumer/ hearthealth/ eating.html; www.dashbwh.harvard.edu/.
78. American College of Sports Medicine's Guidelines for Exercise Testing and Prescription. (2006). American College of Sports Medicine. Philadelphia: Lipicott Williams & Wilkins.
79. Hewyard, VH. (2006). Advanced Fitness Assessment and Exercise Prescription. Champaign, IL: Human Kinetics.
80. Powers SK & Howley ET. (2007). *Exercise Physiology: Theory and Application to Fitness and Performance*, 6th Ed. New York, NY: McGraw-Hill Companies.
81. Brooks G. et al. (1971). Temperature, skeletal muscle, mitochondrial functions and oxygen debt. *American Journal of Physiology* 220: 1053-59.
82. Beaven MC, et al. (2008). Dose effect of caffeine on testosterone and cortisol responses to resistance exercise. *Inter J of Spt Nut and Exer Meta* 18: 131-141.
83. Morgan S. Koren G.Bozzo P. (2013). Is caffeine consumption safe during pregnancy? *Can Fam Physician.* 59(4):361-362. http://www.ncbi.nlm.nih.gov/pmc/articles/PMC3625078/.
84. Santesso N, et al. (2012). Effects of higher versus lower protein diets on health outcomes: a systemic review and meta anaylsis. *European J of Clinical Nut.* 1-9.
85. Yancy WS Jr, et al. (2004). A low carbohydrate, ketogenic diet versus a low-fat diet to treat obesity and hyperlipdemia: a randomized, controlled trial. *Ann Intern Med* 140: 769-777.
86. Denke MA. (2001). Metabolic effects of high-protein, low carbohydrate diets. *The Amer J of Cardio* 88: 59-61.
87. Schuette SA. (1980). Studies of the mechanism of protein induced hypercalciuria in older men and women. *J Nutr* 110: 305-315.
88. Kerstetter JE. (1998). Dietary protein affects intestinal calcium absorption. *Am J Clin Nutr* 68:

859-865.

89. Fellstorm B. (1983). The influence of a high dietary intake of purine-rich animal protein on urinary urate excretion and supersaturation in renal stone disease. *Clin Sci* 64: 399-405.

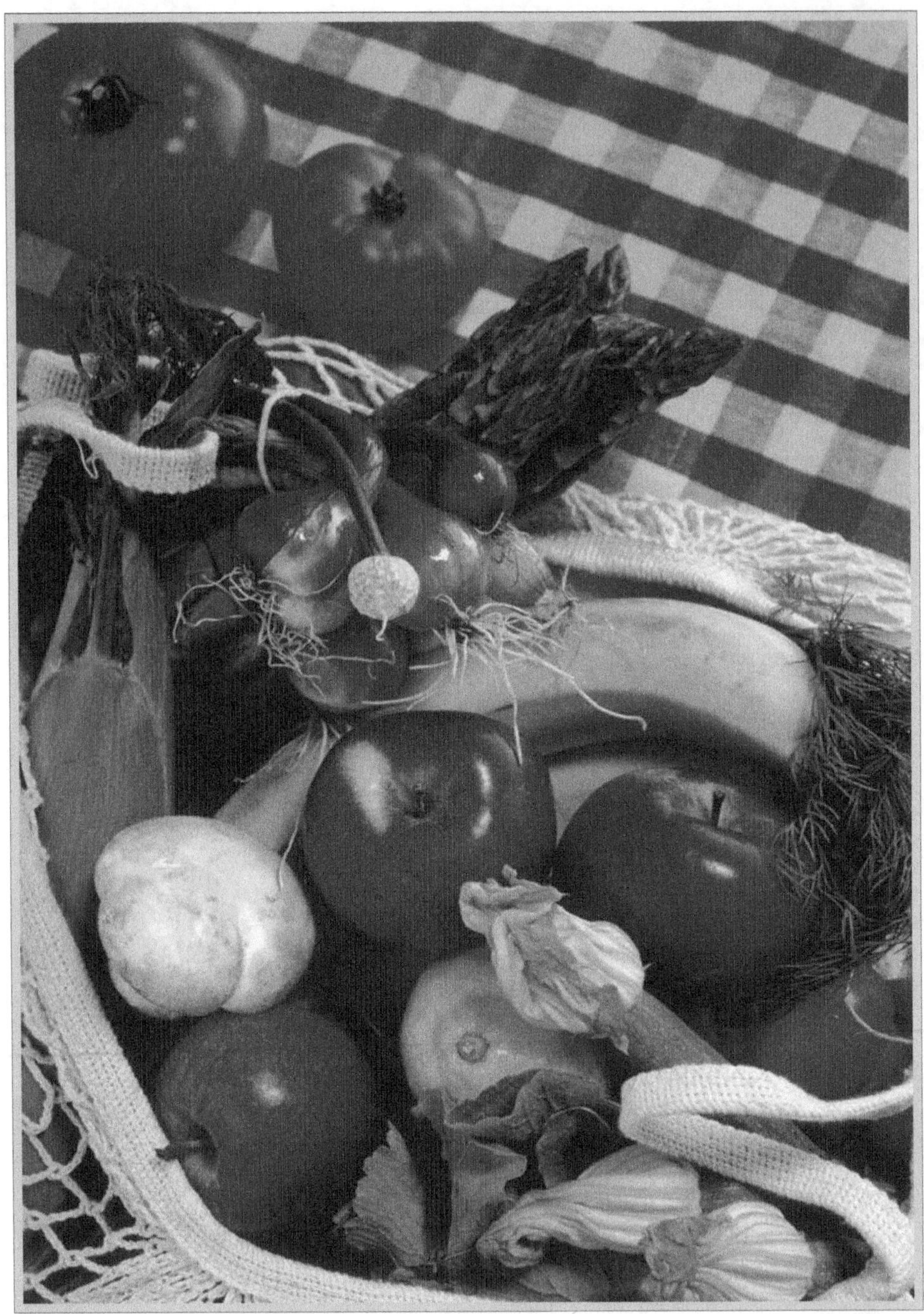

Chapter 6 - Nutrition and Disease

The history of nutrition and health research spans more than five decades. Research in population-based epidemiological studies has helped to clarify some of the roles of diet in preventing and controlling death and disease relating to dietary and lifestyle changes. In this chapter we will discuss some of the major chronic modifiable diseases.

Objectives

After reading and studying this session you should be able to:

1. Discuss the factors associated with all types of diabetes including diagnoses and prevention.
2. Describe the association between diabetes and exercise.
3. Discuss the factors involved in cardiovascular disease, including cholesterol, cholesterol lowering medications, L-carnitine, homocysteine, high sensitivity reactive protein, and coronary calcium scan.
4. Describe the association between cardiovascular disease and exercise.
5. Define and discuss hypertension, including diets associated with reducing hypertension.
6. Describe the association between hypertension and exercise.
7. Discuss factors involved with stroke.
8. Describe the association between stroke and exercise.
9. Discuss the factors involved in cancer risk.
10. Describe the association between cancer and exercise.
11. Define and discuss gastrointestinal disorders.
12. Discuss factors involved with chronic kidney disease.

Introduction

The Food and Agricultural Group of the United Nations (FAO) and World Health Organization met in 2002 and undertook the task of reviewing the scientific data on diet, nutrition, and the prevention of chronic diseases (1). Their findings were not surprising. While many of the diseases associated with age and gender are modifiable, the growing epidemic of chronic diseases is related to diet and lifestyle. Population based studies indicate increased consumption of energy-dense diets high in fat, particularly saturated fat, and low in unrefined carbohydrates. These patterns were found to be in combination with a decline in energy expenditure associated with a sedentary lifestyle. Because of these changes in dietary and lifestyle patterns, chronic diseases — including diabetes mellitus, cardiovascular disease, hypertension and stroke, kidney failure, and certain types of cancer, are becoming increasingly significant causes of death and disease both in developing and newly developed countries, placing additional burdens on already overtaxed national health budgets. What is apparent at the global level is that great changes have swept the entire world since the second half of the twentieth century. In order to achieve the best results in preventing these chronic diseases, national policies must fully recognize the essential role of diet, nutrition, and physical activity.

It has been calculated that, in 2001, chronic diseases contributed approximately 60% of the 56.5 million total reported deaths in the world and approximately 46% of the global burden of disease (125). The proportion of this burden is expected to increase to 57% by 2020 (1). Statistics from the CDC (136) indicate that 7 out of 10 deaths among Americans each year are from chronic diseases. Heart disease, cancer and stroke account for more than 50% of all deaths each year (131). One in every 3 adults is obese (132) and almost 1 in 5 youth between the ages of 6 and 19 is obese (BMI ≥ 95th percentile of the CDC growth chart) (133). Arthritis is the most common cause of disability, with nearly 19 million Americans reporting activity limitations (137). Diabetes continues to be the leading cause of kidney failure, nontraumatic lower-extremity amputations, and blindness among adults, aged 20-74 (134). Excessive alcohol consumption is the third leading preventable cause of death in the U.S., behind diet and physical activity and tobacco (135).

This chapter will concentrate on discussion of some of the major chronic modifiable diseases, including diabetes, cardiovascular disease, hypertension, stroke, cancer, gastrointestinal disorders, and kidney disease, with the goal of educating health and fitness/wellness professionals concerning these modifiable lifestyle changes. All health professionals should be well aware of their scope of practice and refer individuals with symptoms of any of the diseases discussed to the appropriate health care professional.

Diabetes

Diabetes is widely recognized as one of the leading causes of death and disability in the United States. It is the leading cause of kidney failure, non-traumatic lower-limb amputations, and new cases of blindness among adults in the United States. It is a major cause of heart disease and stroke and is the seventh leading cause of death in the United States (2,3,4). According to the 2011 National Diabetes Foundation, 79 million U.S adults 20 years and older had prediabetes, fasting blood glucose levels slightly elevated between 100-125mg/dL (138). Eleven percent of this population has diabetes, which is diagnosed as a fasting blood sugar levels greater than 125mg/dL or A1c greater than or equal to 6.5%. A1c test measures the average blood sugar levels for the past two to three months. Increases in diabetes among US adults continue in both males and females, all ages, all races, all educational levels, and all smoking levels (2,3,4).

Diabetes is a disease in which the body does not produce or properly use insulin. It is associated with long-term complications that affect almost every part of the body (1). The disease often leads to blood vessel and nerve damage which can cause blindness, heart disease, stroke, kidney failure, and amputations. Uncontrolled diabetes can complicate pregnancy, and birth defects are more common in babies born to women with diabetes (1).

In the first stage of diabetes, cells require energy because glucose cannot enter insulin dependent cells. The build up of sugar in the blood can cause an increase in urination by signaling the kidneys to release glucose through the urine, which can lead to large amounts of fluid losses causing dehydration (10). When a person with type 2 diabetes becomes severely dehydrated and is not able to drink enough fluids to make up for the fluid losses, they may develop life-threatening complications (10). As the disease progresses, the high glucose levels in the blood damage red blood cells, nerve cells, cells involved in vision, kidney cells, and heart cells.

The three main types of diabetes include: type 1 diabetes; type 2 diabetes; and gestational diabetes (10).

Type 1 Diabetes

Type 1 diabetes is an autoimmune disease usually diagnosed in children and young adults, and was previously known as juvenile diabetes (10). Type 1 diabetes accounts for about 5 to 10 percent of diagnosed diabetes in the United States (10). It develops most often in children and young adults, but can appear at any age. In type 1 diabetes, the immune system attacks the insulin-producing beta cells in the pancreas and destroys them. The pancreas then produces little or no insulin, thus requiring administration of exogenous insulin several times per day or via an insulin pump (10).

Symptoms of type 1 diabetes usually develop over a short period, although beta cell destruction can begin years earlier. Symptoms include increased thirst and urination, constant hunger, weight loss, blurred vision, and extreme fatigue. If not diagnosed and treated with insulin, a person with type 1 diabetes can lapse into a life-threatening diabetic coma, also known as diabetic ketoacidosis.

At present, scientists do not know exactly what causes the body's immune system to attack the beta cells, but they believe that autoimmune, genetic, environmental factors, and possibly viruses are involved (10).

Type 2 Diabetes

The most common form of diabetes is type 2 diabetes which includes 90 to 95 percent of people with diabetes (10). In type 2 diabetes, either the body does not produce enough insulin or the cells ignore the insulin. This form of diabetes is associated with: older individuals; obese individuals; history of diabetes in the family; previous history of gestational diabetes; physical inactivity; and ethnicity. About 80 percent of people with type 2 diabetes are overweight (2,3,4). When diabetes strikes during childhood, it is routinely assumed to be type 1, or juvenile-onset diabetes. As decreased physical activity and obesity levels increase in children and adolescents, type 2 diabetes (formerly known as adult-onset diabetes) has been reported among U.S. children and adolescents with increasing frequency. Also, studies conducted in Europe showed an increase in the frequency of type 2 diabetes, especially in young children. It is unclear whether the frequency of type 1 diabetes is also increasing among U.S. Youth (12). According to a study by the CDC, it is projected that the number of U.S. youth with type 2 diabetes will increase by 49 percent over the next 40 years (139).

When type 2 diabetes is diagnosed, the pancreas is usually producing enough insulin, but for unknown reasons, the body cannot use the insulin effectively, a condition called insulin resistance (10). After several years, insulin production decreases. The result is the same as for type 1 diabetes—glucose builds up in the blood and the body cannot make efficient use of its main source of fuel. The symptoms of type 2 diabetes develop gradually. Their onset is not as sudden as in type 1 diabetes. Symptoms may include fatigue or nausea, frequent urination, unusual thirst, weight loss, blurred vision, frequent infections, and slow healing of wounds or sores (10).

Gestational Diabetes

Gestational diabetes develops only during pregnancy (10). Like type 2 diabetes, it occurs more often in African Americans, American Indians, Hispanic Americans, and among women with a family history of diabetes. Women who have had gestational diabetes have a 20 to 50 percent chance of developing type 2 diabetes within 5 to 10 years (10). Gestational diabetes is diagnosed based on plasma glucose values measured during the Oral Glucose Tolerance Test (OGTT). Glucose levels are normally lower during pregnancy, so the threshold values for diagnosis of diabetes in pregnancy are lower. If a woman has two plasma glucose values meeting or exceeding any of the following numbers, she has gestational diabetes:

- A fasting plasma glucose level of 95 mg/dL
- A 1-hour level of 180 mg/dL, a 2-hour level of 155 mg/dL
- Or a 3-hour level of 140 mg/dL

Diagnosing Diabetes

The fasting plasma glucose test is the preferred test for diagnosing type 1 or type 2 diabetes (4). It is most reliable when done in the morning. However, a diagnosis of diabetes can be made after positive results on any one of three tests, with confirmation from a second positive test on a different day:

- A random (taken any time of day) plasma glucose value of 200 mg/dL or more, along with the presence of diabetes symptoms
- A plasma glucose value of 126 mg/dl or more after a person has fasted for 8 hours
- An oral glucose tolerance test (OGTT) plasma glucose value of 200 mg/dL or more in a blood sample taken 2 hours after a person has consumed a drink containing 75 grams of glucose dissolved in water

An oral glucose tolerance test is taken in a laboratory or the doctor's office and measures plasma glucose at timed intervals over a 3-hour period. People with pre-diabetes, a state between "normal" and "diabetes," are at risk for developing diabetes, heart attacks, and strokes. However, studies suggest that weight loss, dietary changes and increased physical activity can prevent or delay diabetes, because weight loss and physical activity make the body more sensitive to insulin (10).

A person has impaired fasting glucose (IFG) when fasting plasma glucose is 100 to 125 mg/dl (4,10). This level is higher than normal but less than the level indicating a diagnosis of diabetes. Impaired glucose tolerance (IGT) means that blood glucose during the OGTT is higher than normal but not high enough for a diagnosis of diabetes.

IGT is diagnosed when the glucose level is 140 to 199 mg/dl 2 hours after a person drinks a liquid containing 75 grams of glucose.

Preventing Diabetes

The Diabetes Prevention Program (DPP), a landmark study sponsored by the National Institutes of Health, found that people at increased risk for type 2 diabetes can prevent or delay the onset of the disease by losing 5 to 7 percent of their body weight through increased physical activity and a reduced fat and lower daily caloric intake (5,6).

Small Steps for Big Rewards provides 50 steps for reducing diabetes risk (6):

1. Reduce portion sizes
2. Put less on your plate
3. Keep meat, poultry, and fish servings to about 3 ounces (about the size of a deck of cards)
4. Make less food look like more by serving your meal on a salad or breakfast plate.
5. Try not to snack while cooking or cleaning the kitchen.
6. Try to eat sensible meals and snacks at regular times throughout the day.
7. Make sure you eat breakfast every day.
8. Use broth and cured meats (smoked turkey and turkey bacon) in small amounts. They are high in sodium. Low sodium broths are available in cans and powder.
9. Share your desserts.
10. When eating out, have a big vegetable salad, then split an entree with a friend or have the other half wrapped to go.
11. Stir fry, broil, or bake with non-stick spray or low sodium broth, and try to cook with less oil and butter.
12. Drink a glass of water or other "no-calorie" beverage 10 minutes before your meal to take the edge off your appetite.
13. Select the healthier choice at fast food restaurants. Try grilled chicken instead of the cheeseburger. Skip the french fries or replace the fries with a salad.
14. Listen to music while you eat instead of watching TV (people tend to eat more while watching TV).
15. Eat slowly.
16. Eat a small meal.
17. Teaspoons, salad forks, or child-size utensils may help you take smaller bites and eat less.
18. You don't have to cut out the foods you love to eat, just reduce your portion sizes and eat it them less often.

19. Dance.
20. Show your kids the dances you used to do when you were their age. Turn up the music and jam while doing household chores.
21. Deliver a message in person to a co-worker instead of e-mailing.
22. Take the stairs to your office. Or take the stairs as far as you feel comfortable, and then take the elevator.
23. Make a few less phone calls. Catch up with friends during a regularly scheduled walk.
24. March in place while you watch TV.
25. Park as far away as possible from your favorite store at the mall.
26. Select an exercise video from the store or library.
27. Get off the bus one stop earlier and walk the rest of the way home or to work at least two days a week.
28. Snack on a veggie.
29. Try getting at least one new fruit or vegetable every time you grocery shop.
30. Macaroni and low-fat cheese can be a main dish. Serve it with your favorite vegetable dish and a salad.
31. Try eating foods from other countries. International dishes feature more vegetables, whole grains. and beans and less meat.
32. Cook with a variety of spices instead of salt.
33. Find a water bottle you really like (church or club event souvenir, favorite sports team, etc.) and drink water from it wherever and whenever you can.
34. Always keep a healthy snack with you.
35. Choose veggie toppings like spinach, broccoli and peppers for your pizza.
36. Try different recipes for baking or broiling meat, chicken, and fish.
37. Try to choose foods with little or no added sugar.
38. Gradually work your way down from whole milk to 2% milk to 1% milk until you're drinking and cooking with fat free (skim) milk.
39. Try keeping a written record of what you eat for a week. It can help you see when you tend to overeat or eat foods high in fat or calories.
40. Eat foods made from a variety of whole grains-such as whole wheat bread, brown rice, oats, and whole grain corn-every day. Use whole grain bread for toast and sandwiches; substitute brown rice for white rice for home-cooked meals and when dining out.
41. Don't grocery shop on an empty stomach, and make a list before you go.
42. Read food labels Choose foods with lower fat, saturated fat, calories, and salt.
43. Fruits are colorful and make a welcoming centerpiece for any table. Have a nice chat while sharing a bowl of fruit with family and friends.
44. Slow down at snack time. Eating a bag of low-fat popcorn takes longer than

eating a slice of cake. Peel and eat an orange instead of drinking orange juice.

45. You can exhale, Gail.
46. Don't try to change your entire way of eating and exercising all at once. Try one new activity or food a week.
47. Find mellow ways to relax—try deep breathing, take an easy paced walk, or enjoy your favorite easy listening music.
48. Give yourself daily "pampering time" and honor this time like any other appointment you make... whether it's spending time reading a book, taking a long bath, or meditating.
49. Try not to eat out of boredom or frustration. If you're not hungry, do something else.
50. Honor your health as your most precious gift.

Diabetes and Physical Activity

Physical activity can lower blood glucose levels rapidly. Insulin sensitivity is increased causing cells to better use available insulin to take up glucose. Also, when muscles contract during exercise, they stimulate cells to take up more glucose for energy, independent of insulin activity. This short term lowering of blood glucose levels can cause a person to have hypoglycemia, or low blood glucose levels. People with diabetes should check blood glucose levels prior to and after exercising. To prevent hypoglycemia during exercise (140) people should:

- Eat regular meals
- Have a snack 30 minutes to 2 hours post exercise
- Check blood glucose levels during strenuous activity or prolonged activity
- If blood glucose levels are uncontrolled during exercise, discuss other meal plan changes or possible medication changes with healthcare provider

Vascular problems related to diabetes can cause decreased feeling in lower extremities. People with diabetes may experience unsteady gait and are at a higher risk of developing sores on their feet. Specific exercises may need to be modified to ensure safety and steadiness. Shoes should fit well without rubbing. Socks should help wick moisture and help keep feet dry.

Cardiovascular Disease

Cardiovascular disease refers to the class of diseases that involve the heart or blood vessels (arteries and veins). While the term technically refers to any disease that affects the cardiovascular system, it is usually used to refer to those related to atherosclerosis (arterial disease). These conditions have similar causes, mechanisms, and treatments (10).

Each year heart disease kills more Americans than cancer. Heart disease is the leading cause of death for both men and women (13). Diseases of the heart alone cause 30% of all deaths, with other diseases of the cardiovascular system causing substantial further death and disability (13). About 600,000 people die of heart disease in the United States every year–that's 1 in every 4 deaths (13). Coronary heart disease is the most common type of heart disease, killing more than 385,000 people annually and more than half of the deaths due to heart disease in 2009 were in men (13).

Every year about 715,000 Americans have a heart attack (15). Of these, 525,000 are a first heart attack and 190,000 happen in people who have already had a heart attack (14). Coronary heart disease alone costs the United States $108.9 billion each year (14). This total includes the cost of health care services, medications, and lost productivity.

Epidemiology suggests a number of risk factors for heart disease: age, gender, high blood pressure, high serum cholesterol levels, tobacco smoking, excessive alcohol consumption, family history, obesity, lack of physical activity, psychosocial factors, diabetes mellitus, and air pollution (7). While the individual contribution of each risk factor varies between different communities or ethnic groups, the consistency of the overall contribution of these risk factors is remarkably strong (8,16). About half of Americans (49%) have at least one of these risk factors. Several other medical conditions and lifestyle choices can also put people at a higher risk for heart disease, including (16):

- Diabetes and kidney failure
- Overweight and obesity
- Poor diet
- Physical inactivity
- Excessive alcohol use

Lowering blood pressure and cholesterol are the largest factors in reducing risk of heart disease (16). Currently practiced measures to prevent cardiovascular disease include:

- Eat a low saturated fat, high-fiber diet including whole grains and plenty of fresh fruits and vegetables (at least five portions per day) (17).
- Cease tobacco use and avoid or second-hand smoke (17).

- Limit alcohol consumption to the recommended daily limits consumption of 1-2 standard alcoholic drinks per day. Excessive alcohol intake increases the risk of cardiovascular disease (26).
- Lower blood pressures, if elevated, through the use of anti-hypertensive medications (27).
- Decrease body fat (BMI) if overweight or obese (27).
- Increase daily activity to 30 minutes of vigorous exercise per day at least five times per week (27).
- Decrease psychosocial stress (28). Stress however plays a relatively minor role in hypertension (40).

If the above mentioned preventive measures are not implemented, a physician may prescribe "cholesterol-lowering" medications, such as the statins (43). See discussion below (Cholesterol).

Nutrition and Atherosclerosis

Atherosclerosis is a condition in which an artery wall thickens as a result of the accumulation of fatty materials (29). It is a chronic inflammatory response in the walls of arteries, caused largely by the accumulation of macrophage white blood cells, and promoted by low-density lipoproteins, with inadequate removal of fats and cholesterol from the macrophages by high-density lipoproteins (29).

Atherosclerosis usually begins with the accumulation of soft fatty streaks along the inner arterial walls, especially at branch points (30). Atherosclerotic lesions (plaques) are separated into two broad categories, stable and unstable (32). Stable atherosclerotic plaques, which tend to be asymptomatic, are rich in extracellular matrix and smooth muscle cells. Unstable plaques are rich in macrophages and foam cells and the extracellular matrix (also known as the fibrous cap) is usually weak and prone to rupture (32).

Ruptures of the fibrous cap expose thrombogenic material, such as collagen (33), to the circulation and eventually induce thrombus (clot) formation in the lumen. Upon formation, intraluminal thrombi can occlude (obstruct) arteries outright (i.e. coronary occlusion), but more often they detach, move into the circulation, and eventually occlude or obstruct smaller downstream branches causing thromboembolism. Stroke is often caused by thrombus formation in the carotid arteries) (33).

Complications of advanced atherosclerosis are chronic, slowly progressive, and cumulative. Most commonly, soft plaque suddenly ruptures causing the formation of a thrombus that will rapidly slow or stop blood flow, leading to death of the tissues fed by the artery in approximately 5 minutes (34). This catastrophic event is called an infarction. One of the most common recognized scenarios is called coronary thrombosis of a coronary artery, causing myocardial infarction (a heart attack). The same process in an artery to the brain is commonly called stroke. Another common scenario in very advanced disease is claudication from insufficient blood supply to the legs, typically caused by a combination of both stenosis and aneurysmal segments narrowed with clots (34).

Platelets cause clots to form whenever they encounter injuries in blood vessels. In atherosclerosis, platelets form and aid in the formation of clots (29).

No one is free from atherosclerosis. The important question becomes how far advanced is it, and what can be done to slow or reverse its progression (30).

Cholesterol

Cholesterol levels correlate with risk of heart disease, with a twofold increase in risk between patients with cholesterol levels <180 mg/dl compared to individuals with cholesterol levels > 240 mg/dl (28). Total cholesterol and low-density lipoprotein cholesterol levels are useful markers for determining CVD risk. The following table describes optimum levels for these markers (34,35,36,37).

Total Cholesterol Level	**Category**
Less than 200 mg/dl	Desirable level that indicates lower risk for coronary heart disease. A cholesterol level of 200 mg/dl or higher increases risk
200 to 239 mg/dl	Borderline high
240 mg/dl and above	High blood cholesterol. A person with this level has more than twice the risk of coronary heart disease as someone whose cholesterol is below 200 mg/dl
HDL Cholesterol Level	Category
Men - < 40 mg/dl	Low HDL cholesterol. A major risk factor for heart disease
Women - < 50 mg/dl	Low HDL cholesterol. A major risk factor for heart disease
60 mg/dl and above	High HDL cholesterol. An HDL of 60 mg/dl and above is considered protective against heart disease
LDL Cholesterol Level	Category
< 100 mg/dl	Optimal
100 to 129 mg/dl	Near or above optimal
130 to 159 mg/dl	Borderline high
160 to 189 mg/dl	High
190 mg/dl and above	Very high

Triglyceride Level	Category
< 100 mg/dl	Optimal
< 150 mg/dl	Normal
150 to 199 mg/dl	Borderline high
200 to 249	High
500 mg/dl and above	Very high

Cholesterol ratio is also an important indicator of disease risk and is determined by dividing high-density lipoprotein (HDL, or "good") into total cholesterol. The guidelines indicate maintaining cholesterol ratio 5 to 1 or lower. An optimum ratio is 3.5 to 1. A higher ratio indicates a higher risk of heart disease; a lower ratio indicates a lower risk (30,31).

Cholesterol Lowering Medications

Modern medicine has never been able to explain why some 45—60 percent of patients with hospital admissions for a heart attack have a *"normal level"* of cholesterol (23,48). Even individuals with low-to-normal cholesterol levels may be at risk for a cardiovascular event (23,48). Intensive research is under way to investigate the molecules known to be involved in the process of plaque formation.

Three to four million individuals are taking cholesterol-lowering drugs, and debate on the effectiveness of these medications continues (43). Dr. James M. Wright, a professor at the University of British Columbia and director of the government-funded Therapeutics Initiative was surprised at the collected data for the majority of patients who don't have heart disease (43). He found no benefit of cholesterol lowering medications in people over the age of 65, no matter how much their cholesterol levels declined. He did see a small reduction in the number of heart attacks for middle-aged men taking statins. But even for these men, there was no overall reduction in total deaths or illnesses requiring hospitalization—despite big reductions in "bad" cholesterol (43).

No studies have shown statin cholesterol-lowering drugs to be effective for women at any age, nor for men 69 years of age or older who do not already have heart disease or diabetes (42)." There is a vanishing benefit to lowering cholesterol for healthy adults", states Dr. Wright (43).

According to Dr. Wright, perhaps urging people to switch to a Mediterranean diet or simply to eat more fish is the healthiest choice. In several studies, both lifestyle changes brought greater declines in heart attacks than statins, though the trials were too small to be completely persuasive (41,42). Being physically fit is also important (42).

Other ways to reduce cholesterol levels include (16,17,19):

1. Reduce total dietary fat. Saturated fat is a bigger culprit than dietary cholesterol. Reducing total daily fat intake to 20% of caloric intake, with at least 10% unsaturated fat, appears to be ideal (although very difficult).
2. Reduce dietary cholesterol. Reducing cholesterol intake from 500 to 200 milligrams a day will lower total blood cholesterol by an average of 10 milligrams. However, this response is very variable.
3. Include lots of fiber (oats, beans, fruits and vegetables). Oats have a fiber-rich bran layer that effectively lowers cholesterol; beans, fruits, and vegetables have also been shown to have cholesterol lowering properties.
4. Eat more fish. The oilier fish, such as salmon, mackerel, albacore, and herring, guard against heart disease and hypertension. Eating 2 to 3 meals of fish per week can reduce heart disease risk.
5. Include unsaturated fats. Unsaturated fatty acids have been shown to be heart healthy. These fats can decrease LDL cholesterol, while preserving HDL. Cooking with oils, however, may destroy essential fatty acid activity, and is not as heart healthy as including uncooked sources.
6. Eat fruits and vegetables. A meta-analysis of the latest studies concluded that individuals who consumed the most fruits and vegetables reduced risk of heart disease by 15%. A lower risk of stroke is also associated with higher intake of fruits and vegetables. The lowest risks were associated with consumption of cruciferous vegetables (broccoli, cabbage, cauliflower, brussel sprouts), green leafy vegetables, citrus fruits, and vitamin C rich fruit and vegetables.
7. Decrease caffeine. Caffeine has been shown to increase cholesterol levels; however, accumulated research indicates that this effect is minimized when coffee is brewed from drip coffee makers using filters. The older version of "percolating" coffee for long periods of time produces chemicals known to increase lipid cholesterol levels.
8. Minimize concentrated simple sugars. Concentrated simple sugar intake and other concentrated sweeteners like fructose, corn syrup, and honey, produce a liver enzyme (HMG-CoA reductase) that causes the liver to synthesize more cholesterol (from acetate). Hence, eating sugar can increase cholesterol levels, specifically triglycerides.
9. Limit consumption of processed meats such as bologna, sausages, hotdogs, and salami.

L-Carnitine

"High blood levels of the bacterial by-product of L-carnitine, called trimethylamine *N*-oxide or TMAO, are a warning sign of impending heart attack, stroke, and death, indicates Stanley Hazen of Cleveland Clinic" (39). Hazen's team first linked intestinal microbes to heart disease in 2011, when they spotted TMAO in blood collected from people who later suffered heart attacks, had strokes, or died (40).

Researchers have long reported an association with eating red meat and an increase risk of developing heart disease. One way physicians gauge risk is with blood tests, but tests for cholesterol and other molecules do not explain meat's link to heart disease (39). According to Hazen, "cholesterol, saturated fat and salt account for only a small amount of the risk" (39). Gut bacteria might account for more. In his study, Hazen investigated L-carnitine because the nutrient is structurally similar to a compound that gut microbes can convert to TMAO. Omnivorous human subjects produced more TMAO than did vegans or vegetarians following ingestion of l-carnitine through a microbiota-dependent mechanism (39). Intestinal microbiota may thus contribute to the well-established link between high levels of red meat consumption and CVD risk. Hazen notes, "from the current research, one message is clear, L-carnitine is not good for you. It's not good as a supplement and it's not good in red meat. That's one thing you can take to the bank" (40).

Other researchers note that it is possible that carnitine and TMAO levels in humans are just a marker of red meat intake, not a direct cause of heart disease (126). The data that supports high carnitine levels and/or TMAO are associated with increased heart disease based on correlations not causality. It seems that the saturated fat in red meat is more of risk variable than carnitine and TMAO. More research needs to be done to establish mechanisms and causality in humans (126).

Homocysteine

A molecule called homocysteine has received a lot of attention. Homocysteine is a non-protein, naturally occurring amino acid found in blood plasma. A high level of homocysteine is a powerful risk factor for cardiovascular disease. It is believed to increase the chance of heart disease, stroke, Alzheimer's disease, and osteoporosis. Homocysteine is broken down in the body through two metabolic pathways. The chemical changes that must occur to break down homocysteine require the presence of folic acid (also called folate) and vitamins B^6 and B^{12}. (44). Folic acid is involved in the reaction that converts homocysteine back to another amino acid, methionine. Vitamin B6 and B12 are also involved in the reaction. Initial research indicates that as little as 150 micrograms of folic acid (20 ounces of orange juice) daily can reduce homocysteine levels by 11% within one month (44). However, one study which attempted to decrease the risk by lowering homocysteine was not fruitful (44). This study was conducted on nearly 5000 Norwegian heart attack survivors who already had severe, late-stage heart disease. No study has yet been conducted in a preventive capacity on subjects who are in a relatively good state of health (44).

High-Sensitivity C-Reactive Protein

"Inflammation" is the process by which the body responds to injury or an infection. Laboratory evidence and findings from clinical and population studies suggest that inflammation atherosclerosis is the result of an inflammatory response. The major injurious factors that promote atherogenesis (cigarette smoking, hypertension, atherogenic lipoproteins, and hyperglycemia) are well established. These risk factors give rise to a variety of noxious stimuli that cause the release of chemicals and the activation of cells involved in the inflammatory process. These events are thought to contribute not only to the formation of plaque but may also contribute to its disruption (breaking loose) resulting in the formation of a blood clot. Thus, virtually every step in atherogenesis is believed to involve substances involved in the inflammatory response and cells that are characteristic of inflammation (10).

C-reactive protein (CRP) is one of the acute phase proteins that increase during systemic inflammation (45). It's been suggested that testing CRP levels in the blood may be an additional way to assess cardiovascular disease risk. A more sensitive CRP test, called a highly sensitive C-reactive protein (hs-CRP) assay, is available to determine heart disease risk (45).

A growing number of studies have examined whether hs-CRP can predict recurrent cardiovascular disease, stroke, and death in different settings. High levels of hs-CRP consistently predict recurrent coronary events in patients with unstable angina and acute myocardial infarction (heart attack). Higher hs-CRP levels also are associated with lower survival rates in these patients. Many studies have suggested that after adjusting for other factors, hs-CRP is useful as a risk predictor (44,45). These studies found that the higher the hs-CRP levels, the higher the risk of having a heart attack. In fact, the risk for heart attack in people in the upper third of hs-CRP levels was twice that of those whose hs-CRP level was in the lower third. Studies have also found an association between sudden cardiac death, peripheral arterial disease, and hs-CRP (45,46).

The hs-CRP test accurately detects low concentrations of C-reactive protein to help predict a healthy person's risk of cardiovascular disease (CVD). The American Heart Association and U.S. Centers for Disease Control and Prevention have defined risk groups as follows

(21):

- Low risk: less than 1.0 mg/L
- Average risk: 1.0 to 3.0 mg/L
- High risk: above 3.0 mg/L

The best ways to lower CRP are already known to lower cardiovascular risk. These include diet, exercise, blood pressure control, smoking cessation, and brushing and flossing teeth. Thus, an important role for CRP evaluation is to identify high-risk individuals (even when cholesterol is low) and to motivate them toward heart-healthy interventions (21).

<u>Coronary Calcium Scan</u>

The accumulation of calcium plaque in coronary arteries continues despite aggressive cholesterol reduction with a statin drug (22).

Coronary calcium scoring has become a common test for cardiovascular risk determination (23,47). It was cardiologist Dr. Stephen Seely who wrote, in his treatise entitled *"Is calcium excess in western diet a major cause of arterial disease?"*, that excess calcium intake is a major cause of atherosclerosis in Western countries (24). He contended that young adults need only 300—400 mg of calcium daily, and older adults need even less. In countries where the daily calcium intake is 200—400 mg, arterial diseases are non-existent and blood pressure does not increase with age. After years of debate, the AHA has approved CT scanning for arterial calcification for high-risk individuals (25).

A coronary calcium scan produces a calcium score called an Agatston score. The score is based on the amount of calcium found in the coronary arteries. Scores can be obtained for each major artery and a total score can be calculated (25).

The test is negative if no calcium deposits (calcification) are found in the arteries and indicates low risk of a heart attack in the next 2 to 5 years (25). The test is positive if calcification is found indicating atherosclerosis and coronary heart disease (CHD). The higher the Agatston score is, the more severe the atherosclerosis. (25).

The link between calcium and cardiovascular risk is unclear. Li and colleagues concluded in their investigations of data from the 23,980 Heidelberg cohort that increasing calcium intake from diet might not confer significant cardiovascular benefit, but taking calcium supplements might increase myocardial infarction risk (127). Conversely, Hemelrijuck et al. recently reported that there is no clear link between dietary or supplementary intake of calcium and cardiovascular death in their analysis of

National Health and Nutrition Examination Survey III (128). As a result, the debate on the association between calcium intake and cardiovascular risk continues.

Cardiovascular Disease and Physical Activity

A sedentary lifestyle is one of the 5 major risk factors (along with high blood pressure, abnormal values for blood lipids, smoking, and obesity) for cardiovascular disease, as outlined by the AHA (142). Evidence from many scientific studies shows that reducing these risk factors decreases the chance of having a heart attack or experiencing another cardiac event and reduces the possibility of needing a coronary procedure (bypass surgery or coronary angioplasty).

Regular exercise has a favorable effect on many of the established risk factors for cardiovascular disease. For example, exercise promotes weight reduction and can help reduce blood pressure. Exercise can reduce "bad" cholesterol levels in the blood (low-density lipoprotein level), as well as total cholesterol, and can raise the "good" cholesterol (high-density lipoprotein level). In diabetic patients, regular activity favorably affects the body's ability to use insulin to control glucose levels in the blood. Although the effect of an exercise program on any single risk factor may generally be small, the effect of continued, moderate exercise on overall cardiovascular risk, when combined with other lifestyle modifications (such as proper nutrition, smoking cessation, and medication use), can be dramatic (142).

Hypertension

Hypertension, sometimes called arterial hypertension, is a chronic medical condition in which the blood pressure in the arteries is elevated (50). This requires the heart to work harder than normal to circulate blood through the blood vessels.

Blood pressure is comprised of two measurements, systolic and diastolic, which depend on whether the heart muscle is contracting (systole) or relaxed between beats (diastole) (10). Normal blood pressure at rest is within the range of 80-120mmHg systolic (top reading) and 60-90mmHg diastolic (bottom reading). High blood pressure is said to be present if it is persistently at or above 140/90 mm Hg.

Hypertension is a major risk factor for stroke, myocardial infarction (heart attacks), heart failure, aneurysms of the arteries, peripheral arterial disease, and is a cause of chronic kidney disease (10). Dietary and lifestyle changes can improve blood pressure control and decrease the risk of associated health complications, although drug treatment is often necessary in people for whom lifestyle changes prove ineffective or insufficient (10).

The following table lists Recommended lifestyle changes and potential impacts on blood pressure (50-54):

Modification	Recommendation	Approximate SBP reduction
Reduce weight	BMI < 25 kg/m2 and waist circumference < 94 cm (males) or < 80 cm (females)	1 mm Hg per 1% reduction in weight
Reduce salt intake	< 4 g/day of salt (approximately 1600 mg sodium)	4–5 mm Hg
Increase physical activity	At least 30 minutes physical activity most days of the week	4–9 mm Hg
Modify diet	Consume a diet rich in fruits, vegetables, and low fat dairy products and low in saturated and total fat	8–14 mm Hg
Limit alcohol intake	≤ 2 standard drinks per day	2–4 mm Hg

Dash Modifications

The DASH diet (Dietary Approaches to Stop Hypertension) is a dietary pattern promoted by the National Heart, Lung, and Blood Institute (part of the National Institutes of Health) to prevent and control hypertension (63). The DASH diet is rich in fruits, vegetables, whole grains, and low-fat dairy foods; includes meat, fish, poultry, nuts, and beans; and is limited in sugar-sweetened foods and beverages, red meat, sodium, and added fats. In addition to its effect on blood pressure, it is designed to be a well-balanced approach to eating for the general public. It is now recommended by the United States Department of Agriculture (USDA) as an ideal eating plan for all Americans (63).

The initial Dash study (Dietary Approaches to Stop Hypertension, 1997) was one of the first large research studies that looked at the effects of entire diet, not supplements, on hypertension (69). The eight-week study consisted of 459 adults with normal, high-normal, or high blood pressure. Each participant was randomly assigned to eat one of three diets prepared by DASH dietitians. The Usual Diet (similar to the average American diet) had average levels of fat and cholesterol, and below-average levels of potassium, magnesium, and calcium; the Fruit and Vegetable Diet was identical except that eight to ten servings of fruits and vegetables a day replaced most snacks and sweets which increased potassium, magnesium, and fiber. The third diet, *the combination diet*, cut fat, saturated fat, and cholesterol while upping not only fruits and vegetables, but low-fat dairy foods which increased protein and calcium in addition to potassium, magnesium, and fiber. Calories, alcohol, and sodium were the same in all three diets. The results reported in 1997 were indisputable (69). The combination diet reduced systolic blood pressure by 5.5 points and diastolic blood pressure by 3.0 points. Researchers indicated that there was no way of "teasing out" which nutrients were responsible. But from a public health perspective, it did not matter. What does matter is that a diet rich in fruits and vegetables, with low fat dairy foods, seafood, and only lean meats and poultry, lowers blood pressure dramatically (69).

Dash-Sodium Diet

The same researchers published results from a second study known as the Dash-Sodium study (72). The study consisted of 412 men and women. Participants were randomly assigned to either the DASH diet or a usual diet for 12 weeks. The sodium in both diets was changed every four weeks to one of three levels; a higher intake of 3,300 mg a day, an intermediate intake of 2,400 mg a day, or a lower intake of 1,500 mg a day. The results were startling. On both the DASH and the usual diets, the lower the sodium fell, the lower blood pressures fell. The DASH diet with lowest sodium intake cut blood pressure by an impressive 8.9 points in systolic pressure and 4.5 points in diastolic pressure when compared to the usual diet with the higher sodium intake. This is roughly twice the impact of the usual DASH diet alone. As expected, blood pressure fell more in the people with hypertension than in individuals without hypertension. (55,64,72).

Mediterranean Diet

Oldways, the Harvard School of Public Health, and the European Office of the World Health Organization introduced the classic Mediterranean Diet in 1993 at a conference in Cambridge, MA, along with a Mediterranean Diet Pyramid graphic to represent it visually (124). Details about the pyramid and Mediterranean diet recipes can be found on the Oldways website (124).

The Mediterranean diet is a modern nutritional recommendation inspired by the traditional dietary patterns of southern Italy, Greece, and Spain (56). The principal aspects of this diet include proportionally high consumption of olive oil, legumes, unrefined cereals, fruits, and vegetables, moderate to high consumption of fish, moderate consumption of dairy products (mostly as cheese and yogurt), moderate wine consumption, and low consumption of meat and meat products (56-61).

A 2011 meta-analysis published in the *Journal of the American College of Cardiology* analyzed the results of 50 studies (35 clinical trials, 2 prospective and 13 cross-sectional) covering about 535,000 people to examine the effect of a Mediterranean diet (61). The researchers reported that a Mediterranean diet is associated with lower blood pressure, blood sugar, and triglycerides (60). A meta-analysis published in the *American Journal of Clinical Nutrition* in 2013 compared Mediterranean, vegan, vegetarian, low-glycemic index, low-carbohydrate, high-fiber, and high-protein diets with control diets (62). Researchers concluded that Mediterranean, low-carbohydrate, low-glycemic index, and high-protein diets are effective in improving markers of risk for cardiovascular disease and diabetes (62).

A randomized Spanish trial of diet pattern published in the New England Journal of Medicine (65) in 2013 followed almost 7,500 individuals for a period of over 5 years. Subjects in the research followed one of three different diets. They included either a low fat diet, a Mediterranean diet with 50 ml of extra virgin olive oil daily, or a Mediterranean diet with 30 grams of mixed nuts. The nuts were primarily walnuts which have a high amount of omega-3 fatty acids and vitamin E (65). The results indicated that individuals on a Mediterranean diet supplemented with mixed nuts and olive oil had a 30 percent reduction in risk of having a major cardiovascular event and a 49 percent decrease in stroke risk.

Hypertension and Physical Activity

Epidemiological studies indicate that the relationship between sedentary behavior and hypertension is so strong that the National Heart Foundation (153), the World Health Organization and International Society of Hypertension (155), the United States Joint National Committee on Detection, Evaluation and Treatment of High Blood Pressure, (154) and the American College of Sports Medicine (ACSM)(151) have all recommended increased physical activity as a first line intervention for preventing and treating patients with prehypertension and hypertension. Physical activity is particularly appealing because it has favorable effects on other cardiovascular disease (CVD) risk factors. The 2004 ACSM review of evidence based literature on the relationship between blood pressure and exercise suggests (151):

- Hypertensive individuals should be encouraged to exercise regularly as blood pressure can be reduced for up to 22 hours following a single exercise session. This observation of a reduction in pressure following a single exercise session is called post-exercise hypotension (PEH) (151). The exact cause of PEH is not fully known but the fact that it does occur and lasts for so long in some individuals is part of the rationale for encouraging those with high blood pressure to exercise daily.
- Hypertensive individuals who exercise regularly for several months can expect to see a 5-10 mm Hg reduction in both systolic and diastolic blood pressure readings. However, it is important to note that not all individuals experience these favorable responses. since there is evidence that 25 to 33 percent of hypertensive individuals do not experience PEH. These individuals should still be encouraged to exercise for the other health benefits that they are likely to gain from exercise training.

- Exercise should primarily consist of aerobic activities like brisk walking, jogging, cycling, or swimming. These activities should be performed a minimum of three days per week for 30 to 60 minutes, but could be done daily. The intensity should be in the moderate range, with heart rates representing 40 to 70 percent of heart rate reserve. Resistance training activities should be done two times per week, with an emphasis on lower weight but higher repetitions (8 to 12 per set). Static stretching should be performed during each exercise session to help minimize the risk of musculoskeletal injury.
- Individuals should have their blood pressure checked on a regular basis to make sure their values are being kept within the desirable range. In many cases, individuals will need to be medicated to achieve desirable readings; however, lifestyle modifications, including the adoption of the DASH or Mediterranean diet coupled with regular exercise, should be encouraged. Even if blood pressure is not reduced with exercise training, the hypertensive individual should still exercise to help with weight management, lipid control and improvement in blood sugar control.

Stroke

In the US, over 700,000 strokes occur every year and are responsible for 165,000 deaths annually. Stroke is the second leading cause of death worldwide (129).

A stroke occurs when a clot blocks the blood supply to part of the brain or when a blood vessel in or around the brain bursts. In either case, parts of the brain become damaged or die (66).

About 85% of all strokes are ischemic, in which blood flow to the brain is blocked by blood clots or fatty deposits called plaque in blood vessel linings (73). A hemorrhagic stroke occurs when a blood vessel bursts in the brain. Blood accumulates and compresses the surrounding brain tissue. There are two types of hemorrhagic stroke (73):

- Intracerebral hemorrhage is the most common type of hemorrhagic stroke. It occurs when an artery in the brain bursts, flooding the surrounding tissue with blood.
- Subarachnoid hemorrhage is bleeding in the area between the brain and the thin tissues that cover it.

Transient ischemic attack (TIA) is a "warning stroke" or a "mini-stroke" that results in no lasting damage. Recognizing and treating TIAs immediately can reduce your risk of a major stroke (73). Some factors for stroke cannot be modified by medical treatment or lifestyle changes (67):

- *Age.* Studies show the risk of stroke doubles for each decade between the ages of 55 and 85. But strokes also can occur in childhood or adolescence. Although stroke is often considered a disease of aging, the risk of stroke in childhood is actually highest during the perinatal period, which encompasses the last few months of fetal life and the first few weeks after birth.
- *Gender.* Men have a higher risk for stroke, but more women die from stroke. Men generally do not live as long as women, so men are usually younger when they have their strokes and therefore have a higher rate of survival.
- *Race.* People from certain ethnic groups have a higher risk of stroke. For African Americans, stroke is more common and more deadly—even in young and middle-aged adults—than for any ethnic or other racial group in the United States. Studies show that the age-adjusted incidence of stroke is about twice as high in African Americans and Hispanic Americans as in Caucasians. An important risk factor for African-Americans is sickle cell disease, which can cause a narrowing of arteries and disrupt blood flow. The incidence of the various stroke subtypes also varies considerably in different ethnic groups.
- *Family history of stroke.* Stroke seems to run in some families. Several factors may contribute to familial stroke. Members of a family might have a genetic tendency for stroke risk factors, such as an inherited predisposition for high blood pressure (hypertension) or diabetes. The influence of a common lifestyle among family members also could contribute to familial stroke.

Some of the most important treatable risk factors for stroke are (67):

- ***High blood pressure, or hypertension.*** Hypertension is by far the most potent risk factor for stroke. Hypertension causes a two-to four-fold increase in the risk of stroke before age 80. Some ways to reduce blood pressure include maintaining proper weight; avoiding drugs known to raise blood pressure; eat right, cut down on salt and eat fruits and vegetables to increase potassium; exercise more. A physician may prescribe medicines that help lower blood pressure. Controlling blood pressure also helps avoid heart disease, diabetes, and kidney failure.
- ***Cigarette smoking.*** Cigarette smoking causes about a two-fold increase in the risk of ischemic stroke and up to a four-fold increase in the risk of hemorrhagic stroke. It has been linked to the buildup of fatty substances (atherosclerosis) in the carotid artery, the main neck artery supplying blood to the brain. Blockage of this artery is the leading cause of stroke in Americans. Also, nicotine raises blood pressure; carbon monoxide from smoking reduces the amount of oxygen the blood can carry to the brain; and cigarette smoke makes blood thicker and more likely to clot. Smoking also promotes aneurysm formation. Quitting, at any age, reduces the risk of lung disease, heart disease, and a number of cancers including lung cancer.

- *Heart disease.* Common heart disorders such as coronary artery disease, valve defects, irregular heart beat (atrial fibrillation), and enlargement of one of the heart's chambers can result in blood clots that may break loose and block vessels in or leading to the brain. Atrial fibrillation, which is more prevalent in older people, is responsible for one in four strokes after age 80, and is associated with higher mortality and disability. The most common blood vessel disease is atherosclerosis. Hypertension promotes atherosclerosis and causes mechanical damage to the walls of blood vessels. Physicians treat heart disease by prescribing medication, such as aspirin, to help prevent the formation of clots. Surgery may be recommended to "clean out" a clogged neck artery; or for persons over 50, a physician may recommend aspirin therapy.
- *Warning signs or history of TIA or stroke.* Anyone experiencing *a* TIA should get help at once. Individuals with a previous history of TIA or stroke have a much greater risk of having a stroke than someone who never had one.
- *Diabetes.* In terms of stroke and cardiovascular disease, having diabetes is the equivalent of aging 15 years. Diabetes affects not only the body's ability to use sugar, or glucose, but it also causes destructive changes in the blood vessels throughout the body, including the brain. Also, if blood glucose levels are high at the time of a stroke, then brain damage is usually more severe and extensive than when blood glucose is well-controlled. Hypertension is common among diabetics and accounts for much of their increased stroke risk. Treating diabetes can delay the onset of complications that increase the risk of stroke.
- *Cholesterol imbalance.* Low-density lipoprotein cholesterol (LDL) carries cholesterol (a fatty substance) through the blood and delivers it to cells. Excess LDL can cause cholesterol to build up in blood vessels, leading to atherosclerosis. Atherosclerosis is the major cause of blood vessel narrowing, leading to both heart attack and stroke.
- *Physical inactivity and obesity.* Obesity and inactivity are associated with hypertension, diabetes, heart disease, and stroke. Waist circumference to hip circumference ratio equal to or above the mid-value for the population increases the risk of ischemic stroke three-fold.

Warning signs are clues that the body sends to the brain when oxygen levels decrease. If one or more of these signs of a stroke or "brain attack," occur, don't wait, call a doctor or 911 right away (67)! Warning signs include:

- Sudden numbness or weakness of face, arm, or leg, especially on one side of the body
- Sudden confusion, or trouble talking or understanding speech
- Sudden trouble seeing in one or both eyes
- Sudden trouble walking, dizziness, or loss of balance or coordination

- Sudden severe headache with no known cause

Other danger signs that may occur include double vision, drowsiness, and nausea or vomiting. Sometimes the warning signs may last only a few moments and then disappear. These brief episodes, known as transient ischemic attacks or TIAs, are sometimes called "mini-strokes." Although brief, they identify an underlying serious condition that isn't going away without medical help. Unfortunately, since they clear up, many people ignore them. Don't. Paying attention can save lives (67).

Stroke and Physical Activity

Regular physical activity can improve heart and lung function, raise HDL and lower triglycerides. The American Heart Association recommends 30 minutes of moderately intense aerobic activity at least 5 days per week or 25 minutes of vigorous aerobic activity at least three days per week and moderate to high intensity muscle strengthening activity at least two or more days per week (141).

Cancer

About 1,660,290 new cancer cases are expected to be diagnosed in 2013, and about 580,350 Americans are projected to die of cancer, almost 1,600 people a day (74). Cancer remains the second most common cause of death in the US, accounting for nearly 1 of every 4 deaths (74-78). Anyone can develop cancer. Since the risk of being diagnosed increases with age, most cases occur in adults who are middle aged or older. About 77% of all cancers are diagnosed in persons 55 years of age and older.

A substantial proportion of cancers could be prevented. All cancers caused by cigarette smoking and heavy use of alcohol could be prevented completely. The American Cancer Society estimates that in 2013 about 174,100 cancer deaths will be caused by tobacco use (74-78). The World Cancer Research Fund estimates that about one-quarter to one-third of the new cancer cases expected to occur in 2013 will be related to overweight or obesity, physical inactivity, and poor nutrition, and thus could also be prevented (74-78).

Certain cancers are related to infectious agents, such as human papillomavirus (HPV), hepatitis B virus (HBV), hepatitis C virus (HCV), human immunodeficiency virus (HIV), and Helicobacter pylori (H. pylori); many of these cancers could be prevented through behavioral changes, vaccines, or antibiotics. Many of the more than 2 million skin cancers that are diagnosed annually could be prevented by protecting skin from excessive sun exposure and avoiding indoor tanning (74-78).

In addition to preventing cancer through the avoidance of risk factors, regular screening tests that allow the detection and removal of precancerous growths can prevent cancers of the cervix, colon, and rectum (74-78).

Early detection of cancer, which usually results in less extensive treatment and better outcomes, can also be achieved through screening. Screening is known to reduce mortality for cancers of the breast, colon, rectum, and cervix. A heightened awareness of changes in the breast or skin may also result in detection of these tumors at earlier stages (74-78).

Cancer researchers use the word "risk" in different ways, most commonly expressing risk as lifetime risk or relative risk. Lifetime risk refers to the probability that an individual will develop or die from cancer over the course of a lifetime. In the US, men have slightly less than a 1 in 2 lifetime risk of developing cancer; for women, the risk is a little more than 1 in 3. However, it is important to note that these estimates are based on the average experience of the general population and may over or underestimate individual risk because of differences in exposure (i.e., smoking), and/or genetic susceptibility (74-78).

All cancers involve the malfunction of genes that control cell growth and division. About 5% of all cancers are strongly hereditary, in that an inherited genetic alteration confers a very high risk of developing one or more specific types of cancer. However, most cancers do not result from inherited genes but from damage to genes occurring during one's lifetime. Genetic damage may result from internal factors, such as hormones or the metabolism of nutrients within cells, or external factors, such as tobacco, or excessive exposure to chemicals, sunlight, or ionizing radiation (74-78).

Cancer and Physical Activity

There is convincing evidence that physical activity is associated with a reduced risk of cancers of the colon and breast (143). Several studies have reported links between physical activity and a reduced risk of prostate, lung, and lining of the uterus cancer (143,144). More than 50 studies examining the association between physical activity and colorectal cancer found that adults who increase their physical activity, either in intensity, duration, or frequency, can reduce their risk of developing colon cancer by 30 to 40 percent compared to those who are sedentary regardless of body mass index (143), with the greatest risk reduction seen among those who are most active (144-148). It is estimated that 30 to 60 minutes of moderate to vigorous physical activity per day is needed for a protective effect (147,148). Physical activity may protect against colon cancer and tumor development through its role in energy balance, hormone metabolism, insulin regulation, and by decreasing the time the colon is exposed to potential carcinogens. Physical activity has also been found to alter a number of inflammatory and immune factors, some of which may influence colon cancer risk (143).

Over 60 published studies indicate that physically active women have a lower risk of developing breast cancer than inactive women; the amount of risk reduction achieved through physical activity varies widely (between 20 to 80 percent) (147,148). High levels of moderate and vigorous physical activity during adolescence appear to be especially protective; although evidence suggests that physical activity reduces breast cancer risk in both premenopausal and postmenopausal women (147), A number of studies suggest that the effect of physical activity may be dependent on levels of BMI, with the greatest benefit seen in women in the normal weight range (generally a BMI under 25). Most studies suggest that 30 to 60 minutes per day of moderate-to-high-intensity physical activity is associated with a reduction in breast cancer risk (145,147). Physical activity may prevent tumor development by lowering hormone levels, particularly in premenopausal women; lowering levels of insulin and insulin-like growth factor I (IGF-I), improving the immune response; and assisting with weight maintenance to avoid a high body mass and excess body fat (148).

Studies suggest an inverse relationship between physical activity and incidence of endometrial cancer (145). These studies suggest that women who are physically active have a 20 percent to 40 percent reduced risk (147), with the greatest reduction among those with the highest levels of physical activity. Risk does not appear to vary by age (145). Changes in body mass and changes in the levels and metabolism of sex hormones, such as estrogen, are thought to be the major biological mechanisms between physical activity and endometrial cancer (143).

At least 21 studies have examined the impact of physical activity on the risk of lung cancer (143). These studies suggest an inverse association between physical activity and lung cancer risk, with the most physically active individuals experiencing about a 20 percent reduction in risk (145,147).

Research findings are less consistent about the effect of physical activity on prostate cancer. Research indicates that there is an inverse relationship between physical activity and prostate cancer (145,148). The potential biological mechanisms may be related to changes in hormones, energy balance, insulin-like growth factors, immunity, and antioxidant defense mechanisms (148). One study suggested that regular vigorous activity could slow the progression of prostate cancer in men age 65 or older (150).

Gastrointestinal Disorders

Gastrointestinal Disorders (GI) are digestive disorders that interfere with the workings of the intestine. GI disorder generally fall into two categories — functional and inflammatory (107). Inflammatory bowel disease (109,110) is a group of inflammatory conditions of the colon and small intestine. The major types of inflammatory bowel disease are Crohn's disease and ulcerative colitis (107-109). Irritable bowel syndrome (110) is a disorder that leads to abdominal pain and cramping, changes in bowel movements, and other symptoms. Irritable bowel syndrome is not the same as inflammatory bowel disease (109), which includes Crohn's disease and ulcerative colitis. In IBS, the structure of the bowel is not abnormal (110,111). In this section, we will discuss GI Disorders including celiac disease, IBD, (Crohn's disease, ulcerative colitis), IBS, and conclude with a discussion on GERD.

Celiac Disease

Celiac disease is a chronic inflammatory condition caused by ingestion of dietary gluten (a protein found in wheat, barley, and rye). This inflammation can cause malabsorption of several nutrients, which in turn is related to several deficiency disorders, such as anemia, cancer, and osteoporosis (80). The diagnosis relies on the clinical picture of the patient, serological markers, characteristic findings of small intestinal biopsy, and clinical improvement on a gluten-free diet. Strategies for the diagnosis of celiac disease have changed dramatically within the last 10 years. The advent of serological markers with high sensitivity and specificity is changing understanding of the disease and its prevalence (80).

Symptoms in children are usually associated with the introduction of cereals around the age of 6 months. In young children, there is failure to thrive, diarrhea, vomiting, muscle wasting, abdominal distension, abdominal pain and, occasionally, constipation. In older children, the disease may present as anemia, rickets, short stature, dental enamel defects, poor performance in school, or behavioral disturbances (80). Two to eight percent of children with unexplained short stature presenting to a growth failure clinic have celiac disease (83,84). Treatment of celiac disease may improve growth in those treated before growth is complete (85,86).

The disease in adulthood may be either adult-onset disease or silent disease present since childhood but producing no symptoms. The most common symptoms in adults are abdominal pain, chronic diarrhea, and iron-deficiency anemia. Diarrhea may be absent in 50% of patients and steatorrhea (excess fat in feces) is less common (40%) but indicates more severe disease. Patients with celiac disease may be mistakenly diagnosed as having irritable bowel syndrome. More often celiac disease is diagnosed in asymptomatic patients with iron-deficiency anemia, folate deficiency, abnormal liver tests, or osteoporosis (80).

Celiac disease is frequently associated with iron deficiency (90). Six to ten per cent of patients with iron-deficiency anemia will have celiac disease based on small bowel biopsies (80,81). The disease can also result in vitamin D and calcium malabsorption (90). Fifty per cent of patients with celiac disease have lactose intolerance and may already have a reduced intake of calcium. A significant prevalence of celiac disease has been reported in patients diagnosed with osteopenic bone disease (91). This diminished bone density is associated with an increased risk of fractures (94). A gluten-free diet corrects the bone loss in those with mild disease, and significantly improves it in those with severe malabsorption (95,96).

A gluten-free diet is the only current treatment (79). Dietary restriction is difficult because gluten is not only in wheat, barley and rye, it is also used in many other foods. Careful attention to constantly changing ingredients in commercially prepared foods is necessary, along with careful cooking habits and extremely careful scrutiny while dining out (10).

The U.S. Food and Drug Administration published a regulation defining the term "gluten-free" for voluntary food labeling on August 2, 2013 (177). The FDA was directed to issue the new regulation by the Food Allergen Labeling and Consumer Protection Act (FALCPA), which directed the FDA to set guidelines for the use of the term "gluten-free". It requires that, in order to use the term "gluten-free" on its label, a food must meet all of the requirements of the definition, including that the food must contain less than 20 parts per million of gluten (177). The rule also requires foods with the claims "no gluten," "free of gluten," and "without gluten" to meet the definition for "gluten-free." Food manufacturers have one year to bring their labels into compliance with the new requirements (177).

Inflammatory Bowel Disease - Crohn's Disease

Crohn's disease is a type of inflammatory bowel disease that may affect any part of the gastrointestinal tract from mouth to anus, causing a wide variety of symptoms. The disease was named after gastroenterologist Burrill Bernard Crohn, who, in 1932, described a series of patients with inflammation of the terminal ileum, the area most commonly affected by the illness (117).

The disease primarily causes abdominal pain, diarrhea (which may be bloody if inflammation is at its worst), vomiting (can be continuous), or weight loss but may also cause complications outside the gastrointestinal tract such as skin rashes, arthritis, inflammation of the eye, tiredness, and lack of concentration (107,117). Rectal bleeding may be serious and persistent, leading to anemia. Children with Crohn's disease may suffer delayed development and stunted growth. The range and severity of symptoms varies (121).

There is a genetic association with Crohn's disease. Siblings of affected individuals are at higher risk (118). The disease affects men and women equally and seems to run in some families. Crohn's disease can occur in people of all age groups, but it is more often diagnosed in people between the ages of 20 and 30 (118) and smokers are two times more likely to develop the disease than nonsmokers (119).

Because the symptoms of Crohn's disease are similar to other intestinal disorders, such as irritable bowel syndrome and ulcerative colitis, it can be difficult to diagnose. Ulcerative colitis causes inflammation and ulcers in the top layer of the lining of the large intestine. In Crohn's disease, all layers of the intestine may be involved, and normal healthy bowel can be found between sections of diseased bowel (120).

There is no known pharmaceutical or surgical cure, and treatment options are restricted to controlling symptoms, maintaining remission, and preventing relapse (120). There are no known foods that cause Crohn's disease, and there are no consistent dietary rules to follow that will improve a person's symptoms (121). However, when people are suffering a flare in disease, foods such as bulky grains, hot spices, alcohol, and milk products may increase diarrhea and cramping (118). No special diet has been proven effective for prevention, but it is very important that people who have Crohn's disease follow a nutritious diet and avoid any foods that seem to worsen symptoms.

Nutritional complications are common in Crohn's disease. Deficiencies of proteins, calories, and vitamins may be caused by inadequate dietary intake, intestinal loss of protein, or poor absorption (122).

Treatment may include drugs, nutrition supplements, surgery, or a combination of these options. The goals of treatment are to control inflammation, correct nutritional deficiencies, and relieve symptoms (106-108). The doctor may recommend nutritional supplements, especially for children whose growth has been slowed. Special high-calorie liquid formulas are sometimes used. A small number of patients may need to be fed intravenously for a brief time using a predigested blend of essential nutrients. This procedure can help patients who need extra nutrition temporarily, those whose intestines need to rest, or those whose intestines cannot absorb enough nutrition from food.

Inflammatory Bowel Disease - Ulcerative Colitis

Ulcerative colitis has similarities to Crohn's disease and is another form of IBD. It is an intermittent disease, with periods of expressed symptoms, and periods that are relatively symptom-free. The main symptom of the disease is usually diarrhea mixed with blood. Although the symptoms can sometimes diminish on their own, the disease usually requires treatment to go into remission. Ulcerative colitis has an incidence of 1 to 20 cases per 100,000 individuals per year, and a prevalence of 8 to 246 per 100,000 individuals (116).

Irritable Bowel Syndrome

Irritable Bowel Syndrome (IBS) is one of the most common chronic gastrointestinal illnesses (122). Symptoms of IBS include diarrhea, constipation, abdominal pain, bloating, gas, urgency to defecate, and a feeling of incomplete evacuation after a bowel movement (122). Certain foods and beverages may aggravate symptoms. Some common instigators are fried, fatty and spicy foods; alcohol and caffeine; chocolate; carbonated liquids; dairy products with lactose; sweeteners like sorbitol; wheat products; beans, broccoli and cabbage. Medications and vitamins can also be irritants. Doctors recommend increasing fiber or taking supplements like psyllium (108,110).

Studies have shown that IBS affects 7 to 10 percent of individuals worldwide and its symptoms are reported by 12 percent of Americans. Women are three times more likely than men to develop IBS, and most IBS sufferers experience their first symptoms before their mid-thirties (111).

Gastrointestinal Reflux Disease

Gastroesophageal reflux disease, or GERD, is a chronic condition in which the lower esophageal sphincter allows gastric acids to reflux into the esophagus, causing heartburn, acid indigestion, and possible injury to the esophageal lining. It affects an estimated 5% to 7% of the global population - men, women, and children. Heartburn and/or acid regurgitation experienced weekly has been found to occur in 19.8% of individuals (113-115).

Persistent heartburn is the most frequent, but not the only, symptom of GERD. (The disease may be present even without apparent symptoms.) Although common, GERD often is unrecognized - its symptoms misunderstood. This is unfortunate because it is generally a treatable disease. Serious complications can result if it is not treated properly such as esophageal ulcers, bleeding, loss of dentition, (113-115).

Heartburn is so common that it often is not associated with GERD. All too often, GERD is either self- treated or mistreated (113-115). Treatment usually must be maintained on a long-term basis, even after symptoms disappear. Various methods to treat the disease range from lifestyle measures to the use of medication or surgical procedures. It is essential for individuals who suffer persistent heartburn or other chronic and recurrent symptoms to seek an accurate diagnosis and work with their physician, and to receive the most effective treatment available (113-115). In general, decrease citrus, chocolate, caffeine, mints, spicy foods, fried foods, high fat foods. Other lifestyle changes: exercise, weight loss if necessary, loose fitting clothing, and elevating the head of the bed may help decrease symptoms.

GI Disorders and Physical Activity

Light and moderate exercise is well tolerated and can benefit patients with inflammatory bowel disease and liver disease (156). Physical activity can also improve gastric emptying and lower the relative risk of colon cancer. Severe, exhaustive exercise, however, inhibits gastric emptying, interferes with gastrointestinal absorption, and causes many gastrointestinal symptoms, most notably gastrointestinal bleeding (156).

Chronic Kidney Disease

Chronic kidney disease, or kidney failure, is more common than diabetes - 1 in 7 people have CKD (157). Uncontrolled or prolong diabetes and hypertension are the leading causes, however, obstructions, infections, genetics, race and age are contributors as well. CKD is often known as a silent killer in that the majority of people with kidney failure are unaware and experience common everyday symptoms such weakness, fatigue, loss of appetite, trouble concentrating, swelling, difficulty sleeping and more frequent urination, especially at night (157,158).

CKD is diagnosed through scans, biopsies, and urine and laboratory testing. CKD presents in 5 stages which correlate with a glomerular filtration rate (GFR) or percent kidney function based on blood creatintine levels, age, race and gender (157, 158). A person with normal kidney function can have a GFR or 90-100+ percent. If CKD is diagnosed early dietary and lifestyle interventions can delay or slow down the rate of kidney failure. See the following table.

Stage	GFR	Description
Stage 1	>/=90	Kidney damage, protein in the urine and normal GFR. Assess risk factors: diabetes, hypertension, family history, older age and ethnicity.
Stage 2	60 – 89	Kidney damage and mild decrease in GFR. Have frequent screenings to monitor kidney function.
Stage 3	30-59	Moderate decrease in GFR. May have altered electrolyte levels and require dietary modifications.
Stage 4	15-29	Severe decrease in GFR. Plan for kidney failure treatments.
Stage 5	<15	Renal Replacement Therapy: dialysis or transplant, or end of life planning. Strict renal diet is necessary.

As kidney failure progresses, dietary changes are required to compensate for the reduce excretion of certain nutrients such as protein, potassium, sodium, fluid and phosphorus. These dietary adjustments are laboratory result driven requiring close monitoring by a physician and/or a dietitian (160).

Protein

As kidney disease progress, protein intake may need to be decreased to prevent protein waste from stressing the kidneys. It is important to work with a physician and dietitian to determine exact protein needs.

Potassium

The kidneys are responsible for excreting excess potassium. In kidney disease, potassium levels in the blood can be dangerously low or high. Altered potassium levels in the blood can cause heart arrhythmias. People with kidney disease should consider blood potassium levels before adding high potassium foods such as bananas, melons, dried fruits, oranges, potatoes, avocados, tomatoes, milk and yogurt, salt substitutes and dried beans and peas to the diet.

Sodium

High sodium diets can increase fluid retention causing increases in blood pressure and swelling, which can further kidney damage. Sodium intake should be limited to the American Heart Association guidelines of 1500-2500mg sodium per day.

Fluid

Many people with kidney disease do not need to limit fluid intake. As kidney disease progresses, urine production may decrease requiring limited fluids. The amount of fluid consumed should be individualized.

Phosphorus

Kidneys are involved in bone building process by regulating phosphorus levels in the blood. High phosphorus levels as found in people with kidney disease can increase the risk of chronic kidney disease related mineral bone disease causing calcium to build up in blood vessels, heart, joints, muscles and skin. Dietary phosphates should be limited. Foods high in phosphorus include: dark colas, some powdered drink mixes, brewer's yeast, chocolate, processed meats, dairy products, nuts and nut butter, and dried beans and peas.

Summary

The history of nutrition and health research spans more than five decades. Research in population-based epidemiological studies has helped to clarify some of the roles of diet in preventing and controlling death and disease relating to dietary and lifestyle changes.

Diabetes is widely recognized as one of the leading causes of death and disability in the United States. In 2005–2008, based on fasting glucose or hemoglobin A1c levels, 35% of U.S. adults aged 20 years or older had prediabetes (50% of adults aged 65 years or older). Applying this percentage to the entire U.S. population (2010) yields an estimated 79 million American adults aged 20 years or older with prediabetes. Diabetes is the leading cause of kidney failure, non-traumatic lower-limb amputations, and new cases of blindness among adults in the United States. Diabetes is a major cause of heart disease and stroke. Diabetes is the seventh leading cause of death in the United States. Increases in diabetes among US adults continue in both sexes, all ages, all races, all educational levels, and all smoking levels. The three main types of diabetes include Type 1 diabetes, Type 2 diabetes, and gestational diabetes. The fasting plasma glucose test is the preferred test for diagnosing type 1 or type 2 diabetes (4). It is most reliable when done in the morning. However, a diagnosis of diabetes can be made after positive results on any one of three tests, with confirmation from a second positive test on a different day. The Diabetes Prevention Program (DPP), a landmark study sponsored by the National Institutes of Health, found that people at increased risk for type 2 diabetes can prevent or delay the onset of the disease by losing 5 to 7 percent of their body weight through increased physical activity and a reduced fat and lower calorie diet.

Cardiovascular disease refers to the class of diseases that involve the heart or blood vessels (arteries and veins). While the term technically refers to any disease that affects the cardiovascular system, it is usually used to refer to those related to atherosclerosis (arterial disease). These conditions have similar causes, mechanisms, and treatments. Atherosclerosis is a condition in which an artery wall thickens as a result of the accumulation of fatty materials such as cholesterol and triglyceride (29). It is a syndrome affecting arterial blood vessels, a chronic inflammatory response in the walls of arteries, caused largely by the accumulation of macrophage white blood cells and promoted by low-density lipoproteins (LDL, plasma proteins that carry cholesterol and triglycerides) without adequate removal of fats and cholesterol from the macrophages by functional high-density lipoproteins (HDL). It is commonly referred to as a hardening or furring of the arteries. It is caused by the formation of multiple plaques within the arteries.

Cholesterol levels correlate with risk of heart disease, with two fold increase in risk between patients with cholesterol levels <180 mg/dl compared to individuals with cholesterol levels >240 mg/dl.

Modern medicine has never been able to explain why some 45—60 percent of patients with hospital admissions for a heart attack have a *"normal level"* of cholesterol (23,48). Even individuals with low-to-normal cholesterol levels are at great risk for a cardiovascular event (23-48). Intensive research is under way to investigate the molecules known to be involved in the process of plaque formation. Intensive research is under way to investigate the molecules known to be involved in the process of plaque formation. Three to four million individuals are taking cholesterol-lowering drugs, and debates on the effectiveness of these medications continue (42). No studies have shown statin cholesterol-lowering drugs to be effective for women at any age, nor for men 69 years of age or older, who do not already have heart disease or diabetes.

Scientists have long known that eating red meat increases a person's chances of developing heart disease. One way physicians gauge risk is with blood tests for cholesterol but tests for cholesterol and other molecules don't wholly explain meat's link to heart disease, Hazen says. "Cholesterol, saturated fat and salt only account for a small amount of the risk". Gut bacteria might account for more. In his study, Hazen investigated L-carnitine because the nutrient is structurally similar to a compound that gut microbes can convert to TMAO. Omnivorous human subjects produced more TMAO than did vegans or vegetarians following ingestion of l-carnitine through a microbiota-dependent mechanism. Intestinal microbiota may thus contribute to the well-established link between high levels of red meat consumption and CVD risk.

A molecule called homocysteine has received a lot of attention. Homocysteine is a non-protein, naturally occurring amino acid found in blood plasma. A high level of homocysteine is a powerful risk factor for cardiovascular disease. It is believed to increase the chance of heart disease, stroke, Alzheimer's disease, and osteoporosis. Homocysteine is broken down in the body through two metabolic pathways. The chemical changes that must occur to break down homocysteine require the presence of folic acid (also called folate) and vitamins B^6 and B^{12}. C-reactive protein (CRP) is one of the acute phase proteins that increase during systemic inflammation. It's been suggested that testing CRP levels in the blood may be an additional way to assess cardiovascular disease risk. A more sensitive CRP test, called a highly sensitive C-reactive protein (hs-CRP) assay, is available to determine heart disease risk. Coronary calcium scoring has become a common test for cardiovascular risk determination. A coronary calcium scan produces a calcium score called an Agatston score. The score is based on the amount of calcium found in the coronary arteries. Scores can be obtained for each major artery and a total score.

Hypertension is a major risk factor for stroke, myocardial infarction (heart attacks), heart failure, aneurysms of the arteries, peripheral arterial disease, and is a cause of chronic kidney disease. Dietary and lifestyle changes can improve blood pressure control and decrease the risk of associated health complications, although drug treatment is often necessary in people for whom lifestyle changes prove ineffective or insufficient. The initial Dash study (Dietary Approaches to Stop Hypertension, 1997) was one of the first large research studies that looked at the effects of entire diet, not supplements, on hypertension. The same researchers published results from a second study known as the Dash-Sodium study. The results were startling. The DASH diet with lowest sodium intake cut blood pressure by an impressive 8.9 points in systolic pressure and 4.5 points in diastolic pressure when compared to the usual diet with the higher sodium intake. Researchers of a 2011 meta-analysis examined the effect of a Mediterranean diet on metabolic syndrome reported that a Mediterranean diet is associated with lower blood pressure, blood sugar, and triglycerides. A meta-analysis published in 2013 compared Mediterranean, vegan, vegetarian, low-glycemic index, low-carbohydrate, high-fiber, and high-protein diets with control diets. The research concluded that Mediterranean, low-carbohydrate, low-glycemic index, and high-protein diets are effective in improving markers of risk for cardiovascular disease and diabetes.

In the US, over 700,000 strokes occur every year and are responsible for 165,000 deaths annually. Stroke is the second leading cause of death worldwide. A stroke occurs when a clot blocks the blood supply to part of the brain or when a blood vessel in or around the brain bursts. In either case, parts of the brain become damaged or die.

All cancers caused by cigarette smoking and heavy use of alcohol could be prevented completely. The American Cancer Society estimates that, in 2013, about 174,100 cancer deaths will be caused by tobacco use. The World Cancer Research Fund estimates that about one-quarter to one-third of the new cancer cases expected to occur in the US in 2013 will be related to overweight or obesity, physical inactivity, and poor nutrition.

Gastrointestinal Disorders (GI) are digestive disorders that interfere with the workings of the intestine. GI generally fall into two categories — functional and inflammatory. Celiac disease is a chronic inflammatory condition caused by ingestion of dietary gluten. This inflammation can cause malabsorption of several nutrients, which in turn is related to several deficiency disorders, such as anemia, cancer, and osteoporosis. Gluten is a protein found in wheat, rye, and barley. A gluten-free diet is the only current treatment. Crohn's disease causes abdominal pain, diarrhea (which may be bloody if inflammation is at its worst), vomiting (can be continuous), or weight loss but may also cause complications outside the gastrointestinal tract such as skin rashes, arthritis, inflammation of the eye, tiredness, and lack of concentration. There are no known foods that cause Crohn's disease and there are no consistent dietary rules to follow that will improve a person's symptoms (121). However, when people are suffering a flare in disease, foods such as bulky grains, hot spices, alcohol, and milk products may increase diarrhea and cramping (107). No special diet has been proven effective for prevention, but it is very important that people who have Crohn's disease follow a nutritious diet and avoid any foods that seem to worsen symptoms. Ulcerative colitis has similarities to Crohn's disease and is another form of IBD. It is an intermittent disease, with periods of exacerbated symptoms, and periods that are relatively symptom-free.

Gastroesophageal reflux disease, or GERD, is a chronic condition in which the lower esophageal sphincter allows gastric acids to reflux into the esophagus, causing heartburn, acid indigestion, and possible injury to the esophageal lining. Persistent heartburn is the most frequent - but not the only - symptom of GERD. The disease may be present even without apparent symptoms. A healthy weight can lessen the symptoms of GERD. With the rise of incidences of diabetes and hypertension, chronic kidney disease is becoming more and more popular. Diet and lifestyle changes to better manage diabetes and hypertension can less the risk of developing chronic kidney disease. Improving dietary habits for people with chronic kidney disease can slow the progression of the disease and delay the need for renal replacement therapy.

Physical activity can lower blood glucose levels rapidly. Insulin sensitivity is increased causing cells to better use available insulin to take up glucose. Also, when muscle contract during exercise, it stimulates cells to take up more glucose for energy independent of insulin activity. These short term lowering of blood glucose levels can cause a person to have hypoglycemia, or low blood glucose levels. People with diabetes should check blood glucose levels prior to and after exercising. To prevent hypoglycemia during exercise (140): Eat regular meals; have a snack 30 minutes to 2 hours post exercise; check blood glucose levels during strenuous activity or prolonged activity; if blood glucose levels are uncontrolled during exercise, discuss other meal plan changes or possible medication changes with healthcare provider.

Regular exercise has a favorable effect on many of the established risk factors for cardiovascular disease. For example, exercise promotes weight reduction and can help reduce blood pressure. Exercise can reduce "bad" cholesterol levels in the blood (the low-density lipoprotein [LDL] level), as well as total cholesterol, and can raise the "good" cholesterol (the high-density lipoprotein level [HDL]). In diabetic patients, regular activity favorably affects the body's ability to use insulin to control glucose levels in the blood. Although the effect of an exercise program on any single risk factor may generally be small, the effect of continued, moderate exercise on overall cardiovascular risk, when combined with other lifestyle modifications (such as proper nutrition, smoking cessation, and medication use), can be dramatic (142).

Epidemiological studies indicate that the relationship between sedentary behavior and hypertension is so strong that the National Heart Foundation, (153) the World Health Organization and International Society of Hypertension (155), the United States Joint National Committee on Detection, Evaluation and Treatment of High Blood Pressure, (154) and the American College of Sports Medicine (ACSM)(151) have all recommended increased physical activity as a first line intervention for preventing and treating patients with prehypertension and hypertension. Physical activity is particularly appealing because it has favorable effects on other cardiovascular disease (CVD) risk factors.

There is convincing evidence that physical activity is associated with a reduced risk of cancers of the colon and breast (143). Several studies also have reported links between physical activity and a reduced risk of cancers of the prostate, lung, and lining of the uterus (endometrial cancer). Colorectal cancer has been one of the most extensively studied cancers in relation to physical activity, with more than 50 studies examining this association (143). Many studies have consistently found that adults who increase their physical activity, either in intensity, duration, or frequency, can reduce their risk of developing colon cancer by 30 to 40 percent compared to those who are sedentary regardless of body mass index (BMI), with the greatest risk reduction seen among those who are most active (144-148)). It is estimated that 30 to 60 minutes of moderate to vigorous physical activity per day is needed for a protective effect (147,148). Physical activity may protect against colon cancer and tumor development through its role in energy balance, hormone metabolism, insulin regulation, and by decreasing the time the colon is exposed to potential carcinogens. Physical activity has also been found to alter a number of inflammatory and immune factors, some of which may influence colon cancer risk (143).

Chronic kidney disease, or kidney failure, is more common than diabetes - 1 in 7 people have CKD (157). Uncontrolled or prolong diabetes and hypertension are the leading causes, however, obstructions, infections, genetics, race and age are contributors as well. CKD is often known as a silent killer in that the majority of people with kidney failure are unaware and experience common everyday symptoms such weakness, fatigue, loss of appetite, trouble concentrating, swelling, difficulty sleeping and more frequent urination, especially at night (157,158). CKD is diagnosed through scans, biopsies, and urine and laboratory testing. CKD presents in 5 stages which correlate with a glomerular filtration rate (GFR) or percent kidney function based on blood creatintine levels, age, race and gender (157, 158). A person with normal kidney function can have a GFR or 90-100+ percent. If CKD is diagnosed early dietary and lifestyle interventions can delay or slow down the rate of kidney failure.

Chapter 6 Sample Test

1. What are the factors associated with all types of diabetes including diagnoses and prevention?
2. Describe the association of exercise and diabetes.
3. What are the factors involved in cardiovascular disease including cholesterol, cholesterol lowering medications, L-carnitine, homocysteine, high sensitivity reactive protein, and coronary calcium scan?
4. Describe the association of exercise and cardiovascular disease.
5. Discuss hypertension, including diets associated with reducing hypertension.
6. Describe the association of hypertension and exercise.
7. What are the factors involved with stroke?
8. Describe the association of stroke and exercise.
9. What are the factors involved in cancer risk?
10. Describe the association of cancer and exercise.
11. Define and discuss gastrointestinal disorders?
12. Define the stages of kidney disease and discuss the factors associated with the disease.

References

1. WHO Library Cataloguing-in-Publication Data Joint WHO/FAO Expert Consultation on Diet, Nutrition and the Prevention of Chronic Diseases. (2002).Diet, nutrition and the prevention of chronic diseases: report of a joint WHO/FAO expert consultation, Geneva.
2. Cowie CC, et al. (2009). Full accounting of diabetes and prediabetes in the U.S. population in 1988–1994 and 2005–2006. *Diabetes Care* ;32:287–294.
3. Cowie CC. Rust KF. Byrd-Holt DD. Gregg EW. Ford ES. Geiss LS. Bainbridge KE. Fradkin JE. (2010). Prevalence of diabetes and high risk for diabetes using A1C criteria in the U.S. population in 1988–2006. *Diabetes Care.* 33:562–568.
4. The Expert Committee on the Diagnosis and Classification of Diabetes Mellitus. (2011). Report of the Expert Committee on the Diagnosis and Classification of Diabetes Mellitus. *Diabetes Care.* 34(Suppl. 1):S66–S68. Available at http://care.diabetesjournals.org/content/34/Supplement_1/S62.full.pdf+html
5. National Diabetes Fact Sheet. (2011). Centers for Disease Control. http://www.cdc.gov/diabetes/pubs/factsheet11.htm.
6. Diabetes Prevention Program (DPP) Research Group. (2002). The Diabetes Prevention Program (DPP): description of lifestyle intervention. *Diabetes Care*. 25:2165–2171.
7. Bridget B. Kelly; Institute of Medicine; Fuster, Valentin (2010). *Promoting Cardiovascular Health in the Developing World: A Critical Challenge to Achieve Global Health*. Washington, D.C: National Academies Press.
8. Yusuf S. Hawken S. Ounpuu S, *et al.* (2004). Effect of potentially modifiable risk factors associated with myocardial infarction in 52 countries (the INTERHEART study): case-control study. *Lancet* 364 (9438): 937–52.
9. Whitney, E & Rolfes S. (2013). *Understanding Nutrition,*13th ed. Belmont, CA: Wadsworth, Cengage Learnin (107-108,141-150,586-606)).
10. Ross, C, (Shils) et al. (2012). *Modern Nutrition in Health & Disease, 11th ed.* Philadelphia PA: Lipincott Wilillians & Wilikins (808-875,1069-1095,1171-1193).
11. Lehninger, A. (2013). *Principles of Biochemistry, 6th ed* NY: W H Freeman and Company.
12. Bloomgarden ZT. (2004). Type 2 diabetes in the young: the evolving epidemic. *Diabetes Care.* 27(4):998–1010.
13. Kochanek KD. Xu JQ. Murphy SL. Miniño AM. Kung HC. (2011). Deaths: final data for 2009. *National vital statistics reports*. 60(3).
14. Roger VL. Go AS. Lloyd-Jones DM, et al. (2012). Heart disease and stroke statistics—2012 update: a report from the American Heart Association. *Circulation*. 125(1):e2–220.
15. Heidenreich PA. Trogdon JG. Khavjou OA, et al. (2011). Forecasting the future of cardiovascular disease in the United States: a policy statement from the American Heart Association. *Circulation*. 123:933-44. Epub 2011 Jan 24.
16. CDC. Million Hearts: strategies to reduce the prevalence of leading cardiovascular disease risk factors. United States. (2011). *MMWR*2011;60(36):1248–51.
17. Ignarro LJ. Balestrieri ML. Napoli C. (2007). Nutrition, physical activity, and cardiovascular disease: an update.. *Cardiovascular research.* 73 (2): 326–40.
18. World Heart Federation (2011). World Heart Federation: Cardiovascular disease risk factors. http://www.world-heart-federation.org/cardiovascular-health/cardiovascular-disease-risk-factors/hypertension/.
19. The National Heart, Lung, and Blood Institute (NHLBI). (2011). How To Prevent and Control Coronary Heart Disease Risk Factors - NHLBI, NIH.http://www.nhlbi.nih.gov/health/health-topics/topics/hd/prevent.html.
20. Lonn E. Yusuf S. Arnold MJ. Sheridan P Pogue. Micks M. McQueen MJ. Probstfield J, et al. (2006). Homocysteine Lowering with Folic Acid and B Vitamins in Vascular Disease (PDF). *N*

Engl J Med 354 (15): 1567–77.

21. Ridker, P. (2013). C-Reactive Protein: A Simple Test to Help Predict Risk of Heart Attack and Stroke. Cardiology Patient Page. http://circ.ahajournals.org/content/108/12/e81.full. (accessed 06/12/2013).
22. Cademartir F. (2006). Is calcium the key for the assessment of progression/regression of coronary artery disease? *Heart.* 92(9):1187-1188.
23. Dzugan SA. Smith RA. (2002). Hypercholesterolemia treatment: a new hypothesis or just an accident? *Med Hypotheses.* Volume 59, Issue 6, 12. Pages 751–756.
24. Seely, S. (1991). Is calcium excess in western diet a major cause of arterial disease? *Int J Cardiol.* 33(2):191-198.
25. National Heart Lung and Blood Institute. Diseases and Conditions Index. Coronary Calcium Scan. http://www.nhlbi.nih.gov/health//dci/Diseases/cscan/cscan_whatdoes.html. (Accessed June 12, 2013).
26. Klatsky AL. (2009). Alcohol and cardiovascular diseases. *Expert Rev Cardiovasc Ther* **7** (5): 499–506.
27. McTigue KM. Hess R. Ziouras J. (2006). Obesity in older adults: a systematic review of the evidence for diagnosis and treatment. *Obesity (Silver Spring)* 14 (9): 1485–97.
28. Linden W. Stossel C. Maurice J. (April 1996). Psychosocial interventions for patients with coronary artery disease: a meta-analysis. *Arch. Intern. Med.* 156 (7): 745–52.
29. Maton A. Roshan L. Hopkins J. McLaughlin CW, et al. (1993). *Human Biology and Health.* Englewood Cliffs, NJ: Prentice Hall.
30. Ross R. (1993). The pathogenesis of atherosclerosis: a perspective for the 1990s. *Nature* 362 (6423): 801–9.
31. Ross R.(1999). Atherosclerosis — An Inflammatory Disease. *New England Journal of Medicine* 340 (2): 115–26.
32. Finn AV. Nakano M. Narula J. Kolodgie FD. Virmani R (2010). Concept of vulnerable/unstable plaque. *Arterioscler. Thromb. Vasc. Biol.* 30 (7): 1282–92.
33. Didangelos A. Simper D. Monaco C. Mayr M. (2009). Proteomics of acute coronary syndromes. *Current atherosclerosis reports* 11 (3): 188–95.
34. Executive Summary of Third report of the National Cholesterol Education Program (NCEP) expert panel on detection, evaluation, and treatment of high blood cholesterol in adults (adult treatment panel III). (2002). The National Heart, Lung, and Blood Institute.
35. Third Report of the Expert Panel on Detection, Evaluation, and Treatment of High Blood Cholesterol in Adults (Adult Treatment Panel III)
36. Third Report of the Expert Panel on Detection, Evaluation, and Treatment of High Blood Cholesterol in Adults (Adult Treatment Panel III).http://www.nhlbi.nih.gov/guidelines/cholesterol/index.htm. (accessed May 31, 2012).
37. What is cholesterol? National Heart, Lung, and Blood Institute. http://www.nhlbi.nih.gov/health/health-topics/topics/hbc/. (accessed May 31, 2012).
38. Information about the Update of the Adult Treatment Panel III Guidelines. National Cholesterol Education Program. (2004). http://www.nhlbi.nih.gov/guidelines/cholesterol/upd-info_prof.htm.
39. Koeth RA, et al. (2013). Intestinal microbiota metabolism of l-carnitine, a nutrient in red meat, promotes atherosclerosis. *Nat Med.* 19(5):576-85. doi: 10.1038/nm.3145. Epub 2013 Apr 7.
40. Z. Wang, et al. 2011. Gut flora metabolism of phosphatidylcholine promotes cardiovascular disease. *Nature.* Vol. 472: 57.
41. Marshall, IJ. Wolfe CD. McKevitt C. (2012). Lay perspectives on hypertension and drug adherence: systematic review of qualitative research. *BMJ (Clinical research ed.)* 345: e3953.
42. Dickinson HO. Mason JM. Nicolson DJ. Campbell F. Beyer FR. Cook JV. Williams B. Ford GA. (2006). Lifestyle interventions to reduce raised blood pressure: a systematic review of

randomized controlled trials. *Journal of hypertension* 24 (2): 215–33.

43. Abramson J. Wright JM. (2007). Are lipid-lowering guidelines evidence-based?. *Lancet.* 369: 168-169.
44. Martí-Carvajal AJ. Solà I. Lathyris D. Salanti G. (2009). Homocysteine lowering interventions for preventing cardiovascular events. Cochrane Database of Systematic Reviews 2009, Issue 4. Art. No.: CD006612. DOI: 10.1002/14651858.CD006612.pub2.
45. Danesh J. Wheeler JG. Hirschfield GM. Eda S. Eiriksdottir G. Rumley A. Lowe GD. Pepys MB. Gudnason V. (2004). C-reactive protein and other circulating markers of inflammation in the prediction of coronary heart disease. *N. Engl. J. Med.* 350 (14): 1387–97.
46. Koenig W. (2006). C-reactive protein - a critical cardiovascular risk marker. CRPhealth.com.
47. Cademartir F. (2006). Is calcium the key for the assessment of progression/regression of coronary artery disease? *Heart.* 92(9):1187-1188.
48. Kummerow FA, et al. (2000). The relationship of oxidized lipids to coronary artery stenosis. *Atherosclerosis* 149 (1):181—190.
49. Inflammation, Heart Disease and Stroke: The Role of C-Reactive Protein. (2008). http://www.americanheart.org/presenter.jhtml?identifier=4648. Jan, 2008.
50. Chobanian AV. Bakris GL. Black HR, et al. (2003). Seventh report of the Joint National Committee on Prevention, Detection, Evaluation, and Treatment of High Blood Pressure. *Hypertension* 42 (6):1206–52.
51. Achieving better blood pressure control. (2010). Published in *NPS Prescribing Practice Review.* http://www.nps.org.au/publications/health-professional/prescribing-practice-review/2010/prescribing-practice-review-52.
52. National Heart Foundation of Australia. (2006). Position Statement: The relationships between dietary electrolytes and cardiovascular disease. National Heart Foundation.
53. North of England Hypertension Guideline Development Group. (2004). Essential hypertension: Managing adult patients in primary care. Newcastle upon Tyne: University of Newcastle upon Tyne.
54. National High Blood Pressure Education Program. The Seventh Report of the Joint National Committee on prevention, detection, evaluation, and treatment of high blood pressure. Bethesda: US Department of Health and Human Services, 2003. (accessed 23 July 2010).
55. He FJ. MacGregor GA. Z(2004). Effect of longer-term modest salt reduction on blood pressure. Cochrane Database. *Syst Rev.* CD004937.
56. Capatti A. et al., *Italian Cuisine: A Cultural History*, p. 106.
57. Kushi LH. Lenart EB. Willett WC. (1995). Health implications of Mediterranean diets in light of contemporary knowledge. 1. Plant foods and dairy products. *Am J Clin Nutr.* 61(6 Suppl):1407S-1415S.
58. Kushi LH. Lenart EB. Willett WC. (1995). Health implications of Mediterranean diets in light of contemporary knowledge. 1. Plant foods and dairy products. *Am J Clin Nutr.* 61(6 Suppl):1407S-1415S.
59. Willett WC. (2006). The Mediterranean diet: science and practice. *Public Health Nutr* (1A):105-10.
60. Fung TT. Rexrode KM. Mantzoros CS. Manson JE. Willett WC. Hu FB. (2009). Mediterranean diet and incidence of and mortality from coronary heart disease and stroke in women. *Circulation.* 3;119(8):1093-100.
61. Kastorini CM. Milionis H. Esposito K. Giugliano D Goudevenos J. Panagiotakos D. (2011). "The Effect of Mediterranean Diet on Metabolic Syndrome and its Components". *Journal of the American College of Cardiology* 57 (11):1299–1313
62. Ajala O English P. Pinkney J. (2013). Systematic review and meta-analysis of different dietary approaches to the management of type 2 diabetes. *The American Journal of Clinical Nutrition* 97 (3):505–516.
63. Heller M (2007). *The DASH Diet Action Plan: Based on the National Institutes of Health*

Research, Dietary Approaches to Stop Hypertension. Deerfield, IL: Amidon Press.

64. Moore T, et al. (2001). *The DASH Diet for Hypertension*. New York: Simon & Schuster.
65. Estruch, Ramón et al. (2013). Primary Prevention of Cardiovascular Disease with a Mediterranean Diet. *New England Journal of Medicine*. NEJMoa1200303. Retrieved February 25, 2013.
66. Miniño AM, et al. (2011). Deaths: Final data for 2008 [PDF-2.9M]. *National Vital Statistics Reports*; vol 59 no 10. Hyattsville, MD: National Center for Health Statistics.
67. National Institute of Neurological Disorders and Stroke. National Institutes of Health. NIH Publication No. 11-3440b. http://www.ninds.nih.gov/disorders/stroke/preventing_stroke.htm.
68. Department of Health and Aging. Reduce your risk: new national guidelines for alcohol consumption. Canberra: Australian Government, 2009. (accessed 12 April,2013).
69. Appel, LJ, et al. (1997). Clinical trial of the effects of dietary patterns on blood pressure. DASH Collaborative Research Group. *N Eng J Med,* 336:1117.
70. Conlin PR, et al. (2000). The effect of dietary patterns on blood pressure control in hypertensive patients. *Am J Hyperten:*13(9):945.
71. Steinmertz KA, et al. (1996). Vegetable, fruit and cancer prevention: A review. *J of the Am Dietetic Assoc,* 96:1027-39.
72. Sacks FM, et al. (1995). "Rationale and design of the Dietary Approaches to Stop Hypertension trial (DASH)". *Annals of Epidemiology* (Elsevier) 5 (2): 108–118.
73. Lloyd JD. Adams R. Carnethon M, et al. (2009). Heart disease and stroke statistics—2009 update. A report from the American Heart Association Statistics Committee and Stroke Statistics Subcommittee. *Circulation.* 119:e21-e181.
74. American Cancer Society. Cancer Facts & Figures 2013. Atlanta: *American Cancer Society*. 2013.
75. Zhu L. Pickle LW. Naishadham D, et al. (2012). Predicting US and state-level cancer counts for the current calendar year: part II – evaluation of spatio-temporal projection methods for incidence. *Cancer.* 118(4): 1100-9.
76. Copeland G, Lake A, Firth R, et al. (eds). (2012). Cancer in North America: 2005-2009. Volume Two:Registry-specific Cancer Incidence in the United States and Canada. Springfield, IL: North American Association of Central Cancer Registries, Inc. naaccr.org/Dataand Publications/CINAPubs.aspx.
77. Howlader N. Krapcho M. Neyman N, et al. (2012). SEER Cancer Statistics Review, 1975-2009. *National Cancer Institute.* Bethesda, MD.
78. Chen HS. Portier K. Ghosh K, et al. (2012). Predicting US and State-level counts for the current calendar year: part I – evaluation of temporal projection methods for mortality. *Cancer.* 118(4):1091-9.
79. Ciclitiria, P.J. (2003). Recent advances in celiac disease. *Clinical Medicine*. 3(2);166-169.
80. Abdulkarim AS & Murray JA. (2003). Review article: the diagnosis of celiac disease. *Aliment Pharmacol Ther.*17;987-995.
81. American Dietetic Association: Hot topics: gluten-free diets www.eatright.org/search.aspx? Dec. 2009.
82. Food Labeling Guidance Regulatory Information (gluten-free). http://www.fda.gov/Food/LabelingNutrition/FoodLabelingGuidanceRegulatoryInformation/Topic-SpecificLabelingInformation/ucm265309.htm. Accessed Sept. 8, 2011
83. Rossi TM. Albini CH. Kumar V. (1993). Incidence of celiac disease identified by the presence of serum endomysial antibodies in children with chronic diarrhea, short stature, or insulin-dependent diabetes mellitus. *J Pediatr.* 123(2): 262–4.
84. Tumer L. Hasanoglu A. Aybay C. (2001). Endomysium antibodies in the diagnosis of celiac disease in short-statured children with no gastrointestinal symptoms. *Pediatr Int.* 43(1):71-3.
85. Groll A. Candy DC. Preece MA, et al. (1980). Short stature as the primary manifestation of celiac disease. *Lancet.* 2(8204): 1097–9.

86. Gemme G. Vignolo M. Naselli A, et al. (1999). Linear growth and skeletal maturation in subjects with treated celiac disease. *J Pediatr Gastroenterol Nutr.* 29(3): 339–42.
87. Martelossi S. Torre G. Zanatta M, et al. (1996). Dental enamel defects and screening for coeliac disease. *Pediatr Med Chir.* 18(6): 579–81.
88. Delco F. El-Serag HB. Sonnenberg A. (1999). Celiac sprue among US military veterans: associated disorders and clinical manifestations. *Dig Dis Sci.* 44(5): 966–72.
89. Carroccio A. Iannitto E. Cavataio F, et al. (1998). Sideropenic anemia and celiac disease: one study, two points of view. *Dig Dis Sci.* 43(3): 673–8.
90. Ackerman Z. Eliakim R. Stalnikowicz R, et al. (1996). Role of small bowel biopsy in the endoscopic evaluation of adults with iron deficiency anemia. *Am J Gastroenterol.* 91(10): 2099–102
91. Selby PL. Davies M. Adams JE, et al. (1999). Bone loss in celiac disease is related to secondary hyperparathyroidism. *J Bone Miner Res.* 14(4): 652–7.
92. Lindh E. Ljunghall S. Larsson K, et al. (1992). Screening for antibodies against gliadin in patients with osteoporosis. *J Intern Med.* 231(4): 403–6.
93. Molteni N. Bardella MT. Vezzoli G, et al. (1995). Intestinal calcium absorption as shown by stable strontium test in celiac disease before and after gluten-free diet. *Am J Gastroenterol.* 90(11): 2025–8.
94. Cellier C. Flobert C. Cormier C, et al. (2000). Severe osteopenia in symptom-free adults with a childhood diagnosis of celiac disease. *Lancet.* 355(9206): 806.
95. Vasquez H. Mazure R. Gonzalez D. et al. (2000). Risk of fractures in celiac disease patients: a cross-sectional, case–control study. *Am J Gastroenterol.* 95(1): 183–9.
96. Sategna-Guidetti C. Grosso SB. Grosso S, et al. (2000). The effects of 1-year gluten withdrawal on bone mass, bone metabolism and nutritional status in newly-diagnosed adult coeliac disease patients. Aliment *Pharmacol Ther.* 14(1): 35–43.
97. Corazza GR. Di Sario A,.Cecchetti L, et al. (1996). Influence of pattern of clinical presentation and of gluten-free diet on bone mass and metabolism in adult celiac disease. *Bone.*18(6): 525–30.
98. Schuppan D. (2000). Current concepts of celiac disease pathogenesis. *Gastroenterology.* 119(1);234-242.
99. Mowat I. (1998). Dietary modifications: food dependent autoimmunity in celiac disease. *Gut.* 43(5);599-600.
100. Feighery CF. (1998). Celiac disease: How much of what is toxic to whom? *Gut.* 43(2).164-5.
101. Barera G et al. (2000). Body composition in children with celiac disease and the effects of a gluten- free diet: a prospective case-control study". *Am J Clin Nutr.* 72.71-5.
102. Bateson MC. (2000). Advances in gastroenterology and hepatology. *Postgrad Med J.* 7;328- 332.
103. Mustalahti K, et al. (1999). Osteopenia in patients with clinically silent celiac disease warrants screening. *The Lancet.* 354(9180);744-5.
104. Capristo E et al. (2000). Changes in body composition, substrate oxidation, and resting metabolic rate in adult celiac disease patients after a 1-year gluten-free diet treatment. *Am J Clin Nutr.* 72; 76-81.
105. Kaukinen K, et al. (1999). Wheat starch- containing gluten-free flour products in the treatment of celiac disease and dermatitis herpetiformis. *Scand J Gastroenterol.* 34(2);163-9.
106. Thompson T. (2000). Questionable foods and the gluten-free diet: survey of current recommendations. *JADA.* 100(4);463-5.
107. Baumgart DC. Carding SR. (2007). Inflammatory bowel disease: cause and immunobiology. *The Lancet.* 369 (9573): 1627–40.
108. Baumgart DC. Sandborn WJ (2007). Inflammatory bowel disease: clinical aspects and

established and evolving therapies. *The Lancet.* 369 (9573): 1641–57.

109. Xavier RJ, Podolsky DK (2007). Unraveling the pathogenesis of inflammatory bowel disease.. *Nature* .448 (7152):427–34.
110. Irritable Bowel Syndrome. Bethesda, MD: The National Digestive Diseases Information Clearinghouse; 2007. NIH Publication No. 07-693.
111. Talley NJ. Irritable bowel syndrome. (2010). In: Feldman M, Friedman LS, Brandt LJ, eds. *Sleisenger & Fordtran's Gastrointestinal and Liver Disease.* 9th ed. Philadelphia, Pa: Saunders Elsevier;chap 118.
112. Sun-Young Lee, et al. (2007). Irritable Bowel Syndrome Is More Common in Women Regardless of the Menstrual Phase: A Rome II-based Survey. *J Korean Med Sci.* 22(5): 851–854. http://www.ncbi.nlm.nih.gov/pmc/articles/PMC2693852/
113. DeVault KR. Castell DO. (1999). Updated guidelines for the diagnosis and treatment of gastroesophageal reflux disease. The Practice Parameters Committee of the American College of Gastroenterology. *Am J Gastroenterol* 94 (6): 1434–42.
114. Hershcovici T. Fass R. (2011). Pharmacological management of GERD: where does it stand now?. *Trends in pharmacological sciences* 32 (4): 258–64.
115. Kahrilas, PJ, et al. (2008). American Gastroenterological Association Institute technical review on the management of gastroesophageal reflux disease. *Gastroenterology.* 135(4):1392-1413.
116. Danese S. & Fiocci C. (2011). Ulcerative colitis. The New England Journal of Medicine, 365:1713-1725.
117. Crohn BB. Ginzburg L. Oppenheimer, GD. (2000). Regional ileitis: A pathologic and clinical entity. 1932. *The Mount Sinai journal of medicine, New York* 67 (3): 263–8.
118. Baumgart. Daniel C. Sandborn William J. (2012). Crohn's disease. *The Lancet* 380 (9853): 1590–605.
119. Barrett J, et al. (2008). Genome-wide association defines more than 30 distinct susceptibility loci for Crohn's disease". *Nature Genetics* 40 (8): 955–62.
120. Cosnes J. (2004). Tobacco and IBD: Relevance in the understanding of disease mechanisms and clinical practice. *Best Practice & Research Clinical Gastroenterology* 18 (3): 481–96.
121. Pimentel M, et al. (2000). Identification of a prodromal period in Crohn's disease but not ulcerative colitis. *The American Journal of Gastroenterology* 95 (12):3458–62.
122. Evans J. Steinhart AH. Cohen, Z. McLeod, RS. (2003). Home Total Parenteral Nutrition an Alternative to Early Surgery for Complicated Inflammatory Bowel Disease. *Journal of Gastrointestinal Surgery.* 7 (4):562–6.
123. Brandt LJ, et al. (2009). An evidence-based position statement on the management of irritable bowel syndrome. *Am J Gastroenterology.* 104(suppl):S1-35.
124. Mediterranean Diet Pyramid. Oldways Health Through Heritage. http://oldwayspt.org/resources/heritage-pyramids/mediterranean-pyramid/overview. (accessed 06/13/2013).
125. Resolution WHA55.23. (2002). Diet, physical activity and health. In: Fifty-fifth World Health Assembly, Geneva, 13--18 May 2002. Volume 1. Resolutions and decisions, annexes Geneva, World Health Organization, 2002 (document WHA55/2002/REC/1):28-.3
126. Frei B. Oregon State University Linus Pauling Institute. Carnitine study: A response, April 2013). http://lpi.oregonstate.edu/news/CarnitineStudyResponse.html.
127. Li K, et. al. (2012). Associations of dietary calcium intake and calcium supplementation with myocardial infarction and stroke risk and overall cardiovascular mortality in the Heidelberg cohort of the European prospective investigation into cancer and nutrition study. *Heart* 98(12): 920-925.
128. Hemelrijck et al. (2013). Calicum intake and serum concentration in relation to risk of cardiovascular death in NHANES III. *PloS ONE* 8(4): e61037.
129. Ingall, T. (2004) Stroke-incidence, motallity, morbidity and risk. *J Insur Med* 36(2): 143-152.

130. National Institutes of Health. U.S. National Library of Medicine. Medline Plus. GERD. Heartburn. (accessed 08/07/2013). http://www.nlm.nih.gov/medlineplus/gerd.html.
131. Kung HC, Hoyert DL, Xu JQ, Murphy SL. (2008). Deaths: final data for 2005. National Vital Statistics Reports 2008;56(10). http://www.cdc.gov/nchs/data/nvsr/nvsr56/nvsr56_10.pdf.
132. Ogden CL, Carroll MD, McDowell MA, Flegal KM. (2007). Obesity among adults in the United States—no change since 2003–2004. NCHS data brief no 1. Hyattsville, MD: National Center for Health Statistics; 2007. Available from: http://www.cdc.gov/nchs/data/databriefs/db01.pdf.
133. Ogden CL, Carroll MD, Flegal KM. (2008). High body mass index for age among US children and adolescents, 2003–2006. JAMA. 299:2401–2405.
134. Centers for Disease Control and Prevention. Prevalence of self-reported physically active adults—United States, 2007. MMWR 2008;57:1297–1300. Available from: http://www.cdc.gov/mmwr/preview/mmwrhtml/mm5748a1.htm.
135. Mokdad AH, Marks JS, Stroup DF, Gerberding JL. (2004). Actual causes of death in the United States, 2000. JAMA 2004;291(10):1238–1245.
136. Centers for Disease Control and Prevention. Chronic diseases and health promotion. Updated August 13, 2012. (accessed 08/08/2013). http://www.cdc.gov/chronicdisease/overview/index.htm#ref1.
137. Centers for Disease Control and Prevention. Prevalence of doctor-diagnosed arthritis and arthritis-attributable activity limitation—United States, 2003–2005. MMWR 2006;55:1089–1092. http://www.cdc.gov/mmwr/preview/mmwrhtml/mm5540a2.htm.
138. Center for Disease Control (2006). *Morbidity and Mortality Weekly Report.* (accessed 08/08/2013). http://www.cdc.gov/diabetes/pubs/pdf/ndfs_2011.pdf.
139. Giuseppina Imperatore, James P. Boyle, Theodore J. Thompson, Doug Case, Dana Dabelea, Richard F. Hamman, Jean M. Lawrence, Angela D. Liese, Lenna L. Liu, Elizabeth J. Mayer-Davis, Beatriz L. Rodriguez, Debra Standiford, and for the SEARCH for Diabetes in Youth Study Group. Projections of Type 1 and Type 2 Diabetes Burden in the U.S. Population Aged <20 Years Through 2050: Dynamic modeling of incidence, mortality, and population growth *Diabetes Care December 2012 35:2515-2520; doi:10.2337/dc12-0669.*
140. American Diabetes Association. Blood glucose control and exercise. *Food and Fitness. (accessed 08/08/2013).* http://www.diabetes.org/food-and-fitness/fitness/get-started-safely/blood-glucose-control-and-exercise.html.
141. Symptoms of a heart attach. American Heart Association. (accessed 08/08/2013). http://www.heart.org/HEARTORG/Conditions/911-Warnings-Signs-of-a-Heart-Attack_UCM_305346_SubHomePage.jsp.
142. Myers, J. (2003). Exercise and cardiovascular disease. Circulation. 107:e2-e5. http://circ.ahajournals.org/content/107/1/e2.full.
143. National Institute of Health. National Cancer Institute. Physical activity and cancer. NIH Fact Sheet. (accessed 08/08/2013). http://www.cancer.gov/cancertopics/factsheet/prevention/physicalactivity.
144. Slattery, ML. Physical activity and colorectal cancer. *Sports Medicine* 2004; 34(4): 239–252.
145. IARC Handbooks of Cancer Prevention. *Weight Control and Physical Activity*. Vol. 6. 2002.
146. Ballard-Barbash R, Friedenreich C, Slattery M, Thune L. Obesity and body composition. In: Schottenfeld D, Fraumeni JF, editors. *Cancer Epidemiology and Prevention*. 3rd ed. New York: Oxford University Press, 2006.
147. Lee I, Oguma Y. Physical activity. In: Schottenfeld D, Fraumeni JF, editors. *Cancer Epidemiology and Prevention*. 3rd ed. New York: Oxford University Press, 2006.
148. McTiernan A, editor. *Cancer Prevention and Management Through Exercise and Weight Control*. Boca Raton: Taylor & Francis Group, LLC, 2006.
149. Tardon A, Lee WJ, Delgado-Rodriguez M, et al. Leisure-time physical activity and lung cancer: A meta-analysis. *Cancer Causes and Control* 2005; 16(4):389–397.

150. Giovannucci EL, Liu Y, Leitzmann MF, Stampfer MJ, Willett WC. A prospective study of physical activity and incident and fatal prostate cancer. *Archives of Internal Medicine* 2005; 165(9):1005–1010.
151. Pescatello LS, et al. (2004). American College of Sports Medicine position stand. Exercise and hypertension. Med Sci Sports Exerc. Mar;36(3):533-53.
152. Kokkinos, P, et al. (2000). Exercise and hypertension. Coronary Artery Disease. Vol 11:990102.
153. 5. Exercise is advocated for the Heart Foundation. Hypertension management guide for doctors. 2004, Heart Foundation. Available at: www.heartfoundation.com.au.
154. 6. Joint National Committee on Detection and Treatment of High Blood Pressure. The Sixth Report of the Joint National Committee on Detection, Evaluation, and Treatment of High Blood Pressure. Report V. Arch Intern Med 1997;157:2413–45.
155. 9. World Health Organization/International Society of Hypertension. Prevention of hypertension and associated cardiovascular disease: a 1991 statement. In: Clin Exp Hypertens 1992;333–41.
156. Bi L. Triadafilopoulos G. (2003). Exercise and gastrointestinal function and disease: an evidence-based review or risks and benefits.
157. Centers for Disease Control and Prevention. Diabetes Public Health Resource. National chronic kidney disease fact sheet 2010. (accessed 08/08/2013). http://www.cdc.gov/diabetes/pubs/factsheets/kidney.htm
158. National Kidney Foundation. About chronic kidney disease. (accessed 08/08/2013). http://www.kidney.org/kidneydisease/aboutckd.cfm.
159. The Academy of Nutrition and Dietetics. Evidence Analysis Library. Recommendation summary Chronic Kidney Disease (CKD). (accessed 08/08/2013). http://andevidencelibrary.com/topic.cfm?cat=3929&auth=1
160. National Kidney Disease education Program. Eating right for kidney health tips for people with chronic kidney disease (CKD). NIH publication 11-7405 http://nkdep.nih.gov/resources/eating-right-508.pdf.
161. U.S. Food and Drug Administration. FDA News Release. *FDA defines "gluten-free" for food labeling. (2013). (accessed 08/05/2013). http://www.fda.gov/NewsEvents/Newsroom/PressAnnouncements/UCM363474.htm.*

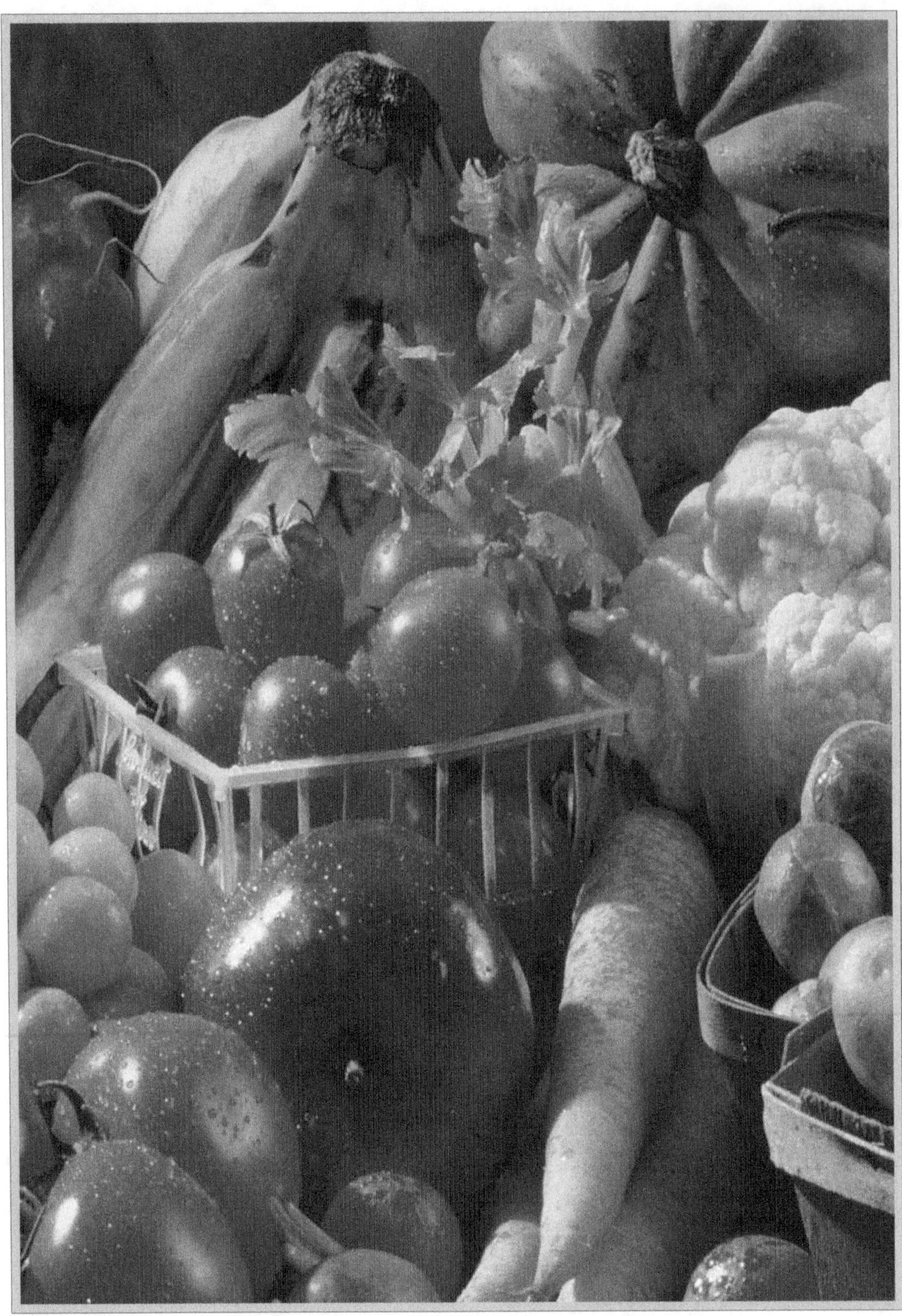

Chapter 7 - Vitamins

In this chapter we will take a more in-depth look at vitamins. Vitamins differ from the energy nutrients in that they are needed in smaller amounts: the energy nutrients are required in gram amounts, while the micronutrients are needed in milligram, microgram and picogram amounts. Vitamins do not provide energy, and they act singly, not as macromolecules. Vitamins include: vitamin A, vitamin C, vitamin D, vitamin E, vitamin K, vitamin B1 (thiamin), vitamin B2 (riboflavin, vitamin B3 (niacin), pantothenic acid, biotin, vitamin B6, vitamin B12, folate (folic acid).

Objectives

After reading and studying this session you should be able to:

1. Discuss water and fat soluble vitamins including roles, food sources, Dietary Reference Intakes, deficiencies, and toxicities.

Introduction

The term vitamin is derived from the root word "vita" meaning essential to life. Vitamins are a group of compounds other than protein, carbohydrates, or fats that cannot be manufactured by the body and are required in small amounts for specific functions of growth, maintenance, reproduction, and repair. They are organic, available in all foods, require no digestion, and are absorbed intact into the bloodstream (1).

The two major categories of vitamins are the water soluble vitamins and the fat soluble vitamins. The water soluble vitamins include all the B vitamins and vitamin C. The fat soluble vitamins are vitamin A, vitamin D, vitamin E, and vitamin K. The body absorbs water soluble vitamins directly into the blood, whereas fat soluble vitamins must be packaged and transported in lipoproteins. In the cells, water soluble vitamins freely circulate while fat soluble vitamins tend to become trapped in the cells associated with fat. Hence, the fat soluble vitamins tend to remain in fat storage sites, are less readily excreted, and more likely to reach toxic levels when consumed in excess (4).

Because vitamins are organic, they are susceptible to destruction by oxygen. The water soluble vitamins, thiamin, riboflavin, and vitamin C are the most vulnerable. Prolonged heating destroys much of these nutrients (1).

Dietary Reference Intakes were discussed in Chapter 1, but a quick review is included here. The *Recommended Dietary Allowance* (RDA) was developed during World War II by a committee established by the National Academy of Sciences in order to investigate issues of nutrition that might "affect national defense" (3). The Recommended Dietary Allowances (RDA) are standards set by scientists studying the individual nutrients and published by the government. These standards include a safety margin and are not "minimum" standards. *The Dietary Reference Intake* (DRI) is a system of nutrition recommendations from the Institute of Medicine (IOM) of the National Academy of Sciences. The DRI system is used by both the United States and Canada and is intended for the general public and health professionals. The current Dietary Reference Intake recommendation is composed of (11):

- Estimated Average Requirements (EAR), expected to satisfy the needs of 50% of the people in that age group based on a review of the scientific literature.
- Recommended Dietary Allowances (RDA), the daily dietary intake level of a nutrient considered sufficient by the Food and Nutrition Board to meet the requirements of 97.5% of healthy individuals in each life-stage and gender group. It is calculated based on the EAR and is usually approximately 20% higher than the EAR.
- Adequate Intake (AI), is where no RDA has been established and the amount

established is somewhat less firmly believed to be adequate for everyone in the demographic group.

- Tolerable upper intake levels (UL), cautions against excessive intake of nutrients (like vitamin A) that can be harmful in large amounts. This is the highest level of daily consumption that current data have shown to cause no side effects in humans when used indefinitely without medical supervision.

Water Soluble Vitamins

The following table summarizes the Dietary Reference Intake (DRI) or adequate intake (AI) for each of the B vitamins and vitamin C (9).

Vitamin	DRI (AI)*	Food Sources (2)	Deficiency	Tolerable Upper Limit
Thiamin, B1	1.2 mg/d men and 1.1 mg/d women	Brewers yeast,grains, whole grains, sunflower seeds, asparagus, potatoes, black-eyed peas, mushrooms, green leafy vegetables	Beriberi disease, damage of nervous system, muscle weakness, CV damage	None established
Riboflavin, B2	1.3 mg/d for men and 1.1 mg/d for women	Milk, milk products, mushrooms, green leafy vegetables, brewer's yeast	Accompanied by other deficiencies Inflammation of the mouth, skin, eyes and GI Tract	None established
Pantothenic Acid, B5	4 to 5 mg/day for adults (AI)	Beef, poultry,whole grains, potatoes, tomatoes, broccoli, (widespread in foods)	Deficiency is rare, GI distress, neurological disturbances, fatigue	None established
Niacin, B3	16 mg/d for men and 14 mg/d for women (NE)	Beef, fish, chicken, brewer's yeast, mushrooms, green leafy vegetables	Pellagra disease, diarrhea, abdominal pain, dermatitis, dementia/ death	35 mg Niacin flush (from large doses)(four times the RDA)
Biotin (also known as vitamin H)	30 ug/d for men and women (AI)	Widespread in foods in small amounts, egg yolks are richest source	Skin rash, hair loss, neurological impairment	None established
Vitamin B6	1.3 mg/d for men and women under 50 years of age and 1.7 mg/d for men over 51 and 1.5 mg/d for women over 51	Banana, brewer's yeast, fish, poultry, green leafy vegetables, chicken, dairy products, whole grain foods	Depression, confusion, abnormal brain wave, convulsions	100 mg/d
Vitamin B12	2.4 ug/d for men and women	Exclusively in animal products	Typically malabsorption not intake, atrophic gastritis, pernicious anemia	None established

Vitamin	DRI (AI)*	Food Sources (2)	Deficiency	Tolerable Upper Limit
Folate (Folic Acid) B9	400 ug/d for both men and women	Dark, green, leafy vegetables, grain products	Macrocytic anemia, aspirin and antacids interfere with absorption	1000 ug/d
Vitamin C	90 mg/d for men and 75 mg/d for women	Fruits, citrus fruits, vegetables	Scurvy disease, bleeding gums, pinpoint hemorrhaging, anemia, infections	2000 mg

The following table summarizes the roles of the B vitamins and Vitamin C.

Vitamin	Metabolic Roles
Thiamin	Part of coenzyme TPP in energy metabolism
Riboflavin	Part of coenzyme FAD and FMN in energy metabolism
Pantothenic Acid	Part of coenzyme A in energy metabolism
Niacin	Part of coenzymes NAD and NADP in energy metabolism
Biotin	Part of coenzyme in energy metabolism (transfer of carbon dioxide)
Vitamin B6	Part of coenzyme used in amino acid and fatty acid metabolism
Vitamin B12	Activates folate; helps synthesize DNA for new cell growth; protects nerve cells
Folate (Folic Acid)	Activates vitamin B12; helps synthesize DNA for new cell growth; protects nerve cells
Vitamin C	Synthesis of collagen, carnitine, hormones, neurotransmitters; antioxidant

In general, supplements containing all eight of the B vitamins are referred to as a vitamin B complex. Many B vitamins are coenzymes. Coenzymes are loosely bound co-factors bound to proteins and required for the proteins biological activity. Co-factors can be considered "helper molecules" that assist in biochemical transformations (2). Without its coenzyme the enzyme cannot function.

Vitamin C acts as an antioxidant. An antioxidants is a substance that can donate electrons to another substance. Substances that have an "unpaired electron" are toxic to the cell. Antioxidants have the capacity to pair with the unpaired electron, thereby rendering it nontoxic.

Thiamin/Riboflavin

Thiamin or vitamin B1, named as the "thio-vitamin" ("sulfur-containing vitamin") is a water-soluble vitamin of the B complex (2). First named *aneurin* for the detrimental neurological effects if not present in the diet, it was eventually assigned the generic descriptor name vitamin B1. Its phosphate derivatives are involved in cellular processes.

The name "riboflavin" (vitamin B2) comes from "ribose", the sugar whose reduced form, ribitol, forms part of its structure, and "flavin", the ring-moiety which imparts the yellow color to the oxidized molecule (2).

Thiamin (vitamin B1) - Roles

Thiamin is part of a coenzyme known as thiamin pyrophosphate-TPP. TPP promotes the conversion of pyruvate to acetyl CoA. Thiamin is also part of nerve cell membranes. Consequently, nervous and muscle tissue require thiamin (2).

Thiamin (vitamin B1) - Deficiency/Toxicity

Deficiencies of thiamin have been reported in malnourished individuals and individuals who derive most of their energy from empty calorie foods and beverages such as alcohol. Prolonged deficiency can result in the disease beriberi. Symptoms of beriberi include muscle weakness in arms and legs, and cardiovascular disease. No adverse effects have been associated with high intakes of thiamin, and no upper level has been established.

Riboflavin (B2) - Roles

Riboflavin (also known as vitamin B2) like thiamin helps enzymes facilitate the release of energy from carbohydrates. The coenzyme forms of riboflavin are FMN (flavin mononucleotide) and FAD (flavin adenine dinucleotide) and are also involved in the energy production. Riboflavin also helps support vision and skin health (2).

Riboflavin (B2) - Deficiency/Toxicity

Riboflavin deficiency (referred to as ariboflavinosis) is often accompanied by deficiencies in other nutrients. Deficiency symptoms include inflammation of the mouth, skin, eyes, and GI tract. No adverse effects have been associated with high intakes and no upper level has been established for this vitamin.

Pantothenic Acid

Pantothenic acid is part of the chemical structure of coenzyme A that forms acetyl CoA. It is involved in more than 100 different steps in the synthesis of lipids, neurotransmitters, steroid hormones and hemoglobin (2).

Pantothenic Acid - Roles

Acetyl CoA is a crossroad molecule of several metabolic pathways, including glucose and fatty acid metabolism. Pantothenic acid is involved in more than 100 different steps in the synthesis of lipids, neurotransmitters, steroid hormones, and hemoglobin (2).

Pantothenic Acid - Deficiency/Toxicity

Deficiency of pantothenic acid is rare. Symptoms include fatigue, GI distress, and neurological problems. No toxic effects have been associated with high intakes, and no upper limit has been established (2).

Niacin

Niacin consists of 2 chemical structures; nicotinic acid and nicotinamide. Nicotinamide is the major form of niacin in the blood, and the body can easily convert nicotinic acid to nicotinamide. The two coenzyme forms of niacin are NAD (nicotinamide adenine dinucleotide) and NADP (the phosphate form of NAD) (4).

Niacin - Roles

Both coenzyme forms of niacin are involved in the metabolism of glucose, fat, and alcohol. Niacin is unique among the B vitamins because the body can make it from the amino acid tryptophan. To make 1 milligram of niacin requires 60 milligrams of dietary tryptophan. This is why niacin requirements are stated in "niacin equivalents", reflecting the body's ability to convert tryptophan to niacin (2).

Niacin - Deficiency/Toxicity

The disease seen in niacin deficiency is pellagra. The symptoms of pellagra are diarrhea, dermatitis, and dementia. Other deficiency symptoms include irritability, loss of appetite, weakness, dizziness, and mental confusion which can progress to dementia. Large doses of niacin are dangerous. In large doses (10 times the RDA), niacin dilates the capillaries and causes a tingling effect known as "niacin flush". Physicians sometimes treat high blood cholesterol by prescribing high doses of niacin. Large pharmacological doses may cause liver damage, peptic ulcers, and possibly diabetes. Symptoms of niacin toxicity include diarrhea, flushing, itching, headaches, nausea, heartburn, fainting, dizziness, and abnormal liver function (4).

Biotin

Biotin, also known as vitamin H is composed of a ureido (tetrahydroimidizalone) ring fused with a tetrahydrothiophene ring (4). Biotin is a coenzyme for carboxylase enzymes, involved in the synthesis of fatty acids, isoleucine, and valine, and in gluconeogenesis (2).

Biotin - Roles

Biotin is a coenzyme that serves as a carbon dioxide carrier. It is involved in the reaction from pyruvate to acetyl CoA (delivering a carbon). It also serves crucial roles in gluconeogenesis, fatty acid synthesis, and the breakdown of certain fatty acids and amino acids (2).

Biotin - Deficiency/Toxicity

Biotin deficiencies are rarely seen but can be induced by eating raw eggs. A protein (avidin) in raw egg white binds biotin and thus prevents its absorption. Studies have shown that more than two dozen egg whites must be consumed daily to produce a deficiency. Cooking denatures this protein and hence cannot bind the biotin. Deficiency symptoms include abnormal heart function, nausea, depression, muscle pain, weakness, fatigue, and hair loss (4). No adverse effects have been seen from high biotin intakes; hence, tolerable upper levels have not been set (2).

Folate

Folate occurs naturally in foods, and folic acid or folacin is the form found in supplements. Folate (and folic acid) is part of the coenzyme that forms DHF (dihydrofolate) and THF (tetrahydrofolate).

Folate - Roles

THF serves as part of an enzyme complex that transfers one carbon compound during metabolism. This transfer helps convert vitamin B12 to one of its coenzyme forms and helps synthesize the DNA required for all rapidly growing cells (as in pregnancy). Foods deliver folate in bound form (folate bound to amino acids). Enzymes in the intestines must hydrolyze the bound folate to monoglutamate form. The complicated system of transporting and converting folates is vulnerable to GI problems. For instance, in alcohol abuse, a folate deficiency rapidly develops and impairs the GI tract. Folic acid and vitamin B12 help cells to multiply. Cells such as red blood cells and the cells that line the GI tract are especially vulnerable to deficiency of these vitamins (2).

Folate - Deficiency/Toxicity

The first symptoms of a deficiency are a type of anemia and GI tract deterioration. Other symptoms include frequent infections, depression, confusion and fatigue. Deficiency during pregnancy can cause birth defects, specifically neural tube defects (4). Folic acid supplementation has been shown to reduce the risk of neural tube defects. Toxicity symptoms include many of the same symptoms seen in deficiency, including birth defects and masking of B12 deficiency symptoms (4).

Vitamin B6

Vitamin B6 occurs in three forms: pyridoxal, pyridoxine, and pyridoxamine. All three forms can be converted to the coenzyme pyridoxal phosphate (PLP) (4).

Vitamin B6 - Roles

Vitamin B6 assists enzymes that metabolize amino acids. PLP has the ability to transfer amino groups, which allows the body to synthesize nonessential amino acids from essential amino acids. PLP is also involved in the conversion of tryptophan to niacin, the conversion of tryptophan to the neurotransmitter serotonin, and the synthesis of heme (2). B6 also influences immune function and steroid hormone activity. Unlike other water soluble vitamins, B6 is stored in muscle tissue (4).

Vitamin B6 - Deficiency/ Toxicity

Deficiency symptoms include weakness, irritability, insomnia, cracked corners of the mouth, and dermatitis. Advanced symptoms include growth failure, impaired motor function, and convulsions. Toxicity symptoms include depression, fatigue, irritability, headaches, numbness, nerve damage, and difficulty walking (4).

Vitamin B12

Vitamin B12 and folate are closely related, and each depends on the other for activation. Vitamin B12 donates a methyl group to activate the folate coenzyme. Vitamin B12 is found exclusively in animal products and its bioavailabilty is greatest from milk and fish (4). Vitamin B12 requires an intrinsic factor for absorption which is synthesized in the stomach. In the stomach this intrinsic factor binds to B12, and the complex is then absorbed by the small intestines.

Vitamin B12 - Roles

Vitamin B12 (also known as cobalamin) regenerates the folate coenzyme. The regeneration of an amino acid, methionine, and the synthesis of genetic material (DNA and RNA) depend on the folate coenzyme and so depend on both folate and vitamin B12. Vitamin B12 is involved in bone cell activity and metabolism, as well as nerve fiber promotion and normal growth.

Vitamin B12 - Deficiency/Toxicity

Most B12 deficiencies are due to inadequate absorption, not intake. Some people inherit a defective gene for the intrinsic factor producing a deficiency. A deficiency can also develop if the stomach has been injured, and the intrinsic factor cannot be produced. One of the first symptoms of B12 deficiency is the anemia due to folate deficiency. Either folate or B12 will clear up the anemia, but if folate is given when B12 is needed, the results are disastrous with devastating neurological symptoms. Folate cures the blood symptoms but not the nerve symptoms.

Since B12 is found exclusively in animal products, strict vegetarians could become deficient in this nutrient. Also, high folate intakes in this group could mask a B12 deficiency. It is therefore essential that strict vegetarians obtain a reliable source of vitamin B12 (11).

Vitamin C

Deficiency of vitamin C produces the disease known as scurvy. While the earliest documented case of scurvy was described by Hippocrates around the year 400 BC, the first attempt to give scientific basis for the cause of this disease was by a ship's surgeon in the British Royal Navy, James Lind (10). Scurvy was common among those with poor access to fresh fruit and vegetables, such as remote, isolated sailors and soldiers. While at sea in May 1747, Lind provided some crew members with two oranges and one lemon per day, in addition to normal rations, while others continued on cider, vinegar, sulfuric acid or seawater, along with their normal rations. In the history of science this is considered to be the first occurrence of a controlled experiment comparing results on two populations of a factor applied to one group only with all other factors the same. The results conclusively showed that citrus fruits prevented the disease. Lind published his work in 1753 in his *Treatise on the Scurvy* (10).

The name "antiscorbutic" was used in the eighteenth and nineteenth centuries as general term for those foods known to prevent scurvy, even though there was no understanding of the reason for this. These foods included: lemons, limes, and oranges; sauerkraut, cabbage, malt, and portable soup (10). It was 1795 before the British navy adopted lemons or limes as standard issue at sea. Limes were more popular as they could be found in British West Indian Colonies, unlike lemons which weren't found in British Dominions, and were therefore more expensive. This practice led to the American use of the nickname "limey" to refer to the British (10).

Vitamin C - Roles

Vitamin C (ascorbic acid) is generally known as an antioxidant and acts as an electron donor for eight different enzymes (12).

Vitamin C helps specific enzymes perform their functions. For example, Vitamin C acts as a co-factor in the formation of the fibrous, structural protein collagen. Collagen strengthens blood vessel walls, forms scar tissue, and is a matrix for bone growth. Vitamin C also helps in the absorption or iron (13).

Vitamin C - Deficiency/Toxicity

Early signs of vitamin C deficiency are difficult to recognize. The gums bleed easily around the teeth, and capillaries under the skin break producing pinpoint hemorrhages. After a month of vitamin C deficiency, scurvy symptoms appear. The skin becomes rough, scaly, and dry. Wounds will not heal because scar tissue will not form. Bone building falters, and the end of long bones become malformed and painful with resulting fractures. Anemia and infections are common. Psychological signs such as hysteria and depression are also common. Sudden death can occur due to massive internal bleeding.

Vitamin C supplements have received widespread publicity in prevention of colds and cancer, which has led to consumption of large doses by a large number of individuals. Side effects of large doses include GI distress and diarrhea. Large amounts of vitamin C in urine obscure results of tests such as glucose and ketones in the diagnosis of diabetes. Large doses have also been shown to affect anticlotting medications. Individuals with kidney disease, gout, or a genetic abnormality that alters the breakdown of vitamin C are prone to producing kidney stones (13).

Fat Soluble Vitamins

Fat soluble vitamins consist of vitamin A, vitamin D, vitamin E, and vitamin K. The following table summarizes the Dietary Reference Intake (DRI) or adequate intake (AI) for each of the fat soluble vitamins (9).

Vitamin	DRI (AI)*	Food Sources (2)	Deficiency	Tolerable Upper Limit
Vitamin A	900 ug/d men and 700 ug/d women	Whole eggs, milk, liver fortified foods (retinol), dark, colored vegetables (beta-carotene).	Infectious diseases, blindness	3000 ug/d
Vitamin D	15 ug/d for men and women	Milk, milk products, (sunlight), egg yolks, oily fish	Rickets disease, osteomalacia, osteoporosis	100 ug/d
Vitamin E	15 mg/d for men and women	Vegetable oils and products made from oils, seeds and nuts	Deficiency is rare, GI distress, neurological disturbances, fatigue	1000 mg/d

Vitamin	DRI (AI)*	Food Sources (2)	Deficiency	Tolerable Upper Limit
Vitamin K	120 ug/d for men and 90 ug/day for women	Green leafy vegetables, oils (gut bacteria make a form of Vitamin K)	Bleeding, osteomalacia,	None established

Vitamin A

In general, there are two categories of vitamin A, depending on whether the food source is from an animal or a plant source (17). Vitamin A found in foods that come from animals is called *preformed* vitamin A and has three different active forms: retinol, retinal, and retinoic acid. Together they are called retinoids. The most usable form of vitamin A is retinol. Retinol can be made into retinal and retinoic acid (other active forms of vitamin A) in the body (17). Sources include liver, whole milk, and some fortified food products.

Vitamin A that is found in colorful fruits and vegetables is called carotenoid. Carotenoids can be made into retinol in the body. The most common carotenoids found in foods that come from plants are beta-carotene, alpha-carotene, and beta-cryptoxanthin (22). Of the 563 identified carotenoids, fewer than 10% can be made into vitamin A in the body (19). Among these, beta-carotene is most efficiently made into retinol (19,20,21). Lycopene, lutein, and zeaxanthin are carotenoids that do not have vitamin A activity but have other health promoting properties (14).

Dietary intake studies suggest an association between diets rich in beta-carotene and vitamin A and a lower risk of many types of cancer (23). A higher intake of green and yellow vegetables or other food sources of beta carotene and/or vitamin A may decrease the risk of lung cancer (14,33). However, a number of studies that tested the role of beta-carotene supplements in cancer prevention did not find them to protect against the disease. In the Alpha-tocopherol Beta-carotene (ATBC) Cancer Prevention Study, more than 29,000 men who regularly smoked cigarettes were randomized to receive 20 mg beta-carotene alone, 50 mg alpha-tocopherol alone, supplements, or both, or a placebo for 5 to 8 years. Incidence of lung cancer was 18% higher among men who took the beta-carotene supplement. Eight percent more men in this group died, as compared to those receiving other treatments or placebo (25). Similar results were seen in the Carotene and Retinol Efficacy Trial (CARET), a lung cancer chemo prevention study that provided subjects with supplements of 30 mg beta-carotene and 25,000 IU retinyl palmitate (a form of vitamin A) or a placebo. This study was stopped after researchers discovered that subjects receiving beta-carotene had a 46% higher risk of dying from lung cancer (26,27). The IOM states that "beta-carotene supplements are not advisable for the general population," although they also state that this advice "does not pertain to the possible use of supplemental beta-carotene as a provitamin A source for the prevention of vitamin A deficiency in populations with inadequate vitamin A" intake (11).

Worldwide, the highest incidence of osteoporosis occurs in northern Europe, a population with a high intake of vitamin A (32). Osteoporosis, a disorder characterized by porous and weak bones, is a serious health problem for more than 10 million Americans, 80% of whom are women. Another 18 million Americans have decreased bone density which precedes the development of osteoporosis. Many factors increase the risk for developing osteoporosis, including being female, thin, inactive, at advanced age, and having a family history of osteoporosis. An inadequate dietary intake of calcium, cigarette smoking, and excessive intake of alcohol also increase the risk (28,29,30). Researchers are now examining a potential new risk factor for osteoporosis: an excess intake of vitamin A. Animal, human, and laboratory research suggests an association between greater vitamin A intake and weaker bones (31,32).

<u>Vitamin A - Roles</u>

Vitamin A is a group of compounds that play an important role in vision, bone growth, reproduction, cell division, and cell differentiation (in which a cell becomes part of the brain, muscle, lungs, blood, or other specialized tissue) (14,15,16). Vitamin A helps regulate the immune system, which helps prevent or fight off infections by making white blood cells that destroy harmful bacteria and viruses (14,15,16). Vitamin A may help lymphocytes (a type of white blood cell) fight infections more effectively. Vitamin A promotes healthy surface linings of the eyes and the respiratory, urinary, and intestinal tracts (17). When those linings break down, it becomes easier for bacteria to enter the body and cause infection. Vitamin A also helps the skin and mucous membranes function as a barrier to bacteria and viruses (15,16,18).

<u>Vitamin A - Deficiency/Toxicity</u>

A deficiency can occur when vitamin A is lost through chronic diarrhea and through an overall inadequate intake, as is often seen in protein-energy malnutrition (15). Low blood retinol concentrations indicate depleted levels of vitamin A which can result from an inadequate intake of protein, calories, and zinc, since these nutrients are needed to make RBP(30). Iron deficiency can also affect vitamin A metabolism. Iron supplements may improve body stores of vitamin A (14). Excess alcohol intake depletes vitamin A stores (14). Vitamin A supplements may not be recommended for individuals who abuse alcohol because their livers may be susceptible to potential toxicity from high doses.

Deficiency symptoms include cessation of bone growth, change in shapes of bones, development of cracks in teeth with a tendency to decay, anemia, plugging of hair follicles forming white lumps. Vitamin A deficiency in pregnancy can lead to birth defects. Deficiency of vitamin A is the major cause of childhood blindness (xerophthalmia) in the world. Blindness progresses first appearing as night blindness (2). Vitamin A deficiency contributes to blindness by making the cornea very dry and damaging the retina and cornea and it diminishes the ability to fight infections. If left untreated, this disease quickly progresses to irreversible blindness. Vitamin A deficiency also increases susceptibility to infectious disease. Children in third world countries given vitamin A supplements recovered faster from pneumonia and other respiratory infections. Vitamin A supplementation also reduces the risk of dying from measles by at least 50% (2).

Deficiency symptoms do not appear until stores are depleted which may take up to a year. Vitamin A deficiency is common in developing countries but rarely seen in the United States. In countries where such deficiency is common and immunization programs are limited, millions of children die each year from complications of infectious diseases such as measles (34).

Vitamin A toxicity affects all body systems and occurs through ingestion of large amounts of preformed vitamin A (animal products) and through supplementation (126). Excessive amounts over time may weaken bones (127). Excessive vitamin A during pregnancy leads to abnormal cell death in the spinal cord which increases risk of birth defects (128).

Vitamin D

Vitamin D is a fat soluble vitamin that is found in food and can also be made through exposure to ultraviolet (UV) rays from the sun. Sunshine is a significant source of vitamin D because UV rays from sunlight trigger vitamin D synthesis in the skin (36,37). Vitamin D exists in several forms, each with a different level of activity. Calciferol is the most active form of vitamin D. Other forms are relatively inactive in the body. Once vitamin D is produced in the skin or consumed in food, it requires chemical conversion in the liver and kidney to form 1,25 dihydroxyvitamin D, the physiologically active form of vitamin D (38).

About 98% to 99% of the milk supply in the U.S. is fortified with 10 micrograms (equal to 400 International Units or IU) of vitamin D per quart. One cup of vitamin D fortified milk supplies one-half of the recommended daily intake for adults between the ages of 19 and 50, one-fourth of the recommended daily intake for adults between the ages of 51 and 70, and approximately 15% of the recommended daily intake for adults age 71 and over. Although milk is fortified with vitamin D, dairy products made from milk, such as cheese and ice creams, are generally not fortified with vitamin D and contain only small amounts. Some ready- to-eat breakfast cereals may be fortified with vitamin D, often at a level of 10% to 15% of the Daily Value.

It can be difficult to obtain enough vitamin D from natural food sources. Consuming vitamin D fortified foods and adequate sunlight exposure are essential for maintaining a healthy vitamin D status. In some groups, dietary supplements may be needed to meet the daily need for vitamin D. In infants, vitamin D requirements cannot be met by human (breast) milk alone (39,54) which usually provides approximately 25 IU vitamin D per liter. Sunlight is a potential source of vitamin D for infants, but the American Academy of Pediatrics (AAP) advises that infants be kept out of direct sunlight and wear protective clothing and sunscreen when exposed to sunlight (56). The American Academy of Pediatrics (AAP) recommends a daily supplement of 200 IU vitamin D for breastfed infants beginning within the first 2 months of life unless they are weaned to receive at least 500 ml (about 2 cups) per day of vitamin D-fortified formula (55). Children and adolescents who are not routinely exposed to sunlight and do not consume at least 2, 8-fluid ounce servings of vitamin D-fortified milk per day are also at higher risk of vitamin D deficiency and may need a dietary supplement containing 200 IU vitamin D. Formula fed infants usually consume recommended amounts of vitamin D because the 1980 Infant Formula Act requires that infant formulas be fortified with vitamin D (55). The minimal level of fortification required is 40 IU vitamin D per 100 calories of formula. The maximum level of vitamin D fortification allowed is 100 IU per 100 calories of formula. This range of fortification produces a standard 20 calorie per ounce formula providing between 265 and 660 IU vitamin D per liter (55).

Vitamin D - Roles

The major biologic function of vitamin D is to maintain normal blood levels of calcium and phosphorus (38,39). By promoting calcium absorption, vitamin D helps to form and maintain strong bones. Active vitamin D functions as a hormone because it sends a message to the intestines to increase the absorption of calcium and phosphorus (38). Vitamin D also works in concert with a number of other vitamins, minerals, and hormones to promote bone mineralization. Research also suggests that vitamin D may help maintain a healthy immune system and help regulate cell growth and differentiation, the process that determines what a cell is to become (38,42,43). Vitamin D sufficiency prevents rickets in children and osteomalacia in adults, two forms of skeletal diseases that weaken bones (40,41).

Vitamin D - Deficiency/Toxicity

Nutrient deficiencies are usually the result of dietary inadequacy, impaired absorption and utilization, increased requirement, or increased excretion. Without vitamin D, bones can become thin, brittle, or misshapen. The classic vitamin D deficiency diseases are *rickets and osteomalacia* (40,41,50).

In children, vitamin D deficiency causes rickets. Rickets is a bone disease characterized by a failure to properly mineralize bone tissue and results in soft bones and skeletal deformities (50,53). Rickets was first described in the mid-17th century by British researcher (50,53). In the late 19th and early 20th century, German physicians noted that consuming 1 to 3 teaspoons (3 teaspoons is equal to 1 tablespoon) of cod liver oil per day could reverse rickets (53). The recommendation to fortify milk with vitamin D made rickets a rare disease in the U.S. for many years. However, rickets has recently reemerged, in particular among African American infants and children (50,53). In 2003, a report from Memphis, Tennessee, described 21 cases of rickets among infants, 20 of whom were African-American (53). Prolonged breastfeeding without vitamin D supplementation is one of the most significant causes of the reemergence of rickets. Additional causes include extensive use of sunscreens and increased use of day-care, resulting in decreased outdoor activity and sun exposure among children (50,53). Rickets is more prevalent among immigrants from Asia, Africa, and Middle Eastern countries for a variety of reasons (50). Among immigrants, vitamin D deficiency has been associated with iron deficiency, leading researchers to question whether or not iron deficiency may impair vitamin D metabolism (50). Immigrants from these regions are also more likely to follow dress codes that limit sun exposure.

In addition, darker pigmented skin converts UV rays to vitamin D less efficiently than lighter skin (50). Melanin is the pigment that gives skin its color. Greater amounts of melanin result in darker skin. The high melanin content in darker skin reduces the skin's ability to produce vitamin D from sunlight. It is very important for African Americans and other populations with dark-pigmented skin to consume recommended amounts of vitamin D. Some studies suggest that older adults, especially women, in these groups are at even higher risk of vitamin D deficiency (51,65). Individuals with darkly pigmented skin who are unable to get adequate sun exposure and/or consume recommended amounts of vitamin D may benefit from a vitamin D supplement.

A deficiency is accurately diagnosed by measuring the concentration of a specific form of vitamin D in blood (44,49). As a fat soluble vitamin, vitamin D requires some dietary fat for absorption. Individuals who have a reduced ability to absorb dietary fat may require vitamin D supplements (66).

Americans age 50 and older are believed to be at increased risk of developing vitamin D deficiency (49). As people age, skin cannot synthesize vitamin D as efficiently, and the kidney is less able to convert vitamin D to its active hormone form. It is estimated that as many as 30% to 40% of older adults with hip fractures are vitamin D insufficient (48). Therefore, older adults may benefit from supplemental vitamin D. Home bound individuals, people living in northern latitudes such as in New England and Alaska, women who wear robes and head coverings for religious reasons, and individuals working in occupations that prevent sun exposure are unlikely to obtain much vitamin D from sunlight. It is important for people with limited sun exposure to consume recommended amounts of vitamin D in their diets or consider vitamin D supplementation (62,63,64).

In adults, vitamin D deficiency can lead to osteomalacia, which results in muscular weakness in addition to weak bones (40,41). Symptoms of bone pain and muscle weakness may indicate vitamin D deficiency, but symptoms may be subtle and go undetected in the initial stages. A deficiency of vitamin D also contributes to osteoporosis by reducing calcium absorption (68). While rickets and osteomalacia are extreme examples of vitamin D deficiency, osteoporosis is an example of a long-term effect of vitamin D insufficiency (69). Adequate storage levels of vitamin D help keep bones strong and may help prevent osteoporosis in older adults, in non-ambulatory individuals (those who have difficulty walking and exercising), in post-menopausal women, and in individuals on chronic steroid therapy (70).

Caffeine may inhibit vitamin D receptors, thus limiting absorption of vitamin D and decreasing bone mineral density. A study found that elderly postmenopausal women who consumed more than 300 milligrams per day of caffeine (which is equivalent to approximately 18 oz of caffeinated coffee) lost more bone in the spine than women who consumed less than 300 milligrams per day (92). However, there is also evidence that increasing calcium intake (for example, adding milk to coffee) can counteract any potential negative effect that caffeine may have on bone loss. More evidence is needed before health professionals can confidently advise adults to decrease caffeine intake as a means of preventing osteoporosis (92).

Vitamin D is among the most likely of the vitamins to have toxic effects (4). Excess Vitamin D raises the concentration of blood calcium (129). Excess blood calcium precipitates formation of kidney stones. Calcification may also harden the blood vessels which is especially dangerous in the major arteries of the heart, lungs, and brain.

Vitamin E

Vitamin E is a fat-soluble vitamin that exists in eight different forms. Each form has its own biological activity, which is the measure of potency or functional use in the body. Alpha-tocopherol is the name of the most active form of vitamin E in humans. It is also a powerful biological antioxidant (98). Vitamin E in supplements is usually sold as alpha-tocopherol acetate, a form of alpha-tocopherol that protects its ability to function as an antioxidant. The synthetic form is labeled "D, L" while the natural form is labeled "D". The synthetic form is only half as active as the natural form (98).

Vitamin E - Roles

Vitamin E has also been shown to play a role in immune function, in DNA repair, and in other metabolic processes (98,99). Antioxidants such as vitamin E are believed to help protect cell membranes against the damaging effects of free radicals. Free radicals may contribute to the development of chronic diseases such as cancer (4). Vitamin E may block the formation of nitrosamines, which are carcinogens formed in the stomach from nitrites consumed in the diet. It also may protect against the development of cancers by enhancing immune function (107). Unfortunately, human trials and surveys that have tried to associate vitamin E intake with incidence of cancer have been generally inconclusive (107).

Vitamin E - Deficiency/Toxicity

A primary deficiency of vitamin E from poor dietary intake is rare. Typically deficiencies are associated with diseases of fat malabsorption such as cystic fibrosis. In deficiency the red blood cells break and spill their contents (erythrocyte hemolysis). This is common in infants born prematurely before the transfer of vitamin E from the mother to the infant which occurs in the last few weeks of pregnancy. Prolonged deficiency causes neuromuscular dysfunction particularly in the spinal cord and retina of the eye. Symptoms include loss of muscular coordination and reflexes and impaired vision and speech.

Vitamin E toxicity is rare because the liver regulates vitamin E concentrations. Extremely high doses may interfere with the blood clotting action of vitamin K and enhance the effects of drugs used to thin blood causing hemorrhaging.

Vitamin K

Worldwide, only a handful of researchers study vitamin K—long known for its critical role in blood clotting. But this vitamin may command a bigger following as its importance to the integrity of bones becomes increasingly clear. According to Sarah Booth at the Jean Mayer USDA Human Nutrition Research Center on Aging at Tufts University in Boston, vitamin K activates at least three proteins involved in bone health (116).

Vitamin K can be obtained from both foods (phylloquinone) and the GI tract synthesizes a form of vitamin k (menaquinone) that the body can use. Phylloquinone is found in some oils, especially soybean oil, and in dark-green vegetables such as spinach and broccoli (118). One serving of spinach or two servings of broccoli provide four to five times the RDA for phylloquinone.

Vitamin K - Roles

The primary role of vitamin K is blood clotting. It is essential for the activation of proteins and calcium involved in the clotting process (4). Vitamin K is also involved in the metabolism of bone proteins. One such protein is the bone-building protein osteocalcin (116). An adequate intake of vitamin K decreases bone turnover and protects against fractures (117). However, according to a study published in the 2008 edition of PloS Medicine vitamin K (5 mg/d) does not protect against age-related decreasing bone density but may protect against fractures and cancers in postmenopausal women taking calcium and vitamin D supplements (121).

Vitamin K - Deficiency/Toxicity

Deficiency of this vitamin causes hemorrhaging. For infants in the U.S. Vitamin K deficiency without bleeding may occur in as many as 50% of infants younger than 5 days old (120). Therefore, the committee on Nutrition of the American Academy of Pediatrics recommends that 0.5 to 10. mg vitamin K be administered to all newborns shortly after birth (120).

Certain drugs such as Warfarin (Coumadin) are administered to prevent formation of clots. These drugs destroy the ability of vitamin K to perform its function in the clotting process (122).

Toxicity is uncommon. Blood clotting studies in humans using 45 mg per day of vitamin K and even up to 135 mg/day (45 mg three times daily) showed no increase in blood clot risk (123). Even doses in rats as high as 25 mg/kg body weight did not alter the tendency for blood-clot formation to occur (124). Unlike the safe natural forms of vitamin K a synthetic form of vitamin K (menadione), is demonstrably toxic. The U.S. FDA has banned this form from over-the-counter sale because large doses have been shown to cause allergic reactions, hemolytic anemia, and cytotoxicity in liver cells (125).

Summary

The term vitamin is derived from the root word "vita" meaning essential to life. Vitamins are a group of organic compounds other than protein, carbohydrates, or fats that cannot be manufactured by the body and are required in small amounts for specific functions of growth, maintenance, reproduction and repair and include: vitamin A, vitamin C, vitamin D, vitamin E, vitamin K, vitamin B1 (thiamin), vitamin B2 (riboflavin), vitamin B3 (niacin), pantothenic acid, biotin, vitamin B6, vitamin B12, folate (folic acid). Vitamins differ from the energy nutrients in that they are needed in smaller amounts. The energy nutrients are required in gram amounts, while the micronutrients are needed in milligram, microgram, and picogram amounts. Vitamins do not provide energy, and they act singly, not as macromolecules. Vitamins are vital to life, are organic, and are available in all foods. They require no digestion and are absorbed intact into the bloodstream.

The two major categories of vitamins are the water soluble vitamins and the fat soluble vitamins. The water soluble vitamins include all the B vitamins and vitamin C. The fat soluble vitamins are vitamin A, vitamin D, vitamin E, and vitamin K. The body absorbs water soluble vitamins directly into the blood, whereas fat soluble vitamins must be packaged and transported in lipoproteins. In the cells, water soluble vitamins freely circulate while fat soluble vitamins tend to become trapped in the cells associated with fat. Hence, the fat soluble vitamins tend to remain in fat storage sites, are less readily excreted, and more likely to reach toxic levels when consumed in excess (4).

Dietary Reference Intakes were discussed in Chapter 1, but a quick review is included here. The *Recommended Dietary Allowance* (RDA) was developed during World War II by a committee established by the National Academy of Sciences in order to investigate issues of nutrition that might "affect national defense" (3). The Recommended Dietary Allowances (RDA) are standards set by scientists studying the individual nutrients and published by the government. These standards include a safety margin and are not "minimum" standards. *The Dietary Reference Intake* (DRI) is a system of nutrition recommendations from the Institute of Medicine (IOM) of the National Academy of Sciences. The DRI system is used by both the United States and Canada and is intended for the general public and health professionals.

The B vitamins are thiamin, riboflavin, pantothenic acid, niacin, biotin, folate (folic acid), B6, and B12. Thiamin (vitamin B1) is part of a coenzyme known as thiamin pyrophosphate-TPP. TPP promotes the conversion of pyruvate to acetyl CoA. Riboflavin also known as vitamin B2, like thiamin helps enzymes facilitate the release of energy from carbohydrates. Pantothenic acid is important as part of CoA. Pantothenic acid is involved in more than 100 different steps in the synthesis of lipids, neurotransmitters, steroid hormones, and the molecule that transports oxygen-hemoglobin. Niacin consists of 2 other chemical structures: nicotinic acid and nicotinamide. Both coenzyme forms are involved in the metabolism of glucose, fat, and alcohol. Large doses of niacin are dangerous. Niacin in large doses (10 times the RDA) dilates the capillaries and causes a tingling effect known as "niacin flush". Biotin plays an important role in metabolism as a coenzyme that serves as a carbon dioxide carrier. This role is critical in the energy cycle (TCA). Deficiency symptoms would include abnormal heart function, nausea, depression, muscle pain, weakness, fatigue, and hair loss.

Folate occurs naturally in foods and folic acid or folacin is the form found in supplements. Folate (and folic acid) is part of the coenzyme forms DHF (dihydrofolate) and THF (tetrahydrofolate). THF helps convert vitamin B12 to one of its coenzyme forms and helps synthesize the DNA required for all rapidly growing cells (as in pregnancy). Folic acid and vitamin B12 help cells to multiply. This function is especially important in cells that have short life spans and must replace themselves rapidly. Cells such as red blood cells and the cells that line the GI tract are especially vulnerable to deficiency of these vitamins. The first symptoms of a deficiency are a type of anemia and GI tract deterioration. Other symptoms include frequent infections, depression, confusion and fatigue. Deficiency during pregnancy can cause birth defects, specifically neural tube defects.

Vitamin B6 assists enzymes that metabolize amino acids. Vitamin B6 occurs in three forms: pyridoxal, pyridoxine, and pyridoxamine. All three forms can be converted to the coenzyme pyridoxal phosphate (PLP). This coenzyme has the ability to transfer amino groups which allows the body to synthesize nonessential amino acids from essential amino acids. Unlike other water soluble vitamins, B6 is stored in muscle tissue. Deficiency symptoms include weakness, irritability, insomnia, cracked corners of the mouth, and dermatitis. Advanced symptoms include growth failure, impaired motor function, and convulsions. The roles of B6 and B12 intertwine because each depends on the other for activation. Vitamin B12 (also known as cobalamin) regenerates the folate coenzyme. The regeneration of an amino acid, methionine, and the synthesis of genetic material (DNA and RNA) depend on the folate coenzyme and so depends on both folate and B12.

In general, supplements containing all eight of the B vitamins are referred to as a vitamin B complex. Many B vitamins are coenzymes. Coenzymes are loosely bound co-factors bound to proteins and required for the proteins biological activity. These proteins are commonly enzymes, and co-factors can be considered "helper molecules" that assist in biochemical transformations (2). The vitamin portion of a coenzyme binds to the enzyme.

Without its coenzyme the enzyme cannot function. Vitamin C acts as an antioxidant. An antioxidant is a substance that can donate electrons to another substance. Substances that have an "unpaired electron" are toxic to the cell. Antioxidants have the capacity to pair with the unpaired electron, thereby rendering it nontoxic.

Fat soluble vitamins consist of vitamin A, vitamin D, vitamin E, and vitamin K. Vitamin A is a group of compounds that play an important role in vision, bone growth, reproduction, cell division, and cell differentiation (in which a cell becomes part of the brain, muscle, lungs, blood, or other specialized tissue). Vitamin A helps regulate the immune system, which helps prevent or fight off infections by making white blood cells that destroy harmful bacteria and viruses. Vitamin D is a fat soluble vitamin that is found in food and can also be made in your body after exposure to ultraviolet (UV) rays from the sun. The major biologic function of vitamin D is to maintain normal blood levels of calcium and phosphorus. By promoting calcium absorption, vitamin D helps to form and maintain strong bones. Vitamin D also works in concert with a number of other vitamins, minerals, and hormones to promote bone mineralization.

Vitamin E exists in eight different forms. Each form has its own biological activity, which is the measure of potency or functional use in the body. Alpha-tocopherol is the name of the most active form of vitamin E in humans. Vitamin E has also been shown to play a role in immune function, in DNA repair, and other metabolic processes. Worldwide, only a handful of researchers study vitamin K—long known for its critical role in clotting but this vitamin may command a bigger following as its importance to the integrity of bones becomes increasingly clear. It activates at least three proteins involved in bone health, says Sarah Booth at the Jean Mayer USDA Human Nutrition Research Center on Aging at Tufts University in Boston. The primary role of vitamin K is blood clotting. It is essential for the activation of proteins and calcium involved in the clotting process. Vitamin K is also involved in the metabolism of bone proteins. Deficiency of this vitamin causes hemorrhaging. For infants in the U.S., Vitamin K deficiency without bleeding may occur in as many as 50% of infants younger than 5 days old. Therefore, the committee on Nutrition of the American Academy of Pediatrics recommends that 0.5 to 10. mg vitamin K be administered to all newborns shortly after birth. Vitamin K toxicity is uncommon. Unlike the safe natural forms of vitamin K a synthetic form of vitamin K (menadione), is demonstrably toxic. The FDA has banned this form from over-the-counter sale in the United States because large doses have been shown to cause allergic reactions, hemolytic anemia, and cytotoxicity in liver cells.

Chapter 7 Sample Test

1. List the major roles for each of the B vitamins and vitamin C.
2. List the major roles for each of the following: Vitamin A, Vitamin D, Vitamin E, and Vitamin K.
3. List two sources for the vitamins listed in question #1.
4. List two sources for the vitamins listed in question #2.
5. Why would it be unwise to take three times the DRI of vitamin D?
6. What advice would you give to a client who tells you that he or she is taking three grams (3000 mg) of vitamin C per day?

References

1. Guyton, A. (1991). *Textbook of Medical Physiology,* 8th ed. Phil: W.B. Saunders Co.
2. Ross, C (Shils) et al. (2012). *Modern Nutrition in Health & Disease, 11th ed.* Philadelphia PA: Lipincott Wilillians & Wilikins (260-415).
3. Harper AE (2003). Contributions of women scientists in the U.S. to the development of Recommended Dietary Allowances. *J. Nutr.* 133 (11): 3698–702.
4. Whitney, E & Rolfes S. (2013). *Understanding Nutrition 13th ed.* Belmont,CA:Wadsworth, Cengage Learnin (297-364).
5. Evans W. Rosenberg AH. (1991). *Biomarkers.* NY: Simon & Schuster.
6. Tucker, K. Plasma vitamin B12 concentrations relate to intake source in the Framingham offspring Study. *Am J of Clin Nutr,* 71(2),514,2000.
7. Recommended Dietary Allowances, 10th ed. Subcommittee on the tenth edition of the RDAs, Food and Nutrition Board Commission on Life Sciences, National Research Council. Washington, DC: National Academy Press, 1989.
8. Liebman, B. Calcium: after the craze. Nutrition Action Healthletter. 21:5, p. 1. 1994.
9. Institute of Medicine, Food and Nutrition Board. Dietary Reference Intakes for Vitamin C, Vitamin E, Selenium and Carotenoids. A report of the Panel on dietary Antioxidants and Related Compounds, Subcommittees on Upper Reference Levels of Nutrients and Interpretation and Uses of Dietary Reference Intakes, and the Standing Committee on the Scientific Evaluation of Dietary Reference Intakes. Washington, D.C, National Academy Press, 2000.
10. Bown. Stephen R. (2003). SCURVY: How a Surgeon, a Mariner and a Gentleman Solved the Greatest Medical Mystery of the Age of Sail". NY: Viking.
11. Dietary Reference Intakes (DRIs): Recommended Intakes for Individuals, Food and Nutrition Board, Institute of Medicine, National Academies, 2004, retrieved 2009-06-09. Includes the 2010 updated recommendations for calcium and vitamin D.
12. Levine M. Rumsey SC., Wang Y. Park JB. Daruwala R (2000). Vitamin C. In Stipanuk MH. *Biochemical and physiological aspects of human nutrition*. Philadelphia: W.B. Saunders. 541–67.
13. McGregor GP. Biesalski HK (2006). Rationale and impact of vitamin C in clinical nutrition. *Curr Opin Clin Nutr Metab Care* 9 (6): 697–703.
14. Gerster H. (1997) . Vitamin A-functions, dietary requirements and safety in humans. *Int J Vitam Nutr Res.* 67:71-90.
15. Ross DA. (1998) . Vitamin A and public health: Challenges for the next decade. *Proc Nutr Soc.* 57:159-65.
16. Harbige LS. (1996). Nutrition and immunity with emphasis on infection and autoimmune disease. *Nutr Health.* 10:285-312.
17. Semba RD. (1998). The role of vitamin A and related retinoids in immune function. *Nutr Rev.* 56:S38-48. [PubMed abstract].
18. de Pee S. West CE. (1996). Dietary carotenoids and their role in combating vitamin A deficiency: A review of the literature. *Eur J Clin Nutr.* 50 Suppl 3:S38-53.
19. Olson JA. Kobayashi S. (1992). Antioxidants in health and disease: Overview. *Proc Soc Exp Biol Med.* 200:245-7.
20. Olson JA. (1996). Benefits and liabilities of vitamin A and carotenoids. *J Nutr.* 126: 1208S-12S.
21. Pavia SA. Russell RM. (1999). Beta-carotene and other carotenoids as antioxidants. *J Am Coll Nutr.* 18:426-33.
22. Bendich A. Olson JA. (1989). Biological actions of carotenoids. *FASEB J.* 3;1927-32.
23. Fontham E. (1990). Protective dietary factors and lung cancer. *Int J Epidemiol.* 9:S32-S42.

24. Rock CL. Jacob RA. Bowen PE. (1996). Update on the biological characteristics of the antioxidant micronutrients: Vitamin C, vitamin E, and the carotenoids. J Am Diet Assoc 1996;96:693-702.
25. Albanes D, et al. (1996). Alpha- tocopherol and beta-carotene supplement and lung cancer incidence in the alpha-tocopherol, beta- carotene cancer prevention study: Effects of base-line characteristics and study compliance. *J Natl Cancer Inst.* 88:1560-70.
26. Redlich CA, et al. (1998). Effect of supplementation with beta-carotene and vitamin A on lung nutrient levels. *Cancer Epidemiol Biomarkers Prev.* 7:211-14.
27. Pryor WA. Stahl W. Rock CL. (2000). Beta carotene: from biochemistry to clinical trials. *Nutr Rev.* 58:39-53.
28. National Institutes of Health. *Osteoporosis prevention, diagnosis, and therapy.* NIH Consensus Statement Online, 2000 March 27-29, 2000:1-36.
29. National Osteoporosis Foundation. *NOF osteoporosis prevention-risk factors for osteoporosis. 2003.* http://www.nof.org/prevention/risk.htm.
30. Binkley N. Krueger D. (2000). Hypervitaminosis A and bone. *Nutr Rev.* 58:138-44.
31. Forsyth KS. Watson RR. Gensler HL. (1989). Osteotoxicity after chronic dietary administration of 13- cis-retinoic acid, retinyl palmitate or selenium in mice exposed to tumor initiation and promotion. *Life Sci.* 45:2149-56.
32. Whiting SJ. Lemke B. (1999). Excess retinol intake may explain the high incidence of osteoporosis in northern Europe. *Nutr Rev.* 57:249-50.
33. Harrison EH. (2005). Mechanisms of digestion and absorption of dietary vitamin A. *Annu Rev Nutr.* 25:5.1-5.18.
34. Rodrigues MI. Dohlman CH. (2004). Blindness in an American boy caused by unrecognized vitamin A deficiency. *Arch Ophthalmol.* 122:1228-9.
35. Office of Dietary Supplements. National Institutes of Health. Vitamin D. http://dietary-supplements.info.nih.gov/factsheets/vitamind.asp. (accessed 06/15/2013).
36. DeLuca HF. Zierold C. (1998). Mechanisms and functions of vitamin D. *Nutr Rev.* 56:S4-10.
37. Reichel H,. Koeffler H. Norman AW. (1989). The role of vitamin D endocrine system in health and disease. N Engl J Med. 320:980-91.
38. van den Berg H. (1997). Bioavailability of vitamin D. *Eur J Clin Nutr.* 51 Suppl 1:S76-9.
39. Institute of Medicine, Food and Nutrition Board. Dietary Reference Intakes: Calcium, Phosphorus, Magnesium, Vitamin D and Fluoride. National Academy Press, Washington, DC, 1999.
40. Goldring SR. Krane S. Avioli LV. (1995). Disorders of calcification: Osteomalacia and rickets. In: LJ D, ed. Endocrinology. 3rd ed. Philadelphia: WB Saunders. 1204-27.
41. Favus MJ. Christakos S. (1996). Primer on the Metabolic Bone Diseases and Disorders of Mineral Metabolism. 3rd ed. Philadelphia, PA: Lippincott-Raven.
42. Holick MF. (2003). Evolution and function of vitamin D. Recent Results. *Cancer Res.* 164:3-28.
43. Hayes CE, Hashold FE, Spach KM, Pederson LB. The immunological functions of the vitamin D endocrine system. Cell Mol Biol 2003;49:277-300.
44. Holick MF. Vitamin D. In: Shils M. Olson J. Shike M. Ross AC, ed. (1999). Modern Nutrition in Health and Disease, 9th ed. Baltimore: Williams and Wilkins.
45. Bowes J. (1998). Church's Food Values of Portions Commonly Used. 17th ed. Philadelphia: Lippincot-Raven.
46. Nutrition Coordinating Center. Nutrition Data System for Research (NDS-R). Version 4.06/3 Minnesota: University of Minnesota, 2003.
47. U.S. Department of Agriculture, Agricultural Research Service. 2003. USDA Nutrient Database for Standard Reference, Release 16. Nutrient Data Laboratory Home Page, http:// www.nal.usda.gov/fnic/foodcomp online.

48. Holick MF. (1994). McCollum Award Lecture, 1994: Vitamin D: new horizons for the 21st century. *Am J Clin Nutr.* 60:619-30.
49. Holick MF. (2002). Vitamin D: the underappreciated D-lightful hormone that is important for skeletal and cellular health. *Curr Opin Endocrinol Diabetes.* 9:87-98.
50. Wharton B. Bishop N. Rickets. *The Lancet.* 2003;362:1389-1400.
51. Nesby-O'Dell S, et al. (2002). Hypovitaminosis D prevalence and determinants among African-American and white women of reproductive age: third National Health and Nutrition Examination Survey, 1988-1994. *Am J Clin Nutr.* 76:187-92.
52. Biser-Rohrbaugh A. Hadley-Miller N. Vitamin D deficiency in breast-fed toddlers. *J of Pediatr Orthaped* 2001;21:508-11.
53. Chesney R. (2003). Rickets: An old form for a new century. Pediatrics International. 45:509-11.
54. Picciano MF. (2001). Nutrient composition human milk. *Pediatr Clin North Am.* 48:53-67.
55. Gartner L. (2003). Greer FR. American Academy of Pediatrics Committee on Nutrition. Prevention of rickets and vitamin D deficiency: new guidelines for vitamin D Intake. *Pediatrics.* 111:908-10.
56. American Academy of Pediatrics committee on Environmental Health. Ultraviolet light: a hazard to children. *Pediatrics* 1999;104:328-33.
57. Fomom SJ. (2002). Reflections on infant feeding in the 1970s and 1980s. *Am J Clin Nutr* 198;46:171- 82.
58. Lips P. (2001). Vitamin D deficiency and secondary hyperparathyriodism in the elderly: consequences for bone loss and fractures and therapeutic implications. Endocrine Rev. 22:477-501.
59. MacLaughlin J. Holick MF. (1985). Aging decreases the capacity of human skin to produce vitamin D3. *J Clin Invest.* 76:1536-38.
60. Holick MF. Matsuoka LY. Wortsman J. (1989). Age, vitamin D, and solar ultraviolet. *Lancet.* 2:1104-5.
61. Need AG. MorrisHA. Horowitz M, Nordin C. (1993). Effects of skin thickness, age, body fat, and sunlight on serum 25-hydroxyvitamin D. *Am J Clin Nutr.* 58:882-5.
62. Webb AR. Kline L. Holick MF. (1988). Influence of season and latitude on the cutaneous synthesis of vitamin D3: Exposure to winter sunlight in Boston and Edmonton will not promote vitamin D3 synthesis in human skin. J Clin *Endocrinol Metab.* 67:373-78.
63. Webb AR. Pilbeam C. Hanafin N. Holick MF. (1990). An evaluation of the relative contributions of exposure to sunlight and of diet to the circulating concentrations of 25-hydroxyvitamin D in an elderly nursing home population in Boston. *Am J Clin Nutr.* 51:1075-81
64. Fairfield KM. Fletcher RH. (2002). Vitamins for chronic disease prevention in adults. *J Am Med Assoc.* 287:3116-26.
65. Harris SS, et al. (2000). Vitamin D insufficiency and hyperparathyroidism in a low income, multiracial, elderly population. *J Clin Endocrinol Metab.* 85:4125-30.
66. Lo CW. Paris PW. Clemens TL. Nolan J. Holick MF. (1985). Vitamin D absorption in healthy subjects and in patients with intestinal malabsorption syndromes. *Am J Clin Nutr.* 42:644-49.
67. Reid IR. (1998). The roles of calcium and vitamin D in the prevention of osteoporosis. Endocrinol Metab Clin North Am 1998;27:389-98.
68. Heaney RP. (2003). Long-latency deficiency disease: insights from calcium and vitamin D. *Am J Clin Nutr.* 78:912-9.
69. Parfitt AM. Osteomalacia and related disorders. In: Avioli LV, Krane SM, etc. *Metabolic bone disease and clinically related disorders.* 2nd ed. Philadelphia: WB Saunders. 1990:329-96.
70. LeBoff MS. Kohlmeier L. Hurwitz S. Franklin J. Wright J. Glowacki J. (1999). Occult

vitamin D deficiency in postmenopausal US women with acute hip fracture. *J Am Med Assoc.* 251:1505-11. [PubMed abstract].

71. Menopausal Hormone Therapy: Summary of a Scientific Workshop. Annals of Internal Medicine 2003;138:361-4.
72. ACOG, Questions and Answers on Hormone Therapy, in American College of Obstetricians and Gynecologists Web site response to the WHI Study Results on Estrogen and Progestin Hormone Therapy 2002. p. 1-8.
73. Chapuy MC. Arlot ME. Duboeuf F. Brun J. Crouzet B. Arnaud S. Delmas PD. Meunier PJ. (I992).Vitamin D3 and calcium to prevent hip fractures in elderly women. *N Engl J Med.* 327:1637-42.
74. Dawson-Hughes B. Harris SS. Krall EA. Dallal GE. Falconer G. Green CL. (1995). Rates of bone loss in postmenopausal women randomly assigned to one of two dosages of vitamin D. *Am J Clin Nutr.* 61:1140-45.
75. Rodriguez-Martinez MA and Garcia-Cohen EC. (2002). Role of Ca2+and vitamin D in the prevention and treatment of osteoporosis. *Pharmacology & Therapeutics.* 93:37-49.
76. Reid IR. (1996). Therapy of osteoporosis: Calcium, vitamin D, and exercise. *Am J Med Sci.* 312:278-86.
77. Chapuy MC. Pamphile R. Paris E. Kempf C. Schlichting M. Arnaud S. Garnere P. Meunier PJ. (2002). Combined calcium and vitamin D3 supplementation in elderly women: confirmation of reversal of secondary hyperparathyroidism and hip fracture risk: the Decalyos II study. *Osteoporosis Int.* 13:257-64.
78. Posner G. Low-Calcemic Vitamin D Analogs (Deltanoids) for Human Cancer Prevention. J. Nutr 2002;132:3802S-3S.
79. Martinez ME and Willett W C. (1998). Calcium, vitamin D, and colorectal cancer: a review of the epidemiologic evidence. *Cancer Epidemiol. Biomark. Prev.* 7:163-68.
80. Garland C, et al. (1985). Dietary vitamin D and calcium and risk of colorectal cancer: a 19-year prospective study in men. *Lancet.* 1:307-9.
81. Holt PR. (1999). Studies of calcium in food supplements in humans. *Ann N Y Acad Sci.* 889:128-37.
82. Langman M and Boyle P. (1998). Chemoprevention of colorectal cancer. *Gut.* 43:578-85.
83. Glinghammar B. Venturi M. Rowland IR. Rafter JJ. (1997). Shift from a dairy product-rich to a dairy product-free diet: Influence on cytotoxicity and genotoxicity of fecal water—potential risk factors for colon cancer. *Am J Clin Nutr.* 66:1277-82.
84. La Vecchia, et al. (1997). Intake of selected micronutrients and risk of colorectal cancer. *Int J Cancer.* 73:525-30.
85. Seth R. (1999). Vitamin D supplementation, 25-hydroxyvitamin D concentrations, and safety. *Am J Clin Nutr.* 69:842-56.
86. Lieberman DA. Prindiville S. Weiss DG. Willett W. (2003). Risk factors for advanced colonic neoplasia and hyperplastic polyps in asymptomatic individuals. *J Am Med Assoc.* 290:2959-67.
87. Buckley LM. Leib ES. Cartularo KS. Vacek PM. Cooper SM. (1996). Calcium and vitamin D3 supplementation prevents bone loss in the spine secondary to low-dose corticosteroids in patients with rheumatoid arthritis. A randomized, double-blind, placebo-controlled trial. *Ann Intern Med.* 125:961-8.
88. Lukert BP and Raisz LG. (1990).Gucocorticoid-induced osteoporosis: Pathogenesis and management. *Annals of Internal Medicine.* 112:352-64.
89. de Sevaux RGL. Hoitsma AJ. Corstens FHM. Wetzels JFM. (2002). Treatment with vitamin D and calcium reduces bone loss after renal transplantation: A randomized study. *J Am Soc Nephrol* 13:1608-14.
90. Buchner DM and Larson EB. (1987). Falls and fractures in patients with Alzheimer-type dementia. *J Am Med Assoc.* 20:1492-5.

91. Sato Y. Asoh T. Oizumi K. (1998). High prevalence of vitamin D deficiency and reduced bone mass in elderly women with Alzheimer's disease. *Bone.* 23:555-7.
92. Rapuri PB. Gallagher JC. Kinyamu HK. Ryschon KL. (2001). Caffeine intake increases rate of bone loss in elderly women and interacts with vitamin D receptor genotypes. *Am J Clin Nutr.* 74:694- 700.
93. Chesney RW. (1989). Vitamin D: Can an upper limit be defined? *J Nutr.* 119 (12 Suppl):1825-8.
94. Vieth R, Chan PR, MacFarlane GD. Efficacy and safety of vitamin D3 intake exceeding the lowest observed adverse effect level. Am J Clin Nutr 2001;73(2):288-94.
95. U.S. Department of Agriculture (USDA) and U.S. Department of Health and Human Services. Nutrition and Your Health: Dietary Guidelines for Americans. 5th ed. USDA Home and Garden Bulleting No. 232, Washington, DC: USDA, 2000. http://www.cnpp.usda.gov/DietGd.pdf.
96. Center for Nutrition Policy and Promotion. United States Department of Agriculture. Food Guide Pyramid, 1992 (revised 1996). http://www.nal.usda.gov/fnic/Fpyr/pyramid.html.
97. NIH Clinical Center Fact Sheets in conjunction with ODS. http://dietary-supplements.info.nih.gov/factsheets/vitamine.asp.
98. Traber MG. Vitamin E. In: Shils ME, Olson JA, Shike M, Ross AC, ed. Modern Nutrition in Health and Disease. 10th ed. Baltimore: Williams & Wilkins, 1999:347-62.
99. Farrell P and Roberts R. Vitamin E. In: Shils M, Olson JA, and Shike M, ed. Modern Nutrition in Health and Disease. 8th ed. Philadelphia, PA: Lea and Febiger, 1994:326-41.
100. U.S. Department of Agriculture, Agricultural Research Service. 2004. USDA National Nutrient Database for Standard Reference, Release 16-1. Nutrient Data Laboratory Home Page, http:// www.ars.usda.gov/ba/bhnrc/ndl.
101. Lonn EM and Yusuf S. (1997). Is there a role for antioxidant vitamins in the prevention of cardiovascular diseases? An update on epidemiological and clinical trials data. *Can J Cardiol.* 13:957-65.
102. Jialal I and Fuller CJ. (1995). Effect of vitamin E, vitamin C and beta-carotene on LDL oxidation and atherosclerosis. *Can J Cardiol.* (11)*:*G:97G-103G.
103. Stampfer MJ. Hennekens CH. Manson JE. Coldi0tz GA. Rosner B. Willett WC. (1993). Vitamin E consumption and the risk of coronary disease in women. *N Engl J Med.* 328:1444-9
104. Knekt P. Reunanen A. Jarvinen R. Seppanen R. Heliovaara M. Aromaa A. (1994). Antioxidant vitamin intake and coronary mortality in a longitudinal population study. *Am J Epidemiol.* 139:1180-9.
105. The Heart Outcomes Prevention Evaluation Study Investigators. Vitamin E supplement and cardiovascular events in high-risk patients. *N Engl J Med.* 342:154-60.
106. Waters DD, et al. (2002). Effects of hormone replacement therapy and antioxidant vitamin supplements on coronary atherosclerosis in postmenopausal women: a randomized controlled trial. *J Am Med Assoc.* 288:2432-40.
107. Weitberg AB and Corvese D. (1997).Effect of vitamin E and beta-carotene on DNA strand breakage induced by tobacco-specific nitrosamines and stimulated human phagocytes. *J Exp Clin Cancer Res.* 16:11-4.
108. Chan JM. Stampfer MJ. Giovannucci EL. (1998). What causes prostate cancer? A brief summary of the epidemiology. *Semin Cancer Biol.* 8:263-73.
109. Graham S. Sielezny M. Marshall J. Priore R. Freudenheim J. Brasure J. Haughey B. Nasca P. Zdeb M. (1992). Diet in the epidemiology of Postmenopausal Breast Cancer in the New York State Cohort. *Am J Epidemiol.* 136:3127-37.
110. Bostick RM. Potter JD. McKenzie DR. Sellers TA. Kushi LH. Steinmetz KA. Folsom AR. (1993). Reduced risk of colon cancer with high intakes of vitamin E: The Iowa Women's Health Study. *Cancer Res.* 15:4230-17.

111. Wu K. Willett WC, et al. (2002). A prospective study on supplemental vitamin E intake and risk of colon cancer in women and men. *Cancer Epidemiol Biomarkers Prev* 2002;11:1298-304.
112. Jacobs EJ, et al. (2002). Vitamin C and vitamin E supplement use and bladder cancer mortality in a large cohort of US men and women. *American Journal of Epidemiology.* 156: 1002-10.
113. Leske MC, et al. (1998). Antioxidant vitamins and nuclear opacities: The longitudinal study of cataract. *Ophthalmology.* 105:831-6.
114. Teikari JM, et al. (1997). Long-term supplementation with alpha-tocopherol. *Acta Ophthalmol Scand.* 75(6):634-40
115. Institute of Medicine, Food and Nutrition board. Dietary Reference Intakes: Vitamin C, Vitamin E, Selenium, and Carotenoids. National Academy Press, Washington, DC, 2000. I and beta-carotene and age-related cataract. Acta Ophthalmol Scand 1997;75:634-40. [PubMed abstract].
116. Booth, S. (2008). Vitamin K - Another good Reason to Eat your Greens. *Agricultural Research.* http://www.ars.usda.gov/ is/AR/archive/jan00/ green0100. htm.
117. Booth SL, et al. (2003). Vitamin K intake and bone mineral density in women and men. *Am J Clin Nutr.* 77:512-516.
118. Agricultural Research Service. National Agricultural Library. USDA Nutrient Database for Standard Reference. Last modified 2011. http://ndb.nal.usda.gov/
119. Suttle JW. Vitamin K. (1984). In: Machlin L, ed. Handbook of Vitamins. New York: NY: Marcel Dekker:147.
120. American Academy of Pediatrics Committee on Fetus and Newborn. (2003). Controversies concerning vitamin K and the newborn. Pediatrics. 112(1 pt 1):191-192.
121. Cheung Am, et al. (2008). Vitamin K supplementation in postmenopausal women with osteopenia (ECKO) trial: A randomized controlled trial. PloS Med. 5(10): e196.
122. Ansell J. Hirsh J. Poller L. Bussey H. Jacobson A. Hylek E (2004). The pharmacology and management of the vitamin K antagonists: the Seventh ACCP Conference on Antithrombotic and Thrombolytic Therap". *Chest* 126 (3 Suppl): 204S–233S.
123. Asakura, et al. (2001). Vitamin K administration to elderly patients with osteoporosis induces no hemostatic activation, even in those with suspected vitamin K deficiency. *Osteoporosis International.* 12 (12): 996–1000.
124. Ronden, et al. (1997). "Modulation of arterial thrombosis tendency in rats by vitamin K and its side chains". *Atherosclerosis* 132 (1): 61–67.
125. Higdon, J. (2008). Vitamin K. Linus Pauling Institute, Oregon State University. Retrieved 2008-04-12.
126. Sheth, A, et al. (2008). Potential liver damage associated with over the counter vitamin supplementation. *Journal of the American Dietetic Association.* 108:1536-1537.
127. Morgan, SL. (2009). Nutrition and bone: it is more than calcium and vitamin D. *Women's health.* 5:727-737.
128. Zhao I, et al. Retinoic acid downregulates microRNAs to induce abnormal development of spinal cord in spnina bifida rat model. *Child's Nervous System.* 24:485-492.
129. Jones C. (2008). Pharmacokinetics of vitamin D toxicity. Am J Clin Nutr. 88:582S-586S.

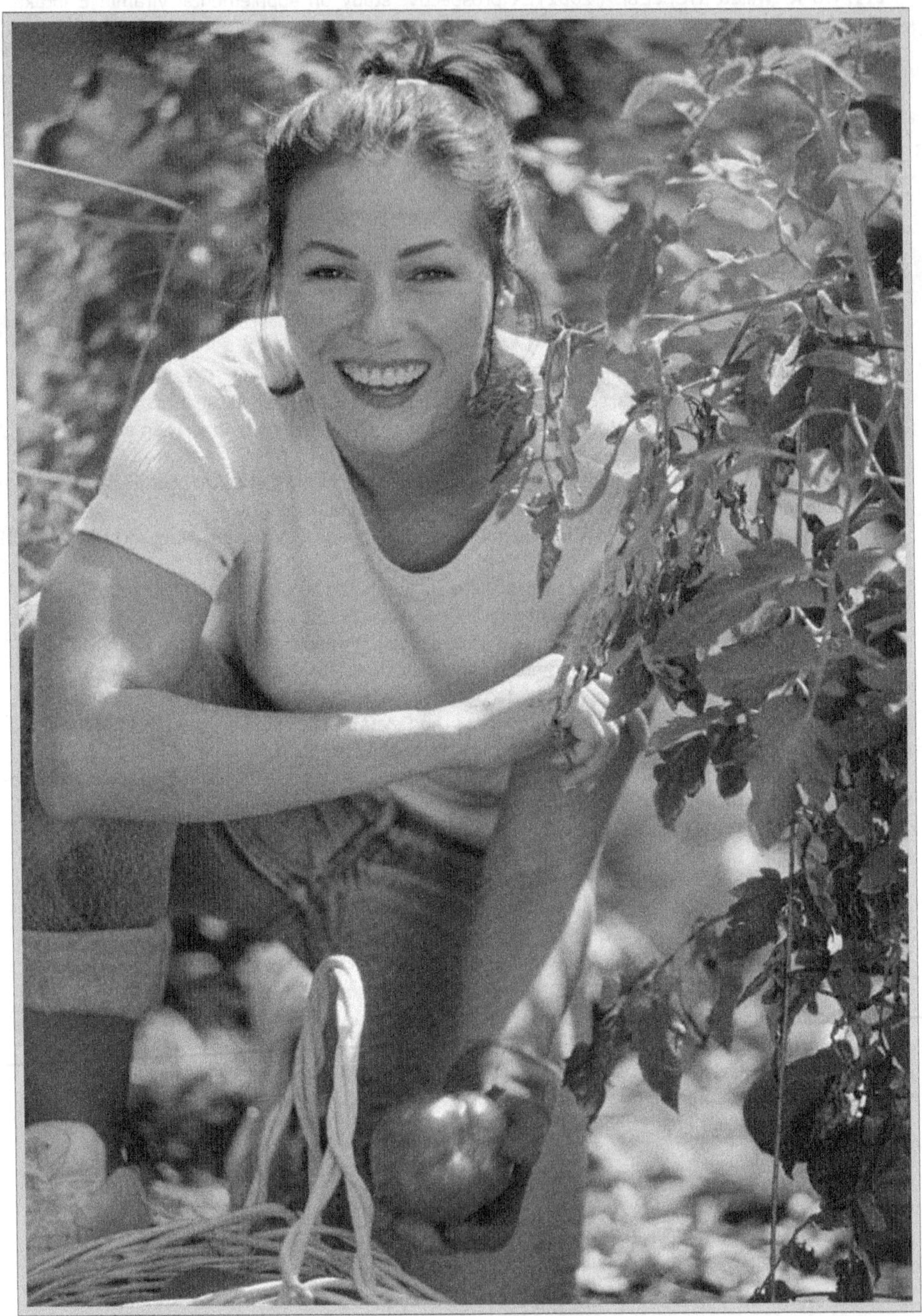

Chapter 8 – Minerals and Water

In this chapter we will we will take an in-depth look at minerals and water. Minerals and water are involved in all aspects of metabolism including catabolic and anabolic reactions.

Objectives

After reading and studying this session you should be able to:

1. Discuss the essential nutrient water including roles, sources, recommendations, deficiencies and toxicities.
2. Discuss the major and trace minerals including roles, food sources, Dietary Reference Intakes, deficiencies, and toxicities.

Introduction

Minerals are inorganic elements essential to life. They act as control agents in body reactions and as cooperative factors in energy production, body building and maintenance of tissues. They retain their identity (they cannot be changed into anything else), and they cannot be destroyed by heat, air, acid, or mixing but can be lost in cooking water (1).

Minerals require no digestion and are absorbed intact from the small intestines. They can become charged particles and can form compounds. Sodium and chloride are a familiar example of a compound i.e., sodium chloride (table salt) (1).

Minerals are divided into two categories - major and trace. The trace minerals are found in smaller amounts in the body, while the major minerals are found in larger amounts. The major minerals are calcium, sodium, chloride, potassium, sulfur, phosphorous and magnesium. The trace minerals are iron, zinc, iodine, selenium, copper, manganese, fluoride, chromium (1).

Some minerals are readily absorbed into the blood, transported freely, and readily excreted by the kidneys. Some minerals require carriers to be absorbed and transported (1).

Water, also an essential nutrient, is by far the most important nutrient to life; it is required in larger amounts than any other nutrient and without it life cannot be sustained beyond a few days (1).

Water

The following table summarizes the Adequate Intake (AI) for water in the adult population (DRI) (18).

Mineral	DRI (AI)*	Sources	Deficiency	Tolerable Upper Limit
Water	3.7 liters/d for men (125.1 ounces) and 2.7 liters/d for women (91.3 ounces)	All beverages, including water, as well as moisture in foods (high moisture foods include watermelon, meats, soups, etc.)	Dehydration, thirst, weakness, exhaustion, delirium	None established

Recommended intakes for water are based on median intakes of generally healthy individuals; hence, individuals can be adequately hydrated at levels below as well as above the AIs. The AIs provided are for total water in temperate climates and normal activities (20 minutes per day) (18). Higher levels of activity and environment increase need more than the recommended intakes (4).

No definitive research exists indicating requirements beyond the AIs. Experts still recommend at least eight glasses of water a day, but that estimate assumes a normal cool, environment, average size, and about 20 minutes of exercise a day (18). Recommendations by AND and ACSM were discussed in chapter 5. They recommend 1.5 liters of fluid per kg body weight loss during exercise. Dehydration (water deficit in excess of 2-3% body mass) decreases exercise performance; thus, adequate fluid intake before, during, and after exercise is important for health and optimal performance (51). The goal of drinking is to prevent dehydration from occurring during exercise. After exercise, approximately 16-24 oz (450-675 ml) of fluid should be consumed for every pound (0.5 kg) of body weight lost during exercise (51).

All sources of food can contribute to total water needs: beverages (including tea, coffee, juices, sodas, and drinking water) and moisture found in foods. Most fruits and vegetables contain up to 90% water, and meats and cheeses can contain 50% (4).

Water-Roles

Water participates in every chemical reaction in the body. Fluids in and around cells remain relatively constant due to the actions of water thereby maintaining homeostasis (4). Water carries nutrients and waste products throughout the body; serves as the solvent for minerals, vitamins, amino acids, glucose, and other small molecules allowing them to participate in metabolic reactions; maintains the structure of molecules such as proteins and glycogen; cushions joints and lubricates eyes, spinal cord, and surrounds the fetus in pregnancy (amniotic fluid); and maintains blood volume and helps regulate body temperature through evaporation from skin.

Water-Deficiency/Toxicity

Dehydration occurs when body water output exceeds water input (4). Fluid loses include urine, lungs (vapor), sweat (skin), and feces. The amount of fluid loss varies considerably, and therefore needs vary considerably. Signs of dehydration include thirst, weakness, exhaustion, delirium, and death. No upper limit has been established because normal functioning kidneys can handle more than 0.7 L (24oz) of fluid per hour. Symptoms of water intoxication include hyponatremia which can result in heart failure and rhabdomyolysis (skeletal muscle tissue injury) which can lead to kidney failure (1).

Major Minerals

The major minerals include calcium, sodium, chloride, potassium, sulfur, phosphorous, and magnesium. The following table summarizes the Dietary Reference Intake (DRI) or adequate intake (AI), food sources, deficiency, and tolerable upper levels for each of the major minerals for the adult population (2).

Mineral	DRI (AI)	Food Sources	Deficiency	Tolerable Upper Limit
Calcium	1000 mg/d for men and women	Milk, milk products, small fish with bones, calcium-set tofu (bean curd), greens, legumes	Stunted growth in children bone loss in adults	2500 mg/d
Sodium	1500 mg/d for men and women (AI)	Table salt, large amounts in processed foods, soy sauce, milk, breads	Hyponatremia from excessive losses not from inadequate intake	2300 mg/d
Chloride	2300 mg/d for men and women (AI)	Table salt, large amounts in processed foods, soy sauce, milk, eggs	Does not occur under normal circumstances	3600 mg/d
Potassium	4700 mg/d for men and women (AI)	All whole foods, meats, milks, fruits, vegetables, grains, legumes	Irregular heartbeat, muscular weakness, glucose intolerance	None established
Sulfate	None established	All protein containing foods	Only when protein intake is inadequate	None established
Phosphorus	700 mg/d for men and women	Animal products (meat, fish, poultry, eggs, milk	Muscular weakness and bone pain	4000 mg/d
Magnesium	400-420 for men and 310-320 for women	Nuts, legumes, whole grains, dark green vegetables, vegetables, seafood	Weakness, confusion, convulsions, bizarre muscle movements	350 mg/d

The following table summarizes the metabolic roles for each of the major minerals.

Mineral	Metabolic Roles
Calcium	Mineralization of bones and teeth; muscle contraction and relaxation; nerve functioning; blood clotting; blood pressure (see discussion below)
Sodium	Maintains normal fluid and electrolyte balance; nerve impulse transmission; muscle contraction
Chloride	Maintains normal fluid and electrolyte balance; is part of hydrochloric acid in the stomach
Potassium	Maintains normal fluid and electrolyte balance; facilitates many bodily reactions; cell integrity; nerve impulse transmission; muscle contraction
Sulfate	Stabilizes shape of proteins by forming di-sulfide bridges; part of biotin, thiamin, and

Mineral	Metabolic Roles
	insulin
Phosphorus	Mineralization of bones and teeth; involved in genetic materials; part of phospholipids; used in energy transfer and buffer systems that maintain acid-base balance
Magnesium	Bone mineralization; building of protein; enzyme action; muscle contraction; nerve impulse transmission; teeth; immune system

Calcium

Calcium is the most abundant mineral in the human body. It is stored in bones and teeth where it functions to support their structure (23). The remaining 1% is found throughout the body in blood, muscle, and the fluid between cells (23).

Dairy foods are the major source of calcium in the diet (3). The U.S. Department of Agriculture recommends that individuals two years and older eat 2-3 servings of dairy products per day (3). A serving is equal to: 1 cup (8 fl oz) of milk; 8 oz of yogurt; 1.5 oz of natural cheese (such as Cheddar); 2.0 oz of processed cheese (such as American). Although dairy products are the main source of calcium in the U.S. diet, other foods also contribute to overall calcium intake. Foods such as Chinese cabbage, kale and broccoli are other alternative calcium sources (3). Although most grains are not high in calcium (unless fortified), they do contribute some calcium to the diet because they are consumed frequently (3). Additionally, there are several calcium-fortified food sources presently available, including fruit juices, fruit drinks, tofu and cereals.

Calcium absorption refers to the amount of calcium that is absorbed from the digestive tract into the body's circulation. Calcium absorption can be affected by calcium status, vitamin D status, age, pregnancy and plant substances in the diet (21). Not all calcium consumed is actually absorbed. Humans absorb about 30% of the calcium in foods, but this varies depending upon the type of food in the diet (24).

The efficiency of absorption decreases as calcium intake increases (24). Net calcium absorption is as high as 60% in infants and young children, who need substantial amounts to build bone (24,27). Absorption decreases to 15%–20% in adulthood and continues to decrease as people age; hence, recommended calcium intakes are higher for females older than 50 years and for both males and females older than 70 years (24,27,28). Vitamin D improves calcium absorption (24).

Phytic acid and oxalic acid, found naturally in some plants, bind to calcium and can inhibit its absorption. Foods with high levels of oxalic acid include spinach, collard greens, sweet potatoes, rhubarb; fiber-containing whole-grain products and wheat bran; beans, seeds, nuts, and soy isolates (24). Research shows that eating spinach and milk at the same time reduces absorption of the calcium in milk (29). In contrast, wheat products (with the exception of wheat bran) do not appear to lower calcium absorption (30).

Some absorbed calcium is eliminated from the body in urine, feces, and sweat. This amount is affected by the following factors:

- Sodium and protein intakes. High sodium and protein intake increases urinary calcium excretion and negatively affects calcium status (31,32). Recent research suggests that high protein intake may increase intestinal calcium absorption, offsetting its effect on calcium excretion so whole body calcium retention remains unchanged (33).
- Caffeine intake. Caffeine is a stimulant which can modestly increase calcium excretion and reduce absorption (34). One cup of regular brewed coffee causes a loss of only 2–3 mg of calcium (32). Moderate caffeine consumption (1 cup of coffee or 2 cups of tea per day) in young women has no negative effects on bone (35).
- Alcohol intake. Alcohol can reduce the absorption of calcium by inhibiting enzymes in the liver that help convert vitamin D to its active form (37). The amount of alcohol required to affect calcium status is unknown.
- Phosphorus intake. The effect of phosphorus on calcium excretion is minimal. Several observational studies suggest that consumption of carbonated soft drinks with high levels of phosphate is associated with reduced bone mass and increased fracture risk. However, the effect is probably due to replacing milk with soda rather than the phosphorus itself (38,39).
- Fruit and vegetable intakes. Metabolic acids produced by diets high in protein and cereal grains increase calcium excretion (40). Fruits and vegetables, when metabolized, shift the acid/base balance of the body towards the alkaline by producing bicarbonate, which reduces calcium excretion. However, it is unclear if consuming more fruits and vegetables affects bone mineral density.

Lactose maldigestion (or "lactase non-persistence") describes the inability of an individual to completely digest lactose, the naturally occurring sugar in milk. Lactose intolerance refers to the symptoms that occur when the amount of lactose exceeds the ability of an individual's digestive tract to break down lactose. Symptoms of lactose intolerance vary from individual to individual depending on the amount of lactose consumed, history of previous consumption of foods with lactose, and the type of meal with which the lactose is consumed (12).

Menopause leads to bone loss because decreases in estrogen production both increase bone resorption and decrease calcium absorption (28,41,42). Annual decreases in bone mass of 3-5% per year are often seen during the years immediately following menopause, with decreases less than 1% per year seen after age 65 (43). Two studies are in agreement that increased calcium intakes during menopause will not completely offset menopausal bone loss (5,6). Hormone replacement therapy (HRT) with estrogen and progesterone helps increase calcium levels and prevent osteoporosis and fractures. Estrogen therapy restores postmenopausal bone remodeling to the same levels as at premenopause, leading to lower rates of bone loss (41). However, because of the potential health risks associated with HRT use, several medical groups and professional societies recommend that postmenopausal women consider using medications, such as bisphosphonates, instead of HRT to prevent or treat osteoporosis (44,45). In addition, consuming adequate amounts of calcium in the diet might help slow the rate of bone loss in all women (44,45).

Calcium - Roles

Calcium is required for muscle contraction, blood vessel contraction and expansion, the secretion of hormones and enzymes, and nervous system function (24). Food calcium never directly affects blood calcium (23). Serum calcium is very tightly regulated and does not fluctuate with changes in dietary intakes; the body uses bone tissue as a reservoir for, and source of, calcium to maintain constant concentrations of calcium in blood, muscle, and intercellular fluids (23).

Bones are living tissues and continue to change throughout life. During childhood and adolescence, bones increase in size and mass (1). Bones continue to add more mass until around age 30, when peak bone mass is reached. Peak bone mass is the point when the maximum amount of bone is achieved. Therefore, it is particularly important to consume adequate calcium and vitamin D throughout infancy, childhood, and adolescence. It is also important to engage in weight-bearing exercise to maximize bone strength and bone density (amount of bone tissue in a certain volume of bone) to help prevent osteoporosis later in life (5,6).

Calcium - Deficiency/Toxicity

Inadequate calcium intake, decreased calcium absorption, and increased calcium loss in urine can decrease total calcium in the body, with the potential of producing osteoporosis and other consequences of chronically low calcium intake. Hypocalcemia can cause numbness and tingling in fingers, muscle cramps, convulsions, lethargy, poor appetite, and mental confusion (1). It can also result in abnormal heart rhythms and even death. Individuals with medical problems that result in hypocalcemia should be under a medical doctor's care and receive specific treatment aimed at normalizing calcium levels in the blood.

Excessively high intakes of calcium can also have adverse effects. Adverse conditions associated with high calcium intakes are hypercalcemia (elevated levels of calcium in the blood), impaired kidney function, and decreased absorption of other minerals (1). Hypercalcemia can also result from excess intake of vitamin D, such as from supplement overuse at levels of 50,000 IU or higher (1). However, hypercalcemia from diet and supplements is rare. Most cases of hypercalcemia occur as a result of malignancy - especially in the advanced stages. Another concern with high calcium intakes is the potential for calcium to interfere with the absorption of other minerals such as iron, zinc, magnesium, and phosphorus (17).

Sodium, Potassium, Chloride

Electrolyte is a "medical/scientific" term for salts, specifically ions. Ions are atoms or molecules that have gained or lost an electron and have an electrical charge. The term electrolyte means that this ion is electrically-charged and moves to either a negative (cathode) or positive (anode) electrode (1):

- ions that move to the cathode (cations) are positively charged
- ions that move to the anode (anions) are negatively charged

Potassium is the body's principal intracellular cation (inside the cell) as opposed to sodium which is the principal cation of the extracellular fluid. Chloride associates with sodium (sodium-chloride) and is the major anion of the extracellular fluid.

Diets rarely lack sodium. Table salt is sodium chloride which contains about 40% sodium. Chloride is never naturally lacking in the diet. It abounds in foods as part of sodium chloride and other salts. Potassium is found in both plant and animal foods.

Sodium, Potassium, Chloride - Roles

The role of electrolytes is to maintain voltages across cell membranes and to carry electrical impulses (nerve impulses, muscle contractions) across the membranes and to other cells (1). Kidneys work to keep the electrolyte concentrations in blood constant despite bodily changes. Without the presence of these electrolytes water would move freely across cell membranes, thus destroying cellular integrity. Hence, electrolytes, through their charge, control water flow into and out of cells.

In addition to being the principal cation of the extracellular fluid and regulating cellular volume, sodium helps maintain acid-base balance and is essential to nerve impulse transmission and muscle contraction. As with glucose, sodium is carefully regulated. Sodium from the intestinal tract reaches the kidneys where the sodium is filtered out of the blood. The kidneys return the blood with an exact amount of sodium required. The amount excreted is generally the same as amount ingested except when sodium levels rise. The kidneys then excrete both the excess water and sodium together (4).

Potassium is involved in maintaining fluid and electrolyte balance and cell integrity. During nerve impulse transmissions and muscle contractions, potassium and sodium reverse places across the cell membrane allowing the cell to quickly pump them back into place. This process is extremely important since it affects all aspect of homeostasis including muscle contraction and heartbeat (4).

Chloride is associated with sodium (sodium-chloride) and is the major anion of the extracellular fluid. Chloride also moves passively across cell membranes and associates with potassium inside cells. So chloride is similar to sodium and potassium in that it also acts as an electrolyte (4).

Sodium, Potassium, Chloride - Deficiency/Toxicity

Deficiency of these nutrients is rare. Deficiency of sodium can occur in dehydration situations such as vomiting, diarrhea, or heavy sweating (23). In normal sweating during exercise, salt losses can safely be replaced later in the day with plain foods (18). Deficiency of chloride has never been seen, and deficiency of potassium is unlikely. However, diets low in fresh fruits and vegetables make it a possibility (18).

Toxicity of sodium produces edema and hypertension, but this is not a problem as long as water needs are met. In sensitive persons, prolonged excess can lead to hypertension. Toxicity of chloride can only result from dehydration due to water deficiency. Toxicity of potassium does not occur from overeating foods high in potassium (4).

The tolerable upper intake level (UL) for sodium is 2300 mg/day per day. More than 95 percent of American men and 90 percent of Canadian men ages 31 to 50, and 75 percent of American women and 50 percent of Canadian women in this age range regularly consume sodium in excess of the UL (18).

Older individuals, African Americans, and people with chronic diseases, including hypertension, diabetes, and kidney disease, are especially sensitive to the blood pressure-raising effects of sodium and should consume less than the upper limit (1). Adults should consume the adequate intake of 4700 mg of potassium per day to lower blood pressure, blunt the effects of sodium, and reduce the risk of kidney stones and bone loss (18).

There is no evidence of chronic excess intakes of potassium in apparently healthy individuals, thus no UL has been established (18).

Sulfur/Sulfate

Sulfate is the oxidized form of sulfur and is the form found in foods (1). Sulfate is found in most foods, and the body obtains sulfur from two sulfur containing amino acids—methionine and cysteine (18).

Sulfur/Sulfate - Roles

Sulfur forms bridges in proteins and is crucial to the contour of protein molecules (1).

Sulfur/Sulfate – Deficiencies/Toxicities

There is no recommended intake for sulfur, no deficiencies are known since needs can be easily met when diets contain protein. Toxicity would occur only when animal proteins are eaten in excess. No upper levels have been established (18).

Phosphorus

Phosphorus is the second most abundant mineral in the body (4). Phosphorus is well absorbed by the intestines and the total body phosphorus pool is regulated by renal excretion. Approximately 85% of the total body phosphate pool is found in bone as hydroxyapatite (4). The remaining amount of phosphate is distributed in blood and soft tissues.

Beans, peas, cereals and nuts contain phytate or inositol phosphate which is resistant to digestion (1). However, phytase from yeast added during leavening of breads, can release some phosphate from phytate. Intestinal microflora can also release phosphate from phytic acid in the colon. Phytase activity from endogenous and exogenous sources can increase the bioavailability of phosphate from plant sources by approximately 50%. Good dietary sources of phosphorous are typically also rich in protein. These foods are mainly milk, meat, nuts, legumes, and grains (4).

Phosphorus - Roles

Phosphorus is a component of bone, teeth, nucleic acids, phospholipids, ATP, and a number of enzymes and coenzymes (1). Phosphorylation/dephosphorylation of cellular compounds is a mechanism for regulating enzyme activity and for transport and storage of compounds. In the blood, phosphate is part of the buffering system (25). Phosphorus is part of DNA and RNA, and is also involved in the energy metabolism. Many enzymes and the B vitamins become active when a phosphate group is added. Phosphate is also part of lipids(phospholipids) (25).

Phosphorus - Deficiency/Toxicity

Phosphorus deficiency caused by inadequate dietary intake does not occur (46). However, chronic and excessive use of anticonvulsants, calcium carbonate supplements, or aluminum hydroxide-containing antacids can decrease phosphate absorption. Hypophosphatemia can also develop in individuals with gastrointestinal malabsorption, diabetes mellitus, hyperparathyroidism, renal dysfunction, or alcoholism. Hypophosphatemia results in bone loss, weakness, and poor appetite. Imbalances in phosphate intake may contribute to negative calcium balance when inadequate intake is accompanied by excessive intake (46).

The upper limit of safety for phosphorus established by the Food and Nutrition Board of the Institute of Medicine is 4000 mg daily for adults (18).

Magnesium

Magnesium is the fourth most abundant mineral in the body and is essential to good health (47). Approximately 50% of total body magnesium is found in bone. The other half is found predominantly inside cells of body tissues and organs. Only 1% of magnesium is found in blood (47).

The center of the chlorophyll molecule (which gives green vegetables their color) contains magnesium hence green vegetables such as spinach are good sources. Some legumes (beans and peas), nuts and seeds, and whole, unrefined grains are also good sources (48). When white flour is refined and processed, the magnesium-rich germ and bran are removed. Bread made from whole grain wheat flour provides more magnesium than bread made from white refined flour. Tap water can be a source of magnesium, but the amount varies according to the water supply (48).

Magnesium - Roles

Magnesium is needed for more than 300 biochemical reactions in the body. It helps maintain normal muscle and nerve function, keeps heart rhythm steady, supports a healthy immune system, and keeps bones strong (50). Magnesium also helps regulate blood sugar levels, promotes normal blood pressure, and is known to be involved in energy metabolism and protein synthesis (50,51). There is an increased interest in the role of magnesium in preventing and managing disorders such as hypertension, cardiovascular disease, and diabetes (47,50,51).

Magnesium - Deficiency/Toxicity

Early signs of magnesium deficiency include loss of appetite, nausea, vomiting, fatigue, and weakness. As magnesium deficiency worsens, numbness, tingling, muscle contractions and cramps, seizures, personality changes, abnormal heart rhythms, and coronary spasms can occur (47,50,51). Severe magnesium deficiency can result in low levels of calcium and/or low levels of potassium in the blood (47).

Even though dietary surveys suggest that many Americans do not consume recommended amounts of magnesium, symptoms of magnesium deficiency are rarely seen in the US (52). For many people, dietary intake may not be high enough to promote an optimal magnesium status (49,52).

Magnesium toxicity is very rare except in certain instances where renal failure prevents urinary excretion (i.e., in the situation where magnesium-containing drugs are given to a patient with renal inabilities) (53). Healthy kidney function excretes magnesium rapidly and efficiently, with little possibility for toxic buildup. Toxicity symptoms include central nervous system depression, skeletal muscle paralysis, and in extreme cases, coma and death. Calcium infusion tends to counteract magnesium toxicity (53). Levels up to 1600 mg daily have proven to produce no side effects as long as there is a balance of at least 50% calcium intake at the same time (53). The UL has been set at 350 mg from non food sources which has been shown to be toxic (48).

Trace Minerals

The trace minerals include iron, zinc, iodine, selenium, copper, manganese, fluoride, chromium, and molybdenum. The following table summarizes the Dietary Reference Intake (DRI) or adequate intake (AI), food sources, deficiency, and upper limits for each of the major minerals for the adult population (4).

Mineral	DRI (AI)	Food Sources (2)	Deficiency	Tolerable Upper Limit (Symptoms)
Iron	8 mg/d for men and 18 mg/d for women (8 mg/d for women over 50)	Red meats, fish, poultry, shellfish, eggs, legumes, dried fruits	Anemia, weakness, fatigue, headaches, impaired cognitive function, impaired immunity, concave nails, pica	45 mg/d (GI distress, iron overload, fatigue, joint pain, skin pigmentation, organ damage)
Zinc	11 mg/d for men and 8 mg/d for women	Protein containing foods (red meats, shellfish, whole grains, fortified	Growth retardation, delayed sexual maturation, impaired immune	40 mg/d (Loss of appetite, impaired immunity, low HDL, copper and iron

Mineral	DRI (AI)	Food Sources (2)	Deficiency	Tolerable Upper Limit (Symptoms)
		foods)	function, hair loss eye and skin lesions	deficiencies)
Iodine	150 ug/d for men and women	Iodized salt, seafood, bread, dairy sources, plants grown in iodine rich soil	Simple goiter, cretinism	1100 ug/d (Underactive thyroid gland, elevated TSH, goiter)
Selenium	55 ug/d for men and women	Seafood, meat, whole grains, fruits and vegetables (depending on soil content)	Predisposition to heart disease (cardiac tissue becomes fibrous – Keshan disease)	400 ug/d (Nail and hair brittleness/loss, irritability, nervous system disorders)
Copper	900 ug/d for men and women	Seafood, nuts, whole grains, seeds, legumes	Anemia, bone abnormalities	10,000 ug/d (Liver damage)
Manganese	2.3 mg/d for men and 1.8 mg/d for women (AI)	Nuts, whole grains, leafy vegetables, tea	Rare (requirements are low and found in all plant foods)	11 mg/d (Nervous system disorders)
Fluoride	4 mg/d for men and 3mg/d for women (AI)	Drinking water (if fluoridated), tea, seafood	Tooth decay	10 mg/d (Pitting and discoloration of teeth)
Chromium	35 ug/d for men and 25 ug/d for women (AI)	Meats (especially liver), whole grains, brewer's yeast	Diabetes-like condition	Not established (none reported)
Molybdenum	45 ug/d for both men and women	Legumes, cereals, nuts	Unknown	2000 ug/d (2 mg/d) (None reported)

The following table summarizes the major functions for each of the trace minerals.

Mineral	Metabolic Roles
Iron	Part of hemoglobin & myoglobin (makes oxygen available in blood and muscle); required for energy metabolism
Zinc	Part of insulin and many enzymes; involved in production of genetic materials; immune reactions; transport of vitamin A; taste perception; wound healing; sperm production; normal fetal development
Iodine	Component of thyroid hormones (regulate growth, development and metabolic rate)
Selenium	Part of an enzyme that prevents oxidation; regulates thyroid hormone
Copper	Helps form hemoglobin; is part of several enzymes
Manganese	Cofactor for several enzymes; bone formation
Fluoride	Maintains bones and teeth; confers decay resistance for teeth
Chromium	Enhances insulin action (may improve glucose tolerance)
Molybdenum	Co-factor for several enzymes

Iron

About 65 to 75 percent of the body's iron is in the blood in the form of hemoglobin and myoglobin (58). Most of the rest is contained in ferritin complexes that are present in all cells but especially in liver cells and the spleen.

The body conserves iron zealously. Storage levels of iron have the greatest influence on iron absorption. Iron absorption increases when body stores are low. When iron stores are high, absorption decreases to help protect against toxic effects of iron overload (56,58).

Once iron is absorbed, it is difficult to excrete so homeostasis is maintained through absorption. Ferritin, an iron storage protein, captures iron from food and stores it in the small intestines (4). When the body needs iron, ferritin releases some of its stores to transferrin, a transport protein, which delivers iron to cells. (4). If the iron is not required, it is carried out when intestinal cells are shed (every 3 to 5 days) and excreted. The liver's stores of ferritin are the primary physiologic source of reserve in the body (56,57).

Iron absorption is also influenced by the type of dietary iron consumed. There are two forms of iron, heme and non-heme. Absorption of heme iron from meat proteins is efficient. Absorption of heme iron ranges from 15% to 35%, and is not significantly affected by diet (59). In contrast, 2% to 20% of non-heme iron in plant foods such as rice, maize, black beans, soybeans, and wheat is absorbed (60).

Non-heme iron absorption is significantly influenced by various food components (1,57-59). One of these methods is to include foods rich in vitamin C in the diet (56). Good sources of vitamin C include citrus fruits and juices, tomatoes, strawberries, melons, dark green leafy vegetables, and potatoes. To have an effect, these foods must be eaten at the same meal as the iron source (56). Another method to improve non-heme iron absorption is to include a source of heme iron (meat) with the meal. Not only will more total iron be eaten, but the percentage of non-heme iron that is absorbed will be greater (56).

Tannins in tea and coffee adversely affect iron availability; while phytates, in some grains, phosphates in cola drinks, and possibly fiber, may interfere with iron absorption (56). Coffee and tea consumption at the time of a meal can significantly decrease iron absorption. Tea can cause iron absorption to drop by 60 percent and coffee can cause a 50 percent decrease in iron uptake.

Iron - Roles

Most of the body's iron is in the proteins hemoglobin (in red blood cells) and myoglobin (in muscle cells). Hemoglobin is the molecule responsible for carrying oxygen to cells, while myoglobin accepts, stores, and releases oxygen in the muscles (56). Iron is also required for the making of amino acids, hormones, and neurotransmitters (1). In addition, iron is involved in reactions within the body that produce energy. Any excess iron is stored in the body as a reserve. Once this reserve is depleted the formation of hemoglobin is affected; red blood cells cannot carry oxygen needed by the cells. When this happens, iron deficiency occurs, and anemia results (56).

<u>Iron - Deficiency/Toxicity</u>

The classic symptoms of iron deficiency are fatigue, weakness, headaches, apathy, pallor, and poor tolerance to cold (56,62,63). Iron deficiency and anemia are not the same. Iron deficiency refers to depleted body iron stores without regard to the degree of depletion or to the presence of anemia. Anemia refers to the severe depletion of iron stores that results in a low hemoglobin concentration (62). Persons with iron deficiency anemia have red blood cells that can't carry enough oxygen from the lungs to the tissues, so energy release is compromised (56, 62, 63).

The greatest need for iron is during growth or periods or blood loss. Young children, adolescents, and pregnant women have increased needs because of the growth taking place during these periods (61). The demands during pregnancy are so large that an iron supplement is recommended for pregnant women. All women of child-bearing age have increased requirements because of the losses from menstruation (61).

The elderly are another group at risk for iron deficiency. Seniors should consume adequate quantities of iron-rich foods and be particularly careful to incorporate vitamin C sources with their meals (56).

Many men and women who engage in regular, intense exercise may have marginal or inadequate iron status (56,64,65). Possible explanations include increased gastrointestinal blood loss after running and a greater turnover of red blood cells. Also, red blood cells within the foot can rupture while running. For these reasons, the need for iron may be 30% greater in those who engage in regular intense exercise (56,64,65).

Toxicity, once rare, is emerging among men in the US (19). Primary hemochromatosis is caused by a hereditary defect that allows iron to be continuously absorbed (19). Secondary hemochromatosis is caused by anemia, alcoholism, and other disorders. Juvenile hemochromatosis and neonatal hemochromatosis are two additional forms of the disease. Juvenile hemochromatosis leads to severe iron overload resulting in liver and heart disease in adolescents and young adults between the ages of 15 and 30. The neonatal form causes rapid iron buildup in a baby's liver that can lead to death (19).

Treatment is simple, inexpensive, and safe. The first step is to rid the body of excess iron. This process is called phlebotomy, which means removing blood the same way it is drawn from donors at blood banks. Based on the severity of the iron overload, a pint of blood will be taken once or twice a week for several months to a year, and occasionally longer. Blood ferritin levels will be tested periodically to monitor iron levels. The goal is to bring blood ferritin levels to the low end of normal and keep them there. Depending on the lab, that means 25 to 50 micrograms of ferritin per liter of serum (19). Once iron levels return to normal, maintenance therapy begins, which involves giving a pint of blood every 2 to 4 months for life. Some people may need phlebotomies more often. An annual blood ferritin test will help determine how often blood should be removed. Regular follow-up with a specialist is also necessary (19).

Zinc

Zinc is an essential mineral that is found in almost every cell. Muscle contains the highest proportion of total body zinc.

Zinc is found in a wide variety of foods (56). Oysters contain more zinc per serving than any other food, but red meat and poultry provide the majority of zinc in the American diet. Other good food sources include beans, nuts, certain seafood, whole grains, fortified breakfast cereals, and dairy products (49,56). Zinc absorption is greater from a diet high in animal protein than a diet rich in plant proteins. Phytates, which are found in whole grain breads, cereals, legumes, and other products, can decrease zinc absorption (56).

<u>Zinc - Roles</u>

Zinc stimulates the activity of approximately 100 enzymes, supports the immune system and wound healing, helps maintain sense of taste and smell, and is needed for DNA synthesis. Zinc also supports normal growth and development during pregnancy, childhood, and adolescence. Zinc associates with insulin in the pancreas; it interacts with platelets in blood clotting; affects thyroid hormone function; and affects behavior and learning performance (56).

<u>Zinc - Deficiency/Toxicity</u>

Zinc deficiency is characterized by growth retardation, loss of appetite, and impaired immune function. In more severe cases, zinc deficiency causes hair loss, diarrhea, delayed sexual maturation, impotence, hypogonadism in males, and eye and skin lesions (49,56,68,69). Weight loss, delayed healing of wounds, taste abnormalities, and mental lethargy can also occur (1,69). Zinc is required for the development and activation of T-cell lymphocytes, a kind of white blood cell that helps fight infection (71). When zinc supplements are given to individuals with low zinc levels, the numbers of T-cell lymphocytes circulating in the blood increase and the ability of lymphocytes to fight infection improves (71).

There is no single laboratory test that adequately measures zinc nutritional status. Medical doctors who suspect a zinc deficiency will consider risk factors such as inadequate caloric intake, alcoholism, digestive diseases, and symptoms such as impaired growth in infants and children (56). Vegetarians may need as much as 50% more zinc than non-vegetarians because of the lower absorption of zinc from plant foods, so it is very important for vegetarians to include good sources of zinc in their diet (56).

Studies show that poor, malnourished children in India, Africa, South America, and Southeast Asia experience shorter courses of infectious diarrhea after taking zinc supplements (72). Amounts of zinc provided in these studies ranged from 4 mg a day up to 40 mg per day and were provided in a variety of forms (zinc acetate, zinc gluconate, or zinc sulfate) (72).

The effect of zinc treatments on the severity or duration of cold symptoms is controversial. A Cochrane review concluded that "zinc (lozenges or syrup) is beneficial in reducing the duration and severity of the common cold in healthy people, when taken within 24 hours of onset of symptoms" (73). The author of another review completed in 2004 also concluded that zinc can reduce the duration and severity of cold symptoms (73). However, more research is needed to determine the optimal dosage, zinc formulation, and duration of treatment before a general recommendation for zinc in the treatment of the common cold can be made (73).

High doses of zinc (more than 50 milligrams) may cause vomiting, diarrhea, headaches, and exhaustion. The upper level for zinc is set at 40 milligrams due to possible interference in copper metabolism at higher levels which can lead to degenerative heart disease (56).

Iodine

Approximately 60% of the total body pool of iodine is stored in the thyroid gland. The remainder is found in the blood, ovaries, and muscle. Thyroid hormone is necessary for regulation of human growth and development (38).

Recommended amounts of iodine can be obtained by eating a variety of foods, including the following (4):

- Fish (such as cod and tuna), seaweed, shrimp, and other seafood, which are generally rich in iodine.
- Dairy products (such as milk, yogurt, and cheese) and products made from grains (like breads and cereals), which are the major sources of iodine in American diets.
- Fruits and vegetables, which contain iodine, although the amount depends on the iodine in the soil where they grew and in any fertilizer that was used.
- Iodized salt, which is readily available in the United States and many other countries. Processed foods, however, such as canned soups, almost never contain iodized salt.

Iodine - Roles

The only known function of iodine involves the synthesis of thyroid hormones (38). These hormones control the body's metabolism and many other important functions. The body also needs thyroid hormones for proper bone and brain development during pregnancy and infancy (38).

Iodine - Deficiency/Toxicity

Iodine deficiency has multiple adverse effects on growth and development and is the most common cause of preventable mental retardation in the world (74). Iodine deficiency disorders result from inadequate thyroid hormone production secondary to insufficient iodine (75,76). During pregnancy and early infancy, iodine deficiency can cause irreversible effects. Cretinism is a condition that develops in the fetus from iodine deficiency during pregnancy (77). This condition is characterized by mental retardation and dwarfism. Neonates are routinely screened for adequate thyroid hormone levels in developed countries and this practice is being adopted in non-developed countries as well (75).

Signs of iodine deficiency include hypothyroidism, lethargy, and weight gain. The clinical presentation of iodine deficiency is goiter. Goiter can also develop from high intakes of goitrogens, naturally occurring substances in foods which decrease iodine availability or interfere with its tissue utilization (74). Dietary sources of goitrogens include cabbage, turnips, rapeseed oil (canola oil), peanuts, cassava, and soybeans. Goitrogens are inactivated by heating, roasting or cooking (74).

High intakes of iodine can cause some of the same symptoms as iodine deficiency—including goiter, elevated TSH levels, and hypothyroidism—because excess iodine in susceptible individuals inhibits thyroid hormone synthesis and thereby increases TSH stimulation, which can produce goiter (56,78). Studies have also shown that excessive iodine intakes cause thyroiditis and thyroid papillary cancer (56,78). Cases of acute iodine poisoning are rare and are usually caused by doses of many grams. Acute poisoning symptoms include burning of the mouth, throat, and stomach; fever; abdominal pain; nausea; vomiting; diarrhea; weak pulse; and coma (56).

The upper limit of safety established for iodine by the Food and Nutrition Board of the Institute of Medicine is 1,100 micrograms daily for adults (56).

Selenium

Selenium exists in two forms: inorganic (selenate and selenite) and organic (selenomethionine and selenocysteine) (79). Both forms can be good dietary sources (80).

Seafood and organ meats are the richest food sources of selenium (1). Other sources include muscle meats, cereals and other grains, and dairy products. The major food sources of selenium are breads, grains, meat, poultry, fish, and eggs (81).

Selenium - Roles

Selenium is a constituent of more than two dozen seleno proteins that play critical roles in reproduction, thyroid hormone metabolism, DNA synthesis, and protection from oxidative damage and infection (79).

Selenium - Deficiency/Toxicity

Marginal intakes may reduce activities of selenium-dependent peroxidases (80,81). Changes in these enzyme activities have been associated with development of Keshan Disease (cardiomyopathy) and Kashin-Beck Disease (chondrodystrophy) in children in selenium-deficient regions of China (80,81). Selenium deficiency can also develop in malnourished patients dependent on enteral or parenteral nutrition for long periods of time (80,81). Muscle pain, weakness, and tenderness have been reported by these patients. Selenium supplementation can correct this type of deficiency. Selenium deficiency is also associated with male infertility and might play a role in Kashin-Beck disease (80,81).

The upper limit of safety for selenium established by the Food and Nutrition Board of the Institute of Medicine is 400 micrograms daily for adults (82). Excessive amounts of selenium (> 750 micrograms/day) can cause nausea, vomiting, diarrhea, loss of hair and nails, tenderness and swelling of the fingers, fatigue, irritability, skin lesions, tooth damage, and nervous system disturbances (82).

Copper

Approximately one third of the total body pool of copper is localized in skeletal muscle. Another third is found in brain and liver. The remaining amount of total body copper is found in bone and other tissues. Since copper is excreted primarily in the bile, diseases of the liver and gall bladder may affect copper balance (85).

Copper is found in organ meats, seafood, nuts, seeds, whole grains, legumes, chocolate, cherries, dried fruits, milk, tea, chicken, and potatoes (56).

Copper - Roles

Copper is a component of enzymes involved in collagen synthesis (1,85). Because of this, connective tissue-rich tissues such as capillaries, scar tissue, and bone matrix are most sensitive to copper status (84). Copper also functions at the catalytic site of the antioxidant enzyme superoxide dismutase. Additionally, the copper-containing plasma protein ceruloplasmin is integral to iron metabolism since it catalyzes oxidation of iron, which is required for its binding to proteins involved in absorption, transport, and storage. The redox potential of copper ions gives it a key role in energy metabolism as a component of the cytochromes that participate in electron transport (85).

Copper - Deficiency/Toxicity

Although severe copper deficiency is rarely observed, marginal copper status is not uncommon (85). Similar to iron, absorption is regulated by an intestinal copper-binding protein that is also involved with mucosal storage of zinc. Consequently, high dose zinc supplements (150 mg/day) can dramatically contribute to copper deficiency by decreasing the amount of protein available to bind copper. High dose vitamin C supplements (1500 mg/day) may also decrease copper absorption because the reduced form of the mineral, which is increased in the presence of vitamin C, is less well-absorbed than the oxidized form (56, 84).

Skeletal abnormalities, reproductive difficulties, impaired nervous tissue function, and changes in hair and skin pigmentation have been observed in severe copper deficiency (56, 84). A role for copper in the maintenance of bone mass has been determined from observations of osteoporosis in preterm infants born with inadequate copper reserves (85,86).

Copper toxicity is unlikely unless exposure to large amounts occurs as a result of industrial contamination or inappropriate use of supplements. Large dose copper supplements (10-20 mg/ day) may contribute to liver damage, abnormalities in red blood cell formation, weakness, and nausea (56).

Copper toxicity is the primary abnormality associated with Wilson's Disease. This inborn error of metabolism initially impacts the central nervous symptom causing tremors, dystonia, dysarthria, dysphagia, chorea, drooling, mental retardation, and lack of coordination (84). Treatment involves a copper-restricted diet and long-term oral penicillin therapy. Penicillin binds copper and reduces its absorption (84).

The upper limit of safety established for copper by the Food and Nutrition Board of the Institute of Medicine is approximately 900 micrograms daily for adults (56).

Manganese

Manganese is a co-factor for enzymes. Wheat germ, nuts, seeds, whole grains, oysters, sweet potatoes, tofu, chocolate, brewed tea, and dark molasses are good sources of manganese (56). Fruits and vegetables such as pineapple, grape juice, and tomato juice provide moderate levels and dairy products and meat provide little manganese (56).

Manganese - Roles

Manganese, a co-factor for enzymes, is involved in hydrolysis, phosphorylation, decarboxylation, transamination, and promotes activities of transferases such as glycosyltransferase and of glutamine synthetase and superoxide dismutase (1, 56).

Manganese - Deficiency/Toxicity

Manganese Deficiency in humans has not been documented but has been induced experimentally in animals (1,56). Poor growth and abnormal reproduction have been observed in rats and mice. No reported cases of manganese toxicity resulting from dietary intake have been reported. Manganese Toxicity has been observed from inhalation of manganese-containing dust by workers in mines and steel mills manifested by adverse effects on the central nervous system (1, 56).

The upper limit of safety for manganese established by the Food and Nutrition Board of the Institute of Medicine is approximately 11 mg daily for adults (1,56).

Chromium

When complexed with organic compounds, chromium is more efficiently absorbed as an inorganic salt (87). Dietary sources of chromium include whole grains, potatoes, oysters, liver, seafood, cheese, chicken, and meat. Brewer's yeast is a rich source of organic chromium complexes. Milled grains and other processed foods have considerably less chromium content than unprocessed (87). Diets composed primarily of processed foods may not provide sufficient amounts of chromium (87). Since chromium is lost in urine, sweat, bile, and hair, excessive physical exercise or tissue injury may also deplete tissue chromium levels (88,89).

Research does not support claims that chromium piccolinate supplements facilitate weight loss, build muscles, or decrease body fat. However, chromium supplementation has been found to improve glucose tolerance in elderly adults who have low blood chromium levels (90).

Chromium - Roles

Chromium was first identified as a component of the "glucose-tolerance factor" which is required for maintenance of normal blood glucose (91-93). As part of this factor, chromium acts synergistically with insulin to facilitate cellular uptake of blood glucose. Chromium may also have a role in other insulin-dependent activities such as protein and lipid metabolism (91-93). Tissue chromium depletion has been observed with age and may be responsible for abnormalities in glucose metabolism that often develop with age (91-93).

Chromium - Deficiency/Toxicity

Chromium deficiency is characterized by insulin resistance, hyperglycemia, and lipid abnormalities. Clinically, this deficiency has only been reported with long-term administration of parenteral nutrition when chromium is not added to the solutions (91-93).

No cases of chromium toxicity from excessive dietary intake have been reported. Chromium administered parenterally in high doses may cause skin irritation. The upper limit of safety for chromium has not been determined due to lack of data on adverse effects (56). The Food and Nutrition Board of the Institute of Medicine recommends intake of chromium should be from food only to prevent high levels of intake (56).

Molybdenum

Milk, dried beans, peas, nuts and seeds, eggs, liver tomatoes, carrots, and meats are good sources of molybdenum (94).

Molybdenum

Molybdenum is a co-factor of aldehyde oxidases which are involved in purine and pyrimidine detoxification (94). Xanthine oxidase is responsible for metabolism of uric acid. Molybdenum may also have a role in stabilizing the unoccupied glucocorticoid receptor (94).

No cases of human molybdenum deficiency have been reported (56,94) and no cases of human molybdenum toxicity have been reported. The upper limit of safety for molybdenum established by the Food and Nutrition Board of the Institute of Medicine is approximately 2,000 micrograms daily for adults (56).

Summary

Minerals are divided into two categories - the major minerals and the trace minerals. The trace minerals are found in smaller amounts in the body, while the major minerals are found in larger amounts. The major minerals are calcium, sodium, chloride, potassium, sulfur, phosphorous, and magnesium. The trace minerals are iron, zinc, iodine, selenium, copper, manganese, fluoride, and chromium.

Water, also an essential nutrient, is by far the most important nutrient to life; it is required in larger amounts than any other nutrient, and without, it life cannot be sustained beyond a few days .

All sources of food can contribute to total water needs: beverages (including tea, coffee, juices, sodas, and drinking water) and moisture found in foods. Most fruits and vegetables contain up to 90% water, and meats and cheeses can contain 50%.

Calcium is the most abundant mineral in the human body. It is stored in bones and teeth where it functions to support their structure. The remaining 1% is found throughout the body in blood, muscle, and the fluid between cells.

Calcium is required for muscle contraction, blood vessel contraction and expansion, the secretion of hormones and enzymes, and sending messages through the nervous system. Food calcium never directly affects blood calcium (23). Serum calcium is very tightly regulated and does not fluctuate with changes in dietary intakes; the body uses bone tissue as a reservoir for, and source of, calcium to maintain constant concentrations of calcium in blood, muscle, and intercellular fluids.

The roll of electrolytes is to maintain voltages across cell membranes and to carry electrical impulses (nerve impulses, muscle contractions) across the membranes and to other cells. Potassium is the body's principal intracellular cation (inside the cell) as opposed to sodium which is the principal cation of the extracellular fluid. Chloride associates with sodium (sodium-chloride) and is the major anion of the extracellular fluid. Diets rarely lack sodium. Table salt is sodium chloride which contains about 40% sodium. Chloride is never naturally lacking in the diet. It abounds in foods as part of sodium chloride and other salts. Potassium is found in both plant and animal foods. Sulfate is the oxidized form of sulfur and is the form found in foods.

Sulfate is found in most foods and the body obtains sulfur from two sulfur containing amino acids—methionine and cysteine. Sulfur forms bridges in proteins and is crucial to the contour of protein molecules. There is no recommended intake for sulfur; no deficiencies are known since needs can be easily met when diets contain protein. Toxicity would occur only when animal proteins are eaten in excess. No upper levels have been established.

Phosphorus is the second most abundant mineral in the body. Phosphorus is well absorbed by the intestines. Approximately 85% of the total body phosphate pool is found in bone as hydroxyapatite. The remaining amount of phosphate is distributed in blood and soft tissues. Phosphorus is a component of bone, teeth, nucleic acids, phospholipids, ATP, and a number of enzymes and coenzymes.

Phosphorylation/dephosphorylation of cellular compounds is a mechanism for regulating enzyme activity and for transport and storage of cell compounds. In the blood, phosphate is part of the buffering system. Phosphorus is part of DNA and RNA, and is also involved in energy metabolism. Many enzymes and the B vitamins become active when a phosphate group is added. Phosphate is also part of lipids—phospholipids.

Magnesium is the fourth most abundant mineral in the body and is essential to good health. Approximately 50% of total body magnesium is found in bone. The other half is found predominantly inside cells of body tissues and organs. Only 1% of magnesium is found in blood, but the body works very hard to keep blood levels of magnesium constant. Magnesium is needed for more than 300 biochemical reactions in the body. It helps maintain normal muscle and nerve function, keeps heart rhythm steady, supports a healthy immune system, and keeps bones strong. Magnesium also helps regulate blood sugar levels, promotes normal blood pressure, and is known to be involved in energy metabolism and protein synthesis. There is an increased interest in the role of magnesium in preventing and managing disorders such as hypertension, cardiovascular disease, and diabetes. Dietary magnesium is absorbed in the small intestines. Magnesium is excreted through the kidneys.

Most of the body's iron is in the proteins hemoglobin (in red blood cells) and myoglobin (in muscle cells). Hemoglobin is the molecule responsible for carrying oxygen to cells, while myoglobin accepts, stores, and releases oxygen in the muscles (56). About 65 to 75 percent of the body's iron is in the blood in the form of hemoglobin, the molecule responsible for carrying oxygen to all cells. Myoglobin, the compound that carries oxygen to the muscle cells, also requires iron. In addition, iron is involved in reactions within the body that produce energy. If iron is lacking in the diet, iron reserves in the body are used. Once this supply is depleted, the formation of hemoglobin is affected. This means red blood cells cannot carry oxygen needed by the cells. When this happens, iron deficiency occurs, and anemia results. Iron is also required for the making of amino acids, hormones, and neurotransmitters.

Zinc is an essential mineral that is found in almost every cell. It stimulates the activity of approximately 100 enzymes. Zinc supports a healthy immune system, is needed for wound healing, helps maintain sense of taste and smell, and is needed for DNA synthesis. Zinc also supports normal growth and development during pregnancy, childhood, and adolescence. Zinc associates with insulin in the pancreas; it interacts with platelets in blood clotting, affects thyroid hormone function, and affects behavior and learning performance.

The only known function of iodine involves the synthesis of thyroid hormones. These hormones control the body's metabolism and many other important functions. The body also needs thyroid hormones for proper bone and brain development during pregnancy and infancy. Approximately 60% of the total body pool of iodine is stored in the thyroid gland. The remainder is found in the blood, ovary, and muscle. Thyroid hormone is necessary for regulation of human growth and development.

Selenium is a constituent of more than two dozen seleno proteins that play critical roles in reproduction, thyroid hormone metabolism, DNA synthesis, and protection from oxidative damage and infection. Selenium exists in two forms: inorganic (selenate and selenite) and organic (selenomethionine and selenocysteine). Both forms can be good dietary sources. Seafood and organ meats are the richest food sources of selenium. Other sources include muscle meats, cereals and other grains, and dairy products.

Copper is a component of enzymes involved in collagen synthesis. Because of this, connective tissue-rich tissues such as capillaries, scar tissue, and bone matrix are most sensitive to copper status. Manganese is a co-factor for enzymes involved in hydrolysis, phosphorylation, decarboxylation, and transamination. It also promotes activities of transferases such as glycosyltransferase and of glutamine synthetase and superoxide dismutase.

Chromium was first identified as a component of the "glucose-tolerance factor" which is required for maintenance of normal blood glucose. As part of this factor, chromium acts synergistically with insulin to facilitate cellular uptake of blood glucose. Chromium may also have a role in other insulin-dependent activities such as protein and lipid metabolism. Tissue chromium depletion has been observed with age and may be responsible for abnormalities in glucose metabolism that often develop with age. Chromium may also have a role in other insulin-dependent activities such as protein and lipid metabolism.

Molybdenum is a co-factor of aldehyde oxidases which are involved in purine and pyrimidine detoxification. Xanthine oxidase is responsible for metabolism of uric acid. Molybdenum may also have a role in stabilizing the unoccupied glucocorticoid receptor.

Chapter 8 Sample Test

1. List two trace minerals, and discuss the roles of each.
2. List two major minerals, and discuss the roles of each.
3. Why would it be unwise to ingest three times the RDA of iron?
4. What are the number of servings of calcium in your diet? What are the recommended number of servings of calcium? Keep a food log again, and determine the number of servings of calcium, fruits, and vegetables in your diet.
5. What advice would you give to a client who tells you that he or she is taking three grams (3000 mg) of calcium per day?

References

1. Ross, C (Shils) et al. (2012). *Modern Nutrition in Health & Disease, 11th ed.* Philadelphia PA: Lipincott Wilillians & Wilikins (102-259).
2. Dietary Reference Intakes for calcium, phosphorous, magnesium, vitamin D and fluoride. (1997). NATIONAL ACADEMY PRESS Washington, D.C. Standing Committee on the Scientific Evaluation of Dietary Reference Intakes Food and Nutrition Board Institute of Medicine. Includes the 2010 updated recommendations for calcium and vitamin D. http://www.nal.usda.gov/fnic/DRI/DRI_Calcium/calcium_full_doc.pdf.
3. Subar AF. Krebs-Smith SM. Cook A. Kahle LL. (1998). Dietary sources of nutrients among US adults. *J Am Diet Assoc.* 98:537-47.
4. Whitney, E & Rolfes S. (2013). *Understanding Nutrition 13th ed.* Belmont,CA:Wadsworth, Cengage Learnin (367-434).
5. Dawson-Hughes B. Dallal GE. Krall EA. Sadowski L. Sahyoun N. Tannenbaum S. (1990). A controlled trial of the effect of calcium supplementation on bone density in postmenopausal women. *N Engl J Med* 1990. 323:878-83.
6. Elders PJ. Lips P. Netelenbos JC, et al. (1994). Long-term effect of calcium supplementation on bone loss in perimenopausal women. *J Bone Min Res.* 9:963-70.
7. Menopausal hormone therapy: Summary of a scientific workshop. (2003). *Ann Intern Med.* 138:361- 364.
8. American College of Obstetricians and Gynecologists. (2002).Questions and answers on hormone therapy. American College of Obstetricians and Gynecologists. http://www.acog.org/from_home/publications/ press_releases/nr08-30-02.cfm.
9. Johnson AO. Semenya JG. Buchowski MS. Enwonwu CO. (1993). Scrimshaw NS. Correlation of lactos maldigestion, lactose intolerance, and milk intolerance. *Am J Clin Nutr.* 57:399-401.
10. Rao DR. Bello H. Warren AP. Brown GE. (1994). Prevalence of lactose maldigestion: Influence and interaction of age, race, and sex. *Dig Dis Sci.* 39:1519-24.
11. Coffin B. Azpiroz F. Guarner F. Mlagelada JR. (1994).Selective gastric hypersensitivity and reflex hyporeactivity in functional dyspepsia. *Gastroenterology.* 107:1345-51.
12. Hertzler SR, Huynh B, Savaiano DA. (1996). How much lactose is "low lactose". *J Am Diet Assoc.* 96:243-46.
13. Marsh AG. Sanchez TV Midkelsen O. Keiser J, Mayor G. (1980). Cortical bone density of adult lacto-ovo- vegetarian and omnivorous women. *J Am Diet Assoc.* 76:148-51.
14. Reed JA. Anderson JJ. Tylavsky FA. (1994). Gallagher JCJ. Comparative changes in radial-bone density of elderly female lacto-ovo-vegetarians and omnivores. *Am J Clin Nutr.* 59:1197S-1202S.
15. Marsano L. and McClain C.J. (1989). Effects of alcohol on electrolytes and minerals. *Alcohol Health & Research World* 13(3):255-260.
16. Burckhardt P. Dawson-Hughes B. Heaney RP. (2001).Nutritional aspects of osteoporosis. *Academic Press.* 17.
17. Spencer H. Menczel J. Lewin I. Samachson J. (1965). Effect of high phosphorus intake on calcium and phosphorus metabolism in man. *J Nutr.* 86:125-32.
18. Dietary Reference Intakes: Electrolytes and Water. *National Academy of Sciences. Institute of Medicine. Food and Nutrition Board.* DRI table for sodium, chloride, potassium, inorganic sulfate and water. http://fnic.nal.usda.gov/dietary-guidance/dietary-reference-intakes/dri-tables.
19. Hemochromatosis. NIH Publication No. 07–4621. (2007). NIH Publication No. 07–4621.
20. Andon MB. Peacock M. Kanerva RL. De Castro JAS. Calcium absorption from apple and orange juice fortified with calcium citrate malate (CCM). J Am Coll Nutr 1996;15:313-16.

21. Heaney RP. Saville PD. Recker RR. (1975). Calcium absorption as a function of calcium intake. *J Lab Clin Med.* 85:881-90.
22. Heaney RP. Recker RR. Hinders SM. (1988). Variability of calcium absorption. *Am J Clin Nutr.* 47:262- 64.23.
23. Schrier RW. (2010). "Does 'asymptomatic hyponatremia' exist?" *Nat Rev Nephrol.* 6 (4):185.
24. Committee to Review Dietary Reference Intakes for Vitamin D and Calcium, Food and Nutrition Board, Institute of Medicine. Dietary Reference Intakes for Calcium and Vitamin D. Washington, DC: National Academy Press, 2010.
25. Rodriquez NR. DiMarco NM. Langley S. (2009). Position of the American Dietetic Association, Dietitians of Canada, and the American College of Sports Medicine: Nutrition and athletic performance. *J Am Diet Assoc.* 109(3):509-527 [homepage on the Internet]. c2012. Available from: http://journals.lww.com/acsm-msse/Fulltext/2009/03000/Nutrition_and_Athletic_Performance.27.aspxPrev Chronic Dis. 2006 October; 3(4): A129. Published online 2006 September 15. PMCID: PMC1784117.
26. Sawka M. Burke L. Eicher R, et al. (2007). Exercise and fluid replacement. *Med Sci Sports Exerc.* 39(2):377-390.[homepage on the Internet]. c2012. Available from: http://www.acsm-msse.org.
27. National Institutes of Health. Optimal calcium intake. NIH Consensus Statement: 1994;12:1-31.
28. Heaney RP. Recker RR. Stegman MR. Moy AJ. (1989). Calcium absorption in women: relationships to calcium intake, estrogen status, and age. *J Bone Miner Res.* 4:469-75.
29. Weaver CM. Heaney RP. (1991). Isotopic exchange of ingested calcium between labeled sources: evidence that ingested calcium does not form a common absorptive pool. *Calcif Tissue Int.* 49:244-7
30. Weaver CM. Heaney RP. Martin BR. Fitzsimmons ML. (1991). Human calcium absorption from whole-wheat products. *J Nutr.* 121:1769-75.
31. Weaver CM. Proulx WR. Heaney RP. (1999). Choices for achieving adequate dietary calcium with a vegetarian diet. *Am J Clin Nutr.* 70:543S-8S.
32. Heaney RP. (1996). Bone mass, nutrition, and other lifestyle factors. *Nutr Rev.* 54:S3-S10.
33. Kerstetter JE. O'Brien KO. Caseria DM. Wall DE. Insogna KL. (2005). The impact of dietary protein on calcium absorption and kinetic measures of bone turnover in women. *J Clin Endocrinol Metab.* 90(1):26-31.
34. Barrett-Connor E. Chang JC. Edelstein SL. (1994). Coffee-associated osteoporosis offset by daily milk consumption. *JAMA.* 271:280-3.
35. Massey LK. Whiting SJ. Caffeine, urinary calcium, calcium metabolism, and bone. J Nutr 1993;123:1611-4.
36. Hirsch PE. Peng TC. Effects of alcohol on calcium homeostasis and bone. In: Anderson J, Garner S, eds. Calcium and Phosphorus in Health and Disease. Boca Raton, FL: CRC Press, 1996:289-300.
37. U.S. Department of Agriculture. Results from the United States Department of Agriculture's 1994-96 Continuing Survey of Food Intakes by Individuals/Diet and Health Knowledge Survey, 1994-96.
38. Calvo MS. (1993). Dietary phosphorus, calcium metabolism and bone. *J Nutr.* 123:1627-33.
39. Heaney RP. Rafferty K. (2001). Carbonated beverages and urinary calcium excretion. *Am J Clin Nutr.* 74:343-7.
40. Fenton TR. Eliasziw M. Lyon AW. Tough SC. Hanley DA. (2008). Meta-analysis of the quantity of calcium excretion associated with the net acid excretion of the modern diet under the acid-ash diet hypothesis. *Am J Clin Nutr.* 88(4):1159-66.
41. Breslau NA. (1994). Calcium, estrogen, and progestin in the treatment of osteoporosis. *Rheum Dis Clin North Am.* 20:691-716.
42. Gallagher JC. Riggs BL. (1980). Deluca HF. Effect of estrogen on calcium absorption and

serum vitamin D metabolites in postmenopausal osteoporosis. *J Clin Endocrinol Metab.* 51:1359-64.

43. Daniels CE. (2001). Estrogen therapy for osteoporosis prevention in postmenopausal women. *Pharmacy Update-NIH* (2001;March/Apri).l
44. Kirschstein R. (2003). Menopausal hormone therapy: summary of a scientific workshop. *Ann Intern Med.* 138:361-4.
45. American College of Obstetricians and Gynecologists. (2004). Frequently Asked Questions About Hormone Therapy.
46. Bugg NC. Jones JA. (1998). Hypophosphataemia. Pathophysiology, effects and management on the intensive care unit. *Anaesthesia.* 53(9):895-902.
47. Rude RK. (1998). Magnesium deficiency: A cause of heterogeneous disease in humans. *J Bone Miner Res.* 13:749-58.
48. Institute of Medicine. Food and Nutrition Board. Dietary Reference Intakes: Calcium, Phosphorus, Magnesium, Vitamin D and Fluoride. National Academy Press. Washington, DC, 1999.
49. U.S. Department of Agriculture, Agricultural Research Service. 2011. USDA National Nutrient Database for Standard Reference, Release 24. Nutrient Data Laboratory Home Page, http://www.ars.usda.gov/ba/bhnrc/ndl.
50. Saris NE. Mervaala E. Karppanen H. Khawaja JA. Lewenstam A. (2000). Magnesium: an update on physiological, clinical, and analytical aspects. *Clinica Chimica Acta.* 294:1-26.
51. Wester PO. (1987). Magnesium. *Am J Clin Nutr.* 45:1305-12.
52. Vormann J. (2003). Magnesium: nutrition and metabolism. *Molecular Aspects of Medicine.* 24:27-37.
53. Xing JH and Soffer EE. (2001). Adverse effects of laxatives. *Dis Colon Rectum.* 44:1201-9.
54. Institute of Medicine. Food and Nutrition Board. Dietary Reference Intakes: Calcium, Phosphorus, Magnesium, Vitamin D and Fluoride. National Academy Press. Washington, DC, 1999.
55. U.S. Department of Agriculture, Agricultural Research Service. (2003). USDA National Nutrient Database for Standard Reference, Release 16. Nutrient Data Laboratory Home Page, http:// www.nal.usda.gov/fnic/foodcomp.
56. Institute of Medicine. Food and Nutrition Board. Dietary Reference Intakes for Vitamin A, Vitamin K, Arsenic, Boron, Chromium, Copper, Iodine, Iron, Manganese, Molybdenum, Nickel, Silicon, Vanadium and Zinc. Washington, DC: National Academy Press, 2001.
57. Miret S. Simpson RJ. McKie AT. (2003). Physiology and molecular biology of dietary iron absorption. *Annu Rev Nutr.* 23:283-301.
58. Bothwell TH. Charlton RW. Cook JD. Finch CA. (1979). Iron Metabolism in Man. St. Louis: Oxford: Blackwell Scientific.
59. Monson ER. (1988). Iron and absorption: dietary factors which impact iron bioavailability. *J Am Dietet Assoc.* 88:786-90.
60. Tapiero H. Gate L. Tew KD. (2001). Iron: deficiencies and requirements. *Biomed Pharmacother.* 55:324-32.
61. CDC Recommendations to prevent and control iron deficiency in the United States. (1998). Centers for Disease Control and Prevention. *MMWR Recomm Rep.* 47:1-29.
62. Haas JD. Brownlie T 4th. (2001). Iron deficiency and reduced work capacity: a critical review of the research to determine a causal relationship. *J Nutr.* 131:691S-6S.
63. Bhaskaram P. (2001). Immunobiology of mild micronutrient deficiencies. Br J Nutr. 85:S75-80.
64. Clarkson PM and Haymes EM. (1995). Exercise and mineral status of athletes: calcium, magnesium, phosphorus, and iron. *Med Sci Sports Exerc.* 27:831-43.
65. Raunikar RA. Sabio H. (1992). Anemia in the adolescent athlete. *Am J Dis Child.* 146:1201-5.

66. Sandstead HH. (1994). Understanding zinc: recent observations and interpretations. *J Lab Clin Med.* 124:322-7.
67. Solomons NW. (1998). Mild human zinc deficiency produces an imbalance between cell-mediated and humoral immunity. *Nutr Rev.* 56:27-8.
68. Prasad AS. Zinc: an overview. Nutrition 1995;11:93-9.
69. Maret W. Sandstead HH. (2006). Zinc requirements and the risks and benefits of zinc supplementation. *J Trace Elem Med Biol.* 20:3-18.
70. Beck FW. Prasad AS. Kaplan J. Fitzgerald JT. Brewer GJ. (1997). Changes in cytokine production and T cell subpopulations in experimentally induced zinc-deficient humans. *Am J Physiol.* 272:E1002-7.
71. Shankar AH. Prasad AS. (1998). Zinc and immune function: the biological basis of altered resistance to infection. *Am J Clin Nutr.* 68:447S-63S
72. Black RE. (1998). Therapeutic and preventive effects of zinc on serious childhood infectious diseases in developing countries. *Am J Clin Nutr.* 68:476S-9S.
73. Singh M. Das RR. (2011). Zinc for the common cold. Cochrane Database Syst Rev. 16;2:CD001364.
74. The Lancet (2008). *Iodine deficiency—way to go yet. The Lancet* 372 (9633): 88 (editorial) (accessed 06/28/2013).
75. Zimmermann MB. (2009). Iodine deficiency. *Endocr Rev.* 376-408.
76. Zimmermann MB, Jooste PL, Pandav CS. (2008). Iodine-deficiency disorders. *Lancet.* 4;372(9645):1251-1262.
77. *Robbins and Cotran - Pathologic basis of disease 8/E.* (2004). Philadelphia, PA: Sauders Elsevier.
78. Pennington JA. (1990). A review of iodine toxicity reports. J Am Diet Assoc. 90(11):1571-1581.
79. Sunde RA. Selenium. In: Bowman B, Russell R, eds. Present Knowledge in Nutrition. 9th ed. Washington, DC: International Life Sciences Institute; 2006:480-97
80. Sunde RA. Selenium. In: Bowman B, Russell R, eds. Present Knowledge in Nutrition. 9th ed. Washington, DC: International Life Sciences Institute; 2006:480-97.
81. Sunde RA. Selenium. In: Coates PM, Betz JM, Blackman MR, et al., eds. *Encyclopedia of Dietary Supplements.* 2nd ed. London and New York: Informa Healthcare; 2010:711-8.
82. Institute of Medicine, Food and Nutrition Board. Dietary Reference Intakes: Vitamin C, Vitamin E, Selenium, and Carotenoids. National Academy Press, Washington, DC, 2000.
83. Turnlund J. (1998). Human whole-body copper metabolism. Am J Clin Nutr. 67,5:9605-9645
84. Uauy R. (1998). Genetic and environmental determinants of copper metabolism. Am J Clin Nutr. 67:951Sb-1102S.
85. Uauy R, et al. (1998). Essentiality of copper in humans. Am J Clin Nutr. 67:952s-959s.
86. Linder MC, et. al. Copper transport. Am J Clin Nutr. 67:965s-971s/
87. Anderson RA. Bryden NA. Polansky MM. (1992). Dietary chromium intake: freely chosen diets, institutional diets and individual foods. *Biol Trace Elem Res.* 32:117-21.
88. Anderson R. (1994). *Stress Effects on Chromium Nutrition in Humans and Animals, 10th Edition.* Nottingham University Press, England.
89. Lukaski HC. Bolonchuk WW. Siders WA. Milne DB. (1996). Chromium supplementation and resistance training: effects on body composition, strength and trace element status of men. *Am J Clin Nutr.* 63:954-65.
90. Althuis MD. Jordan NE. Ludington EA. Wittes JT. (2002). Glucose and insulin responses to dietary chromium supplements: a meta-analysis. *Am J Clin Nutr.* 76:148-55.
91. Mertz W. (1969). Chromium occurrence and function in biological systems. *Physiol Rev.* 49:163-239.
92. Mertz W. (1993). Chromium in human nutrition: a review. *J Nutr.* 123:626-33.
93. Mertz W. (1998). Interaction of chromium with insulin: a progress report. *Nutr Rev.* 56:174-

7.
94. Sardesai VM. (1993). Molybdenum: an essential trace element. *Nutr Clin Pract* 8 (6): 277–81.
95. Simpson M. Howard T. ((2011). Selecting and effectively using hydration for fitness. *American College of Sports Medicine.* ACSM Consumer Information Committee. http://www.acsm.org/docs/brochures/selecting-and-effectively-using-hydration-for-fitness.pdf.

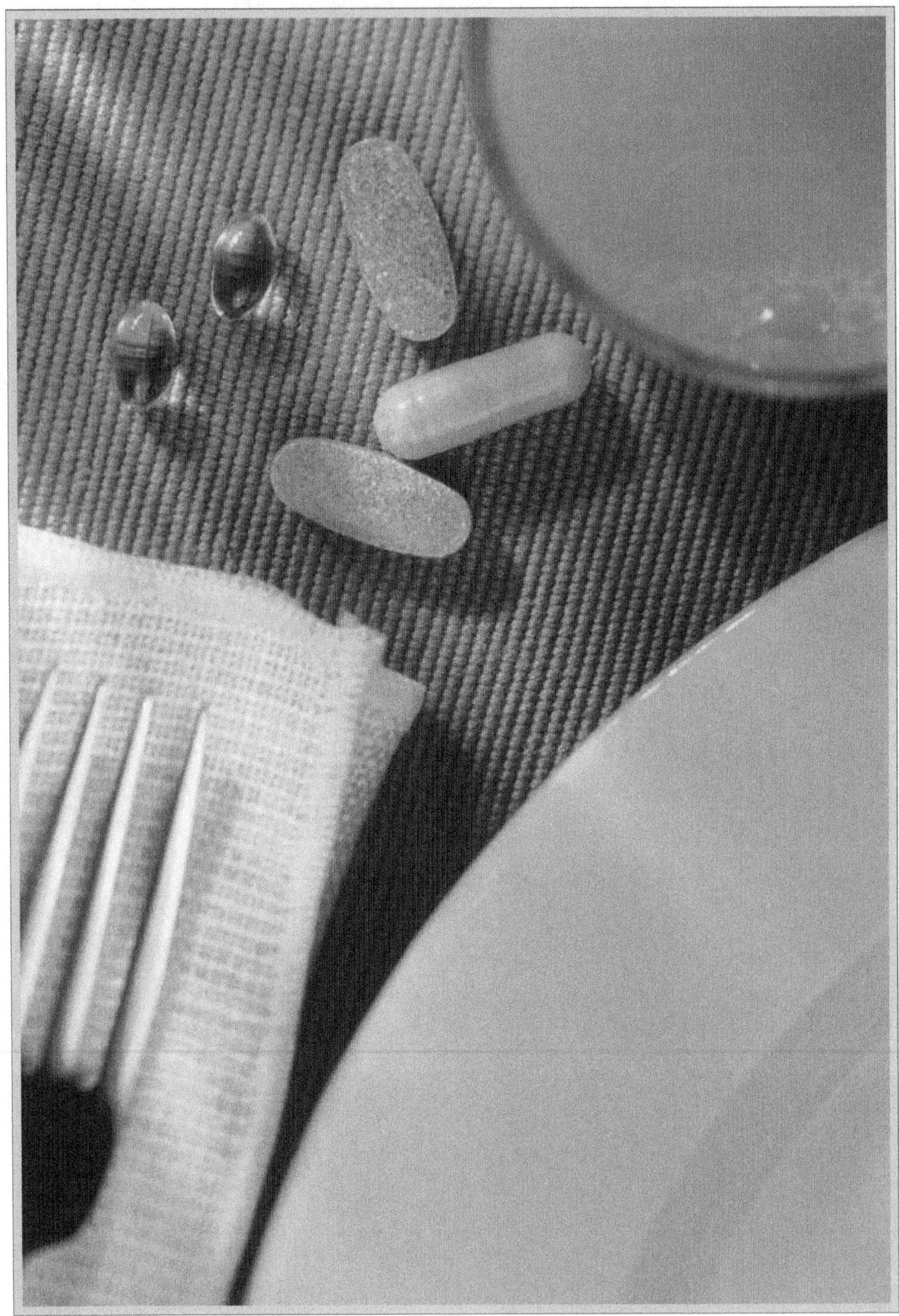

Chapter 9 - Complementary and Alternative Medicine

The information presented in this chapter will focus on alternative medicine therapies. Our discussion will center on the category of dietary supplements. This chapter begins with a discussion on background information including definitions and regulations of supplements. This chapter includes an in-depth look at categories of supplements (botanicals, vitamins and minerals, ergogenic aids, weight loss supplements), as well as a discussion of supplement "verification" programs and points to consider before ingesting a supplement. Discussion will conclude with position stands by national organizations concerning use of supplements and the role of health and fitness professionals with regard to their use.

Objectives

After reading and studying this chapter you should be able to:

1. Discuss the origins of the National Center for Complementary and Alternative Medicine (NCCAM) and classifications of "Complementary health".
2. Explain natural based therapies (supplements) in light of the Dietary Supplement Health and Education Act of 1994 including health claims, labeling regulations, good manufacturing practices, standardization, and safety.
3. Discuss the role of the Office of Dietary Supplements (ODS).
4. Describe each of the four categories of supplements - botanicals, vitamins and minerals, ergogenic aids, and weight loss supplements.
5. Discuss independent supplement verification programs.
6. Identify points to consider before ingesting a dietary supplement.
7. Discuss the position stand by the Academy of Nutrition and Dietetics and the American College of Sports Medicine, The National Athletic Trainers' Association, the International Olympic Committee, and the American Academy of Sports Dietitians and Nutritionists on use of supplementation.

Introduction

Many Americans, nearly 40 percent, use health care approaches developed outside of mainstream Western, or conventional medicine (2). When describing non-mainstream health approaches people often use the words "alternative" and "complementary" interchangeably, but the two terms refer to different concepts (2):

- "Complementary" generally refers to using a non-mainstream approach together with conventional medicine.
- "Alternative" refers to using a non-mainstream approach in place of conventional medicine.

True alternative medicine is not common. Most people use non-mainstream approaches along with conventional treatments, and the boundaries between complementary and conventional medicine overlap and change with time. For example, guided imagery and massage, both once considered complementary or alternative, are used regularly in some hospitals to help with pain management (2).

Non-mainstream health care approaches may also be considered part of integrative medicine or integrative health care. For example, cancer treatment centers with integrative health care programs may offer services such as acupuncture and meditation to help manage symptoms and side effects for patients who are receiving conventional cancer treatments such as chemotherapy (2).

Several facts about this growing trend on "integrative health care" include (2):

- Many individuals, health care providers, and health care systems are integrating various practices with origins outside of mainstream medicine.
- The integrative trend is growing among providers and health care systems.

What is the science behind these non-mainstream approaches? Advocates claim strong science exists and complain about the slow moving and overly cautious FDA, while scientists argue that Congress is advocating for unproven therapies rather than subjecting new treatments to evaluation. In many instances, a lack of reliable data makes it difficult for people to make informed decisions about using these therapies (2).

NCCAM

The National Center for Complementary and Alternative Medicine (NCCAM) is the Federal Government's lead agency for scientific research on complementary and alternative medicine (CAM). They are one of the twenty-seven institutes and centers that make up the National Institutes of Health (NIH) within the U.S. Department of Health and Human Services (1). The mission of NCCAM is to explore complementary and alternative healing practices in the context of rigorous science, train CAM researchers, and disseminate authoritative information to the public and professionals (2).

The origin of NCCAM began in 1992, when Senator Tom Harkin (D-Iowa), convinced bee pollen had cured his allergies, assigned $2 million of his discretionary funds to establish the Office of Unconventional Medicine, renamed the Office of Alternative Medicine (OAM) (2). Funds for OAM increased annually and in 1998 increased to $19.5 million. Also in 1998, Senator Harkin won a decisive battle when the NIH opened a new office - the National Center for Complementary and Alternative Medicine (NCCAM) - with a $50 million budget (2). As a sign that NCCAM was indeed a scientific entity to be dealt with, the renowned Dr. Stephen E. Straus was appointed the first director on October 6, 1999 (7). When interviewed, Dr. Straus made it clear that the office would perform rigorous scientific studies and that the public and companies with vested interests in new alternative therapies "will have to accept that research may show that some new therapies will not be good; some therapies will not be safe; and some therapies will not be any more effective than present alternatives" (7).

NCCAM Classifications

NCCAM generally uses the term "complementary health approaches" when discussing the practices and products they research. NCCAM categorizes complementary health approaches into two subgroups - dietary supplements and mind body practices. Some approaches may not neatly fit into either of these groups—for example, the practices of traditional healers, Ayurveda medicine from India, traditional Chinese medicine, homeopathy, and naturopathy (1).

Dietary Supplements

This group includes a variety of products, such as herbs (subcategory of botanicals), vitamins and minerals, amino acids, enzymes, and/or other ingredients. They are widely marketed, readily available to consumers, and sold as dietary supplements. Interest in and use of supplements have grown considerably in the past few decades. According to the 2007 National Health Interview Survey (NHIS) 17.7 percent of American adults had used a nonvitamin/nonmineral natural product in the past year (8). These products were the most popular complementary health approaches among both adults and children (8).

Mind-Body Practices

Mind and body practices include a large and diverse group of procedures. Acupuncture is a technique in which practitioners stimulate specific points on the body by inserting thin needles through the skin. Massage therapy includes many different techniques in which practitioners manually manipulate the soft tissues of the body (2).

Most meditation techniques, such as mindfulness meditation or transcendental meditation, involve ways in which a person learns to focus attention. Movement therapies include a broad range of Eastern and Western movement-based approaches. Relaxation techniques, such as breathing exercises, guided imagery, and progressive muscle relaxation, are designed to produce the body's natural relaxation response (2).

Spinal manipulation is practiced by health care professionals such as chiropractors, osteopathic physicians, naturopathic physicians, physical therapists, and some medical doctors. Practitioners perform spinal manipulation by using their hands or a device to apply a controlled force to a joint of the spine (2).

Tai chi and qi gong are practices from traditional Chinese medicine that combine specific movements or postures, coordinated breathing, and mental focus. The various styles of yoga used for health purposes typically combine physical postures or movement, breathing techniques, and meditation. Other examples of mind and body practices include healing touch and hypnotherapy (2).

According to the 2007 National Health Interview Survey, several mind and body practices ranked among the top complementary health approaches used by adults (8), which included deep breathing, meditation, chiropractic and osteopathic manipulation, massage, yoga, progressive relaxation, and guided imagery (2).

The amount of research on mind and body approaches varies widely depending on the practice. For example, acupuncture, yoga, spinal manipulation, and meditation have been studied extensively and some of these practices hold promise in pain management, whereas other practices have had little research to date (2).

In the next section we will limit our discussion to dietary supplements. Mind-body practices will be discussed only as they relate to weight loss practices under the category of supplements.

Supplements

To reiterate the NCCAM classification, natural products, consist of botanicals, vitamins and minerals, amino acids, enzymes and/or other ingredients. They are widely marketed, readily available to consumers, and sold as dietary supplements.

Background

Use of dietary supplements is common among the U.S. adult population. Over 40% used supplements in 1988–1994, and over one-half in 2003–2006 (8). According to the 2007 National Health Interview Survey, which included questions on Americans' use of dietary supplements (not including vitamins and minerals), 17.7 percent of American adults had used these types of products in the past 12 months. National Health and Nutrition Examination Survey (NHANES) data collected from 2003 to 2006 that covered all types of dietary supplements indicate that 53 percent of American adults took at least one dietary supplement, most commonly multivitamin/multimineral supplements (taken by 39 percent of all adults) (137).

A major reason for this explosion is the passage of the Dietary Supplement Health and Education Act of 1994 (DSHEA) by Congress (1). Before 1994, The Food and Drug Administration regulated dietary supplements to ensure that they were safe and wholesome and that their labeling was truthful and not misleading. Ensuring safety involved evaluation of all new ingredients, including those used in dietary supplements (5).

President Clinton, on October 25, 1994, signed the DSHEA "acknowledging that millions of consumers believe dietary supplements offer health benefits and that consumers want a greater opportunity to determine whether supplements may help them" (3). With the passage of the DSHEA, supplement manufacturers were given "carte blanche" to market supplements without regulation. The Council of Responsible Nutrition, an organization of manufacturers of dietary supplements hailed this act as a "landmark change". This legislation was a landmark change! (6).

Before 1994, the original definition of a supplement was a product that contained one or more of the essential nutrients (7). After DSHEA, the definition of a supplement was changed to any product intended for ingestion as a supplement to the diet (7). This definition now includes liquid, pill, capsule, or tablet forms of vitamins, minerals, herbs, botanicals and other plant derived substances, amino acids and concentrates, metabolites, constituents, and extracts of these substances (4). Again, according to the FDA, dietary supplements are not drugs. The FDA definition of a drug is an article, which may or may not be derived from plants that is intended to diagnose, cure, mitigate, treat, or prevent disease (4). Before marketing, drugs must undergo *clinical* studies to determine their effectiveness, safety, possible interactions with other substances, and appropriate dosages. The FDA reviews these data and authorizes usage before marketing. Under DSHEA, Congress amended the Federal Food, Drug, and Cosmetic Act (FD&C Act) to include provisions that apply only to dietary supplements and dietary ingredients of dietary supplements (4). As a result of these provisions, dietary ingredients used in dietary supplements are no longer subject to the premarket safety evaluations required of other new food ingredients or for new uses of old food ingredients (7).

The FDA notes that under the DSHEA supplements are no longer regulated like other products such as drugs, additives, cosmetics, foods (animal and human), medical devices, and radiation emitting consumer products (microwaves) (4). The FDA warns that dietary supplements are not replacements for conventional diets (14). The FDA also warns that it must not be assumed that "all natural" means safe, (poisonous mushrooms are all natural); it must not be assumed that what is stated on the label is actually in the bottle; and just because the accompanying literature makes claims about the safety and health advantages of the supplement, it must not be assumed that these claims are true (4).

Office of Dietary Supplements (ODS)

The Dietary Supplement Health and Education Act of 1994 (Public Law 103-417, DSHEA), authorized the establishment of the Office of Dietary Supplements (ODS) at the National Institute of Health (NIH) (3). The ODS was created in 1995 within the Office of Disease Prevention (ODP), Office of the Director (OD), NIH. DSHEA defined the purpose and responsibilities of ODS as follows (3):

- To explore more fully the potential role of dietary supplements as a significant part of the efforts of the United States to improve health care.
- To promote scientific study of the benefits of dietary supplements in maintaining health and preventing chronic disease and other health-related conditions.
- To conduct and coordinate scientific research within NIH relating to dietary supplements.
- To collect and compile the results of scientific research relating to dietary supplements, including scientific data from foreign sources.
- To serve as the principal adviser to the Secretary and to the Assistant Secretary for Health and provide advice to the Director of NIH, the Director of the Centers for Disease Control and Prevention, and the Commissioner of the Food and Drug Administration on issues relating to dietary supplements.

One of the purposes in creating the ODS was to promote scientific research in the area of dietary supplements. Dietary supplements may have an impact on the prevention of disease and on the maintenance of health (4). Although vitamin and mineral supplements have been available for decades, their health effects have been the subject of scientific research only within the last 15-20 years. Considerable research on the effects of botanical and herbal supplements has been conducted in Asia and Europe where plant products have a long tradition of use (18). The overwhelming majority of these supplements, however, have not been studied using modern scientific techniques. Nor have they been extensively studied in population groups that may be at risk for chronic diseases (18). For many reasons, therefore, it is important to enhance research efforts to determine the benefits and risks of dietary supplements (4).

Definitions/Regulations

As defined by Congress (Dietary Supplement Health and Education Act) a dietary supplement is a product, other than tobacco, that (3):

- Is intended to supplement the diet
- Contains one or more dietary ingredients or their constituents including vitamins, minerals, botanicals (herbs), amino acids
- Is intended to be taken by mouth as a pill, capsule, tablet, or liquid
- Is labeled on the front panel as being a dietary supplement

Supplement ingredients sold in the United States before October 15, 1994, are not required to be reviewed by the FDA for their safety before they are marketed because they are presumed to be safe based on their history of use by humans (3,9). For a new dietary ingredient the manufacturer must notify the FDA of its intent to market the supplement containing the new dietary ingredient and provide information on how it determined that reasonable evidence exists for safe human use of the product. FDA can either refuse to allow new ingredients into or remove existing ingredients from the marketplace for safety reasons (3,9).

Although dietary supplements are regulated by the FDA as foods, they are regulated differently from other foods and from drugs. Classification as a dietary supplement is typically determined by the information that the manufacturer provides on the product label or in accompanying literature (3). There are no provisions in the DSHEA for FDA to "approve" dietary supplements for safety or effectiveness before they reach the consumer. Once a dietary supplement is marketed, FDA has to prove that the product is not safe in order to restrict its use or remove it from the market (3).

Claims

Drug manufacturers may claim that their product will diagnose, cure, mitigate, treat, or prevent a disease. Such claims cannot be made for dietary supplements.

The label of a dietary supplement or food product may contain one of three types of claims (3):

- Health claims describe a relationship between a food, food component, or dietary supplement ingredient, and reducing risk of a disease or health-related condition.
- Nutrient content claims describe the relative amount of a nutrient or dietary substance in a product.
- A structure/function claim is a statement describing how a product may affect the organs or systems of the body, and it cannot mention any specific disease. Structure/function claims do not require FDA approval but the manufacturer must provide FDA with the text of the claim within 30 days of putting the product on the market. Product labels containing such claims must also include a disclaimer that reads, "This statement has not been evaluated by the FDA. This product is not intended to diagnose, treat, cure, or prevent any disease."

Supplement Label

The FDA requires that the following information appear on the dietary supplement label (3):

- Name of product (including the word "supplement" or a statement that the product is a supplement)
- Net quantity of contents
- Name and place of business of manufacturer, packer, or distributor
- Directions for use

The supplements facts panel must include:

- Serving size, list of dietary ingredients, amount per serving size (by weight), percent of Daily Value (%DV), if established
- If the dietary ingredient is a botanical, the scientific name of the plant or the common or usual name standardized in the reference *Herbs of Commerce, 2nd Edition* (2000 edition) and the name of the plant part used
- If the dietary ingredient is a proprietary blend (i.e., a blend exclusive to the manufacturer), the total weight of the blend and the components of the blend in order of predominance by weight
- Nondietary ingredients such as fillers, artificial colors, sweeteners, flavors, or binders; listed by weight in descending order of predominance and by common name or proprietary blend

It is difficult to determine the quality of a dietary supplement product from its label. While the FDA has labeling criteria for supplements, under DSHEA there is no way to enforce it. The degree of quality control depends on the manufacturer, the supplier, and others in the production process (3).

Good manufacturing Practices (GMPs)

In 2007, the FDA issued Good Manufacturing Practices (GMPs) for dietary supplements (10). GMPs are a set of requirements and expectations by which dietary supplements must be manufactured, prepared, and stored to ensure quality (10). The current good manufacturing practices (CGMPs) final rule will require that proper controls are in place for dietary supplements so that they are processed in a consistent manner, and meet quality standards (9.) The CGMPs apply to all domestic and foreign companies that manufacture, package, label or hold dietary supplements, including those involved with the activities of testing, quality control, packaging and labeling, and distributing them in the U.S. The rule establishes CGMPs for industry-wide use necessary to require that dietary supplements are manufactured consistently as to identity, purity, strength, and composition. The requirements include provisions related to: the design and construction of physical plants that facilitate maintenance, cleaning, proper manufacturing operations, quality control procedures, testing final product or incoming and in process materials, handling consumer complaints, and maintaining records. To limit any disruption for dietary supplements produced by small businesses, the rule has a staggered three-year phase-in for small businesses (10). The final CGMPs became effective in June 2008 for large companies. Companies with less than 500 employees had until June 2009 and companies with fewer than 20 employees had until June 2010 to comply with the regulations. It remains unclear how effective the issued GMPs are and level of compliance.

Standardization

Standardization is a process that manufacturers may use to ensure batch-to-batch consistency of their products. In some cases, standardization involves identifying specific chemicals that can be used to manufacture a consistent product. The standardization process also provides a measure of quality control (3,11).

Dietary supplements are not required to be standardized in the United States (3,11). In fact, no legal or regulatory definition exists in the United States for standardization as it applies to dietary supplements. Because of this, the term "standardization" may mean many different things. Some manufacturers use the term standardization incorrectly to refer to uniform manufacturing practices. Following a recipe is not sufficient for a product to be called standardized. Therefore, the presence of the word "standardized" on a supplement label does not necessarily indicate product quality.

Safety

Dietary supplements are not required by federal law to be tested for safety and effectiveness before they are marketed and the amount of scientific evidence available for supplement ingredients varies widely (3,11). Some ingredients in dietary supplements have been carefully evaluated. For example, scientists know that calcium and vitamin D are important for keeping bones strong and reducing bone loss. Other supplements, such as many herbal products, need more study to determine their value (3,11).

In 2010, the Department of Health and Human Services (HHS) reported that the FDA has worked with the industry to recall more than 190 dietary supplement products that contained potentially harmful ingredients, more 40 of the products were marketed for weight loss and more than 80 marketed for body building (116). Most notably, the products contained FDA-approved drug products, such as synthetic steroids. In a separate statement, the FDA issued a letter of concern to the supplement industry citing 300 tainted product alerts (92,118). An investigation by the US Government Accountability Office found that from 2008-2011 the FDA received 6,307 reports of health problems (adverse event reports, AER) from dietary supplements (117). Of the 6,307 reports: 53% resulted in unspecified important medical events of a serious nature; 29% resulted in hospitalization; 20% resulted in serious injury or illnesses; 8% resulted in a life threatening condition; and 2% resulted in death (117). (Because each AER can report multiple outcomes percentages of outcomes should not be totaled). However, it is important to note the number of AER is greatly under-reported. Consumers may not be voluntarily reporting these events to the FDA. During the same period, poison centers received over 1,000 more reports of AER linked to dietary supplements than did the FDA (117).

Supplement Categories

In this next section we will discuss each of the following natural product/supplement categories:

- Plant based supplements (botanicals)
- Vitamin and mineral supplements
- Ergogenic aids
- Weight loss supplements

Botanicals

A botanical is a plant or plant ingredient valued for medicinal properties, flavor, and/or scent. Products made from botanicals that are used to maintain or improve health may be called herbal products, botanical products, or phytomedicines. To be classified as a dietary supplement, a botanical must meet the definition of a supplement previously described (18).

Botanicals are sold in many forms: as fresh or dried products; liquid or solid extracts; and tablets, capsules, powders, and tea bags. For example, fresh ginger root is often found in the produce section of food stores; dried ginger root is sold packaged in tea bags, capsules, or tablets; and liquid preparations made from ginger root are also sold. A particular group of chemicals or a single chemical may be isolated from a botanical and sold as a dietary supplement, usually in tablet or capsule form (18).

Common preparations include teas, decoctions, tinctures, and extracts. A tea, also known as an infusion, is made by adding boiling water to fresh or dried botanicals and steeping them. The tea may be drunk either hot or cold. Some roots, bark, and berries require more forceful treatment to extract their desired ingredients. They are simmered in boiling water for longer periods than teas, making a decoction, which also may be drunk hot or cold. A tincture is made by soaking a botanical in a solution of alcohol and water. Tinctures are sold as liquids and are used for concentrating and preserving a botanical. They are made in different strengths that are expressed as botanical-to-extract ratios (i.e., ratios of the weight of the dried botanical to the volume or weight of the finished product). An extract is made by soaking the botanical in a liquid that removes specific types of chemicals. The liquid can be used as is or evaporated to make a dry extract for use in capsules or tablets (18).

Many people believe that products labeled "natural" are safe. This is not necessarily true because the safety of a botanical depends on many things, such as its chemical makeup, how it works in the body, how it is prepared, and the dose used (18).

The action of botanicals range from mild to powerful (potent). Mild botanicals, such as chamomile and peppermint, are usually taken as teas to aid digestion and are generally considered safe. Some mild botanicals may have to be taken for weeks or months before their full effects are achieved. Valerian may be effective as a sleep aid but it is rarely effective after just one dose. It may take up to 14 days of use before effects are seen. In contrast, a powerful botanical produces a fast result. Kava is reported to have an immediate and powerful action affecting anxiety and muscle relaxation (18).

The dose and form of a botanical preparation also play important roles in its safety. Teas, tinctures, and extracts have different strengths. The same amount of a botanical may be contained in a cup of tea, a few teaspoons of tincture, or an even smaller quantity of an extract. Also, different preparations vary in the relative amounts and concentrations of chemical extraction from the whole botanical. For example, peppermint tea is generally considered safe to drink, but peppermint oil is much more concentrated and can be toxic if used incorrectly (18).

It is difficult to determine the quality of a botanical dietary supplement product from its label. The degree of quality control depends on the manufacturer, the supplier, and others in the production process. Scientists use several research approaches to evaluate botanical dietary supplements for their potential health benefits and safety risks (18). See Chapter 10 for further discussion concerning research approaches.

The Office of Dietary Supplements has developed "fact sheets" for the following botanicals (19): Acai, Aloe Vera, Astragalus, Bilberry, Bitter Orange, Black Cohosh, Butterbur, Cat's Claw, Chamomile, Chasteberry, Cinnamon, Cranberry, Dandelion, Echinacea, Essiac/Flor-Essence, European Elder, Evening Primrose Oil, Fenugreek, Feverfew, Flaxseed, Garlic, Ginger, Ginkgo, Ginseng, Goldenseal, Grape Seed Extract, Green Tea, Hawthorn, Hoodia, Horse Chestnut, Kava, Lavender, Licorice Root, Milk Thistle, Mistletoe, Noni, PC-SPES, Peppermint Oil, Red Clover, Sage, Saw Palmetto, Soy, St. John's Wort, Tea, Thunder God Vine, Turmeric, Valerian, Yohimbe.

Vitamins – Minerals

Many forms of vitamin, mineral, and food based supplements are sold in individual and combined forms (3). Scientific evidence shows that some dietary supplements are beneficial for overall health and for managing some health conditions (68). For example, calcium and vitamin D are important for keeping bones strong and reducing bone loss; folic acid decreases the risk of certain birth defects; and omega-3 fatty acids from fish oils might help some people with heart disease. Other supplements need more study to determine their value (17). To reiterate, the U.S. Food and Drug Administration (FDA) does not determine whether dietary supplements are effective before they are marketed (3).

Many sources of information on individual dietary supplements are available (1-4,9-15) and will not be itemized here. See Chapter 8 and 9 for details concerning vitamins and minerals. The joint position statements by the Academy of Nutrition and Dietetics, Dietitians of Canada (DC), and American College of Sports Medicine (ACSM), the International Olympic Committee, the National Athletic Trainers' Association, and the American Academy of Sports Dietitians and Nutritionists on the use of dietary supplements is discussed in a later section.

Ergogenic Aids

Ergogenic aids are any external influences which can positively affect physical or mental performance (21,22). Ergogenic aids can be as simple as water used before and after exercising, to carbohydrates and proteins for energy, to something as advanced as anabolic steroids (17).

Numerous ergogenic aids that claim to enhance sports performance are used by amateur and professional athletes (20). Approximately 50 percent of the general population have reported taking some form of dietary supplements, while 76 to 100 percent of athletes in some sports use them (20). New products with ergogenic claims appear on the market almost daily and most are classified as supplements. This indicates that the contents of the product and the claims on the label have not been evaluated by the FDA and may have no scientific basis (20). Hence, they should be used with caution and only after careful product evaluation for safety, efficacy, potency, and legality (17). A qualified sports dietitian and, in particular, the Board Certified Specialist in Sports Dietetics in the United States, should provide individualized nutrition direction and advice after a comprehensive nutrition assessment (17).

Water

The most important ergogenic aid for athletes is water. Preventing dehydration during exercise is one of the most effective ways to maintain exercise capacity. Exercise performance can be significantly impaired when 2% or more of body weight is lost through sweat. Weight loss of more than 4% of body weight during exercise can lead to heat illness, heat exhaustion, heat stroke, and possibly death (23). Athletes should not depend on thirst because they typically do not get thirsty until they have lost a significant amount of fluid through sweat. Athletes should weigh themselves prior to and following exercise and consume approximately 16-24 oz (450-675 ml) of fluid for every pound (0.5 kg) of body weight lost during exercise (51).

Carbohydrates/Proteins

One of the best ergogenic aids available for athletes and active individuals alike is carbohydrate. Research has identified carbohydrate as an ergogenic aid that can prolong exercise (16, 22). Additionally, ingesting a small amount of carbohydrate and protein 30-60 minutes prior to exercise and use of sports drinks during exercise can increase carbohydrate availability and improve exercise performance. Finally, ingesting carbohydrate and protein immediately following exercise can enhance carbohydrate storage and protein synthesis (16, 21,22).

Amino Acids

Theoretically, amino acid supplementation during intense training may help minimize protein degradation and thereby lead to greater gains in fat-free mass. However, the science indicates otherwise (71,72). Amino acids require carriers to enter cells. Large doses of an individual amino acid can create a demand for a carrier thereby limiting the absorption of another amino acid. Toxicity of single amino acids in animal studies raises concerns about their use in humans (67). Large doses of branched-chain amino acids can raise plasma ammonia concentrations which can be toxic to brain cells. Branched chain amino acids may be beneficial in disease states (liver disease) but are otherwise not recommended (93,94).

Anabolic Steroids

"Anabolic steroids" is the name for synthetic variants of the male sex hormone testosterone. The scientific term for these compounds is *anabolic-androgenic steroids:* "anabolic" refers to muscle-building; and "androgenic" refers to male sexual characteristics (24, 29).

Anabolic steroids can be legally prescribed to treat conditions resulting from steroid hormone deficiency, such as delayed puberty, as well as diseases that result in loss of lean muscle mass. But athletes, bodybuilders, and others obtain these drugs illegally in an attempt to enhance performance and/or improve their physical appearance (24, 29).

Anabolic steroids have three mechanisms of action (25):

- Anticatabolic effects reverse the actions of glucocorticoids and help metabolize ingested proteins thereby converting a negative nitrogen balance into a positive one.
- Anabolic effects directly induce skeletal muscle synthesis.
- A "steroid rush (a state of euphoria) and decreased fatigue occurs that allows the athlete to train harder and longer.

Early studies used physiological doses, or doses two to three times these amounts, with mixed results. More controlled, recent reviews have concluded that anabolic steroids do indeed cause increased strength and muscle mass (25,26). A randomized, double-blind, 10-week study of 40 men examined the effect of supraphysiological testosterone doses (26). The participants were divided into four groups: those given a placebo with or without weight training, and those given 600-mg testosterone with or without weight training. Diet and training times were controlled. Fat-free mass, muscle size and strength increased more than placebo in both groups taking testosterone than in the groups taking placebo. The subjects in the exercise plus testosterone group had a 9 percent increase in mass and 23 percent increase in bench-press strength, compared with 3 percent and 9 percent in the subjects in the exercise plus placebo group (26).

Abuse of anabolic steroids has shown to lead to aggression and other psychiatric problems (27,32,33). Many users report feeling good while on steroids; however, extreme mood swings can occur, including manic-like symptoms and anger ("roid rage") that may lead to violence (27,32,33). Users may also suffer from paranoid jealousy, extreme irritability, delusions, and impaired judgment stemming from feelings of invincibility (27,32,33).

Steroid abuse can lead to serious health problems. Consequences that have been linked to steroid abuse include kidney impairment or failure; damage to the liver; and cardiovascular problems including enlargement of the heart, high blood pressure, and changes in blood cholesterol (even in young people) (34,35). Steroid use also causes severe acne and fluid retention and the following age and gender specific factors (34,35):

- For *men*—shrinkage of the testicles (testicular atrophy), reduced sperm count or infertility, baldness, development of breasts (gynecomastia), increased risk for prostate cancer (34,35).
- For *women*—growth of facial hair, male-pattern baldness, changes in or cessation of the menstrual cycle, enlargement of the clitoris, deepened voice (36).
- For *adolescents*—stunted growth due to premature skeletal maturation and accelerated puberty changes, and risk of not reaching expected height (37).
- In addition, people who inject steroids run the risk of contracting or transmitting HIV/AIDS or hepatitis (24).

Withdrawal symptoms occur when anabolic steroid use is stopped. Withdrawal symptoms include: mood swings, fatigue, restlessness, loss of appetite, insomnia, reduced sex drive, and steroid cravings (31). One of the most dangerous withdrawal symptoms is depression which can sometimes lead to suicide attempts. Research has found that some steroid abusers turn to other drugs such as opioids to counteract the negative effects of withdrawal (31).

Creatine

Creatine monohydrate accounts for about $400 million in annual sales in the United States alone (39). Athletes in the former Soviet Union may have been ingesting creatine to enhance performance as early as the 1970s (40). The popularity of creatine increased substantially in the early 1990s by the revelation that Olympic gold medal winners Linford Christie and Sally Gunnell used creatine (38). In addition, scientific publications reported that dietary creatine supplementation could increase muscle creatine stores (41) and improve the performance of brief, high-power exercise (42).

Many research articles have been published on creatine, but its efficacy as an ergogenic aid still remains controversial (38).

Creatine is a non-essential compound that can be obtained in the diet or synthesized by the liver, pancreas, and kidneys (43). It exists in free and phosphorylated forms (i.e., phosphocreatine or PCr). Approximately 95% of the body's creatine is stored in skeletal muscle where it acts as an energy buffer. During times of increased energy demand, phosphocreatine (PCr) donates its phosphate to adenosine diphosphate (ADP) to produce adenosine triphosphate (ATP) (43). Exercise tasks like sprinting and weight lifting rely heavily on the ATP-PCr energy system (43). It is the only fuel system in the muscles that can produce energy at sufficiently high rates to accomplish these tasks. But the ATP-PCr energy system lasts for only seconds before PCr stores are depleted. Consequently, it has been hypothesized that people who increase their muscle creatine levels by ingesting creatine supplements have a greater energy reserve available to support this type of activity (44). In addition to increasing muscle creatine stores, creatine supplementation may increase phosphocreatine resynthesis (44), although this has not been consistent (45).

Roughly 300 studies have been carried out to test the effects of creatine on exercise performance and a definitive answer to the question "Does creatine work" is still not completely clear to scientists (38). Although reports have been inconclusive the data suggest that creatine loading can improve performance in high-intensity exercise lasting less than 30 seconds (38). Studies reporting creatine benefits for resistance training exercise are consistent in demonstrating positive effects (38). It appears likely that creatine allows some athletes to train with higher work loads. Even though blinding should be a standard in these studies, there are often confounding variables that can affect the outcome of an investigation (i.e., difficult matching a placebo, training history, diet, etc.) (38).

Also meta-analyses have been conducted in an attempt to compare results of many studies in an unbiased manner; however, there are several limitations to this approach (38):

- The criteria for selection of studies are subjective and differ among investigators.
- A problem of potentially biased sampling of studies exists because small sample sizes may have lead to erroneous positive results.

- Many studies finding no effect are never published. It is interesting to note that no studies reported negative effects of creatine supplementation on performance (unless it was secondary to an increase in body weight)(38).
- Small sample sizes, characteristic of most of the studies of creatine effects could over represent or under represent subjects who are predisposed to increase their muscle creatine levels in response to creatine supplementation (38). There is a large inter-subject variability in muscle creatine changes in response to supplementation. Certain individuals may possess a gene variant that allows them to store more creatine in their muscles. Ethical issues arise if only some individuals experience a benefit, such as whether these individuals have an unfair advantage in sport performance (48).

The research and use of creatine supplementation has grown beyond athletic performance. Scientists have been investigating the potential benefits of creatine supplementation in individuals with Parkinson's disease and Huntington's disease (119-123). In addition, preliminary clinical studies suggest creatine supplementation may help lower triglycerides and lower homocysteine levels (123-125). While the results are promising, more research is needed.

Caffeine

Caffeine occupies a unique position in the sports world. It is an inherent part of the diet of many athletes. While it is common to equate caffeine with coffee, it should be noted that rarely is coffee the vehicle used in research studies. Therefore, it may be misleading to equate the two because coffee contains hundreds of additional chemicals (51).

Caffeine appears to be taken up by all tissues of the body, making it difficult to independently study the effects on the central nervous system, the muscles, and fat tissue in exercising humans. It is also apparent that different mechanisms are probably responsible for performance enhancement in different types of exercise (51,53).

In the athletic arena, caffeine is a controlled or restricted drug. Urinary levels of greater than 12 mc/ml following competitions are considered illegal by the International Olympic Committee (IOC) (51). An athlete can consume a very large amount of caffeine before reaching this limit. A 70 kg person could drink about three or four mugs or six regular size cups of drip-percolated coffee approximately 1 hour before exercise; exercise for 1 to 1.5 hours, and produce a subsequent urine sample that would only approach the urinary caffeine limit (53). A caffeine level above 12 mc/ml suggests that an individual has deliberately taken caffeine in the form of tablets or suppositories in an attempt to improve performance. Not surprisingly, only a few athletes have been caught with illegal caffeine levels during competitions (52).

Well-controlled studies have established that moderate doses of caffeine ingested one hour prior to exercise enhance the performance of certain types of endurance exercise in the laboratory (53,4,56). Moderate caffeine doses produce urinary caffeine levels well below the allowable limit, as determined by the IOC (53,56,58,59). These results are specific to well-trained elite or recreational athletes. There is little information on the performance and metabolic effects of caffeine in recreationally active or untrained subjects (60).

It has been suggested that caffeine ingestion may lead to poor hydration status prior to and during exercise. However, two studies reported no changes in core temperature, sweat loss, or plasma volume during exercise following caffeine ingestion (61,62). A recent report also demonstrated that urine volumes and body hydration status during exercise were unaffected by caffeine ingested in a fluid replacement drink (63).

The possible benefits of caffeine in large doses must be weighed against adverse effects such as stomach upset, nervousness, irritability, headaches, and diarrhea (67).

<u>Energy Drinks</u>

"Energy drinks" are beverages that contain caffeine, taurine, vitamins, herbal supplements, and sugar or sweeteners and are marketed to improve energy, weight loss, stamina, athletic performance, and concentration (95,96,97). Energy drinks are available in 140 countries and are the fastest growing beverage in the US market; in 2011, sales topped $9 billion (98). Half of the energy drink market consists of children 12 years old, adolescents 12–18 years old, and young adults 19 –25 years old (95).

Energy drinks have no therapeutic benefit, and many ingredients are understudied and not regulated (96). The known and unknown pharmacology of agents included in such drinks, combined with reports of toxicity, raises concern for potentially serious adverse effects. Future research should aim to understand the effects in at-risk populations. Toxicity surveillance should be improved, and regulations of energy drink sales and consumption should be based on appropriate research (96).

<u>Energy Bars</u>

Today, anyone who feels the need for a nutritional boost might ingest an energy or meal-replacement bar. There are literally hundreds of choices (66). Some are high in calories, mainly from sugar and fat. Some resemble candy bars with a few extra nutrients. Some bars are high in carbohydrates, some are high protein bars. Other bars are breakfast bars, meal replacement bars, diet bars, even brain bars that claim to improve memory. When choosing a bar consumers should consider:

- Is this a meal replacement? If so, Look for bars containing at least 300 calories and 10 grams of protein. Try to keep added sugars under 4 grams and saturated fat under 4 grams.
- In general select bars with at least 2 to 3 grams of fiber and remember to read the ingredient list.
- If weight is an issue, look for a bar with fewer than 150 calories and set a limit of one bar per day.
- Bars can be pricey, ranging from $1.50 to $3.50 per bar. A less expensive alternative is a snack of peanut butter with graham crackers. It has the same calories, protein, carbs and fat that are found in some energy bars at a fraction of the cost (67).

Most nutritionists emphasize that even when consuming energy bars they should not crowd out whole foods from the diet (17). For a quick snack try eating fruits such as apples or bananas. Before an athletic competition, a bagel or graham crackers can produce a response in blood glucose levels similar to energy bars, and they cost a lot less (67).

Weight Loss Supplements

The National Center for Complementary and Alternative Medicine's summary report indicates that most dietary supplements marketed for weight loss have not been proven effective and some have been proven to be dangerous (65). Below is a summary of some of the weight loss supplements evaluated by NCCAM (65).

<u>Acai</u>

Acai berry products have been marketed as folk or traditional remedies for weight-loss and anti-aging purposes. No definitive scientific evidence exists to support these claims; no independent studies have been published in peer-reviewed journals; and there is no definitive scientific evidence based on studies in humans to support the use of acai berry for any health-related purpose. There is little reliable information about the safety of acai as a supplement. It is widely consumed as an edible fruit or as a juice. People who are allergic to acai or to plants in the *Arecaceae* (palm) family should not consume acai.

<u>Bitter Orange</u>

Bitter orange has been used in traditional Chinese medicine for nausea, indigestion, and constipation. Current uses are for heartburn, loss of appetite, nasal congestion, and weight loss. Overall, only a few small studies of bitter orange have been published and the evidence is insufficient to support the use for any health purpose.

Many herbal weight-loss products now use concentrated extracts of bitter orange peel in place of ephedra. The U.S. Food and Drug Administration banned ephedra because it raises blood pressure and is linked to heart attacks and strokes (65). There is currently little evidence that bitter orange is safer than ephedra. Bitter orange contains the chemical synephrine, which is similar to the main chemical in ephedra. There have been reports of fainting, heart attack, and stroke in healthy people after taking bitter orange supplements alone or combined with caffeine. People who should avoid bitter orange supplement are individuals that have a heart condition or high blood pressure, or are taking medications such as MAO inhibitors (antidepressant), caffeine, or other herbs/supplements that speed up heart rate. Because lack of evidence that safety exists, pregnant women or nursing mothers should avoid products that contain bitter orange.

Ephedra

Ephedra has been used for more than 5,000 years in China and India to treat conditions such as colds, fever, flu, headaches, asthma, wheezing, and nasal congestion. Ephedra was used as an ingredient in dietary supplements for weight loss, increased energy, and enhanced athletic performance. According to the FDA, there is little evidence of ephedra's effectiveness, except for short-term weight loss. However, the increased risk of heart problems and stroke far outweighs any benefits. An NCCAM-funded study that analyzed phone calls to poison control centers found a higher rate of side effects from ephedra compared to other herbal products (65). Other studies and systematic reviews found an increased risk of heart, psychiatric, and gastrointestinal problems, as well as high blood pressure and stroke (65).

Between 1995 and 1997, the FDA received more than 900 reports of possible ephedra toxicity (99). Serious adverse events such as stroke, heart attack, and sudden death were reported in 3 cases. Using ephedra may worsen many health conditions such as cardiovascular disease, kidney disease, diabetes, and may cause seizures in otherwise healthy people (99). Taking ephedra can also result in anxiety, difficulty urinating, dry mouth, headache, heart damage, high blood pressure, irregular heart rhythms, irritation of the stomach, kidney stones, nausea, psychosis, restlessness, sleep problems, and tremors (99).

In 2004, the FDA banned the sale of dietary supplements containing ephedra (99). The FDA found that these supplements had an unreasonable risk of injury or illness, particularly cardiovascular complications, and a risk of death. The ban does not apply to traditional Chinese herbal remedies or to products like herbal teas regulated as conventional foods (99).

Green Tea

Green tea and green tea extracts have traditionally been used to prevent and treat a variety of cancers (including breast, stomach, and skin cancers), for mental alertness, weight loss, lowering cholesterol levels, and protecting skin from sun damage (100). A 2012 Cochrane review of 18 studies in overweight or obese adults found that the weight loss was statistically not significant and not likely to be clinically important (100). Green tea is safe for most adults when used in moderate amounts. There have been some case reports of liver problems in people taking concentrated green tea extracts (100). The problems do not seem to be connected with green tea infusions or beverages. Green tea and green tea extracts contain caffeine, but it would take a lot of green tea to reach toxicity (100). Caffeine can cause insomnia, anxiety, irritability, upset stomach, nausea, diarrhea, or frequent urination in some people. Green tea extract contains small amounts of vitamin K, which can make anticoagulant drugs, such as warfarin, less effective (65).

Sibutramine

FDA laboratories found more than 100 weight-loss products illegally marketed as dietary supplements that contained sibutramine, the active ingredient in the prescription weight-loss drug Meridia (115). In 2010, Meridia was withdrawn from the market after studies showed that it was associated with an increased risk of heart attack and stroke (115).

Mind and Body Approaches

There is considerable interest and growing scientific evidence that meditation and yoga may be useful in supporting behavior change and healthier lifestyles, including weight-loss and weight management programs (65).

Mindfulness meditation is a type of meditation that uses various approaches, such as attention on breathing, to develop increased awareness. The physiological effects include reduced stress, and control of emotions and cravings. To date, there are only a few studies on the effects of mindfulness as a component of weight-loss programs. A 2013 systematic review and meta-analysis indicates that attentive eating is likely to influence food intake and may aid in weight loss or maintenance. Meditation is considered to be safe for healthy people (101). There is a concern, and there have been rare reports, that meditation could cause or worsen symptoms in people who have certain psychiatric problems (101).

Yoga is a mind and body practice with origins in ancient Indian philosophy. The various styles of yoga typically combine physical postures, breathing techniques, and meditation or relaxation (102). Research on the effectiveness of yoga as an intervention for weight loss is limited and varies in quality. A 2013 review of the current evidence found that yoga can be effective in promoting weight loss (102). A pilot study of a 3-month yoga program for adults at high risk for developing type 2 diabetes suggests that yoga would be a possible risk reduction option and that yoga holds promise as an approach to reducing cardio-metabolic risk factors (103).

Overall, those who practice yoga have a low rate of side effects, and the risk of serious injury from yoga is low (65,102). However, certain types of stroke as well as pain from nerve damage are among the rare possible side effects of practicing yoga (65, 102). Women who are pregnant and people with certain medical conditions, such as high blood pressure, glaucoma should consult with their healthcare provider before starting a yoga program (65, 102).

Acupuncture describes procedures involving the stimulation of points on the body using a variety of techniques (104). The acupuncture technique that has been most often studied involves penetrating the skin with thin, solid, metallic needles that are manipulated by the hands or by electrical stimulation. Not much research has been conducted on the effects of acupuncture for weight loss. A 2012 study in obese adults, who had just completed a behavioral weight-loss program, compared an acupressure technique with a control intervention comprised of social-support group meetings for weight maintenance (104). The primary analysis of the study showed no significant difference in weight regain between the acupressure and control groups. In another study, researchers examined the effect of auricular acupuncture on obese women compared with sham acupuncture (105). Researchers found no statistical difference in body weight, body mass index, and waist circumference between the acupuncture group and placebo (105). Relatively few complications have been reported from the use of acupuncture; however, it can cause potentially serious side effects if not delivered properly by a qualified practitioner.

Verification Programs

Several independent organizations offer quality testing of dietary supplements and allow products that pass their tests to display seals of approval (3). These seals of approval provide assurance that the product was properly manufactured, contains the ingredients listed on the label, and does not contain harmful levels of contaminants; however, these verification programs do not guarantee that a product is safe or effective. Organizations that offer this quality testing include:

- ConsumerLab.com
- NSF International
- U.S. Pharmacopeia

ConsumerLab.com

ConsumerLab.com (CL), founded in 1999 by Dr. Tod Cooperman, has independently tested over 2,000 products (106). It publishes results of its tests at ConsumerLab.com which receives over 2.5 million visits per year. Products tested are purchased independently by ConsumerLab.com at the retail level (stores, mail order, online, etc.). CL does not accept product samples from manufacturers for product reviews, and CL may select samples at any time during the year (to avoid sampling bias). Products are selected to reflect popular brands in the market as well as a selection of smaller brands. Blind tests are conducted by academic and commercial laboratories selected for their expertise in the type of testing needed for each product. These facilities are generally FDA inspected, follow GLP (good laboratory practice) protocols, are accredited by outside groups, and/or participate in method validation programs (106).

ConsumerLab.com has been criticized because it tests only one sample and also "sells" its seal of approval to manufacturers that wish to have their product tested. ConsumerLab.com scientists counter this criticism by obtaining samples from retail stores and not from the manufacturer directly (106).

NSF International Dietary Supplement Certification

Since 1944, NSF International, an independent, not-for-profit organization, has been testing products. The letters do not actually stand for any specific words. They were derived from the founding name dating back to the 1940s, which was the National Sanitation Foundation (107). The name was changed to NSF International in the early 1990s when the National Sanitation Foundation and NSF Testing Labs were merged (107).

The NSF Mark can be found on millions of consumer, commercial, and industrial products today. Products evaluated and certified by NSF International include bottled water, food equipment, home water treatment products, home appliances, plumbing and faucets, and even pool and spa components (107). NSF became involved in the testing of dietary supplements because of the growth of the diet industry and the fact that these products do not receive the same regulation as prescription or over the counter drugs (107). The NSF Mark provides the consumer with assurance that the product has been thoroughly and independently tested.

To help minimize the risk that a dietary supplement or sports nutrition product contains a substance banned by one of the major sports organizations, NSF developed the Certified for Sport™ program (108). Under this program, products are tested to ensure they contain the identity and quantity of dietary ingredients declared on the product label. In addition, the program helps ensure the product does not contain unacceptable quantities of contaminants for the recommended serving size listed on the product label. Exceeding recommended serving sizes may increase risk, so athletes should be sure to follow the serving size instructions indicated for the product (108). NSF developed this program to meet the growing demand of athletes, coaches, and all of those concerned about banned substances in sports. The program certifies that participating manufacturers and their products meet NSF's stringent independent certification process guidelines (108).

The certification program certifies products and inspects facilities for a range of substances, including: stimulants, narcotics, steroids, diuretics, beta-2-agonists, beta blockers, masking agents, and other substances (108). The list of banned substances for which testing is performed is updated regularly based on the scientific ability to detect a banned substance and through input from the international sports community (108).

U.S. Pharmacopeia Dietary Supplement Verification Program

United States Pharmacopeia (USP) is an independent, not-for-profit organization and the official standard-setting body for medicine. Its standards are enforceable by the FDA. While not a government entity, USP works closely with government agencies, ministries, and regulatory agencies to help provide standards of identity, strength, quality, and purity that safeguard the supply of medicines, dietary supplements, and food ingredients. USP standards are recognized in a variety of U.S. federal legislation. USP's drug standards are specified in the adulteration and misbranding provisions of the Federal Food, Drug, and Cosmetic Act; the Dietary Supplement Health and Education Act (DSHEA) misbranding provision has a role for USP's dietary supplement standards; and more than

200 FDA regulations incorporate USP food ingredient standards (109).

Unlike drugs (which are required by law to be tested by USP), supplement manufacturers can "voluntarily" request to have their products tested. The USP Verified Dietary Supplement Mark is awarded to finished dietary supplements that pass USP's comprehensive verification processes. Manufacturers can display the mark on the label of USP Verified products. The mark represents that USP has rigorously tested and verified the supplement to assure: what's on the label is in fact in the bottle; all the listed ingredients in the declared amount; the supplement does not contain harmful levels of contaminants; the supplement will break down and release ingredients in the body; the supplement has been made under good manufacturing practices (109).

Points to Consider

Dietary supplements are intended to supplement the diet not to replace the balance of a variety of foods important to health. Before ingesting any dietary supplements consumers should consider the following points.

Is It Safe?

Many supplements contain active ingredients that can have strong effects in the body. Consumers should be alert to the possibility of unexpected side effects, especially when taking a new product. The term "natural" does not mean safe and is a very subjective term. Do not assume that this term ensures wholesomeness or safety.

Supplements are most likely to cause side effects or harm when taken instead of prescribed medicines or when people take many supplements in combination (3). Some supplements can increase the risk of bleeding, or if a person takes them before or after surgery, they can affect the person's response to anesthesia (3). Dietary supplements can also interact with certain prescription drugs in ways that might cause problems. For example (3):

- Vitamin K can reduce the ability of the blood thinner Coumadin to prevent blood from clotting.
- St. John's Wort can speed the breakdown of many drugs (including antidepressants and birth control pills) and thereby reduce these drugs' effectiveness.
- Antioxidant supplements, like vitamins C and E, might reduce the effectiveness of some types of cancer chemotherapy.

Some ingredients found in dietary supplements are added to a growing number of foods, including breakfast cereals and beverages (3,67). As a result, consumers may be ingesting more of these ingredients. Taking more than required can raise risk of side effects. For example, getting too much vitamin A can cause headaches and liver damage, reduce bone strength, and cause birth defects. Excess iron causes nausea and vomiting and may damage the liver and other organs (3,67).

Most dietary supplements have not been tested for safety in pregnant women, nursing mothers, or children (3, 67). Hence caution should be taken during pregnancy, nursing, and should not be given to children (beyond a basic multivitamin/mineral product).

There are about 65,000 dietary supplements on the market consumed by more than 150 million Americans (64). Of the 465 drugs subject to a Class 1 recall in the U.S. between 2004 and 2012, 237 (51%) were dietary supplements (64, 110). To reiterate, these supplements accounted for more than half the Class 1 drugs recalled by the FDA. This means they contain substances that could cause serious health problems or even death (64). The majority of those recalled supplements were bodybuilding, weight loss, or sexual enhancement products that contain unapproved medicinal ingredients, including steroids. Almost one-quarter of the substances were manufactured outside of the United States which does not require adherence to good manufacturing practices (64, 110).

When the FDA learns of an adulterated dietary supplement, it is required to contact the manufacturer to trace the source of the product and initiate a recall (12, 64). However, a recent investigation by the Office of the Inspector general determined that the FDA does not possess accurate contact information for 20 percent of supplement manufacturers (64). The FDA has recently introduced a number of initiatives aimed at mitigating the impact of the most common adulterated supplements; however, despite these initiatives, products subject to Class I recalls continue to be readily available for sale.

Anyone that suspects a serious reaction from a dietary supplement should inform their health care provider. He or she may report the experience to the FDA and to the dietary supplement manufacturer (by using the contact information on the product label) (111).

If Safe, Is It Effective?

We have already discussed effectiveness in previous sections. To reiterate, unknown variables in published research include age, gender, activity level, and interactions with other supplements or drugs. Be wary of results claiming a "quick fix" that depart from scientific research and established dietary guidance (3,12). Consumers should learn to spot false claims: "If something sounds too good to be true, it probably is." Some examples of false claims on product labels include: Quick and effective cure-all; can treat or cure disease; "totally safe"; all natural; definitely no side effects; limited availability; no-risk, money-back guarantees; or requires advance payment (3). It is critical to skeptically evaluate studies on substances and supplements. While this is a daunting task, it is imperative as health professional to be able to understand the proposed mechanism, suggested use, identify poor research design, and inappropriate extrapolation of results (92). More information on research and design principles will be discussed in Ch. 10.

Is It Required?

If the supplement is deemed safe and effective, does it provide health benefits for the individual consumer. In many instances, the answer is "no". Often it's the "allure" of added health benefits that entice consumers. However, in some cases, supplementation may be wise if nutrient need is not meet through food. These informed decisions should be made using reliable resources and a stepwise process, including consulting with qualified health professionals.

What Are the Side Effects?

Most consumers of supplements (or drugs) do not believe that they will suffer the side effects; they assume it's always someone else that suffers the side effects), but consumers must ask themselves the following questions concerning side effects:

- What are the side effects? All chemicals have side effects. Some may not seem serious, such as dehydration or dry mouth, but dry mouth and dehydration can have serious consequences.
- What are the percentages of individuals that suffer the known consequences? Five percent of individuals experiencing dry mouth is less severe than 5% experiencing chronic conditions, such as loss of eyesight.
- Am I willing to risk the possibility of suffering the consequences? Some of the consequences can be minor, while others can be very serious. Also, there are often unknown side effects and consequences.
- What is the proper dose to minimize side effects? In many instances, this may not be known.
- How, when, and for how long will I need to ingest the supplement?

To Multivitamin or Not

Should healthy adults be taking a daily multivitamin? For those who eat a healthy diet, a multivitamin may have little to no benefit and in some cases may do harm.

The Iowa Women's Health Study concluded that the use of common dietary vitamins and mineral supplements may be associated with increased total mortality (126). The strongest association to total mortality in this study was supplemental iron (126). Another study published in the Journal of the American Medical Association concluded that treatment with beta carotene, vitamin A and vitamin E may increase mortality (127). A study out the National Cancer Institute reported that men who took a high dose of zinc that lead to chronic zinc oversupply were at greater risk of prostate cancer than men who did not take any zinc supplementation (128). Another study reported an association between multivitamin use and an increase risk of breast cancer (129). Critics of these studies claim that the associations are weak because these studies didn't exclude participants that were sick or consider the duration of supplement use and that high doses of any supplement could cause harm (130). Conversely, there are studies that have shown no risk of mortality, increased risk of breast cancer, cardiovascular disease or cancer when taking a multivitamin (131,132,133). A study published in the American Journal of Clinical Nutrition, reported that multivitamin use was inversely associated with myocardial infarction (134).

Because of the conflicting results of these studies and lack of randomized trials, many scientists believe there is not enough to recommend for or against taking a multivitamin (130,135). However, the argument for taking a multivitamin continues because the supplements can provide essential micronutrients to those that do not eat a healthy diet (130). Although according to a 2012 report from the Centers for Disease Control and Prevention's Division of Laboratory Sciences in the National Center for Environmental Health, fewer than 10 percent of the American population suffered from nutritional deficiencies (112). Researchers collected data from blood and urine samples provided by participants in the CDC's National Health and Nutrition Examination Survey between 1999 and 2006 (112).

"These findings are a snapshot of our nation's overall nutrition status," explained Christopher Portier, director of CDC's National Center for Environmental Health (113). "Measurements of blood and urine levels of these nutrients are critical because they show us whether the sum of nutrient intakes from foods and vitamin supplements is too low, too high, or sufficient" (113).

"You get your nutrients through your food," states Alice Lichtenstein, DSc, senior scientist and director of the Cardiovascular Nutrition Laboratory at the Jean Mayer U.S. Department of Agriculture (USDA) Human Nutrition Research Center on Aging at Tufts University and the author of a position paper on the usefulness of multivitamins (114). "That doesn't make a multivitamin just redundant, it could make it dangerous", states Dr. Lichtenstein (114). A large surplus of supplemental folate may have an adverse effect on colon cancer, and other research has found a relationship between folic acid supplements and prostate and breast cancers, as well (114). An overabundance of vitamin A can manifest in accelerated bone loss (114).

With 40% of US adults reporting use of a multivitamin, the debate and research needs to continue to determine the relationships between vitamins, minerals, and chronic disease (130,136). What does become clear through these investigations, is the decision to take a multivitamin (or any supplement) should not be made lightly and that the "food first" approach appears to be best.

Position Stands

The following discussion centers on the position of national organizations concerning the use of supplements. Included are the position stands of the American College of Sports Medicine (ACSM), the Academy of Nutrition and Dietetics (AND), the International Olympic Committee (IOC), the National Athletic Trainers' Association (NATA), the Collegiate & Professional Sports Dietitians Association (CPSDA), and the American Academy of Sports Dietitians and Nutritionists (AASDN).

Position Stand of the AND and ACSM

In general, no vitamin or mineral supplements are required if an athlete is consuming adequate energy from a variety of foods to maintain body weight. Supplementation recommendations unrelated to exercise, such as folic acid for women of childbearing potential, should be followed. A multivitamin /mineral supplement may be appropriate if an athlete is dieting or eliminating food groups, etc. Single-nutrient supplements may be appropriate for a specific medical or nutritional reason (iron supplements to correct iron deficiency anemia) (17).

The Academy of Nutrition and Dietetics and the American College of Sports Medicine have classified ergogenic aids into one of four categories (17):

1. Those that perform as claimed
2. Those that may perform as claimed but for which there is insufficient evidence of efficacy at this time
3. Those that do not perform as claimed
4. and those that are dangerous, banned, or illegal and, therefore, should not be used

According to the AND and the ACSM, ergogenic aids that perform as claimed include creatine; caffeine; sports drinks, gels and bars; sodium bicarbonate; protein and amino acid supplements. See discussion concerning protein and amino acid supplements, creatine, caffeine, energy drinks, and energy bars (17). Sodium bicarbonate may be an effective ergogenic aid as a blood buffer (role in acid–base balance and prevention of fatigue), but its use is not without unpleasant adverse effects such as diarrhea.

AND states that current evidence indicates protein and amino acid supplements are no more or no less effective than food when energy is adequate for gaining lean body mass (71,72). Although widely used, protein powders and amino acid supplements are a potential source for illegal substances such as nandrolone, which may not be listed on the ingredient label (72).

The ACSM and the AND indicate that groups who are at risk (including athletes on severe energy-restricting diets, and perhaps those following vegetarian diets), may benefit from taking a low-dose, multivitamin and mineral supplement, or from including micronutrient-fortified, liquid meal replacement supplements in their diet (17). The AND and the ACSM have concluded that, "athletes should be counseled regarding the appropriate use of ergogenic aids". Such products should only be used after careful evaluation for safety, efficacy, potency, and legality" (73, 74).

Position Stand of the International Olympic Committee

The IOC recognized and evaluated two micronutrients in its latest consensus statement, namely antioxidants and vitamin D supplementation. Antioxidants have been popular in literature and research studies. There are arguments for and against the use of these by athletes (69) Arguments that support antioxidant supplementation propose that these micronutrients are able to decrease the reactive oxygen species that forms during exhaustive exercise (69). These arguments suggest that some athletes do not consume a healthy diet that contains antioxidant food groups, such as whole grains, fruits, vegetables, nuts and seeds (69). On the other hand, it is believed that although exercise can promote oxidative stress, there is no evidence to support the theory that this exercise-induced oxidative stress is detrimental to human health or performance; or that participation in regular exercise increases the body's own ability to produce endogenous antioxidants. If energy requirements are met, and the athlete is able to ingest all of the various dietary antioxidants, additional supplementation is NOT warranted; also, toxic levels may impair muscle functioning and reduce training adaptations to exercise (69). In light of the above controversy, the IOC recommends that athletes not consume antioxidant supplements and caution should be exercised with the use of single-nutrient, high-dose antioxidant supplements (69).

The IOC also indicates vitamin D supplementation is not supported by a strong body of evidence. Vitamin D can accumulate in the body and cause toxic side-effects such as nausea, vomiting, poor appetite, constipation, weakness, weight loss, mental confusion, irregularities in cardiac rhythm and calcification of soft tissues, all of which would negatively impact exercise performance and general health (69). Current guidelines are opposed to vitamin D supplementation, unless it is medically warranted. Because vitamin D and calcium metabolism are so closely linked, athletes should be sure to obtain adequate levels of calcium from dietary sources (69)."

The IOC strongly discourages the indiscriminate or widespread use of supplements, especially in terms of acute or long-term effects on health, positive doping outcomes and possible detrimental effects on exercise performance (75,76). Often, supplements either contain little or no active ingredient or too much of certain toxic nutrients. They may also contain harmful impurities, such as lead, broken glass, and animal feces because of poor manufacturing practices (75,76). The majority of products on the market fail to reach expected standards (74,75). Other involved risks include inaccurate labeling, failure to declare the ingredients on the label, and cross-contamination of supplements (75,76).

Position Stand of the National Athletic Trainers' Association

The NATA has published the following recommendations for Athletic Trainers when evaluating literature associated with performance nutrition and dietary supplements (77). The NATA advises Athletic Trainers that the keys to good health and successful athletic performance are a carefully designed, healthful, and nutritionally balanced diet and well-developed training program; there is no "quick fix" or shortcut to success (77). When an athlete is considering use of a dietary supplement, several questions should be investigated: Is it safe, is it legal, and will it work? As allied health professionals, Athletic Trainers must be ready to educate athletes in the areas of safety, efficacy, and regulation. This is especially true when the Athletic Trainer is asked to serve as the primary evaluator in accordance with NCAA regulations (92). Another objective of the NATA's position stance is to promote a "food first" philosophy (92).

The Collegiate & Professional Sports Dietitians Association (CPSDA)

The CSPSD is a national not for profit organization founded in 2009, comprised of registered dietitians who specialize in sports nutrition on a full time basis ("Sports RDs"). Sports RDs are employed primarily by major college athletic departments, professional sports teams, U.S. Olympic governing bodies and the U.S. military. CPSDA Board of Directors recommends a standard feeding protocol for athletes at all levels of participation as follows:

- Fuel athletes throughout the day with healthy whole foods to ensure adequate energy availability, speed recovery, restore energy, and repair muscle damage after exercise. Athletes must have easy and open access to planned meals and recovery snacks throughout the day to replace nutrients, fluids, electrolytes, and energy utilized during activity in order to replenish energy, facilitate recovery, repair muscle damage, mediate inflammation, and stimulate immune function. Athletes in all phases of training require feedings of nutrient rich whole foods in frequent intervals and, as necessary, safe dietary supplements to replace expended nutrients and electrolytes, enhance immune function, and achieve optimal body composition. Smaller but more frequent feedings of nutritious whole foods throughout the day improve mental as well as physical performance, thereby contributing to academic and athletic performance. A Training Table planned meals for athletes in a dining hall is a learning lab where athletes receive ongoing education that underscores the measurable benefits of a healthy lifestyle and where athletes experience proper nutrition as the best defense against banned performance enhancing substances. College athletes in particular, whether or not they receive financial aid to assist with tuition, housing and/or food, should be given equal access to whole foods throughout the day to ensure full restoration of nutrients, fluids, and electrolytes expended in activity to speed recovery, stimulate immune function, reduce inflammation, and fully replace energy stores. CPSDA recommends and supports a simple rule that would allow institutions to feed all athletes within their respective budgets as institutional staff deems appropriate for the benefit of the health, well-being, and performance of the athletes.

The American Academy of Sports Dietitians and Nutritionists (AASDN)

Health/wellness and fitness professionals, including Athletic Trainers', are aware that the endorsement or sale of prescription and over-the-counter medications is beyond their scope of practice. What is not clear is their role in the endorsement or sale of nutritional supplements. Marketing by the supplement industry has convinced professionals and consumers that supplements, unlike drugs, have no side effects, are "all natural," and are therefore "safe". However, consumers are ingesting combinations of supplements and supplements with prescription and non-prescription drugs, without any regard to side effects, interactions, and complications. Therefore, it is the position of the American Academy of Sports Dietitians and Nutritionists (AASDN) that endorsement or sale of nutritional supplements by health/wellness and fitness professionals (other than licensed nutritionists/dietitians) constitutes an unsafe practice and is in violation of the professional code of conduct held by all health/wellness and fitness professionals to "do no harm". Endorsement or sale of nutritional products must come directly from the consumer's physician or a Registered /Licensed Dietitian.

Summary

Many Americans, nearly 40 percent, use health care approaches developed outside of mainstream Western, or conventional medicine. When describing non-mainstream health approaches people often use the words "alternative" and "complementary" interchangeably, but the two terms refer to different concepts:

- "Complementary" generally refers to using a non-mainstream approach together with conventional medicine.
- "Alternative" refers to using a non-mainstream approach in place of conventional medicine.

True alternative medicine is not common. Most people use non-mainstream approaches along with conventional treatments, and the boundaries between complementary and conventional medicine overlap and change with time. For example, guided imagery and massage, both once considered complementary or alternative, are used regularly in some hospitals to help with pain management. Non-mainstream health care approaches may also be considered part of integrative medicine or integrative health care. For example, cancer treatment centers with integrative health care programs may offer services such as acupuncture and meditation to help manage symptoms and side effects for patients who are receiving conventional cancer treatments such as chemotherapy.

Several facts about this growing trend on "integrative health care" include:

- Many individuals, health care providers, and health care systems are integrating various practices with origins outside of mainstream medicine.
- The integrative trend is growing among providers and health care systems.

What is the science behind these non-mainstream approaches? Advocates claim strong science exists and complain about the slow moving and overly cautious FDA, while scientists argue that Congress is advocating for unproven therapies rather than subjecting new treatments to evaluation. In many instances, a lack of reliable data makes it difficult for people to make informed decisions about using these therapies.

The National Center for Complementary and Alternative Medicine (NCCAM) is the Federal Government's lead agency for scientific research on complementary and alternative medicine (CAM). They are one of the twenty-seven institutes and centers that make up the National Institutes of Health (NIH) within the U.S. Department of Health and Human Services. The mission of NCCAM is to explore complementary and alternative healing practices in the context of rigorous science, train CAM researchers, and disseminate authoritative information to the public and professionals.

The origin of NCCAM began in 1992, when Senator Tom Harkin (D-Iowa), convinced bee pollen had cured his allergies, assigned $2 million of his discretionary funds to establish the Office of Unconventional Medicine, renamed the Office of Alternative Medicine (OAM). Funds for OAM increased annually and in 1998 increased to $19.5 million. Also in 1998, Senator Harkin won a decisive battle when the NIH opened a new office - the National Center for Complementary and Alternative Medicine (NCCAM) - with a $50 million budget. As a sign that NCCAM was indeed a scientific entity to be dealt with, the renowned Dr. Stephen E. Straus was appointed the first director on October 6, 1999. When interviewed, Dr. Straus made it clear that the office would perform rigorous scientific studies and that the public and companies with vested interests in new alternative therapies "will have to accept that research may show that some new therapies will not be good; some therapies will not be safe; and some therapies will not be any more effective than present alternatives.

The Dietary Supplement Health and Education Act of 1994 (Public Law 103-417, DSHEA), authorized the establishment of the Office of Dietary Supplements (ODS) at the National Institute of Health (NIH). The ODS was created in 1995 within the Office of Disease Prevention (ODP), Office of the Director (OD), NIH. One of the purposes in creating the ODS was to promote scientific research in the area of dietary supplements. Dietary supplements can have an impact on the prevention of disease and on the maintenance of health.

Dietary supplements are not required to be standardized in the United States. In fact, no legal or regulatory definition exists in the United States for standardization as it applies to dietary supplements. Because of this, the term "standardization" may mean many different things. Some manufacturers use the term standardization incorrectly to refer to uniform manufacturing practices. Following a recipe is not sufficient for a product to be called standardized. Therefore, the presence of the word "standardized" on a supplement label does not necessarily indicate product quality.

Several independent organizations offer quality testing of dietary supplements and allow products that pass their tests to display seals of approval (3). These seals of approval provide assurance that the product was properly manufactured, contains the ingredients listed on the label, and does not contain harmful levels of contaminants; however, these verification programs do not guarantee that a product is safe or effective. Organizations that offer this quality testing include: U.S. Pharmacopeia, ConsumerLab.com, and NSF International.

Dietary supplements are intended to supplement the diet not to replace the balance of a variety of foods important to health. Before ingesting any dietary supplements consumers should consider the following points. Many supplements contain active ingredients that can have strong effects in the body. Consumers should be alert to the possibility of unexpected side effects, especially when taking a new product. The term "natural" does not mean safe and is a very subjective term. Do not assume that this term ensures wholesomeness or safety. Supplements are most likely to cause side effects or harm when taken instead of prescribed medicines or when people take many supplements in combination. Some supplements can increase the risk of bleeding, or if a person takes them before or after surgery, they can affect the person's response to anesthesia. Most dietary supplements have not been tested for safety in pregnant women, nursing mothers, or children. Hence caution should be taken during pregnancy, nursing, and should not be given to children (beyond a basic multivitamin/mineral product). There are about 65,000 dietary supplements on the market consumed by more than 150 million Americans. Of the 465 drugs subject to a Class 1 recall in the U.S. between 2004 and 2012, 237 (51%) were dietary supplements. To reiterate, these supplements accounted for more than half the Class 1 drugs recalled by the FDA. This means they contain substances that could cause serious health problems or even death. The majority of those recalled supplements were bodybuilding, weight loss, or sexual enhancement products that contain unapproved medicinal ingredients, including steroids. Almost one-quarter of the substances were manufactured outside of the United States which does not require adherence to good manufacturing practices.

Americans, on balance, are sufficiently nourished with essential vitamins and minerals like Vitamins A and D and folate, according to a new report from the Centers for Disease Control and Prevention's Division of Laboratory Sciences in the National Center for Environmental Health. In fact, fewer than 10 percent of the American population suffered from nutritional deficiencies, according to the research.

The IOC recognized and evaluated two specific micronutrients in its latest consensus statement, namely antioxidants and vitamin D supplementation. Arguments that support antioxidant supplementation propose that these micronutrients are able to decrease the reactive oxygen species that forms during exhaustive exercise. On the other hand, it is believed that although exercise can promote oxidative stress, there is no evidence to support the theory that this exercise-induced oxidative stress is detrimental to human health or performance; or that participation in regular exercise increases the body's own ability to produce endogenous antioxidants. In light of the above controversy, the IOC recommends that athletes not consume antioxidant supplements and caution should be exercised with the use of single-nutrient, high-dose antioxidant supplements. The IOC strongly discourages the indiscriminate or widespread use of supplements, especially in terms of acute or long-term effects on health, positive doping outcomes and possible detrimental effects on exercise performance (75,76). Often, supplements either contain little or no active ingredient or too much of certain toxic nutrients. They may also contain harmful impurities, such as lead, broken glass, and animal feces because of poor manufacturing practices (75,76). The majority of products on the market fail to reach expected standards (74,75). Other involved risks include inaccurate labeling, failure to declare the ingredients on the label, and cross-contamination of supplements (75,76).

The CSPSD is a national not for profit organization founded in 2009, comprised of registered dietitians who specialize in sports nutrition on a full time basis ("Sports RDs"). Sports RDs are employed primarily by major college athletic departments, professional sports teams, U.S. Olympic governing bodies and the U.S. military. CPSDA Board of Directors recommends a standard feeding protocol for athletes at all levels of participation. Health/wellness and fitness professionals, including Athletic Trainers', are aware that the endorsement or sale of prescription and over-the-counter medications is beyond their scope of practice. What is not clear is their role in the endorsement or sale of nutritional supplements. Marketing by the supplement industry has convinced professionals and consumers that supplements, unlike drugs, have no side effects, are "all natural," and are therefore "safe". However, consumers are ingesting combinations of supplements and supplements with prescription and non-prescription drugs, without any regard to side effects, interactions, and complications. Therefore, it is the position of the American Academy of Sports Dietitians and Nutritionists (AASDN) that endorsement or sale of nutritional supplements by health/wellness and fitness professionals (other than licensed nutritionists/dietitians) constitutes an unsafe practice and is in violation of the professional code of conduct held by all health/wellness and fitness professionals to "do no harm". Endorsement or sale of nutritional products must come directly from the consumer's physician or a Registered /Licensed Dietitian.

Chapter 9 Sample Test

1. Define "Complementary health approaches," and discuss the role NCCAM plays.
2. Summarize details concerning the origins of the National Center for Complementary and Alternative Medicine (NCCAM), and list the classifications of "Complementary health".
3. Define and discuss natural based therapies (supplements) in light of the Dietary Supplement Health and Education Act of 1994 including health claims, labeling regulations, good manufacturing practices, standardization, and safety.
4. When was the Office of Dietary Supplements formed and what is its role?
5. List the four categories of supplements, and provide examples of each.
6. List three independent supplement verification programs, and provide details of each program.
7. List four points to consider before ingesting a dietary supplement.
8. Create a table listing the position stand on vitamin/mineral supplementation and use of ergogenic aids by the following organizations: the Academy of Nutrition and Dietetics and the American College of Sports Medicine, The National Athletic Trainers' Association, the International Olympic Committee, and the American Academy of Sports Dietitians and Nutritionists on use of supplementation.

References

1. U.S. Department of Health and Human Services. NIH. NCCAM. NCCAM Facts-at-a-Glance and Mission. (accessed June 24, 2013). http://nccam.nih.gov/about/ataglance.
2. U.S. Department of Health and Human Services. NIH. NCCAM. Complementary, alternative, or integrative health: What's in a name? http://nccam.nih.gov/health/whatiscam. NCCAM Pub No. D347 Date Created: October 2008 Last Updated: May 2013.
3. Office of Dietary Supplements. National Institutes of Health. Dietary Supplements: what you need to know. Reviewed: June 17, 2011. (accessed 06/28/2013). http://ods.od.nih.gov/HealthInformation/DS_WhatYouNeedToKnow.aspx
4. U.S. Food and Drug Administration. Dietary Supplement Health and Education Act of 1994. Regulatory Information. Updated 2009. (accessed 06/28/2013. http://www.fda.gov/RegulatoryInformation/Legislation/FederalFoodDrugandCosmeticActFDCAct/SignificantAmendmentstotheFDCAct/ucm148003.htm.
5. U.S. Food and Drug Administration. Federal Food, Drug, and Cosmetic Act (FD&C Act). Updated 2011. (accessed 06/28/2013). http://www.fda.gov/RegulatoryInformation/Legislation/FederalFoodDrugandCosmeticActFDCAct/default.htm.
6. Council for Responsible Nutriton. DSHEA Summary and Analysis. (accessed 06/28/2013). http://www.crnusa.org/leg.html#dshea.
7. Aronson, A. et al. Frontline. The alternative fix. PBS Video. (2004). FRL 72203. (production of WGBH Boston). 2003. Walters, B. What's Really in the Bottle. ABC/20-20, Dec. 2005.
8. Centers for Disease Control and Prevention. National Center for Health Statistics. Data Briefs. (Updated May, 2011). http://www.cdc.gov/nchs/data/databriefs/db61.htm.
9. U.S. Food and Drug Administration. Guidance for Industry: Current Good Manufacturing Practice in Manufacturing, Packaging, Labeling, or Holding Operations for Dietary Supplements; Small Entity Compliance Guide. (2010). Small entity compliance guide. http://www.fda.gov/Food/GuidanceRegulation/GuidanceDocumentsRegulatoryInformation/DietarySupplements/ucm238182.htm#I.
10. U.S. Food and Drug Administration. (2007).Overview of the Implementation of the Current Good Manufacturing Practices for Dietary Supplements Guidance for Industry.
11. Office of Dietary Supplements. (2011). National Institutes of Health. Dietary Supplements. http://ods.od.nih.gov/factsheets/DietarySupplements-HealthProfessional/
12. U.S Food and Drug Administration. Dietary Supplements. Updated 05/21/2013. (accessed 06/29/2013. http://www.fda.gov/Food/DietarySupplements/default.htm.
13. USDA National Agriculture Library. Food and Nutrition Information Center. Updated 06/28/2013.
14. Medline Plus. U.S. National Library of Medicine. NIH. Updated Jan. 2013. http://www.nlm.nih.gov/medlineplus/druginformation.html
15. PubMed. National Center for Biotechnology Information, U.S. National Library of Medicine 8600 Rockville Pike, Bethesda MD, 20894 USA. http://www.ncbi.nlm.nih.gov/pubmed/?term=dietary+supplements.
16. Kreider R, et al. (2010). ISSN exercise & sport nutrition review: research & recommendations. *Journal of the International Society of Sports Nutrition*. 7 doi:10. 1186/1550-2783-7-7.
17. Rodriquez NR. DiMarco NM. Langley S. (2009). Position of the American Dietetic Association, Dietitians of Canada, and the American College of Sports Medicine: Nutrition and athletic performance. *J Am Diet Assoc.* 109(3):509-527 [homepage on the Internet]. c2012. Available from: http://journals.lww.com/acsm-msse/Fulltext/2009/03000/ Nutrition_and_Athletic_Performance.27.aspxPrev Chronic Dis. 2006 October; 3(4): A129.

Published online 2006 September 15. PMCID: PMC1784117.

18. Office of Dietary Supplements. National Institutes of Health. Botanical Dietary Supplements. Reviewed June 24, 2011. http://ods.od.nih.gov/factsheets/BotanicalBackground-HealthProfessional/.
19. Office of Dietary Supplements. National Institutes of Health. Botanical Supplement Fact Sheets. Reviewed June 2011. http://ods.od.nih.gov/factsheets/list-Botanicals/.
20. Ahrendt DM. (2001). Ergogenic aids: Counseling the Athlete. Am Fam Physician. 63(5):913-923.
21. Leutholtz B. Kreider R. (2001). Exercise and Sport Nutrition. In *Nutritional Health*. Edited by Wilson T, Temple N. Totowa, NJ: Humana Press. 207-39.
22. Kreider R. Leutholtz B. Katch F. Katch V. (2009). *Exercise & Sport Nutrition.* Santa Barbara: Fitness Technologies Press.
23. Maughan RJ. Noakes TD. (1991). Fluid replacement and exercise stress. A brief review of studies on fluid replacement and some guidelines for the athlete. *Sports Med.* 12(1):16-31.
24. National Institute on Drug Abuse. Drug facts. Revised July 2012. NIH Pub: 06-3721. http://www.drugabuse.gov/publications/drugfacts/anabolic-steroids
25. Haupt HA. Rovere GD. (1984). Anabolic steroids: a review of the literature. *Am J Sports Med.* 12:69–84.
26. Bhasin S. Storer TW. Berman N, Callegari C. Clevenger B. Phillips J, et al. (1996). The effects of supraphysiologic doses of testosterone on muscle size and strength in normal men. *N Engl J Med.* 335:1–7.
27. Bahrke MS. Yesalis CE. Wright JE. (1996). Psychological and behavioral effects of endogenous testosterone and anabolic-androgenic steroids: an update. *Sports Med* 22(6):367–390.
28. Berning JM. Adams KJ. Stamford BA. (2004). Anabolic steroid usage in athletics: facts, fiction, and public relations. *J Strength Conditioning Res* 18(4):908–917, 2004.
29. Blue JG. Lombardo JA. (1999). Steroids and steroid-like compounds. *Clin Sports Med* 18(3):667–689.
30. Bronson FH. Matherne CM. (1997).Exposure to anabolicandrogenic steroids shortens life span of male mice. *Med Sci Sports Exerc* 29(5):615–619.
31. Brower KJ. (1997). Withdrawal from anabolic steroids. *Curr Ther Endocrinol Metab* 6:338–343.
32. Daly RC, et al. (2003). Neuroendocrine and behavioral effects of high-dose anabolic steroid administration in male normal volunteers. *Psychoneuroendocrinology* 28(3):317–331.
33. Pope HG Jr. Kouri EM. Hudson MD. (2002). Effects of supraphysiologic doses of testosterone on mood and aggression in normal men: a randomized controlled trial. *Arch Gen Psychiatry* 57(2):133–140.
34. Su T-P, et al. (1993). Neuropsychiatric effects of anabolic steroids in male normal volunteers. *JAMA* 269(21):2760–2764.
35. Sullivan ML. Martinez CM. Gennis P. Gallagher, EJ. (1998). The cardiac toxicity of anabolic steroids. *Prog Cardiovasc Dis* 41(1):1–15.
36. Gruber AJ. Pope HG Jr. (2000). Psychiatric and medical effects of anabolic-androgenic steroid use in women. *Psychother Psychosom* 69:19–26.
37. Elliot D. Goldberg L. (1996). Intervention and prevention of steroid use in adolescents. *Am J Sports Med* 24(6):S46–S47.
38. Rawson ES, et al. (2003). SSE#91: Scientifically debatable: Is creating worth its weight. 16 (4).
39. American Academy of Pediatrics (2001). News Release: Though not recommended, young athletes use creatine to improve performance. http://pediatrics.aappublications.org/content/108/2/421.abstract. Accessed 12/16/03.
40. Kalinski, M. I. (2003). State-sponsored research on creatine supplements and blood doping in elite Soviet sport. *Perspect. Biol. Med.* 46, 445-451.

41. Harris, RC. Söderlund K. & Hultman E. (1992). Elevation of creatine in resting and exercised muscle of normal subjects by creatine supplementation. *Clin. Sci.* 83, 367-374.
42. Greenhaff P L. Casey A. Short AH. Harris R. Söderlund K. & Hultman, E. (1993). Influence of oral creatine supplementation of muscle torque during repeated bouts of maximal voluntary exercise in man. *Clin. Sci.* 84, 565-571.
43. Walker JB (1979). Creatine: biosynthesis, regulation, and function. *Adv. Enzymol. Relat. Areas Mol. Med.* 50, 177-242
44. Greenhaff PL. Bodin, K..Söderlund K. & Hultman, E. (1994). Effect of oral creatine supplementation on skeletal muscle phosphocreatine resynthesis. *Am. J. Physiol.* 266, E725-730.
45. Vandenberghe K. Van Hecke P. Van Leemputte M. Vanstapel F. & Hespel, P. (1999). Phosphocreatine resynthesis is not affected by creatine loading. *Med. Sci. Sports Exerc.* 31, 236-242.
46. Branch JD. (2003). Effect of creatine supplementation on body composition and performance: a meta-analysis. *Int. J. Sport Nutr. Exerc. Metab.* 13, 198-226.
47. Nissen SL. & Sharp R L (2003). Effect of dietary supplements on lean mass and strength gains with resistance exercise: a meta-analysis. *J. Appl. Physiol.* 94, 651-659.
48. Terjung R L, et al. (2000). American College of Sports Medicine roundtable. The physiological and health effects of oral creatine supplementation. *Med. Sci. Sports Exerc.* 32, 706-71.
49. Greenwood, M., et al. (2003). Creatine supplementation during college football training does not increase the incidence of cramping or injury. *Mol. Cell. Biochem.* 244, 83-88.
50. Poortmans JR Francaux M. (1999). Long-term creatine supplementation does not impair renal function in healthy athletes. Med Sci Sports Exerc 1999;31: 1108-10.
51. Graham TE. Spriet LL. (1996). Caffeine and Exercise Performance. Gatorade Sports Science Institute. SSE#60 (9):1.
52. Delbecke FT. and M. Debachere. (1984). Caffeine: use and abuse in sports. *Int. J. Sports Med.* 5:179-182.
53. Graham TE and LL Spriet. (1991). Performance and metabolic responses to a high caffeine dose during prolonged exercise. *J. Appl. Physiol.* 71:2292-2298.
54. Graham TE and LL Spriet. (1995). Metabolic, catecholamine and exercise performance responses to varying doses of caffeine. *J. Appl. Physiol.* 78:867-874.
55. Graham TE. Rush JWE and M.H. VanSoeren. (1994). Caffeine and exercise: metabolism and performance. Can. *J. Appl. Physiol.* 2:111-138.
56. Spriet, LL, et al. (1992). Caffeine ingestion and muscle metabolism during prolonged exercise in humans. *Am. J. Physiol.* 262 (Endocrinol. Metab.):E891-E898.
57. Graham TE, et al. (1995). Caffeine Vs. coffee: coffee isn't an effective ergogenic aid. *Med. Sci. Sports Exerc.* 27:S224.
58. Bangsbo J, et al. (1992). Acute and habitual caffeine ingestion and metabolic responses to steady-state exercise. *J. Appl. Physiol.* 72:1297-1303.
59. VanSoeren MH, et al. (1993). Short term withdrawal does not alter caffeine-induced metabolic changes during intensive exercise. *FASEB J.* 7:A518. (Abstract).
60. Chesley A. Hultman E. Spriet LL. (1994). Variable effects of caffeine on muscle glycogenolysis in recreationally active subjects during intense aerobic exercise. *Can. J. Appl. Physiol.* 19:10P.
61. Falk B. R Burstein. J Rosenblum. Y Shapiro. E Zylber-Katz, and N. Bashan. (1990). Effects of caffeine ingestion on body fluid balance and thermoregulation during exercise. *Can. J. Physiol. Pharmacol.* 68:889-892.
62. Gordon, N.F., et al. (1982). Effects of caffeine on thermoregulatory and myocardial function during endurance performance. *S. Afr. Med.* J. 62:644-647.
63. Wemple RD. DR Lamb, and AC Blostein. (1994). Caffeine ingested in a fluid replacement beverage during prolonged exercise does not cause diuresis. *Med. Sci. Sports Exerc.* 26:S204. (Abstract).

64. Harel Z, et al. (2013). The Frequency and Characteristics of Dietary Supplement Recalls in the United States. *JAMA Intern Med.* 173(10):929-930.
65. U.S. Department of Health & Human Services. NCCAM. (2013).Weight Loss and Complementary practices: What the science says. *NCCAM Clinical Digest.* June 2013. http://nccam.nih.gov/health/providers/digest/weightloss-science?nav=upd.
66. Trubo R. (2002). Nutrition bars: Healthy or hype. MedicineNet.com. Medically updated Jan. 20, 2004. (accessed 06/29/2013). http://www.medicinenet.com/script/main/art.asp?articlekey=51787.
67. Whitney, E & Rolfes S. (2013). *Understanding Nutrition 13th ed.* Belmont, CA: Wadsworth, Cengage Learning.
68. Ross C. (Shils) et al. (2012). *Modern Nutrition in Health & Disease, 11th ed.* Philadelphia PA: Lipincott Wilillians & Wilikins.
69. Powers S. Nelson WB. Larson-Meyer E. (2011). Antioxidant and Vitamin D supplements for athletes: sense or nonsense? *J Sports Sci.* 29(S1):S47-S55.
70. Burke L. (2006). Supplements and sports foods. In: Burke L, Deakin V, editors. *Clinical Sports Nutrition.* Sydney, Australia: McGraw-Hill; 2006. p. 485-579.
71. Phillips SM Moore DR. Tang J. (2007). A critical examination of dietary protein requirements, benefits, and excesses in athletes. *Int J Sports Nutr Exer Metab.* 17:S58–S76.
72. Tipton KD. Witard OC. (2007). Protein requirements and recommendations for athletes: relevance of ivory tower arguments for practical recommendations. *Clin Sports Med.* 26:17–36.
73. Coyle E, Jeukendrup A, Wagenmakers A, Saris W. Fatty acid oxidation is directly regulated by carbohydrate metabolism during exercise. Am J Physiol. 1997;273:E268–75.
74. Donahoo W, Levine J, Melanson E. Variability in energy expenditure and its components. Curr Opin Clin Nutr Metab Care. 2004;7:599–605.
75. Maughan RJ. Greenhaff PL. Hespel P. (2011). Dietary supplements for athletes: emerging trends and recurring themes. *J Sports Sci.* 29(S1):S57-S66.
76. Maughan RJ, Depiesse F, Geyer H, et al. The use of dietary supplements by athletes. J Sports Sci. 2007;25 Suppl 1:S103-S113.
77. Buell, JL, et al. (2013). National Athletic Trainers' Association Position Statement: Evaluation of dietary supplements for performance nutrition. *Journal of Athletic Training.* 48(1):124–13. doi: 10.4085/1062-6050-48.1.16.
78. Bergstrom J, Hermansen L, Hultman E, Saltin B. Diet, muscle glycogen, and physical performance. Acta Physiol Scand. 1967;71(2):140–150.
79. Sherman WM, Brodowicz G, Wright DA, Allen WK, Simonsen J, Dernbach A. Effects of 4 h preexercise carbohydrate feedings on cycling performance. Med Sci Sports Exerc. 1989;21(5):598–604.
80. Sherman WM, Peden MC, Wright DA. Carbohydrate feedings 1 h before exercise improves cycling performance. Am J Clin Nutr. 1991;54(5):866–870.
81. Jacobs KA, Sherman WM. The efficacy of carbohydrate supplementation and chronic high-carbohydrate diets for improving endurance performance. Int J Sport Nutr. 1999;9(1):92–115.
82. Jeukendrup AE, Aldred S. Fat supplementation, health, and endurance performance. Nutrition. 2004;20(7–8):678–688.
83. Jeukendrup AE. Carbohydrate intake during exercise and performance. Nutrition. 2004;20(7–8):669–677.
84. Ivy JL, Goforth HW Jr, Damon BM, McCauley TR, Parsons EC, Price TB. Early postexercise muscle glycogen recovery is enhanced with a carbohydrate-protein supplement. J Appl Physiol. 2002;93(4):1337–1344.
85. Hawley JA, Tipton KD, Millard-Stafford ML. Promoting training adaptations through nutritional interventions. J Sports Sci. 2006;24(7):709–721.

86. Office of Dietary Supplements. Dietary Supplement Health and Education Act of 1994. http://ods.od.nih.gov/about/dshea_wording. aspx. Accessed April 5, 2012.
87. Green GA, Catlin DH, Starcevic B. Analysis of over-the-counter dietary supplements. Clin J Sport Med. 2001;11(4):254–259.
88. Consumer Lab. About ConsumerLab.com and product tests. http:// www.consumerlab.com/aboutcl.asp. Accessed March 18, 2011.
89. 22. US Food and Drug Administration. Beware of fraudulent "dietary supplements." http://www.fda.gov/forconsumers/consumerupdates/ucm246744.htm. Accessed March 15, 2011.
90. World Anti-Doping Agency. World Anti-Doping code. http:// www.wadaama.org/en/World-Anti- Doping-Program/Sports-and-Anti-Doping-Organizations/The-Code/. Accessed July 14, 2010.
91. National Collegiate Athletic Association. NCAA banned substances. http://www.ncaa.org/wps/wcm/connect/public/NCAA/Healthþandþ Safety/DrugþTesting/Resources/NCAAþbannedþdrugsþlist. Accessed April 18, 2011.
92. National Collegiate Athletic Association. 2011–12 NCAA Division I manual. http://www.ncaapublications.com/productdownloads/D112. pdf. Accessed April 18, 2011.
93. Takeshita S, et al. (2009). A snake enriched with oral branched-chain amino acids prevents a fall in albumin in patients with liver cirrhosis. Nutrition Research. 29:89-93.
94. Kawaguchi T, et al. (2008). Branched-chain amino acid enriched supplementation improves insulin resistance in patients with chronic liver disease. Int J of Molecular Medicine. 105-112.
95. Seifert SM, et al. (2011). Health effects of energy drinks on children, adolescents, and young adults. Pediatrics. 127:511.
96. Lee J. Energy drinks vs. sports drinks: know thy difference. Available at: http:// speedendurance.com/2009/07/09/ energy-drinks-vs-sports-drinks-know-thydifference. Accessed January 17, 2011.
97. McCarthy M. Overuse of energy drinks worries health pros. Available at: www. usatoday.com/sports/2009-07-01- Drinks_N.htm. Accessed January 17,2011.
98. Nitzke S, Tanumihardjo S, Salomon J, Coleman G. Energy drinks, sports drinks, and other functional/enhanced beverages are often a waste of money. Available at: www.uwex.edu/ces/wnep/specialist/nfl/ mmpdfs/0810.pdf#page1.
99. U.S. Food and Drug Administration. Final rule declaring dietary supplements containing ephedrine alkaloids adulterated because they present an unreasonable risk. *Federal Register*. 2004;69(28):6788–6854.
100. Jurgens TM. Whelan AM. Killian L. Doucette S. Kirk S. Foy E. (2012). Green tea for weight loss and weight maintenance in overweight or obese adults. *Cochrane Summaries*. Published Online 2012. Assessed as up-to-date: 2012. DOI: 10.1002/14651858.CD008650.pub2.
101. Robinson E, et al. (2013). Eating attentively: A systematic review and meta-analysis of the effect of food intake memory and awareness on eating. *Am J Clin Nutr.* 2013 Apr;97(4):728-42. doi: 10.3945/ajcn.112.045245. Epub 2013 Feb 27.
102. Rioux JG. Ritenbaugh C. (2013). Narrative review of yoga intervention clinical trials including weight-related outcomes. *Altern Ther Health Med.* 2013 May-Jun;19(3):32-46.
103. Yang K, et al. (2011). Utilization of 3-month yoga program for adults at high risk for type 2 diabetes: a pilot study. *Evid Based Complement Alternat Med.* 257891. doi: 10.1093/ecam/nep117. Epub 2011 Jan 9.
104. Elder C, et al. (2012). Randomized trial of tapas acupressure technique for weight loss maintenance. *BMC Complementary and Alternative Medicine* 2012, 12:19 doi:10.1186/1472-6882-12-19.
105. Chung-Hua Hsu, Chi-Jung Wang, Kung-Chang Hwang, Tzung-Yan Lee, Pesus Chou, and Hen-Hong Chang. (2009). *Journal of Women's Health.* 18(6): 813-818. doi:10.1089/jwh.2008.1005.

106. Cooperman T. ConsumerLab.com. http://www.consumerlab.com/aboutcl.asp, (accessed 07/01/2013.
107. NSF International . What do the letters stand for. http://www.nsf.org/regulatory/services/faq_general.asp. (accessed 07/01/2013).
108. NSF International. Certified for Sport. http://www.nsf.org/consumer /athletic_banned_substances/index.asp?program=AthleticBanSub (accessed 07/01/2013).
109. U.S. Pharmacopeial Convention. Legal Recognition of USP Standards. (accessed 07/01/2013). http://www.usp.org/about-usp/legal-recognition.
110. Katz MH, et al. (2013). How can we know if supplements are safe if we do not know what is in them?"*JAMA Int Med. 173(10):928. doi:10.1001/jamainternmed.2013.415.*
111. U.S. Food and Drug Administration. How consumers can report an adverse event or serious problem to FDA. Updated: 06/05/2013. (accessed 07/01/2013). http://www.fda.gov/ Safety/MedWatch/HowToReport/ucm053074.htm.
112. Second National Report on Biochemical Indicators of Diet and Nutrition in the U.S. Population. Executive Summary. (2012). National Center for Environmental Health Division of Laboratory Sciences. http://www.cdc.gov/nutritionreport/pdf/ExeSummary Web_032612.pdf#zoom=100. (accessed 07/02/2013).
113. Shepherd R. (2012, April 2). "CDC Announces People In The US Have Healthy Vitamin And Mineral Levels." *Medical News Today*. Retrieved from http://www.medicalnewstoday.com/articles/243649.php.
114. Melnick M. (2012). Should you take a multivitamin? The Huffington Post. (accessed 07/02/2013). http://www.huffingtonpost.com/2012/08/01/should-you-take-a-multivitamin_n_1725380.html.
115. U.S. Food and Drug Administration. (2013). 6 Tip-offs to Rip-offs: Don't Fall for Health Fraud Scams. *Consumer Updates.http://www.fda.gov/ForConsumers/ConsumerUpdates/ ucm341344.htm.*
116. Hamburg MA. (2010). FDA, Silver Springs, MD. Retrieved: http://www.fda.gov/downloads/Drugs/ResourcesForYou/Consumers/BuyingUsingMedicineSafely/MedicationHealthFraud/UCM236985.pdf.
117. US Food and Drug Administration. News release: tainted products marketed as dietary supplements potentially dangerous. http://www.fda.gov/NewsEvents/Newsroom/PressAnnouncements/ucm236967.
118. United States Government Accountability Office. (2013). Dietary supplements: FDA may have opportunities to expand its use of reported health problems to oversee products. GAO-13-244.
119. Adhihetty PJ, Beal MF. (2008) Creatine and its potential therapeutic value for targeting cellular energy impairment in neurodegenerative diseases. *Neuromolecular Med.*10(4):275-90.
120. Bender A, Koch W, Elstner M, et al., (2006). Creatine supplementation in Parkinson disease: a placebo-controlled randomized pilot trial. *Neurology* 67(7):1262-4.
121. Bender A, Samtleben W, Elstner M, Klopstock T. (2008). Long-term creatine supplementation is safe in aged patients with Parkinson disease. *Nutr Res.* Mar;28(3):172-8.
122. Hass CJ, Collins MA, Juncos JL. (2007) Resistance training with creatine monohydrate improves upper-body strength in patients with Parkinson disease: a randomized trial. *Neurorehabil Neural Repair* 21(2):107-15.
123. University of Maryland Medical Center. Creatine: Retrived: http://umm.edu/health/medical/altmed/supplement/creatine#ixzz2YYibwWmy.
124. Korzun WJ. (2007). Oral creatine supplements lower plasma homocysteine concentrations in humans. *Clin Lab Sci.* 17(2):102-6.
125. Cornelissen VA, Defoor JG, Stevens A, Schepers D, Hespel P, Decramer M, Mortelmans L, Dobbels F, Vanhaecke J, Fagard RH, Vanhees L. (2010). Effect of creatine supplementation

as a potential adjuvant therapy to exercise training in cardiac patients: a randomized controlled trial. *Clin Rehabil.* 2010 Nov;24(11):988-99.

126. Mursu J, Robien K, Harnack LJ, Park K, Jacobs DR, Jr. (2011) Dietary Supplements and Mortality Rate in Older Women: The Iowa Women's Health Study. *Arch Intern Med* 171:1625-33.
127. Bjelakovic G, Nikolova D, Gluud LL, Simonetti RG, Gluud C. (2007). Mortality in randomized trials of antioxidant supplements for primary and secondary prevention: systematic review and meta-analysis. *JAMA* 297:842-57.
128. Leitzmann MF, Stampfer MJ, Wu K, Colditz GA, Willett WC, Giovannucci EL. (2003). Zinc supplement use and risk of prostate cancer. *J Natl Cancer Inst.* 95:1004-7.
129. Larsson SC, Akesson A, Bergkvist L, Wolk A. (2010). Multivitamin use and breast cancer incidence in a prospective cohort of Swedish women. *Am J of Clin Nut* 91(5): 1268-72.
130. Harvard School of Public Health. Nutrition insurance policy: a daily multivitamin. Retrieved July 8, 2013: http://www.hsph.harvard.edu/nutritionsource/multivitamin/.
131. Macpherson H, Pipingas A, Pase MP. (2013). Mutilvitamin-multimineral supplementation and mortality: a meta-analysis of randomized controlled trails. *Am J of Clin Nut* 97(2): 437-44.
132. Chan AL, Leung HW, Wang SF. (2011). Multivitamin supplement use and risk of breast cancer: a meta analysis. *Ann Pharmacother* 45(4): 476-84.
133. Park SY, Murphy SP, Wilkens LR, Henderson BE, Kolonel LN. (2011). Multivitamin use and the risk of mortality and cancer incidence: the multiethnic cohort study. *Am J Epidemiol* 173(8): 906-14.
134. Rautianinen S, Akesson A, Levitan EB, Morgenstern R, Mittleman MA, Wolk A. (2010). Multivitamin use and the risk of myocardial infarction: a population-based cohort of Swedish women. Am J Clin Nutr 92(5): 1251-6.
135. National Institutes of Health State-of-the-Science Conference Statement: multivitamin/mineral supplements and chronic disease prevention. *Am J Clin Nutr.* 2007;85:257S-64S.
136. Gahche J, Bailey R, Burt V, et al. (2011). Dietary supplement use among U.S. adults has increased since NHANES III (1988–1994). Hyattsville, MD.
137. U.S. Department of Health and Human Services. NCCAM. Using dietary supplements wisely. Updated March 2013. (accessed 08/11/2013). http://nccam.nih.gov/health/supplements/wiseuse.htm

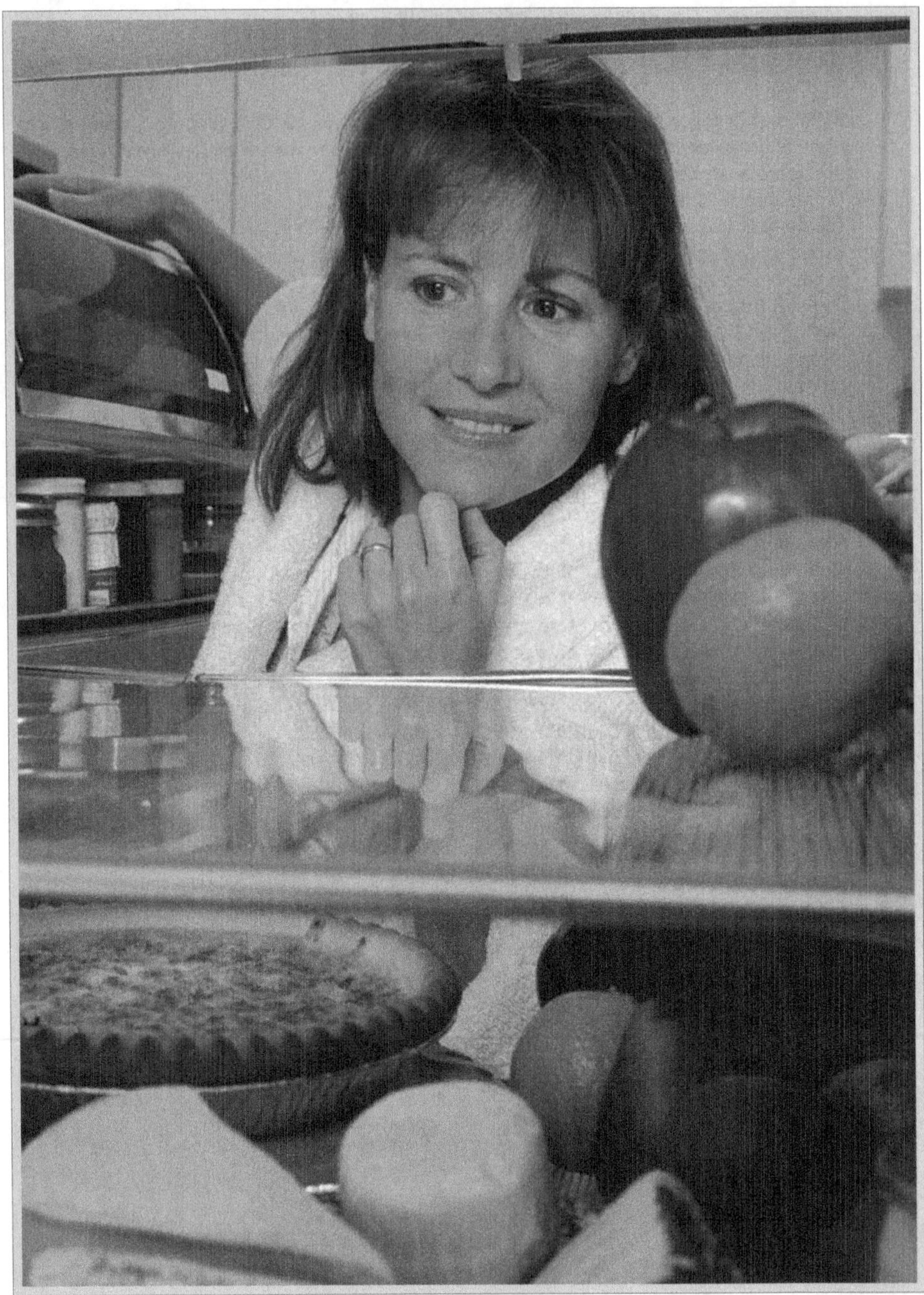

Chapter 10 - Nutrition Research

The revolution in genetics, patent protections for bio-engineered molecules, laws strengthening intellectual property rights, and licensing and patenting of results from federally-sponsored research have created new incentives for scientists, clinicians, and academic institutions to join forces with for-profit industry in an unprecedented array of entrepreneurial activities. In this chapter discussion will focus on current trends in nutrition research, steps involved in critical analysis of research and discussion of reputable nutrition resources.

Objectives

After reading and studying this chapter you should be able to:

1. Define and discuss "bias" in research, and discuss "conflicts of interest" as it relates to research. Define and discuss the two types of "conflicts of interest".
2. Define the Bayh-Dole Act, and describe how it changed federally sponsored research.
3. Discuss the steps involved in critical analysis of research in nutrition.
4. List reputable resources for obtaining sound, scientific nutrition information.

Introduction

While many professionals are involved in research, many more read the results of research and apply it to the real world. Therefore, it is vitally important to be able to critically analyze research to determine if the methods and results are valid.

When conducting research, scientists follow what is known as the "scientific method" (1). This method relies on identifying and researching a problem to be solved or asking a specific question to be answered. The next step is to formulate a possible solution to the problem or an answer to the question (hypothesis) and make a prediction that can be tested through research. A study design is decided upon, the research is completed, and the data is collected. The data must then be analyzed and the results interpreted. The original hypothesis is either supported by the data or is not supported. Scientists typically raise more questions so future research projects always exist (1).

The findings from research studies are typically submitted to a board of reviewers composed of other scientists from other institutions within the same discipline who rigorously evaluate the study to assure that the scientific method was followed (1). This process is known as "peer-review". Findings are considered preliminary until other scientists confirm or disprove them through other studies (replication). The findings are not accepted by the research community until they are replicated many times by other researchers (1).

Bias

The scientific method minimizes bias. Bias is defined as any tendency which prevents unprejudiced consideration of a question (2,3). In research, bias occurs when error is introduced into sampling or testing by selecting or encouraging one outcome or answer over others (3). Some degree of bias is nearly always present in a published study and can occur at any phase of the research project, including the study design, data collection, data analysis, and publication. Interpretation of bias cannot be limited to a simple yes or no. Instead, reviewers of the literature must consider the degree to which bias was prevented by proper study design, implementation, and conclusion (4). For clinical trials and randomized controlled trials, monitoring by a monitoring board (Data and Safety Monitoring Board) may be required. Vigilance is always necessary (4).

Conflict of Interest

Researchers have a tradition of free inquiry and free exchange of ideas. As stated in the position statement of the American Society of Gene Therapy on financial conflicts of interest, researchers are "united in the shared purpose to create knowledge, to critique existing knowledge, and to disseminate knowledge (5)." A conflict of interest involves the abuse of the trust that people have in research (5). A relationship based on trust is necessary with colleagues, the government, the study sponsors, and the public. A conflict of interest can damage an entire project which is why conflicts of interest are so serious (5).

As defined by Fishbach (Responsible Conduct of Research from Columbia University) a conflict of interest is a situation in which financial or other personal considerations have the potential to compromise (or bias) judgment and objectivity (11):

> "An apparent conflict of interest is one in which a reasonable person would think that the professionals judgment is likely to be compromised. A potential conflict of interest involves a situation that may develop into an actual conflict of interest. It is important to note that a conflict of interest exists whether or not decisions are affected by a personal interest; a conflict of interest implies only the potential for bias, not a likelihood. It is also important to note that a conflict of interest is not considered research misconduct since the definition for misconduct is currently limited to fabrication, falsification, and plagiarism (11)."

There are many varieties of conflicts of interest. They all involve the use of a person's authority for personal and/or financial gain. Conflicts of interest can involve individuals as well as institutions, and individuals may have conflicts on both an individual and an institutional level (6).

Other conflicts of interests include conflicts of commitment (effort, obligations) (6). A conflict of effort occurs when the time spent on an activity competes with the time expected to be spent on teaching, research, etc. (6). Some universities, for example, have policies allowing 20% of a faculty member's effort, or one day a week, for outside activity (11). Another type of conflict, conscience, occurs when personal beliefs influence objectivity. For example, a scientist may have a particular political or religious view that influences his or her view of the scientific merit of a study (11).

Conflicts of interest are divided into two categories, intangible - those involving academic activities and scholarship; and tangible - those involving financial relationships.

Intangible Conflicts of Interest - Academic/Intellectual

Bradley, et al. (7) state that "Academic scientists have special responsibilities to disseminate knowledge, maintain academic standards, critique the current state of knowledge, synthesize existing knowledge, and to apply this knowledge to solve problems

(7)." An academic conflict of interest can occur if an individual: interferes with the peer-review process; responds positively to a manuscript because it favors a method in which he/she has a personal interest; or acts to delay the publication of a competitor's manuscript in order to strengthen his or her own chances for publication or funding (7).

Blumenthal, et al., studied publication practices and found that not only are negative results less likely to be published but that even positive findings are withheld if it is perceived as advantageous for the authors (8). In one study, 20% of researchers reported delaying publication of results for their own advantage (8). These statistics indicate that the drive for recognition can be overwhelming, especially if a future position or livelihood depends on achievements (8).

Bias and loss of objectivity can not only damage the entire research study but can also lead to injury and harm to study participants (11). Two such examples in the history of research ethics include: The Tuskegee Study of Syphilis in the Negro Male (1932-1972); and the Willowbrook Hepatitis Studies (1963-1966) (9,10).

The Tuskegee Syphilis Study, conducted by the Public Health Service, enrolled hundreds of black males who were infected with syphilis. Despite published research indicating that penicillin was an acceptable treatment for syphilis, the researchers purposely withheld the antibiotic from their subjects. By the time the study was stopped in 1973, many men had become ill or died without being well informed of the risks and benefits of the study. Staten Island's Willowbrook State School for the Retarded conducted a study (1956 to 1972) using mentally retarded children as its subjects. Investigators infected these children with a hepatitis virus in order to document its effects on the body and its reactions to potential vaccines. The investigators in both studies were so caught up in the scientific aspects of their projects that they ignored the welfare of the participants in the study.

More recent headlines have called attention to conflicts of interest even at notable institutions such as the University of Pennsylvania (14), the Fred Hutchinson Cancer Center (15), and St. Elizabeth's Medical Center (16) in Boston. In these situations there were deaths attributed to the research.

Intangible conflicts of interest are problematic and pervasive throughout research, but tangible conflicts of interest may destroy the integrity of science itself (11).

Tangible Conflicts of Interest – Financial

Financial conflicts of interest are considered tangible because they can be seen and measured. While they appear easier to deal with than intangible conflicts of interest they are pervasive and difficult to interpret (11).

Since 1980 with the passage of the Bayh-Dole Act, there has been a change within the research community where commercialization of biomedical research has become accelerated. Research and development by pharmaceutical companies increased 24 fold in 25 years (1977 to 2002), and these companies alone spent more on research and development than the total 2002 NIH operating budget of $24 billion (18). The number of physicians involved in drug studies increased by 60% during a five-year span (17). In the same time period, the proportion of trials conducted in academic medical centers dropped from 80% to 40% (17).

Before 1980, the federal government retained the rights to research and discoveries of the investigators it funded. At the same time, biotech companies were having difficulty obtaining licenses to manufacture and market their discoveries, and the research enterprise was not thriving. Congress responded in 1980 by passing the Bayh-Dole Act which (12):

- Permits recipients of federal funds to obtain the title to inventions they develop and to transfer the technology to the private sector
- Requires federally funded researchers to obtain a patent for products developed in order to obtain commercial opportunities
- Requires federally funded researchers to report to the National Institutes of Health (NIH) on the use of their discoveries

The Bayh-Dole Act (12), in essence, removed the ban on academic entrepreneurship and allowed researchers to take an active role in the private applications of their research. This enabled researchers and universities to benefit significantly from the shared royalties. Ultimately, many universities have thrived on these relationships; "...among companies that sponsor academic research, 58% require their investigators to withhold results for more than six months to give them time to apply for a patent or to provide a lead over competitors..." (11). Potential or actual financial conflicts of interest are the unintended consequences of the Bayh-Dole Act.

On the other side of these financial conflicts of interest is the need for manufacturers to publish research and determine the safety and efficacy of their products. This reality means that they have to fund research, which in their defense, is a double edge sword. Manufacturers/companies are often criticized for not having evidenced-based support and/or criticized for funding the research that supports their products. As a result, it is important to not automatically discredit the research that is funded by the manufacturer, but to read with a healthy dose of skepticism, which is wise to do with most literature. In addition, these funding sources provide many academic institutions with financial resources to enhance the academic learning environment, such as purchasing lab equipment.

Another caveat with private funding, is that the contracts between the manufacturer and the researcher often have a clause that if the findings of the investigation are not favorable to the product the researcher is unable to publish or discuss those results.

Unfortunately, because of these conflict-of-interest the trust and morale standard is often compromised.

Scientists Behaving Badly

Scientists Behaving Badly was published in Nature (June, 2005). Martinson, et. al. surveyed several thousand scientists based in the United States and funded by the National Institutes of Health (NIH) and asked them to report their own behavior. Their findings revealed a range of very questionable practices. The result of this research suggests that "regular misbehaviors present greater threats to the scientific enterprise than those caused by high-profile misconduct cases such as fraud" (57). To assure anonymity, the survey responses were never linked to respondents' identities. Of the 3,600 surveys mailed to mid-career scientists, 3,409 were deliverable and 1,768 yielded usable data, giving a 52% response rate. Survey respondents were asked to report in each case whether or not ('yes' or 'no') they themselves had engaged in the specified behavior during the past three years. Overall, 33% of the respondents said they had engaged in at least one of the top ten misbehaviors during the previous three years. Among mid-career respondents, this proportion was 38%; in the early-career group, it was 28%. The research investigators believe that reliance on self reports actually underestimated the questionable behaviors despite assurances of anonymity. "It is now time for the scientific community to consider which aspects are most amenable to change, and what changes are likely to be the most fruitful in ensuring integrity in science," state the research authors (57)."

Federal Conflict-of-Interest Regulations

In 1985, responding to the change created by the Bayh-Dole Act, the US Public Health Service, which includes the NIH and the National Science Foundation (NSF), enacted regulations entitled *Responsibility of Applicants for Promoting Objectivity in Research* (19).

These regulations require institutions to establish standards and procedures that ensure that the design, conduct, or reporting of research is not biased by any conflicting financial interests of the investigator. The key components of these regulations include (19):

- The institution has the primary responsibility to develop its own internal policies and procedures. The institution is required to review disclosure of significant financial interest and manage conflicts of interest.
- Investigators are required to disclose significant financial interest to the institution.
- The institution is required to report to the federal funding agency if it believes significant financial interest could affect the research.
- "Investigators" are those individuals responsible for the design, conduct, or reporting of research, and the investigator's spouse and dependent children are included in the definition.

Many professional societies and associations have set up internal review boards (IRB) to develop policies to deal with the enacted federal regulations (11). However, many IRB members have equity interests in companies sponsoring studies that they are reviewing. Federal regulations require that members recuse themselves from voting on protocols if they or their families have any financial interests that could influence the deliberations on a protocol (11).

While disclosure is seen by many as the best means to manage conflicts of interest, there are others like Dr. Marcia Angell, Senior Lecturer of Social Medicine at Harvard Medical School, who believe that financial conflicts can never be managed (21). Dr. Angell states that, "clinical researchers must be able to design and conduct studies in an unbiased and objective manner that is free from conflicts caused by significant financial involvement with the commercial sponsors of the research. In this case, the only sure safeguard is for the investigator to have absolutely no financial relationships with entities that support his or her research." This approach has often been referred to as "zero tolerance (21)".

"*Significant* financial interest" as defined by *Responsibility of Applicants for Promoting Objectivity in Research* (19) is anything of monetary value that could include salary or payment for services from an <u>outside institution</u>, including equity (stock) interests, and any intellectual-property rights. Limits for equity interest for the investigator and his/her spouse and dependent children can not exceed $10,000 in value which does not represent more than 5% ownership in any single entity (19). In 1998, the FDA issued its final rule requiring disclosure by investigators of financial interests below $25,000, which is considered a more realistic and reasonable total (19). "*Significant* financial interest" does not include salary, royalties, or other remuneration from the investigator's <u>home institution</u>; or income from seminars, lectures, or teaching sponsored by public or nonprofit entities; or income from service on advisory committees or review panels for public or nonprofit entities (19).

Journals increasingly are requiring that authors list the companies that fund their research. Often, these lists are very long, indicating that researchers have many ties to industry. Concomitantly, investigators have concerns with privacy when having to disclose their financial relationships and these concerns may act as deterrents to disclosure. Some researchers are worried that preoccupation with financial conflicts of interest will have a negative effect on disclosure and will promote websites that act as "conflict-of-interest police" such as the Center for Science in the Public Interest – Integrity in Science - website (22).

The extent of these growing university-industry ties is "huge". Bekelman and his colleagues found that approximately two-thirds of academic institutions hold equity interests in start-up companies that sponsor research and that industry sponsorship is significantly associated with both pro-industry research conclusions and restrictions on publications and data sharing (23).

Managing Conflicts of Interest

It is clear that conflicts of interest are here to stay! Intangible and tangible conflicts of interest will always exist.

In 2012, Fang and colleagues published a detailed review of the 2,047 retracted biomedical and life-science research articles indexed by PubMed (26). Of the articles retracted, 67.4% of the restrictions were because of misconduct, which includes fraud or suspected fraud (43.3%), duplicate publications (14.2%) and plagiarism (9.8%), miscellaneous reasons or unknown causes accounted for the reminder (26). Even after the articles are retracted, it is common for these articles to still be referenced in other articles (26). This highlights the importance of always tracking down the primary source. As the investigators of this study point out, "given that most scientific work is publicly funded and that retractions because of misconduct undermine science and its impact on society, the surge of retractions suggests a need to reevaluate incentives driving this phenomenon (26)." The investigators also list possible solutions, which include: using checklists by authors and reviewers, improved training in logic, enhanced statistics, more focus on ethics, database for scientific misconduct, uniform guidelines for retractions, and a new reward system for science (26, 58).

Bekelman, et al. state that "most conflicts of interest created by academic-industry relationships are real, consequential, but tolerable, so long as they are managed to contain risks while preserving benefits. We must be vigilant against conflicts of interest that lead to bias and loss of objectivity. The enterprise of research depends on it (23)."

Critical Analysis of Current Research

This section will look at each of the major classifications of research design. Given the current research environment and the difficulty of managing conflicts of interest it is vitally important for all professionals (and consumers) to be able to critically analyze research to determine if the results are valid and reproduced in an "unbiased" manner. Findings are considered preliminary until other scientists confirm or disprove them through other studies (replication). The findings are not accepted by the research community until they are replicated many times by other researchers from different institutions.

Study Design

The two major types of study designs are descriptive and analytical (28,29). The following table summarizes the different types of descriptive studies and outlines the limitations associated with each type of study.

Descriptive	Definition	Example	Limitations
Descriptive: Correlational	General characteristics (exposures) with a disease in whole populations	Per capita consumption of meat and increased rates of colon cancer in women	Used to form a hypothesis; no way of knowing if results relate to individuals or other determinants in meat
Descriptive: Case Studies	Characteristics of individuals with a disease	Five young homosexual men with pneumonia previously seen only in older people	Indicates an association but no evidence concerning cause
Descriptive: Cross Sectional	Frequency of disease in individuals compared to age, gender, socioeconomic and lifestyle variables	Health Interview Survey periodically collects info from 100,000 US people and disease frequency is calculated. Low levels beta-carotene associated with cancer	Does not provide information on whether or not the exposure (low beta-carotene) was related to the cause of the disease (cancer)

Descriptive Studies

Descriptive studies are concerned with describing general characteristics of associations with a disease (smoking and lung cancer). *Descriptive* studies focus on whole populations or individuals (28,29).

- Correlational descriptive studies (also known as population studies) refer to associations of whole populations (28,29). Correlation should not infer cause and effect. For example, humans have toe nails, finger nails, and die.

Inferring cause and effect would suggest that finger nails and toe nails kill. Absurd, yes. But many individuals in the media and in science are making such "absurd" leaps. Another example of such a leap was a correlational descriptive study suggested a link between meat consumption and colon cancer (31). When looking at large populations of women in different countries and meat consumption, this study found a direct relationship between meat consumption and increased risk for colon cancer in women. Correlational studies are useful in formulating a hypothesis but are limited because they only look at population averages. There is no way of knowing if women who develop colon cancer even eat meat. People with high meat consumptions may also have diets high in saturated fat or low in fiber which can be a contributing factor for the increased rate of disease.

- Descriptive case reports and case series *describe* characteristics of one or a number of individuals with a given disease. For example, in 1980 five young, previously healthy homosexual men were diagnosed with a type of pneumonia seen only in older men and women whose immune systems were suppressed (32). This unusual circumstance suggested that these individuals suffered from an unknown disease (now known as AIDS). This type of study design indicates an association, but there is no indication of cause.
- The cross sectional survey is a third type of *descriptive* study. Individuals are asked to complete surveys with respect to personal and demographic characteristics. The frequency of diseases is then compared to age, gender, socioeconomic, and lifestyle variables. For example, individuals with cancer often have lower serum beta-carotene levels than healthy individuals of the same age and gender(41). However, there is no way of knowing if the low beta-carotene levels are due to the cancer or to the dietary changes associated with the debilitating effects of the disease.

The following table summarizes the different types of analytical studies and outlines the limitations associated with each of these designs.

Analytical	**Definition**	**Example**	**Limitations**
Analytical: Observational (case control)	Group with the disease (case) under study are compared to group without the disease (control)	Bladder cancer and artificial sweeteners. One group with bladder cancer compared to a group without the disease with respect to artificial sweeteners	Does not provide information as to whether the variable (artificial sweeteners) was responsible for the cancer
Analytical: Observational (cohort)	Study groups are classified on presence or absence of exposure and followed to	See below	See below

Analytical	Definition	Example	Limitations
	determine development of disease		
Analytical: Observational (cohort - retrospective)	Looks back in time at people who were diagnosed with a disease and people not diagnosed. The 2 groups are compared as to what they ate before diagnosis.	Study links caffeine to pancreatic cancer. Individuals with pancreatic cancer and individuals without the cancer are asked questions about caffeine intake and results are compared	Indicates association but includes recall bias and contains confounding variables (not the caffeine but other chemicals in coffee or coffee drinkers may not eat fruits and vegetables)
Analytical: Observational (cohort - prospective)	Data is collected on a large group of people for an extended period of time and disease frequency is determined	Honolulu-Asia Aging Study. Asian men followed for five years. Tofu associated with premature aging of the brain	Associations may be due to other factors. Men who ate the most tofu came from poorer families which may have affected brain function
Analytical: Clinical Trials	Researchers randomly assign large groups of people without a specific disease to either a treatment or a control group	HERS. Trial indicated that 4 years of hormone replacement therapy did not reduce risk of heart disease in women.	Results do not indicate underlying cause. Was it the design of the study or are there no "heart" benefits of hormone replacement therapy

Analytical Studies

Analytical studies differ from descriptive studies in that the comparison is explicit; i.e., the investigator assembles groups of individuals for the specific purpose of systematically determining whether or not the risk of disease is different for individuals exposed or not exposed to the factor of interest (28,29). Analytical studies are classified as observational or intervention studies (clinical trials).

Analytical observational studies include case-control studies or cohort studies (retrospective or prospective studies) (28,29).

- In a case-control study, a group who has a certain disease is compared to a group without the disease. For example, participants in a study examining the effects of artificial sweeteners and cancer were interviewed to obtain information on their history of consumption of foods with artificial sweeteners (34,35) One group consisted of people without cancer, and the other consisted of hospitalized patients with cancer (34). The investigators found a similar proportion of individuals who had used artificial sweeteners among both groups.
- In an analytical cohort study, groups of individuals are classified on the basis of the presence or absence of exposure and then followed for a specified period of time to determine the development of the disease (28,29). These studies can be retrospective or prospective in

nature.

- A retrospective analytical cohort study looks back in time. It involves contacting people who were recently diagnosed with a disease (pancreatic cancer) and similar people who were not diagnosed with the same disease. Both groups are asked questions concerning the exposure (caffeine) (33). Some studies may collect blood samples or other information about possible causes of the disease. Scientists then analyze the data to see if individuals with the disease ate differently than the group without the disease with respect to the exposure (33). Retrospective studies are the only way to study rare diseases since they do not require a lot of people or a long period of time (28,29). These studies are able to focus on a specific disease and food or lifestyle that may affect the disease; *they are a first step in establishing a relationship between a certain disease and a food or chemical.* Examples of headlines from such studies are: "Study links caffeine to increased pancreatic cancer" (33); or "Study links use of aspartame to brain tumors (35)." Retrospective studies can be inaccurate and may contain confounding variables (other variables that may be responsible for the observed effect). Known confounding variables can be adjusted for. In the above example of caffeine and pancreatic cancer, smoking is a known confounding variable; i.e., a larger percentage of coffee drinkers smoke, hence smoking must be controlled for in the study design. There may be unknown variables that produced the increased incidence of cancer, not the caffeine (coffee drinkers may not eat as many fruits and vegetables). Another serious flaw with this type of design is that it is difficult to establish what people ate in previous years and there is a potential for what is known as recall bias in which people with a diagnosed disease are more apt to investigate their disease and may report differently than people without the disease (28,29).
- A prospective analytical cohort study is one in which data is collected on a large group of people for an extended time period, and disease frequency is determined. Examples of prospective studies include: The Nurses Health Study (36,37) which began in 1977 and includes over 120,000 female nurses; the Framingham Heart Study which is now in its third generation and began with 6,000 men and women (38). In this type of study, there is no recall bias because data is collected before the disease develops. Individuals are asked questions concerning their present habits; hence, the data is apt to be more

accurate. Data can be collected periodically, and more than one disease can be studied (36). However, associations may be due to confounding factors. Hence, results from this type of study must be viewed as preliminary.

Analytical clinical trials randomly assign hundreds or thousands of people without a specific disease to either a treatment group or a control group (27).

- Double-blind clinical trials are designed to test the effect of a substance by using experimental and control groups in which neither the subjects nor the investigators know which treatment or substance is being administered to which group (27). The purpose of a double-blind study is to eliminate the risk of bias by researchers and the participants which could distort the results. A double-blind study may be augmented by a cross-over experiment, in which experimental subjects unknowingly become control subjects, and vice versa (27). The groups are followed for several years, and the disease rate in each group is compared. In this type of study, the researchers decide how much of the nutrient will be given to the treatment group versus the control group, which ensures that there is a sizable difference between the groups. There is no confounding because a trial randomly assigns people to one group.
- Clinical trials take into account the "placebo effect". Placebo effect is the measurable, observable, or felt improvement in health not attributable to treatment (39,40). Some believe the placebo effect is psychological, due to a belief in the treatment, or to a subjective feeling of improvement. In other words, if people believe a product will work, there is a distinct possibility that it will. For over 500 Danish physicians who responded to a questionnaire, placebo use was as high as 86% among general practitioners, 54% among hospital-based physicians, and 41% among private specialists (41). In Chicago, 45% of 231 internists admitted to using placebo (44). Dr. Irving Kirsch, a psychologist at the University of Connecticut, analyzed 39 studies (between 1974 and 1995) of depressed patients treated with drugs, psychotherapy, or a combination of both. He found that 50% of the drug effect is due to the placebo response (39). When placebos were given for pain management, the pain relief followed the same path as an active drug. The peak relief came about an hour after administration for both the placebo and drug (40). Hence, in scientific research the placebo effect must be controlled for if the results are to be attributed to the study hypothesis. These studies are relatively easy to interpret.

The limitations associated with clinical trials are that they are expensive to conduct, and if the trial fails, it's hard to know why. Was it the dose, the population studied, the trial period, or the sample size? In a 1996 trial, researchers reported unexpected findings when increased lung cancer risk was found in the beta-carotene group versus the control group (41). Beta-carotene was chosen because results from observational studies indicated that people who ate more carotene-rich fruits and vegetables had a lower risk of lung cancer. It is not known why this specific trial produced such unexpected results. Perhaps it is something else in beta-carotene rich foods that prevent cancer (41)!

Questions to be Answered

Below are points for all professionals and consumers alike to consider when analyzing research (51-53):

1. Study elements. Each element of a study should be examined (51). Do the research author's qualifications include a degree of knowledge in nutrition? Is the research well written, and does the abstract offer a clear overview including the research problem, sample size, methodology, duration, findings, and recommendations? Is the target population clearly defined? Do the researchers provide a review of previous literature, or is the research based on a new hypothesis? Did the researchers observe the results themselves, or did they rely on self reports from program participants? Did the results indicate statistically significant findings? Are the findings linked back to the literature review? Was the hypothesis supported or null/void? Also, the study must begin with unbiased assumptions, populations, etc.
2. Study design. What is the study design, and what are the limitations associated with the type of study? The limitations of the study should be described in the discussion section of the study.
3. Peer-review. The scientific study under discussion should be published in a peer-reviewed journal. Peer review refers to the process by which the editors of a journal ask experts in a study's subject to review the study to ensure it was conducted appropriately. If the study was poorly designed or comes up short, it is usually not published. Studies that come from less trustworthy sources (such as non peer-reviewed journals or websites) should be questioned. However, peer-review is not a guarantee that the research is unbiased as discussed in the section on conflicts of interest. The scientific peer review process is an attempt to supply quality scientific research through the evaluation by qualified experts of research findings for competence, significance, and originality and to reduce the

dissemination of misinformation and confusion (61-63). While the peer review process is widely accepted and the standard in the research community, criticisms continue and include the presence of bias, inability to detect major flaws, unnecessary delays in publications, and inability to uncover misconduct (61). It is important to recognize that the peer review process cannot ensure that an article is truthful; it can only claim that it is worth publishing (61, 64). While there are difficulties and flaws with the method, a review process is necessary in attempt to limit fraudulent studies and maintain a level of professional standard for work that has been properly scrutinized by experts (61). Consequently, the process needs to be continuously evaluated and adapted to the changing environment (61).

4. Previous research. Credible research disseminates new findings in the context of previous research. A single study on its own provides limited information, but if a body of literature supports a finding, it increases confidence in the findings.
5. Are there conflicts of interest? Who paid for the study? Was the study funded by the same company that sells the product being touted as a new life saving discovery?
6. Control group. To obtain reliable data, the study should be a controlled, double blind study in which the subjects (and persons actually involved in distributing the product) are not informed as to whether they are given the actual product being tested or a placebo. Without a control group, there is no way of knowing if the product is actually producing the wanted results or if other variables within the group caused the wanted results.
7. Statistical analysis. For someone without a strong statistical background, it can be very difficult to understand and interpret the statistical reporting in research. However, when statistical significance is reported, it is vital to be able to examine the analysis even closer. While it is the responsibility of the investigators and review board to determine if the appropriate analysis was used and reported, we cannot always rely on all of the results to be reported. We must ask the questions, "are the differences big enough to have real meaning", "is there practical significance?" For example, when statistical significance is reported, it is important that the effect size is reported. The definition of effect size is an objective and standardized measure of the magnitude of the observed effect (59). The effect size is vital in expressing the importance of the research finding and is intrinsically linked to sample size, probability level and statistical power (ability of a test to detect an effect of a particular size/field). An in depth review of statistics is well beyond the scope of this text. Fortunately, there are many great resources available. One excellent resource for more information on statistics is Dr. Will Hopkins' Sports Science site: http://www.sportsci.org/. While the site

primarily uses examples from exercise and sport science, the principles apply to all empirical sciences.

8. Applicability. Does the research make sense? For example, even if coffee does adversely affect the nervous system, do you drink enough of it to see any negative effects?
9. Research or news! Remember, if a headline professes a new remedy for a nutrition-related topic, it may well be a research based piece of news, but more often than not, it is designed to catch the attention of an unsuspecting consumer. Find the original journal article to see if it really supports the conclusions being drawn in the news report.
10. Population groups. Even when the research is well designed, duplicated, and safety issues have been answered, the results are typically applicable to one group. Were the subjects men or women; athletes, or sedentary individuals; were they healthy individuals, or individuals with diseases such as diabetes, cancer, or HIV? Results should never be "extrapolated" to include other groups.

In 2005, Dr. John Ioannidis, currently a professor of medicine and statistics at Stanford University, wrote an excellent article published in PloS Medicine discussing why most published research findings are false (65). In the essay, Dr. Ioannidis discusses that there is an increasing concern that most current published research findings are false, and the probability that a research finding is true may depend on the study's power, bias, number of other studies on the same question, and the ratio of true to no relationships among the variables researched in a given area of study (65). The essay goes on to identify six corollaries that make a research finding less likely or more likely to be true. A research finding is more likely to be true if:

1. Large studies, like randomized controlled trials with large sample sizes, were completed.
2. The findings are supported by large effect sizes.
3. There are subsequent studies that confirm the findings.
4. A strict adherence to a standardized approach to conducting and reporting, this also applies when the outcomes are straightforward (death vs. scales); more diversity among the designs, definitions, outcomes and analytical modes increases the likelihood that the finds are not true,
5. There is no financial, other interest or prejudices.
6. The area of research is not "hot"; this concept is often describe as the Proetus phenomenon, which is the fast sequential research that provides extreme alternating research claims and opposite refutations (65, 66). As readers, the assumptions about biases are subjective but useful in interpreting the results and keeping the findings in context (65). Scientific research is a noble and difficult pursuit, and by recognizing the limitations, we avoid undermining the "research

enterprise" (67).

The Victoria Transport Policy Institute provides an easy to read guideline for evaluating research quality: http://www.vtpi.org/resqual.pdf.

When researching nutrition information on websites consider the following criteria for discerning if the site is valid (54):

1. Use multiple sites, especially government sites, such as the Centers for Disease Control and Prevention (www.cdc.gov) and the Food and Drug Administration (www.fda.gov), as well as the sites of nationally recognized nutrition- or health-related associations such as the Academy of Nutrition and Dietetics (www.eatright.org) and American Heart Association (www.americanheart.org). It is important to note that these organizations are not without bias and conflict of interest. For example, the Academy of Nutrition and Dietetics, the world's largest organization for food and nutrition professionals, has corporate sponsorships from Abbott Nutrition, The Coca-Cola Company, National Diary Council, General Mills, Kellogg Company, McCormick, Pepsico, SOYJOY, Truvia, and Unilever (60).
2. Rely primarily on sites that are managed or reviewed by a group of qualified health professionals. "Blogs" might be fun but are not necessarily reliable.
3. Look for the Health on the Net symbol at the bottom of the main page of the website. The Health on the Net Foundation is a nonprofit, international organization that promotes the HONcode, a set of principles for standardizing the reliability of health information on the Internet. Currently, website sponsors are not required to follow HONcode standards. For more information about HONcode, you can visit the organization's website (www.hon.ch/).
4. Do not trust information at a site that does not indicate valid sources, such as well respected peer-reviewed scientific journals or nationally-recognized universities or medical centers. Contributing authors and their credentials should be identified; when they are, perform an online search of the scientific journals, as well as the authors' names and credentials, to determine their validity.
5. Do not trust a site that includes attacks on the trustworthiness of the medical or scientific establishment.
6. Avoid sites that provide online diagnoses and treatments. Be wary of commercial sites (.com) with links to government sites or the sites of well-known medical, nutrition, or scientific associations. An unreliable site can be linked to reliable sites without having received their endorsements.
7. Avoid providing your personal information at the site because its confidentiality may not be protected.

The following table summarizes several studies using the above techniques.

Research	Poortmans J. (ref # 47) Long term oral creatine consumption/ renal function	Westman E, et al. (ref #48) Effect of 6 month adherence to low-carb diet	Nieman DC, et al. (ref #49) New handhed device for measuging RMR	Utter A, et al. (ref # 50) Evaluation of air displacement for assessing body composition	Watzl B, et al. (ref #55) Fruit and vegetable concentrate lowers homocysteine in men
Study Design	Descriptive	Descriptive	Descriptive	Descriptive	Descriptive
Design Details	Eight men and 1 woman self reporting of creatine ingestion for one to five years	Fifty-one individuals on low-carbohydrate diet with no caloric restrictions	RMR measured in 63 subjects, ages 21 to 69, using the Body Gem	Body composition measured using Bod Pod and compared to hydrostatic weighing	Concentration of homocysteine measured in 32 men
Peer-Review	Yes – Medicine in Science & Sports (ACSM Journal)	Yes – American Journal of Medicine	Yes – Journal of the Academy of Nutrition and Dietetics	Yes – Medicine in Science & Sports (ACSM Journal)	Yes – Human Nutrition and Metabolism (makers of study capsules blew the whistle) independent, non-biased research has been done
Limitations	Small sample; self reporting; only one measure of renal function	Self reported; physical activity uncontrolled; modest results could be contributed to exercise	Body Gem was compared to Douglas Bag; no other measurements were included	Hydrostatic weighing has a large margin of error.	Concentration used was "enriched" with beta-carotene, ascorbic acid, vitamin E and folic acid"
Conflicts of Interest	Unknown	Unlimited grant by Atkins group to Duke Univ; Atkins group trained research staff	Research paid for by makers of Body Gem	Research paid for by makers of Bod Pod	Research paid for makers of Juice Plus
Control	Yes – 85 sedentary males (self reported)	No	No	No	No
Results /Applicability	No renal damage reported	Individuals lost modest amount of weight; on average 1500 calories and were eaten; participants were given an	No differences found in RMR between Douglas Bag and Body Gem	Bod Pod produced similar results to hydrostatic weighing	Plasma homocysteine was reduced

		appetite suppressant			
Replication	Other small, similar design studies	Other similar design studies	No independent, non-biased research has been done	No independent, non-biased research has been done	No independent, non-biased research has been done

In the first example researchers looked at the effects of oral creatine supplementation in young healthy athletes (47). The sample size was small. Eight men and 1 woman were recruited and asked how often, how much, and how long they had been ingesting creatine. The amount of reported intake ranged from one to eighty grams per day. One person reported taking creatine for 5 years, but the article does not indicate how much creatine that person consumed. The results indicate that there were no detrimental effects of creatine supplementation. This study, published in the ACSM journal is of such poor quality and design one has to wonder how it was approved by ten peer-reviewers.

Adherence to a low carb diet in the next example shows how research can be not only funded by a for-profit organization but also implemented by the organization (48). The research for this project was funded by an unlimited grant from the Atkins Group and Duke University staff members were actually trained by the Atkins Group. Participants in this research project were given an appetite suppressant and added nutrients known to reduce cholesterol levels, biasing the results.

The next two examples describe research completed at the university level examining the accuracy of newly developed equipment by several manufacturers (49,50). In the first example, resting metabolic rate was measured in 63 men using a hand held device called the Body Gem (49). Results indicated that the Body Gem was as accurate as the Douglas Bag method. In the second example, body composition was measured in 66 NCAA Division 1 college wrestlers using the Bod Pod (50). Results indicated that the Bod Pod was as accurate as hydrostatic weighing. One has to ask, "are these devices really as accurate as the results claim"? Typically, confidence levels are low when the group that manufacturers the product also evaluates it!

The final example provides details of a research project in which the product being tested was not the product being used in the research. German manufacturers of the research product "blew the whistle" on the research authors by publishing a letter to the editor of Human Nutrition and Metabolism indicating that the study product was "enriched" (51).

As these examples indicate, peer-reviewed research, even at the university level, is suspect in today's research environment. Professionals have an obligation to critically evaluate all research before reporting or accepting the results.

Reputable Resources

Below is a list of nutrition sources that can be trusted to provide minimally biased research and also addresses conflicts of interest (11):

- US Department of Agriculture Food and Nutrition Information Center. The USDA site http://fnic.nal.usda.gov has more than twenty-five hundred links to dietary, nutrition, diet and disease, weight and obesity, food-safety and food-labeling, packaging, dietary supplement, and consumer question sites. Using this interactive site, you can find tips and resources on how to eat a healthy diet and a food planner, among other sections.

1. The Academy of Nutrition and Dietetics (AND). The AND promotes scientific evidenced-based, research-supported food and nutrition information on its website, http://www.eatright.org. It is focused on informing the public about recent scientific discoveries and studies, weight-loss concerns, food safety topics, nutrition issues, and disease prevention.
2. Department of Health and Human Services. The HHS website, HealthFinder.gov, provides credible information about healthful lifestyles and the latest in health news. A variety of online tools assist with food-planning, weight maintenance, physical activity, and dietary goals. You can also find healthful tips for all age groups, tips for preventing disease, and on daily health issues in general.
3. Centers for Disease Control and Prevention. The Centers for Disease Control and Prevention (http://www.cdc.gov) distributes an online newsletter called *CDC Vital Signs*. This newsletter is a valid and credible source for up-to-date public health information and data regarding food, nutrition, cholesterol, high blood pressure, obesity, teenage drinking, and tobacco usage.
4. Dietitians of Canada. Dietitians of Canada, http://www.dietitians.ca/, is the national professional association for dietitians. It provides trusted nutrition information to Canadians and health professionals.
5. Health Canada. Health Canada, http://www.hc-sc.gc.ca/index-eng.php, is the Federal department that helps Canadians improve their health. Its website also provides information about health-related legislation.
6. Universities. Several universities have excellent health letters that may be accessed on line. These health letters summarize the latest nutrition data. In most instances these universities, along with Center for Science in the Public Interest, agree on the latest nutrition research findings. It is this "consensus", along with multiple research studies indicated similar results which provides credence to the reported results. As evidence accumulates, scientists begin to integrate the findings which then become accepted among the nutrition

community. Over the years, the picture of what is "true" gradually changes, and dietary recommendations are then reviewed and changed.

7. Associations. Associations such as the American Heart Association, the American Cancer Society, and the American Diabetes Society have helpful information for populations with these diseases. American College of Sport Medicine and National Strength and Conditioning Association have helpful information on sports nutrition.
8. Medline/PubMed Resources Guide: An excellent place to start a search for peer-reviewed literature.
9. Google Scholar: Provides for a literature search across many disciplines and includes theses, books, abstracts, and articles.

Summary

While many professionals are involved in research, many more read the results of research and apply it to the real world. Therefore, it is vitally important to be able to critically analyze research to determine if the methods and results are valid. When conducting research, scientists follow what is known as the "scientific method". Bias is defined as any tendency which prevents unprejudiced consideration of a question. The scientific method minimizes bias.

A conflict of interest involves the abuse of the trust that people have in research. A relationship based on trust is necessary with colleagues, the government, the study sponsors, and the public. A conflict of interest can damage an entire project which is why conflicts of interest are so serious.

A conflict of interest is a situation in which financial or other personal considerations have the potential to compromise (or bias) judgment and objectivity. Conflicts of interest are divided into two categories: intangible - those involving academic activities and scholarship; and tangible - those involving financial relationships. An academic conflict of interest can occur if an individual: interferes with the peer-review process; responds positively to a manuscript because it favors a method in which he/she has a personal interest; or acts to delay the publication of a competitor's manuscript in order to strengthen his or her own chances for publication or funding. Financial conflicts of interest are considered tangible because they can be seen and measured. While they appear easier to deal with than intangible conflicts of interest they are pervasive and difficult to interpret. Since 1980 (with the passage of the Bayh-Dole Act), there has been a change within the research community where commercialization of biomedical research has become accelerated. Research and development by pharmaceutical companies increased 24 fold in 25 years (1977 to 2002), and these companies alone spent more on R. & D. than the total 2002 NIH operating budget of $24 billion. "The number of private practice physicians involved in drug studies increased by 60% over a five-year span. Conversely, the proportion of trials conducted in academic medical centers dropped from 80% to 40% over the same time period." In 1985, responding to the change created by the Bayh-Dole Act, the US Public Health Service, which includes the NIH and the National Science Foundation (NSF) enacted regulations entitled *Responsibility of Applicants for Promoting Objectivity in Research*. These regulations require institutions to establish standards and procedures that ensure that the design, conduct, or reporting of research is not biased by any conflicting financial interests of the investigator.

It is clear that conflicts of interest are here to stay! Intangible and tangible conflicts of interest will always exist. A detailed review of 2,047 biomedical and life-science research articles indexed by PubMed revealed that only 21.3% of retractions were attributable to error. In contrast, 67.4% of retractions were attributed to misconduct; including 43.4% from fraud or suspected fraud; 14.4% due to duplicate publication; and 9.8% were attributed to plagiarism. Bekelman, et al. State that "most conflicts of interest created by academic-industry relationships are real, consequential, but tolerable, so long as they are managed to contain risks while preserving benefits. We must be vigilant against conflicts of interest that lead to bias and loss of objectivity. The enterprise of research depends on it".

Given the current research environment and the difficulty of managing conflicts of interest it is vitally important for all professionals (and consumers) to be able to critically analyze research to determine if the results are valid and reproduced in an "unbiased" manor. Findings are considered preliminary until other scientists confirm or disprove them through other studies (replication). The findings are not accepted by the research community until they are replicated many times by other researchers from different institutions. The two major types of study designs are descriptive and analytical. *Descriptive* studies are concerned with describing general characteristics of associations with a disease (smoking and lung cancer). *Descriptive* studies focus on whole populations or individuals. *Analytical* studies differ from descriptive studies in that the comparison is explicit; i.e. the investigator assembles groups of individuals for the specific purpose of systematically determining whether or not the risk of disease is different for individuals exposed or not exposed to the factor of interest. Double-blind clinical trials are designed to test the effect of a substance by using experimental and control groups in which neither the subjects nor the investigators know which treatment or substance is being administered to which group. The purpose of a double-blind study is to eliminate the risk of bias by researchers and the participants which could distort the results. A double-blind study may be augmented by a cross-over experiment, in which experimental subjects unknowingly become control subjects, and vice versa.

Points for all professionals and consumers alike to consider when analyzing research include: Study elements - each element of a study should be examined; What is the study design and what are the limitations associated with the type of study; is the journal peer-reviewed; is there previous research supporting the evidence; what is the extent of bias and conflicts of interest; is there a control group and which groups are included (applicability); is it research or news? Several examples using these techniques are available in table form in this chapter. Reputable resources are also available in this chapter.

Chapter 10 Sample Test

1. What is the scientific method? Discuss its applicability in today's current research environment.
2. What does conflict of interest refer to? What are the two types of conflicts of interest; and what impact does conflicts of interest have on research in today's environment?
3. Define the Bayh-Dole act, and describe how it changed federally sponsored research.
4. List the steps involved in critical analysis of research, and provide examples.
5. List reputable resources for obtaining sound, scientific, minimally biased research.
6. Analyze a recent research paper using the steps involved in critical analysis.

References

1. Newton. (1999). Rules for the study of natural philosophy. Newton Book 3, *The System of the World*. pp.794–6,
2. Dictionary.com; http://dictionary.reference.com/browse/bias. (accessed 07/06/2013).
3. Merriam-Webster.com; http://www.merriam-webster.com/dictionary/bias. (accessed 07/06/2013).
4. Gerhard T. (2008). Bias: Considerations for research practice. *Am. J. Health. Syst. Pharm.* 2008;65:2159–2168.
5. American Society of Gene Therapy. (2000). Policy of The American Society of Gene Therapy on Financial Conflict of Interest in Clinical Research. Retrieved 2003 May 28 from http://www.asgt.org.
6. Bradley SG. (2000). Managing Conflicting Interests, p. 136. In: Magrina FL, editor. Scientific Integrity: An Introductory Text with Cases. Washington, DC: American Society for Microbiology.
7. Bradley SG. (2000). Managing Conflicting Interests, p. 144. In: Magrina FL, editor. Scientific Integrity: An Introductory Text with Cases. Washington, DC: American Society for Microbiology; 2000, pp. 131-157.
8. Blumenthal D. Campbell E. Anderson M. Causino N. Louis K. (1997). Withholding Research Results in Academic Life Science. Evidence from a National Survey of Faculty [Comment]. *JAMA.* 277(15): 1224-1228.
9. Tuskegee Study of Untreated Syphilis in the Negro Male. Tuskegee Study - Timeline". *NCHHSTP*. CDC. 2008-06-25. (accessed 07/16/2013).
10. Hevesi, Dennis. (2010). Robert W. McCollum, Dean of Dartmouth Medical School, Dies at 85. *The New York Times.*The took these kids and took blood samples from them and simply injected the diseases into their bodies. (accessed 07/06/2013).
11. Fishbach R. Plaza J. (2004). Columbia Center for New Media Teaching & Learning (CCNMTL) Responsible Conduct of Research. Columbia University. http://ccnmtl.columbia.edu/projects/rcr/rcr_conflicts/foundation/index.html. (accessed 07/03/2013).
12. Indiana University Libraries. The Bayh-Dole Act of 1980 Digital Collections. Last updated: 9/19/2011. ast updated: 9/19/2011. (accessed 07/02/2013).
13. Fanelli D (2009) How Many Scientists Fabricate and Falsify Research? A Systematic Review and Meta-Analysis of Survey Data. *PLoS ONE* 4(5): e5738. doi:10.1371/journal.pone. 0005738.
14. Sanders E. (2003). Researcher Wilson to Step Down as IHGT Head. The Daily Pennsylvanian. http://ccnmtl.columbia.edu/projects/rcr/rcr_conflicts/misc/Ref/UPENN_IHGT.pdf (accessed 07/06/2013).
15. Uninformed Consent: What patients at "The Hutch" weren't told about the experiments in which they died. Seattle Times, Local News, Sunday, March 11, 2001.
16. Hilts PJ. (2000). A Second Death Linked to Gene Therapy. *The New York Times on the Web.* May 4, 2000; Science.
17. Nelson DK. (2002). Conflict of Interest: Researchers in Amdur and Bankert ed. *Institutional Review Board: Management and Function*: Sudbury, MA. pp.197-203.
18. Bodenheimer T. (2000). Uneasy Alliance -- Clinical Investigators and the Pharmaceutical Industry. *N Engl J Med.* 342(20): 1539-1544.
19. Objectivity in Research. *NIH Guide*, Volume 24, Number 25, July 14, 1995.
20. Government Printing Office. (1999). Title 21 Food and Drug. http://www.gpo.gov/fdsys/pkg/CFR-1999-title21-vol1/content-detail.html.
21. Angell M. (2000). Is Academic Medicine for Sale? *N Engl J Med.* 342(20): 1516 – 1518.

22. Integrity in Science Database. Monitoring, exposing and opposing conflicts. http://www.cspinet.org/integrity/ (accessed 07/06/2013).
23. Bekelman JE, Li Y. (2003). Scope and Impact of Financial Conflicts of Interest in Biomedical Research. *JAMA.* 289(4): 454-465.
24. Blumenthal D. (1996). Ethics issues in academic-industry relationships in the life sciences: the continuing debate. *Acad Med.* 71(12):1287-90.
25. Zimmerman M. SnowB. (2012). Essentials of nutrition: A functional approach. Creative Commons. http://2012books.lardbucket.org/books/essentials-of-nutrition-a-functional-approach/index.html.
26. Fang, F. Steen R. Casadevall A. (2012). Misconduct accounts for the majority of retracted scientific publications. *PNAS.* doi: 10.1073/pnas.1212247109.
27. Double-bind study. Medical Dictionary. Farlex. http://medical-dictionary.thefreedictionary.com/double-blind+study (accessed 07/06/2013.
28. Blair RC. & Taylor, RA (2008). *Biostatistics for the health sciences (1st ed.).* Upper Saddle River, NJ: Pearson Prentice Hall.
29. Forthofer, R. N., Lee, E. S., & Hernandez, M. (2007). *Biostatistics: A guide to design, analysis, and discovery (2nd ed.).* Amsterdam: Elsevier Academic Press.
30. Hennekins CH, Buring JE. 1987. *Epidemiology in Medicine*. Boston,MA: Little, Brown and Company.
31. Armstrong BK, et al. 1975. Environment factors and cancer incidence and mortality in different countries. *Int J Cancer*,15:617.
32. Center for Disease Control. 1981. *Pneumocystic* pneumonia—Los Angeles. *M.M.W.R.*,30:250.
33. LaVecchiaC ,et al. 1987. Coffee consumption and risk of pancreatic cancer. *Int J Cancer,*40(3);309- 13.
34. Bosetti C, et al. (2009). Artificial sweeteners and the risk of gastric, pancreatic, and endometrial cancers in Italy. *Cancer Epidemiol Biomarkers Prev*. (8):2235-8. doi: 10.1158/1055-9965.EPI-09-0365.
35. Gurney JG, et al. 1997. Aspartame consumption in relation to childhood brain tumor risk. *J Natl Cancer Inst*,89(14):1072-4.
36. The Nurses' Health Study. http://www.channing.harvard.edu/nhs/. (accessed 07/06/2013).
37. Hennekens CH, et al. (1979). Use of permanent hair dyes and cancer among registered nurses. *Lancet.* 1390-93.
38. Framingham Heart Study. http://www.framinghamheartstudy.org/. (accessed 07/06/2013).
39. Kirsh, I, Sapirstein, G. Listening to Prosac but hearing placebo: A meta-analysis of antidepressant medication. Prevention & Treatment. Vol 1, June 1998.
40. Talbot, M. The Placebo Prescription. New York Times Magazine, January 9, 2000.
41. Hróbjartsson A, Norup M. The use of placebo interventions in medical practice-a national questionnaire survey of Danish clinicians. Eval Health Prof. 2003;26(2):153–65.
42. Prior A, et al. 2000. Beta carotene: from biochemistry to clinical trials. Nutrition Review, 58(2pt1):39-53 Review.
43. The Writing Group for the PEPI Trial. 1995. Effects of estrogen or estrogen/progestin regimens on heart disease risk factors in postmenopausal women. The Postmenopausal Estrogen/Progestin Interventions (PEPI) Trial. *JAMA*,273(3):199-208.
44. Sherman R, Hickner J. Academic physicians use placebos in clinical practice and believe in the mind-body connection. J Gen Intern Med. 2008;23(1):7–10. [PMC free article] [PubMed]
45. Grostein, F, et al. 1997. Postmenopausal hormone therapy and mortality. New Eng J of Med, 336(25)1769-75.
46. Reader M. O'Connell B, et.al. (2002). Glycemic and insulinemic response of subjects with type 2 diabetes after consumption of three energy bars. *Journal of the ADA*. Vol 102,8:1139.

47. Poortmans JM, et al. (1999). Long-term oral creatine supplementation does not impair renal function in healthy athletes. Med & Sci in Sports & Exercise. 0195-993108-1108.
48. Westman E. Yancy W, et.al. (2002). Effect of 6-month adherence to a very low carbohydrate diet program. *Am. J Med.* 113:30-36.
49. Nieman DC, et al. (2003). A handheld device for measuring resting metabolic rate and oxygen consumption. (2003). *J Amer Diet Assoc.* 103(5):588-592.
50. Utter A. Gross F, et al. (2003).Evaluation of Air Displacement for Assessing Body Composition of Collegiate Wrestlers. *Medicine & Science in Sports & Exercise.* 35(3):500-505.
51. Coughlan M. Cronin P. Ryan F. (2007). Step by step guide to critiquing research. School of Nursing and Midwifery. University of Dublin, Trinity College, Dublin.http://lancashirecare.files.wordpress.com/2008/03/step-by-step-guide-to-criti-research-part-1-quantitative-reseawrch.pdf.
52. Denzin N.K. Lincoln, Y.S. (Eds.) (1994). *Handbook of Qualitative Research.* Thousand Oaks, CA: Sage Publications Inc
53. Law M, et al. (1998) Guidelines for critical reivew form – qualitiative studies. http://fhs.mcmaster.ca/rehab/ebp/pdf/qualguidelines.pdf.
54. Evaluating Nutrition Information. Chapter 2. McGraw-Hill Higher Education. mcgraw-hill.com/sites/dl/free/0073522716/.../chapter02.pdf. (accessed 07/07/2013).
55. Watzl B. Bub A. (2003). Fruit and vegetable concentrate of vitamin supplement? *J. Nutr. 133 no. 11 3725.*http://jn.nutrition.org/cgi/content/full/133/11/3725.
56. Grady, D, et al. 2000. Postmenopausal hormone therapy increases risk for venous thromboem- bolic disease. Ann Intern Med, 132(9):690-696.
57. Martinson C. Anderson MS. de Vries R. Scientists behaving badly. *Nature.* 435:737-738 (9 June 2005). doi:10.1038/435737.http://www.nature.com/nature/journal/v435/n7043/full/435737a.html.
58. Casadevall A, Fang FC. (2012). Reforming science: Methodological and cultural reforms. *Infect Immun.* 80:891–896.
59. Field A. (2005). *Discovering Statistics Using SPSS, 2nd Ed.* Thousands Oaks, CA. SAGE Publications Inc.
60. Academy of Nutrition and Dietetics. Who are the academy's corporate sponsors? http://www.eatright.org/corporatesponsors/.
61. Benos DJ, et al. (2007). The ups and downs of peer review. *Adv Physiol Edu* 31:145-152.
62. Brown T. (2006). Sense about science. *Peer Review and the Acceptance of New Scientific Ideas.*
63. Macrina FL. (2005). Authorship and peer review. In: *Scientific Integrity: Text and Cases in Responsible Conduct of Research* (3rd ed.), edited by Macrina FL. Washington, DC: ASM.
64. Couzin J. (2006). Stem cells and how the problems eluded peer reviewers and editors. *Science* 311: 23–24.
65. Ioannidis JPA. (2005). Why most published research findings are false. *PLoS Med* 2(8): 696-701.
66. Ioannidis JP, Trikalionas TA. (2005). Early extreme contradictory estimates may appear in published research: The proteus phenomenon in molecular genetics research and randomized trials. *J Clin Epidemiol* 58: 543-549.
67. Ioannidis JPA. (2007). Why most published findings are false: Author's reply to goodman and Greenland. PLoS Medicine 4(6): 1132-1133.

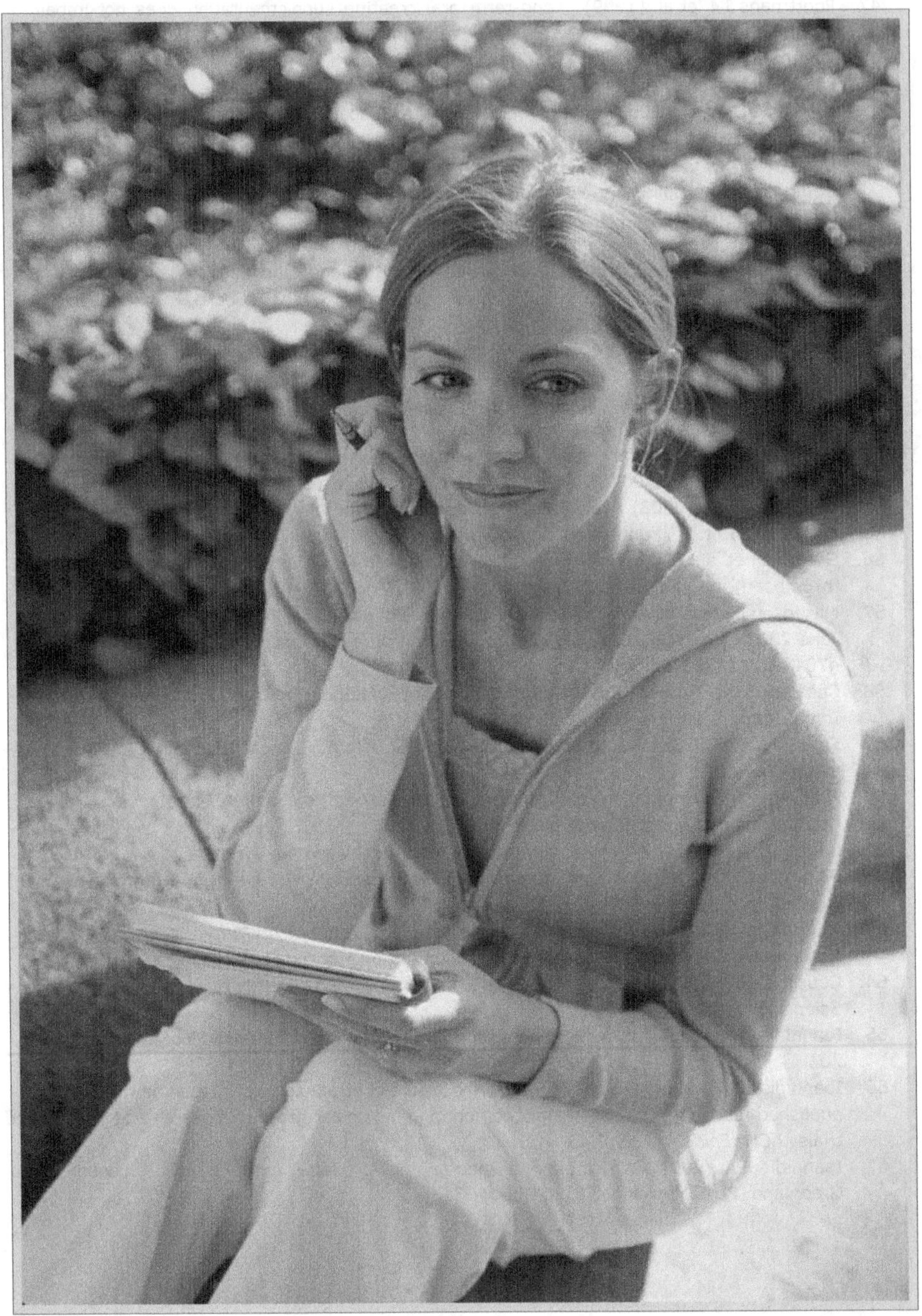

Chapter 11 - Prerequisites

This chapter will focus on prerequisites to implementing a nutrition program including legal considerations, discussion of a professional scope of practice, and a working knowledge of how to "coach" individuals into choosing healthy lifestyle changes.

Objectives

After reading and studying this chapter, you should be able to:

1. Discuss the difference between a dietetic program and a sports nutrition degree program including legal status of each.
2. Define licensure laws and legal issues involved with implementing a nutrition program.
3. Discuss a scope of practice for implementing a safe and effective nutrition program.
4. Discuss coaching skills necessary to motivate individuals to make healthy lifestyle changes including the Stages of Readiness to Change, questioning, understanding the change process, and the SMART rule for goal setting.

Introduction

Legal and professional controversies exist concerning unlicensed nutrition professionals implementing nutrition programs. Forty-six states have laws that regulate the profession of dietetics and nutrition which restrict nutrition practice by non-licensed professionals (1,2). According to the Academy of Nutrition and Dietetics (AND), the purpose of licensure is to protect the public from harm by non-qualified individuals practicing nutrition (4). The Academy of Nutrition and Dietetics has strong lobbying groups that are instrumental in passage of these laws. However, many licensure laws are ambiguous, skewed and politically motivated. These laws contain language that is difficult to interpret with clauses aimed at intimidating non-licensed professionals from disseminating nutrition information; these same laws include clauses that allow employees of health food stores to discuss nutrition with absolutely no qualifications whatsoever. Also, there are no limitations on writing nutrition and diet books that contain erroneous, unscientific, and even dangerous information.

Hence, the first step in implementation of any nutrition program by professionals other than licensed dietitians/nutritionists requires a thorough understanding of nutrition licensure laws.

Legal Considerations

More than 600 undergraduate and graduate didactic, dietetic technician, and supervised practice programs exist in the U.S. (3). Dietitians have a degree in clinical nutrition and must obtain advanced education for recognition in specialty fields such as renal nutrition, pediatric nutrition, certified diabetes educator, certified nutrition support clinician, sports dietetics practice, gerontological nutrition practice and oncology nutrition practice (4). The basic educational requirement in a dietetics program is a bachelor's degree with a major in dietetics, foods and nutrition, food service systems management, or a related area. Students take courses in foods, nutrition, institution management, chemistry, biology, microbiology, and physiology. Other courses are business, mathematics, statistics, computer science, psychology, sociology, and economics (4). Individuals with the RD credential have fulfilled these requirements, possess at least a bachelor's degree (about half of RDs hold advanced degrees), have completed a supervised practice program, and have passed a registration examination, in addition to maintaining continuing education requirements for recertification (4).

All dietetics programs are clinical in nature and do not require completion of sports nutrition course work. Dietitians wishing to enter the sports nutrition field are not required to obtain further eduction. The AND does offer a Sports Dietetics certification program. Individuals that successfully complete the requirements for this certification earn the title of Board Certified Specialists in Sports Dietetics (CSSD). Requirements for specialty certification include: Current Registered Dietitian (RD); maintenance of the RD status for a minimum of two years from the original examination date; documentation of 1,500 hours of specialty practice experience as an RD within the past five years; documentation of 1,000 hours of specialty practice experience as an RD within the past five years by the date the application (4).

A master's degree program in sports nutrition combines the fields of health and nutrition with fitness. Students learn ways to prevent injuries and provide treatment through nutrition programs. Master's degree graduates can obtain positions that focus on athletic performance and prevention of chronic diseases. A sports nutrition master's degree program teaches students how to measure metabolism, develop menus and create nutritional programs in order to prevent or accommodate injuries. Students also learn to customize specific training needs to improve physical performance in athletics (7).

A masters degree in sports nutrition from a reputable university does not afford the same legal rights as a dietitian even though the individual with the masters degree in sports nutrition is clearly qualified to implement a sports nutrition program. Individuals who have earned a Masters Degree in sports nutrition from a reputable university cannot "sit in" for the Board Certified Specialists in Sports Dietetics (CSSD) exam (only RDs can take the exam); hence, they can not achieve the same legal status unless first obtaining a clinical dietetics degree.

An article by Michael Ellsberg appeared in Forbes Magazine (April, 2012) concerning an attempt by the Academy of Nutrition and Dietetics (formerly ADA) to limit market competition in nutrition counseling (8). According to Mr. Ellsberg, "through a series of bills the Academy of Nutrition and Dietetics appears to be gaining legal control over who may provide nutrition counseling in a professional context". The article brought to light an AND document describing the AND strategy to limit competition for its members (8). The article raises the question: "should consumers have access to a wide array of different nutrition counseling choices/philosophies, among a wide array of professionals with differing credentials, or should the AND have strong legally-enforced say in who may or may not compete with the specific group of nutrition professionals it represents" (8)? The article goes on to include the following quote from the AND document: *"Simply put, governments more strictly regulate the work of and qualifications for dietitians than it does for nutritionists, and competitors are explicit about their intention to exploit this dietetics/nutrition distinction. An array of competitors is already providing would-be clients with personalized health education and nutritional counseling in growth areas such as prevention and wellness and in private practice careers. The required and necessary skill set of RDs competing with these other nutrition professionals may not necessarily be the same that clinical dietitians, but RDs cannot cede this expanding market to others who clearly intend to provide nutrition services."*

The Academy issued a rebuttal response in which Pepin Tuma, director of regulatory affairs is quoted as saying: "The (Forbes) article references CDR's Competition Study document, which outlines the structure and importance of our efforts. This document was intended for internal purposes only". The rebuttal by Tuma clearly states that AND never attempted to limit nutrition counseling (9)! The following statement is taken directly from the rebuttal:

> "In fact, there is not a single dietetics licensure law in the country that would prohibit licensed chiropractors, pharmacists, nurses, personal trainers, or acupuncturists from providing nutritional counseling (9)."

This statement appears to be a grievous deception. For example, Liz Lipski, who has a Ph.D. in clinical nutrition and an MS in nutrition, but who does not have a Registered Dietitian credential, was told by the North Carolina Board of Dietetics/Nutrition that she could not practice nutrition in that state (10). On April 20, 2011, the North Carolina Board of Dietetics/Nutrition denied Liz Lipski, PhD, CCN, CHN the right to practice as a nutritionist in North Carolina (10). Specifically, she was asked to return to college and take several semesters worth of undergraduate courses common for those studying to be Registered Dietitians, but which were not on her program of study as a nutritionist (10). Rather than return to the undergraduate level as a Ph.D, she sold her home, uprooted herself and her family, and took her practice to Virginia. Lipski writes on her site: The ADA has been skillful in creating licensing requirements that legally prevent highly qualified nutrition professionals from practicing in North Carolina. We decided to move where I have accepted a job as the national sales manager for a top clinical laboratory (10).

Jim Turner, chair of the board of Citizens for Health, and a veteran of state regulatory fights against AND-supported licensure laws, stated (8): "What's fascinating about this situation is that the AND structure actually excludes some of the most nutrition-educated people in the country from being able to provide nutrition information. You can have a master's in nutrition or even a Ph.D. and not qualify for the ADA recognition. So you have people who are well-qualified in nutrition, who are not allowed to exchange that information with consumers, because they don't have a legally recognized scope of practice. That's a tragic, unfortunate result of these laws (8)."

In the next section, we will define state licensure laws and discuss ways in which professionals can include nutrition services while still adhering to the strictest laws. In this next section, wellness professionals refers to individuals that practice health in the context of a healthy balance of the mind, body, and spirit that results in an overall feeling of well-being (16) and excludes licensed dietitians/nutritionists. Fitness professionals refers to both health related and skilled related fitness professionals. Athletic Trainers' refers to individuals that meet the requirements of a state licensing board and qualifications set by the Board of Certification. Athletic Trainers' are under the direction of a physician and are recognized by the American Medical Association, and are in good standing with the Board of Certification and in good standing with their state licensing board (17). A medical condition is a broad term that includes all diseases and disorders (15).

State Licensure Laws

Some states have licensure laws that define the range of practice for someone using the designation "nutritionist"; in other states, virtually anyone can call himself or herself a "nutritionist" regardless of education or training; and some states have very "strong" licensure laws requiring state licensing (4).

State licensure regulations fall into the following categories: licensure, statutory certification, or registration. These terms are defined as (4):

- Licensure - statutes include an explicitly defined scope of practice and performance of the profession (nutrition/weight management) is illegal without first obtaining a license from the state. Hence, it is illegal to provide nutrition or weight management in these states without a license. There is a provision, however, that allows a person to provide weight control services provided the program is developed and monitored by a licensed professional; and provided the individual does not change the program.
- Statutory Certification - limits use of particular titles to persons meeting predetermined requirements, while persons not certified can still practice the occupation or profession. Individuals in these states may provide weight management and nutrition services without being licensed; however, individuals may not use the term dietitian or licensed dietitian without adequate credentials.
- Registration - is the least restrictive form of regulation. Unregistered persons are permitted to practice the profession. Individuals in these states may provide weight management and nutrition services without being licensed.

Illinois is one example of a state with a "licensure" law. In 1991, Illinois passed *The Dietetic and Nutrition Services Practice Act,* which regulates and defines the scope of practice in nutrition and includes (5):

- "Any person who practices, offers to practice, attempts to practice, or holds oneself out to practice dietetics or nutrition counseling without being licensed under this Act shall, in addition to any other penalty provided by law, pay a civil penalty to the Department in an amount not to exceed $5000 for each offense as determined by the Department.

- Exemptions: Any person licensed in the state of Illinois under any other ACT engaging in the practice for which he or she is licensed; the practice of nutrition services by a person who is employed by the U.S. government; any person providing oral nutrition information as an *operator or employee of a health food store or business that sells health products, including dietary supplements, food, or food materials, or disseminating written nutrition information in connection with the marketing and distribution of those products; the practice of nutrition services by any person who provides weight control services provided the nutrition program has been reviewed by, consultation is available from, and no program change can be initiated without prior approval by, an individual licensed under this ACT,* a dietitian or nutrition counselor licensed in another state that has licensure requirements to be at least as stringent as the requirements by this ACT, or a registered dietitian. The Illinois law goes on to itemize other details not relevant to this discussion.

Note the exemption in the Illinois state licensure law that allows employees of a health food store to disseminate information on dietary supplements, or food and food materials without any stated qualifications.

Connecticut is an example of a state with a "certification" regulation. Under this law, persons not certified can still practice the occupation or profession of nutrition but may not use particular titles, such as dietitian, certified dietitian, or licensed dietitian (6).

While states such as CT allow non-licensed professionals to provide weight management and nutrition services, for legal reasons it is recommended that all wellness/fitness professionals work with a licensed nutrition professional. As health fitness/wellness professionals, we take an oath to do no harm. Providing nutrition services without adequate professional supervision could result in harm; and while it may be legal in some states, an individual could be held liable if an incident occurred due to inaccurate or damaging advice.

As defined by the Center for Nutrition Advocacy, nutrition is not the sole purview of any single profession but is a tool-set skillfully used by a wide variety of trained professionals to improve the health of those they serve (19). The Center for Nutrition Advocacy (CNA) is an initiative of the Certification Board for Nutrition Specialist (CBNS), the certifying body for the Certified Nutrition Specialist (CNS®) and the Certified Nutrition Specialist –

Scholar^{SM} (CNS-S^{SM}) credentials. The CNS is the most frequently recognized, non-dietetics credential, with its credential and/or examination recognized in the regulatory frameworks of 13 state and territories. The CNS is not to be confused with other non-regulatory certifications such as the AASDN Nutrition Specialist, the NASM Fitness Nutrition Specialist, Physician Nutrition Specialist, or Specialist in Fitness Nutrition Certification by ISSA.

The AASDN Nutrition Specialist Certification is the only non-regulatory nutrition certification program that includes all materials used by certificants including documents and scripted programs. The AASDN Nutrition Specialist program is also the only non-regulatory nutrition certification program that includes unlimited sports dietitian support. Hence, The AASDN Nutrition Specialist Certification program standards provide safe, effective and legal programs to the public.

Scope of Practice

The American Academy of Sports Dietitians and Nutritionists (AASDN) has undertaken the task of developing a more specific nutrition scope of practice for AASDN Nutrition Specialists (NS). This scope of practice is applicable to all fitness/wellness health professionals that partner with qualified, licensed professionals but is specific to AASDN certified professionals. The goal of this document is to provide AASDN certificants with clear, concise, and professional standards for inclusion of nutrition education. These guidelines are aimed at clarifying issues and adherence to all state nutrition licensure laws.

The AASDN Nutrition Scope of Practice for AASDN Nutrition Specialists:

<u>Standard 1 - Declarations and Definitions</u>

"AASDN" refers to the American Academy of Sports Dietitians & Nutritionists. "Board" refers to the AASDN Credentialing Commission Board members. "Wellness professionals" refers to individuals that practice health in the context of a healthy balance of the mind, body, and spirit that results in an overall feeling of well-being (16) and excludes licensed dietitians/nutritionists. "Fitness professional" refers to both health related and skilled related fitness professionals. "Athletic Trainers'" refers to individuals that meet the requirements of a state licensing board and qualifications set by the Board of Certification. Athletic Trainers' are under the direction of a physician and are recognized by the American Medical Association; and are in good standing with the Board of Certification and their state licensing board (17). "Nutrition Specialist" refers to a person who has successfully completed the AASDN Nutrition Specialist program and is a member in good standing with the AASDN Credentialing Commission. A "medical condition" is a broad term that includes all diseases and disorders (15). The "profession" refers to the profession of nutrition in conjunction with wellness programming. "Licensed professional" refers to a licensed dietitian/nutritionist.

Standard 2: Code of Ethics

Individuals that engage in the practice of nutrition in conjunction with fitness/wellness programming shall adhere to the AASDN Code of Ethics. The Code provides guidance for decision-making concerning ethical matters and serves as a means for self-evaluation and reflection regarding the ethical practice of nutrition in conjunction with fitness/wellness programming.

1. Accurately communicate and provide educational services equitably to all individuals regardless of social or economic status, age, gender, race, ethnicity, national origin, religion, disability, diverse values, attitudes, or opinions.
2. Be accountable for individual non-medical judgments and decisions about health and fitness, nutrition, preventive, rehabilitative, education, and/or research services.
3. Maintain high quality professional competence through continued study of the latest research in nutrition and health and fitness as provided through respected, reliable sources.
4. Be expected to conduct educational activities in accordance with recognized legal, scientific, ethical, and professional standards.
5. Respect and protect the privacy, rights, and dignity of all individuals by not disclosing health and fitness, nutrition, and or research information unless required by law or when confidentiality jeopardizes the health and safety of others.
6. Call attention to unprofessional services that result from incompetent, unethical, or illegal professional behavior.
7. Contribute to the ongoing development and integrity of the profession by being responsive to, mutually supportive of, and accurately communicating academic and other qualifications to colleagues and associates in the field.
8. Participate in the profession's efforts to establish high quality services by avoiding conflicts of interest and endorsements of products and supplements.
9. Participate in and encourage critical discourse to reflect the collective knowledge and be proactive within the exercise and nutrition profession to protect the public from misinformation, incompetence, and unethical acts.
10. Provide interventions grounded in a theoretical framework supported by research that enables a healthy lifestyle.

Standard 3: Practice of nutrition in conjunction with fitness/wellness programming

The practice of nutrition education in conjunction with fitness/wellness programming by AASDN Nutrition Specialists shall include a variety of educational activities/documents but only when created by, reviewed by, and/or in consultation with an AASDN licensed dietitian/nutritionist. No program/document change can be initiated without prior approval by an AASDN licensed dietitian/nutritionist. No program/document can be modified or altered in any way without approval by an AASDN licensed dietitian/nutritionist. The AASDN Nutrition Specialist, in conjunction with the AASDN licensed professional, may provide clients with educational information through lectures, articles, and classes. The AASDN Nutrition Specialist, in conjunction with the AASDN licensed professional, may utilize AASDN approved documents with the apparently healthy, exercising population. Nothing in this standard authorizes the AASDN Nutrition Specialist to "diagnose" disease or make nutritional recommendations for individuals requiring special dietary needs. Nothing in this standard authorizes the AASDN Nutrition Specialist to provide such services without direct approval and in consultation with an AASDN licensed dietitian/nutritionist. The AASDN Nutrition Specialist **cannot** provide nutrition services to individuals with medical conditions without direct oversight and in consultation with an AASDN licensed dietitian/nutritionist.

Standard 4: Educational Requirements

The practice of nutrition in conjunction with the AASDN Nutrition Specialist shall include a variety of educational requirements prior to practice which includes successful completion of the AASDN Nutrition Specialist Certification; and all certificants must be members in good standing with the AASDN Credentialing Commission.

Standard 5: Nutritional Product Endorsement and Sales

AASDN does not endorse any particular supplements or brand of supplements. It is beyond the scope of practice for Nutrition Specialists to recommend or suggest the use of any nutrition supplementation (vitamin, mineral, herbal, ergogenic, or weight loss). Any such recommendations must come directly from the client's physician or a licensed dietitian. The Nutrition Specialist shall refrain from endorsement of, or sales of, supplements and products containing supplement on the label. Such endorsement or sales constitutes a conflict of interest and is beyond the scope of practice of a non-licensed professional

Standard 6: Professional Responsibility and Competence

The AASDN Nutrition Specialist that has attained the AASDN Nutrition Specialist Certification who is in good legal and professional standing with all academic and certificate programs may implement programs that have been created by an AASDN licensed dietitian/nutritionist when working with the apparently, healthy exercising population. It is the responsibility of the AASDN Nutrition Specialist to be aware of specific statues in his/her state as well as understanding his/her professional standard of care and limitations in working with at risk populations or individuals with medical conditions. The AASDN Nutrition Specialist shall practice only within the boundaries of their competence as defined by their academic training, hands-on experience, professional certification, and in conjunction with a licensed dietitian/nutritionist. When indicated, the AASDN Nutrition Specialist professional shall monitor his/her effectiveness and take steps including, but not limited to, continuing education to maintain a reasonable level of awareness of current scientific and professional information.

Choosing a Licensed Professional

Choosing a qualified professional to oversee nutrition programs is of utmost importance. It must not be assumed that all dietitians have the appropriate background to provide this service. As discussed previously, a person may hold a master's degree in sports nutrition from a respected and reputable university but does not have the same legal rights as a licensed dietitian/nutritionist even though the individual with the masters degree in sports nutrition may be equally or more qualified to implement a sports nutrition program. Therefore it is important to interview potential licensed professionals to determine educational background, experience in nutrition program development, and experience in sports nutrition counseling.

Certification

The decision to pursue professional certification is an important step in being recognized as a competent practitioner in one's chosen discipline. The benefits of earning a certificate or certification in nutrition include: increasing level of expertise in the field of nutrition; adding a credential to list of credentials; providing additional services to help individuals be more successful; and increasing earning capacity. The first step when seeking a certificate or certification in nutrition is to decide on a regulatory program (such as an RD or CNS®). When seeking a nutrition certification from a non-regulatory program, research the program to confirm that it: adheres to all state licensure laws; possesses a defined scope of practice; offers continuous support by a qualified, licensed professional; and that the program provides mechanisms for the safety of the public.

Program Materials

As previously discussed, due to current licensure laws the practice of nutrition in conjunction with wellness programming can include a variety of services but again only when created by, reviewed by, and/or in consultation with a licensed dietitian/nutritionist.

Also, no program change can be initiated without prior approval by the licensed dietitian/nutritionist. The fitness/wellness health professional, in conjunction with the licensed dietitian/nutritionist, may provide clients with the following nutrition information: educational information through lectures, articles, and classes; energy calculations; and pre-approved menu plans for the apparently healthy, exercising population, including children and older individuals that have no medical conditions. It must be clear that the fitness/wellness health professional is not qualified to "diagnose" disease or make nutritional recommendations for individuals with medical conditions requiring special dietary needs. Again, a medical condition is a broad term that includes all diseases and disorders (15). The fitness/wellness health professional cannot provide nutrition services to individuals with medical conditions (18), without direct oversight and in consultation with a licensed dietitian/nutritionist.

State litigation is ever evolving as it relates to providing nutrition information. At present, six states currently have activity in this area: Arizona, Michigan, New Jersey, New York, North Carolina, and Washington. Visit http://nutritionadvocacy.org/laws-state for updates.

Coaching Skills

Many of us have heard about coaching at some point in our career. There are business coaches, career coaches, relationship coaches; there are coaches available for almost any personal or professional pursuit. What exactly is coaching? The definition is a powerful concept: Coaching is a co-creative partnership between a qualified coach and a willing client that supports the client through desired life changes. The key to this definition is the term "co-creative." In coaching, you are not the expert in your client's life. You work with your client to discover solutions to their wellness challenges as they emerge through discussion and exploration.

Coaching is very different from athletic or personal training, nutrition consulting, or traditional therapy or counseling. In personal training, athletic training, or nutrition consulting sessions, you are the expert, you have the information or answers, and you educate your client by passing on that information or those answers. The client is more like a sponge waiting to soak up your expertise, not a creative partner who is equally involved in the informing process.

For example, a nutrition consultant will review a client's food diary and make a list of possible areas for improvement, such as reducing saturated fat intake. The nutrition consultant would then decide that the client's next session would be geared toward educating the client about saturated fat and its health effects, in hopes that the client would see the benefit in reducing the amount of saturated fat she eats. A coach, on the other hand, would take note of the elevated intake of saturated fat and then ask the client what, if anything, he/she is willing to change about it. If the client did not identify the need to change that part of his/her lifestyle, the coach might ask if the client were open to being educated about the effects of saturated fat. However, if the client declined receiving the information, nothing further would be done at that time. The coach could broach the topic again at an appropriate time when the client expressed an interest in making healthy changes regarding fat intake.

Remember, whether you work in the field of nutrition or fitness, you are endowed with knowledge that many of your coaching clients will seek as they set wellness goals. As a coach, how then do you determine the appropriate time to provide the wellness expertise that your client needs? The answer is easy: you only provide information that your client requests in relation to goals. If the client needs specific information about cholesterol, you can provide that. If your client expresses a desire to work with a trainer, and you are a trainer, you can offer your services. Any requests for your expertise must come from the client, and they must be spelled out in the weekly coaching goals. Therefore, wellness coaches wear two hats; their serve as a coach, and when called upon to provide wellness direction, an educator.

Remember, in life coaching, the coach does not have a high level of expertise in the wellness arena. If a client wants help with health related issues, the clients must set goals to seek out and retain help from wellness experts, such as yourself. In wellness coaching, you are the referred professional, and this gives you a special opportunity to be more involved in your client's progress.

Counseling Versus Coaching

Carol Ballard, Psy.D, counselor and director of a collegiate counselor center, provides insight into the similarities and distinctions between coaching and counseling: "Coaching and counseling are allied fields that share the goal of helping clients achieve lives of greater health and fulfillment. Both counselors and coaches help clients set measurable, attainable goals. Both teach the skills necessary for achieving the goals, and both provide support and encouragement while clients work toward their goals."

A major difference is the client population. Coaches work with clients who are reasonably healthy and well-functioning and wish to augment their well-being through achieving certain personal or professional goals. Goals may be specific to wellness or performance or may be more broadly aimed at achieving greater life satisfaction through, for example, changes in career or lifestyle. The work is focused on the present and its influence on the future. The work is also typically brief and designed to accomplish the client's goals relatively quickly. "Improvement" and "enhancement" are hallmarks of coaching.

Counselors also work with such clients and, when they do, there can be considerable overlap between coaching and counseling. However, counselors also work with clients who have some degree of impairment in functioning, ranging from mild to severe, and this is when counseling enters areas not included in coaching. For example, along with various other aspects of their work with these clients, counselors may see a connection between the clients' present and past and may help clients explore early family relationships, previous traumatic experiences, or other aspects of the past in order to aid them in resolving present-day concerns. Counselors frequently help clients to deal with troubling thoughts and feelings, developmental concerns, and relationship issues. Such work may take considerable time, even extending to months or years. "Healing" and "recovery" are hallmarks of counseling.

Coaching	**Counseling**
Helps clients	Helps clients
Helps clients enhance functioning	Helps clients enhance or regain functioning
Helps clients set and work towards goals	Helps clients set and work towards goals
Emphasizes careful, intense listening	Emphasizes careful, intense listening
A more casual, collaborative approach	A more formal, structured approach
Deals with clients who are healthy but want to improve in certain areas or meet specific goals	May deal with clients who have serious mental or emotional disorders
Maintains focus on the client's goals	Can move between guidance and therapy as needed
External focus – deals with measurable behaviors	Often includes focus on internal aspects such as thought and emotion
Focuses on the present and the immediate future	Often explores the effect of the past on the present
May appeal to clients as more "health related"	May have a "mental illness" stigma for some clients
Less well-known to the average person	More familiar to most people; more likely to be paid for by insurance
Personal Trainer (20)	Wellness Coach
Presents as the expert	Presents as a facilitator
Primarily instructs/didactic in nature	Primarily listens
Corrects a problem	Builds on strengths/self efficacy
Provides a solution	Assists with overcoming ambivalence

Not all of these distinctions are cast-iron. For example, many therapists avoid the formal hierarchical relationship of counselor as expert and client as uninformed seeker and conversely, many coaches may be quite structured in their approach. Both coaching and counseling provide valuable services. Which modality would best fit a client's needs depends on such factors as the issue or goal to be addressed, the client's financial and other resources, and the availability of services. It also depends on the client's understanding of the differences and similarities between the two and the clients expectation of what would best help meet current goals. At different times, the same individual may benefit from both coaching and counseling. So, if it seems that there are more similarities than differences, that is probably the case. In fact, coaching could be seen as a subset of counseling. As coaching continues to evolve as a profession, its strengths and its distinctions from counseling will become more familiar to the average consumer of services, making it easier for clients to choose the right modality when help is needed.

Listening

Listening is an "art." It requires you to silence the expert in your brain, and focus on what's being said by the client. When listening, first, connect fully with the client. In order to do this, you must believe in your client's ability to effect change as he/she takes steps toward goal achievement. Next, you must be "present." You must not think, plan, or wonder while the client is speaking: your job is just to listen. It's surprising what you can hear people say when your history, knowledge, and assumptions are put aside. Finally, keep in mind that silence is valuable in many coaching moments. Give clients time to process questions and information, and arrive at their own conclusions. Remember, in successful coaching, the client has the answers. The coach is simply a partner that supports a willing client through desired lifestyle changes.

Stages of Readiness to Change

A successful coaching business is built around successful and enthusiastic clients. However, clients are only successful when they are ready to make changes. It's very likely that 90% of the potential clients will be ready to change something; that's why they sought your help in the first place. However, some individuals might not understand that coaching actually requires them to take action. Some individuals perceive receiving information as action; but clients cannot remain idle afterward and then blame others for their unhealthy condition (12). Therefore, assessing whether or not an individual is ready to change is of the utmost importance when interviewing/screening a potential client. The fitness/wellness professional must be diligent about weeding out clients who really are not ready to take responsibility for their choices and actions (12).

The Stages of Readiness to Change, made famous by Dr. James Prochaska, is a useful tool in determining if a person is ready to make lifestyle changes (14). The steps in this model include the following stages: precontemplation, contemplation, preparation, action, maintenance, and the relapse/recycling stage.

Precontemplation Stage

The precontemplation stage is the stage in which a client is not yet ready to change. The client may deny that there is a problem (My doctor told me to exercise, but some people who don't exercise are still healthy); blame someone else for the problem (It's my spouse's fault that I can't stick to an exercise program); or blame themselves (I can't make any positive changes in my life). Most often, the problem is identified by a doctor, family member, or friend. Offering a fitness prescription at this stage is contraindicated. It will merely frustrate you and place you into a no-win situation.

It's easy to identify clients who are not ready to change. When you begin communicating with the potential client, ask, "What seems to be the matter that you'd like to change?" An individual unwilling to make changes will respond with a number of excuses to take the responsibility for his/her condition off of his/her own shoulders. Listen for blame shifting in the response. Clients unwilling to change may blame circumstances, lack of time, occupation or other people in his/her life for their condition. You can feel comfortable saying to this person, "I hear you are frustrated with your situation, but unless you can take the responsibility for your current habits and situation, I can't help you. Can you tell me what you can do to change your current situation to make it better for your health?" Pose the question, and then let the client think about it. If he/she comes up with some solid answers that reveal that indicate a personal need to change some things, then there is a glimmer of hope. If you hear the blame game from the beginning, the potential client is probably not a potential client at all.

Contemplation Stage

Clients in the contemplation stage weigh the costs and benefits of lifestyle modification. For example, the client may be considering starting an exercise program, but he/she is unsure if the long-term benefits (health, weight management) outweigh the short-term costs (time, finances). This stage is also characterized by ambivalence; a desire to change is accompanied by fear and doubt that changes will actually work. This client can be educated about the potential for change, the causes of the fear, (i.e. failed past attempts to maintain an exercise program), and the concept of practicing until something fits. This client may well be a great client after a bit more understanding about the process of change.

Preparation Stage

This stage is characterized by the client's asking for advice on what to do in order to make healthy lifestyle changes. Watch for self-motivational statements such as, "I need to do something." In this stage, the client becomes less defensive and more willing to discuss modification of current behavior. This is the window of opportunity. This is where a fitness prescription devised with the help of the client becomes beneficial.

Clients in the preparation stage intend to initiate change within a month's time. This is where intentions become observable behavior changes. For example, a client in this stage may have decided to join the gym next month and have begun to visit various health clubs. The preparation stage is a rewarding experience for coaches because clients are beginning to take charge of their health.

Action Stage

The action stage is that wonderful stage where we see behaviors that indicate positive lifestyle changes. The client is investing time and energy into reaching his/her goals. For example, the client has begun to attend the gym regularly. However, during the action stage clients are at the greatest risk of relapse. Our role in this stage is to reinforce and affirm the client's commitment to change. If the client has been a partner in developing the plan, he or she is more likely to adhere to the plan and make it work. We may need to modify the fitness prescription if the client experiences areas of difficulty.

Maintenance Stage

Maintenance is helping the client to maintain positive lifestyle changes. Strategies in this stage may require different strategies than those used in the Action Stage. Ambivalence may reappear at this stage. Some clients may need to mourn the loss of old bad habits. They are aware of the old habits as being unhealthy (the midnight refrigerator raids), but there is still a need to mourn the loss. They may also need to take steps to reduce the occurrence of relapses into old behavior patterns. Clients may need to anticipate situations that could lead to relapse and arm themselves with coping strategies in advance. They may also need to make changes within their environment to ensure continued success. Support and reaffirmation during the maintenance stage is critical.

Relapse and Recycling

Any change in behavior takes with it the possibility of relapsing into old, established behaviors. The key to success is helping the client to understand that relapse is a part of developing permanent behavior changes. It is important that we don't add to the client's guilt over relapsing into old behaviors. Our role is to help them analyze stumbling blocks and reframe the experience as a learning tool. Helping the client navigate through this stage requires that we assist them in coping with feelings of failure. We go back to the preparation stage with them and renegotiate a plan. What was it that worked for them in the past, and what didn't? What small changes can be made to reinforce self-efficacy?

Questioning

Questioning is an effective way to evaluate what stage of change a client is at (12). Questions to ask include:

1. Are you able to make changes?
2. Why is now the time to change?
3. Is it possible to try new habits?
4. Is it impossible or just difficult to change?
5. What will changing do for you?
6. What will happen if you don't change?

The first answer must be yes, or some indication of willingness to try. The second answer must contain a personally relevant reason, something that is emotionally meaningful to the client. They may give you an external reason at first (such as "My doctor told me to"). Keep asking the question, stressing, "Why do YOU feel it's time to change?" Your goal is to see if they have a real, internal reason for changing. The third answer must be YES. The fourth answer must be "just difficult!" If he/she says "impossible," he/she is not ready to change. The fifth answer must be evaluated by the coach. Is the reason realistic? We must listen for any grandiose ideas of major life improvements coming from small body-centered changes. Listen to what the client says, and decide if this is the kind of client you can work with or not. If the expected outcomes seem far-fetched to you, ask the client if the expected results are realistic, and challenge the client until expectations become more realistic. The sixth answer must be free of all-or-nothing thoughts, like suicide. In such cases, referral to a psychologist may be recommended. Listen for emotionally charged answers, such as "I might not live to see my granddaughter graduate high school, and I don't want that!"

If an emotion stemming from a personally powerful and relevant reason for change is driving the decision, the client can likely do the work that a coaching relationship involves.

As you can see, the client is part of the reason coaching works. When a potential client comes to you verbalizing that they want to change and asking what he/she needs to do, then you have the makings for a beautiful coaching relationship. The desire to change is the first key to making changes that stick. In a successful coaching relationship, the client: truly wants to make life changes; accepts responsibility for choices, actions, and consequences; is not afraid to try; understands that failure is not a personal flaw; and learns to change thinking patterns and habits.

The next major key to success is a willingness on the client's part to take responsibility for actions. In so doing, the client can't be afraid to try new methods. The client can't continue to believe that a failed plan is an indication of failure as a person. Nothing could be further from the truth. Trying and failing are part of making life changes, and the client must be willing to keep moving forward.

Finally, in order to make lasting changes in a client's life, both the coach and client must understand that a complete change in the way the client thinks must occur. A client feels the ramifications of acting and thinking in unhealthy, unproductive ways. For example, if a client believes he/she is a failure and that nothing will ever work, he/she is right! If the client believes he/she can try anything, and that is bound to succeed at some point, he/she is also right! As coaches, it's our job to make it very clear that what the client thinks will truly shape reality. It's the client's job to believe in their own capacity to succeed in healthy changes.

Understanding the Change Process

As humans, we are mammals with survival instincts. These innate instincts are imbedded within us to keep us alive, and one of the keys to staying alive in any environment is knowing what's coming. If you can predict what will happen when certain actions take place, you can control the outcome of such actions in your favor. This is why the process of change is difficult for most clients. The fear of the unknown sets in, as they are stepping into unchartered waters.

At a young age, we, like all animals, learn how to act by imitating our parents and those people we are exposed to in our early years. As a baby human, we can be exposed to habits and actions from our parents that are not healthy or conducive to our well-being; and unfortunately, we don't know enough at that age to differentiate between healthy and unhealthy habits. The result: we take everything we are shown, and we adopt it as our own. Only later, as thinking adults, can we choose healthier habits based on what we want our lives, bodies, and futures to be like (12). As adults, we know the outcomes of the habits we've been practicing for years and years; and these habits, although unhealthy and unproductive, are safe and predictable and easy for us to do. This is where our "comfort zone" lies.

Unlike animals who act clearly on the instinct that will keep them alive, we humans can choose actions at any time that clearly act against our own survival. People eat too much, drink too much, and let their bodies go to waste. As coaches, we have to remind our clients that they can and should choose habits and outcomes that bring them closer to their desired outcomes. If something isn't working in a client's life, the client must be able to see that it is a choice to change the actions that lead to that outcome. For example, if the client's family overate, and the client adopted poor eating habits that lead to excess weight gain, he/she needs to choose to learn and incorporate healthier habits that will lead to weight loss, if that truly is the goal. Coaching focuses on present and future actions. Adult clients must understand that it is possible to change any habit they have ever learned: it just takes work and time. The coaching relationship is a safe, effective place to undertake such work.

To reiterate, the process of change can be scary and difficult for clients. Therefore, when our clients are starting the change process, we have to help them control their environment as much as possible so they can feel safe in making healthy changes. For example, if stress triggers a desire to eat ice cream, and the habit we'd like to form is that stress triggers a desire to go for a walk, we must either remove the habitual outcome, (the ice cream), or reduce /eliminate the habitual stimulus for eating ice cream, (the stress). Not all stress can be eliminated from anyone's life. However, some types of stress can be reduced, and this is what we can help the client work to reduce.

Part of changing a client's environment includes enlisting support outside of the coaching relationship. It is critical for the client to be surrounded by family and friends who support the changes he/she is making. Because you as a coach understand the change process, you can help the client explain to her loved ones the type of support he/she needs: unconditional belief in her ability to change, and undying enthusiasm for her intended success. When a coach models this type of support, clients usually can recruit effective helpers outside of the coaching relationship. As their circle of support grows, the change process becomes easier; their potential for lasting change increases; and the likelihood for over-reliance on the coach decreases.

A client's reason for going through this difficult process must have some sort of emotionally charged reward attached to it. People make a majority of their choices based on their feelings, not based on fact or rational arguments. This is true in advertising, and it's true in life! For example, the marketing team that Goodyear hired understood that people make decisions based on emotions. Their advertisement included babies and puppies, which elicit warm emotions in most of us. They also represent things that we feel a need to protect. The goal: consumers will remember the pleasant feelings they felt while viewing Goodyear commercials, and they will assume that because the advertisement had babies and puppies riding on their tires that the product must be safe. The reasoning is emotional not rational; in fact, another brand of tires might be exactly as safe or even safer!

The process of change plays on the same emotional response that advertising does. Facts or logic don't necessarily matter: it's emotion that counts! It's that strong feeling that will carry them through the tough times when relapse is a real danger.

Related to that is the client's perception of the costs and benefits of making the change. The perceived or projected benefits of making the change must outweigh the perceived costs of making the change. For example, the desire to feel confident in a swimsuit on the beach, and the projected positive outcomes attached to that image, must far outweigh the perceived difficulties or costs in actually making the changes necessary to achieve that desired goal. If eating smaller portions, limiting alcohol consumption, and greatly increasing exercise are deemed to be more costly for the client than the perceived joy of achieving the swimsuit goal, the client will not put the effort forth to achieve the goal.

If change is so difficult, how can we as coaches instill the confidence in our clients that they can change? The answer to this dilemma is practice! The more they do something, the better or more efficient they get at doing it. The client practices the behavior change once and then repeats over and over again until it becomes as natural as brushing their teeth or answering the phone when it rings. A supportive coaching environment allows clients to feel safe and supported as they try new habits that support their desired outcome, and make adaptations according to what works for them.

Remember, although the change process is difficult for clients, smart coaches only work with clients who are ready to change.

SMART Rule

Modifying habits requires an understanding of the parameters involved in goal setting. We need to help clients set goals and objectives that are reasonable and not overwhelming; and they must follow the SMART Rule (15).

S stands for specific—the goal must be specific. If the goal is too broad, it will be beyond achievement.

M stands for measurable—the goal must be measurable. One can set goals, but if they are not measurable there is no way of knowing if that goal has been achieved.

A stands for "A value"—the goal must be important and of value to the client. If not important, then it will not be accomplished. For example, a client losing weight for a spouse will not work. The client must set a goal that is important to him or her.

R stands for realistic—the goal must be realistic. For a person who is 50% body fat, achieving 20% body fat in 6 months is unrealistic and will only frustrate the client.

T stands for time frame—all goals must have a deadline. If no deadline exists, then there is no incentive to achieve the goal.

The first step in goal setting is to set long term goals (i.e. achieve a healthy body in one or two years). When long term goals have been agreed upon, the next step is to set short range goals which are still reasonable and measurable, (one month to three months). For example, losing one to three percent fat per month is the standard or average fat loss. This goal is reasonable, measurable, specific, and has a time frame.

Once the short term goals are set, the next step is to create a calendar that specifically identifies the daily tasks required to accomplish the short term goal. For example, on the calendar, the client can summarize daily exercise, and daily food totals. At the end of the time period, the fitness professional can review the calendar with the client. While this task is arduous and time consuming, it provides valuable feedback and produces the wanted results. If the calendar showed that exercise was sparse and extra calories were consumed every day from high caloric foods, the client would discover the reason why she didn't lose any weight.

Supporting

The final major component of coaching is supporting. Those in the wellness profession already have had practice supporting clients, but the following six points detail how to support your client to ensure their coaching experience is successful.

First, you as a coach must have unconditional positive regard for the client. This means that, while you don't necessarily like what the client is doing to herself with her unhealthy actions, you unfailingly believe that he/she is a good person and that he/she has the power to live the life he/she always wanted. Your enthusiasm for your client's ability to change must be contagious! When clients come to you, they will most likely be convinced of their imminent failure. If you show that you believe in them from the start, they will learn to believe in themselves too.

Next, you must demonstrate a genuine interest in your client's goal achievement. As the coach, you must be as highly invested in your client's success as he/she is. Show your client that you are invested by staying present when he/she speaks to you. Focus solely on what the client is saying and how he/she is feeling at any given moment; never lose yourself in your own thoughts or feelings. This requires practice. In the end and you will begin to feel what it is truly like to hear and care about what your clients are going through as they wade through the murky waters of change.

Part of showing you care is holding your client accountable for his/her choices and actions. If he/she lets her weekly goals go unaccomplished or starts blaming and making excuses for missed opportunities to try new actions, don't let those moments slip by unnoticed! Coaching requires that you call your client on his/her dropped goals. Ask the client what he/she thought would happen by not following goal action steps, and ask what they experienced as a result. Holding clients accountable shows that you care. It communicates that you want them to have every opportunity to succeed, and you know that the client can't succeed if he/she doesn't try the new actions that he/she set out to try.

Along with trying and succeeding are two very important points that clients seem to forget about: praise and celebration. Praise your clients when they try something new, and celebrate with them when they find an action that works for them. Most wellness clients have tried diets in the past. Diets never work because they are someone else's plan being imposed on a whole diverse group of people. Therefore clients will likely be used to trying plans that fail. Hence, celebrate every single success no matter how small. Every action that helps lead our clients to a healthier long-term habit should be praised and celebrated. Positive reinforcement does wonders in the process of lifestyle change.

What happens when clients seem to be heading in a positive direction, and suddenly something triggers a relapse? How do we respond as coaches? Supporting and positive reinforcement is just as important in times of relapse.

When life events trigger unwanted emotions, a common response is to reach for the first thing that brings comfort and takes the disease away. For our clients, these are usually the unhealthy habits they have been working so successfully toward erasing from their lives, such as alcohol or high-fat foods. This reversion to old unhealthy habits is called relapse, and if we can help our clients understand its cause, we can then help them avoid the destructive thoughts and actions that usually come after it.

It helps to remind clients that they are human; they are not perfect, and in no way were they ever meant to be. Explain to clients that change is not a linear process; it takes many ups and downs to finally attain a positive, forward-moving trend in behavior over time. It's persistence and a general trend toward a healthier lifestyle that matters in the long run. They might take 2 steps forward and one step back every single day for months on end, but in the end they will still be moving forward.

If relapses continue consistently, the coach must reevaluate the client's readiness to change. Ask the client the following questions:

1. What do you perceive is the greatest obstacle to your success right now?
2. What needs to happen in order for you to succeed?
3. What can he/she do to make the road less bumpy?
4. Is he/she really ready to give up her dream just because it's difficult?
5. What can you, as her coach, assist her with during this difficult time?

Listen for blame in the client's answers. Remind the client of his/her emotionally charged vision. Stick to this line of questioning until your client realizes that he/she did, indeed, come to you to make changes, and he/she is going to move forward with those changes regardless of the obstacles faced along the way.

Your coaching duties are called into overtime play during relapse, and the results can be just the breakthrough your client needed to advance by leaps and bounds. As a coach, you provide a very important outlet for the client's thoughts and feelings surrounding a relapse. Remember your role: Stay present; listen, question and support! Always believe 100% in your client's ability to make positive changes.

Summary

Legal and professional controversy exists concerning populations that can and should implement nutrition programs. Forty-six states have laws that regulate the profession of dietetics and nutrition. However these laws are ambiguous, skewed and politically motivated. They contain language that is difficult to interpret with clauses aimed at intimidating non-licensed professionals from disseminating nutrition information but include clauses that allow employees of health food stores to discuss nutrition with absolutely no qualifications whatsoever. Also, there are no limitations on writing nutrition and diet books. State licensure and state certification are entirely separate and distinct from registration or certification by the Commission on Dietetic Registration; however, the Academy of Nutrition and Dietetics have strong lobbying groups that are instrumental in passage of these laws. Hence, the first step in implementation of any nutrition program by professions other than licensed dietitians requires a thorough understanding of these laws.

A master's degree program in sports nutrition combines the fields of health and nutrition with fitness. A Masters Degree in sports nutrition from a reputable university does not afford the same legal rights as a dietitian with a bachelor's degree even though the individual with the Masters Degree in sports nutrition is clearly more qualified to implement a sports nutrition program. Individuals who have achieved a masters degree in sports nutrition from a reputable university cannot "sit in" for the Board Certified Specialists in Sports Dietetics (CSSD) exam (only RDs can take the exam); hence, they cannot achieve the same legal benefits unless first obtaining a clinical dietetics degree.

An article by Michael Ellsberg appeared in Forbes Magazine (April, 2012) concerning an attempt by the Academy of Nutrition and Dietetics (formerly ADA) to limit market competition in nutrition counseling. According to Mr. Ellsberg, "through a series of bills the Academy of Nutrition and Dietetics appears to be gaining legal control over who may provide nutrition counseling in a professional context". The Academy issued a rebuttal response in which Pepin Tuma, director of regulatory affairs, was interviewed by the author and is quoted: "The (Forbes) article references CDR's Competition Study document, which outlines the structure and importance of our efforts. This document was intended for internal purposes only". The rebuttal by Tuma clearly states that ADA never attempted to limit nutrition counseling! "In fact, there is not a single dietetics licensure law in the country that would prohibit licensed chiropractors, pharmacists, nurses, personal trainers, or acupuncturists from providing nutritional counseling." This statement appears to be a grievous deception since several national cases exist indicating otherwise.

Some states have licensure laws that define the range of practice for someone using the designation "nutritionist"; in other states, virtually anyone can call himself or herself a "nutritionist" regardless of education or training; and some states have very "strong" licensure laws. State licensure regulations fall into the following categories: licensure; statutory certification; or registration. For the previously discussed reasons, all fitness professionals should provide a program under the direction of a licensed dietitian or provide a program that has been created by, reviewed by, in consultation with, or directly approved by a sufficiently qualified, licensed dietitian/nutritionist.

As defined by the Center for Nutrition Advocacy, nutrition is not the sole purview of any single profession, but is a tool-set skillfully used by a wide variety of trained professionals to improve the health of those they serve (19). The Center for Nutrition Advocacy (CNA) is an initiative of the Certification Board for Nutrition Specialist (CBNS), the certifying body for the Certified Nutrition Specialist (CNS®) and the Certified Nutrition Specialist - Scholar℠ (CNS-S℠) credentials. The CNS is the most frequently recognized, non-dietetics credential, with its credential and/or examination recognized in the regulatory frameworks of 13 state and territories. The CNS is not to be confused with other non-regulatory certifications such as the AASDN Nutrition Specialist, the NASM Fitness Nutrition Specialist, Physician Nutrition Specialist, or Specialist in Fitness Nutrition Certification by ISSA.

The AASDN Nutrition Specialist Certification is the only non-regulatory nutrition certification program that includes all materials used by certificants including documents and scripted programs. The AASDN Nutrition Specialist program is also the only non-regulatory nutrition certification program that includes unlimited sports dietitian support. Hence, The AASDN Nutrition Specialist Certification program standards provide safe, effective, and legal programs to the public.

The American Academy of Sports Dietitians and Nutritionists (AASDN) has undertaken the task of developing a more specific nutrition scope of practice for AASDN Nutrition Specialists (NS) and AASDN Nutrition Managers (NM). This scope of practice is applicable to all fitness/wellness health professionals that partner with qualified, licensed professionals but is specific to AASDN certified professionals. The goal of this document is to provide AASDN with clear, concise, and professional standards for inclusion of nutrition education. These guidelines are aimed at clarifying issues and adherence to all state nutrition licensure laws.

Choosing a qualified professional to oversee nutrition programs is of utmost importance. It must not be assumed that all dietitians have the appropriate background to provide this service. As discussed previously, a person may hold a master's degree in sports nutrition from a respected and reputable university but does not have the same legal rights as a licensed dietitian/nutritionist even though the individual with the

Masters Degree in sports nutrition may be equally or more qualified to implement a sports nutrition program. Therefore, it is important to interview potential licensed professionals to determine educational background, experience in nutrition program development, etc.

The decision to pursue professional certification is an important step in being recognized as a competent practitioner in one's chosen discipline. The benefits of earning a certificate or certification in nutrition include: increasing level of expertise in the field of nutrition; adding a credential to list of credentials; and increasing earning capacity. The first step when seeking a certificate or certification in nutrition is to decide on a regulatory program (such as an RD or CNS®). When seeking a nutrition certification from a non-regulatory program be sure that the program adheres to all state licensure laws; possesses a defined scope of practice; offers continuous support by a qualified, licensed professional; and that the program provides mechanisms for the safety of the public.

Working with clients requires a working knowledge of coaching skills. This section provided basic principles of coaching. The definition is a concisely worded description of this powerful concept: coaching is a co-creative partnership between a qualified coach and a willing client that supports the client through desired life changes. The key to this definition of coaching is the term "co-creative." In coaching, you are not the expert in your client's life. You work with your client to discover solutions to their wellness challenges as they emerge through discussion and exploration. Therefore, coaching is very different from athletic or personal training, nutrition consulting, or traditional therapy or counseling.

Carol Ballard, Psy.D, counselor and director of a collegiate counselor center, provides insight into the similarities and distinctions between coaching and counseling: "Coaching and counseling are allied fields that share the goal of helping clients achieve lives of greater health and fulfillment. Both counselors and coaches help clients set measurable, attainable goals. Both teach the skills necessary for achieving the goals, and both provide support and encouragement while clients work toward their goals."

A major difference is the client population. Coaches work with clients who are reasonably healthy and well-functioning and wish to augment their well-being through achieving certain personal or professional goals. Goals may be specific to wellness or performance or may be more broadly aimed at achieving greater life satisfaction through, for example, changes in career or lifestyle. The work is focused on the present and its influence on the future. The work is also typically brief and designed to accomplish the client's goals relatively quickly. "Improvement" and "enhancement" are hallmarks of coaching.

Smart coaches only choose to work with clients who are ready to change. In the initial client screening process, the fitness/wellness professional will want to be diligent about weeding out clients who really are not ready to take responsibility for their choices and actions. A successful coaching business is built around successful and enthusiastic clients.

CHAPTER 11 - SAMPLE TEST

1. What is the difference between dietetics programs and sports nutrition master degree programs? What is the legal status of each?
2. How can health professionals incorporate nutrition programs while still adhering to state licensure laws?
3. What is coaching?
4. What is the difference between coaching and counseling?
5. List the *Stages of Readiness to Change* and provide details of each stage.
6. What does the "change process" refer to?
7. What is the "SMART" rule and how is it used?

References

1. States with laws that regulate the practice of dietetics. Academy of Nutrition and Dietetics. http://www.eatright.org/HealthProfessionals/content.aspx?id=7092. (accessed 07//08/2013).
2. Comnmission on Dietetic Resigstration. State licensure. http://cdrnet.org/state-licensure. (accessed 07/08/2013).
3. Coordinated programs in dietetics. (2013). Academy of Nutrition and Dietetics. http://www.eatright.org/ACEND/content.aspx?id=74.
4. Definition of Terms. Academy of Nutrition and Dietetics. Updated 1/2013. Quality Scope of Dietetics Practice Framework Sub-Committee of the Quality Management Committee Definition of Terms List Updated 7/2011. ID=6442451086 Size=1050 KB
5. Professions and Occupations (225ILCS30) Dietetic and Nutrition Services Practice Act. http://ilga.gov/legislation/ilcs/ilcs3.asp?ActID=1297&ChapAct=225%A0ILCS %A030/&ChapterID=24&ChapterName=PROFESSIONS+AND+OCCUPATIONS&ActName=Dietetic+and+Nutrition+Services+Practice+Act. (accessed 07//08/2013).
6. CT Department of Public Health. Regulation and Licensure. Health Professionals. http://www .ct.gov/dph/cwp/view.asp?a=3115&q=468182&dphNav=| (accessed 07/08/2013).
7. Masters degree programs in sport nutrition. Education Portal. http://education-portal.com/masters_degree_sport_nutrition.html. (accessed 07/08/2013).
8. Ellsberg, M. (2012). Is the American Dietetic Association attempting to limit market competition in nutrition counseling? Forbes Magazine. http://www.forbes.com /sites/michaelellsberg/2012/04/05/american-dietetic-association/.
9. Tuma, PA. (2012). ADA Responds to Forbes. Food Management. http://food-management.com/news-amp-trends/ada-responds-forbes.
10. Lipski L. (2011). Liz Lipski's quest to practice as a nutritionist in North Carolina. http://lizappeal.com/. (accessed 07/08/2013).
11. AASDN Candidate Scope of Practice includingNational Nutrition Scope of Practice (2011). http://aasdn.org/documents/candidatehandbook.pdf.
12. Pentz J, Hauber, S. *Nutrition for Professionals.* LMA Publishing: Boston, MA. 8th ed: chapter 11. www.lifestylemanagement.com. Updated 2012.
13. Diseases & Conditions. Centers for Disease Control and Prevention. http://www.cdc.gov/diseasesconditions/az/a.html. (accessed 07/08/2013).
14. Prochaska,JO. CC DiClimente. (1984). *The transtheoretical approach: Crossing traditional boundariesof therapy.* Homewood, IL:Dow Jones/Irwin.
15. Doran, G. T. (1981). There's a S.M.A.R.T. way to write management's goals and objectives. *Management Review.* Volume 70, Issue 11(AMA FORUM), pp. 35–36.
16. Zimmer, Ben (2010-04-16). Wellness. *The New York Times.* (accessed 07/14/2013). http://www.nytimes.com/2010/04/18/magazine/18FOB-onlanguage-t.html?_r=0.
17. Definition of health related fitness – is this popular term being used correctly. (accessed 074/15/2013). http://www.sensible-health-related-fitness.com/definition-of-health-related-fitness.html.
18. Recognition of obesity as a disease. American Medical Association House of Delegates. (accessed 07/14/2013). http://media.npr.org/documents/2013/jun/ama-resolution-obesity.pdf.
19. Center for Nutrition Advocacy. Center Mission and Vision. (accessed 07/29/2013). http://nutritionadvocacy.org/about-us.
20. Frates EP, Moore MA, Lopez CN, and McMahon GT. (2011). Coaching for behavior change in physiatry. Am J Phys Med Rehabil 90: 1074–1082.

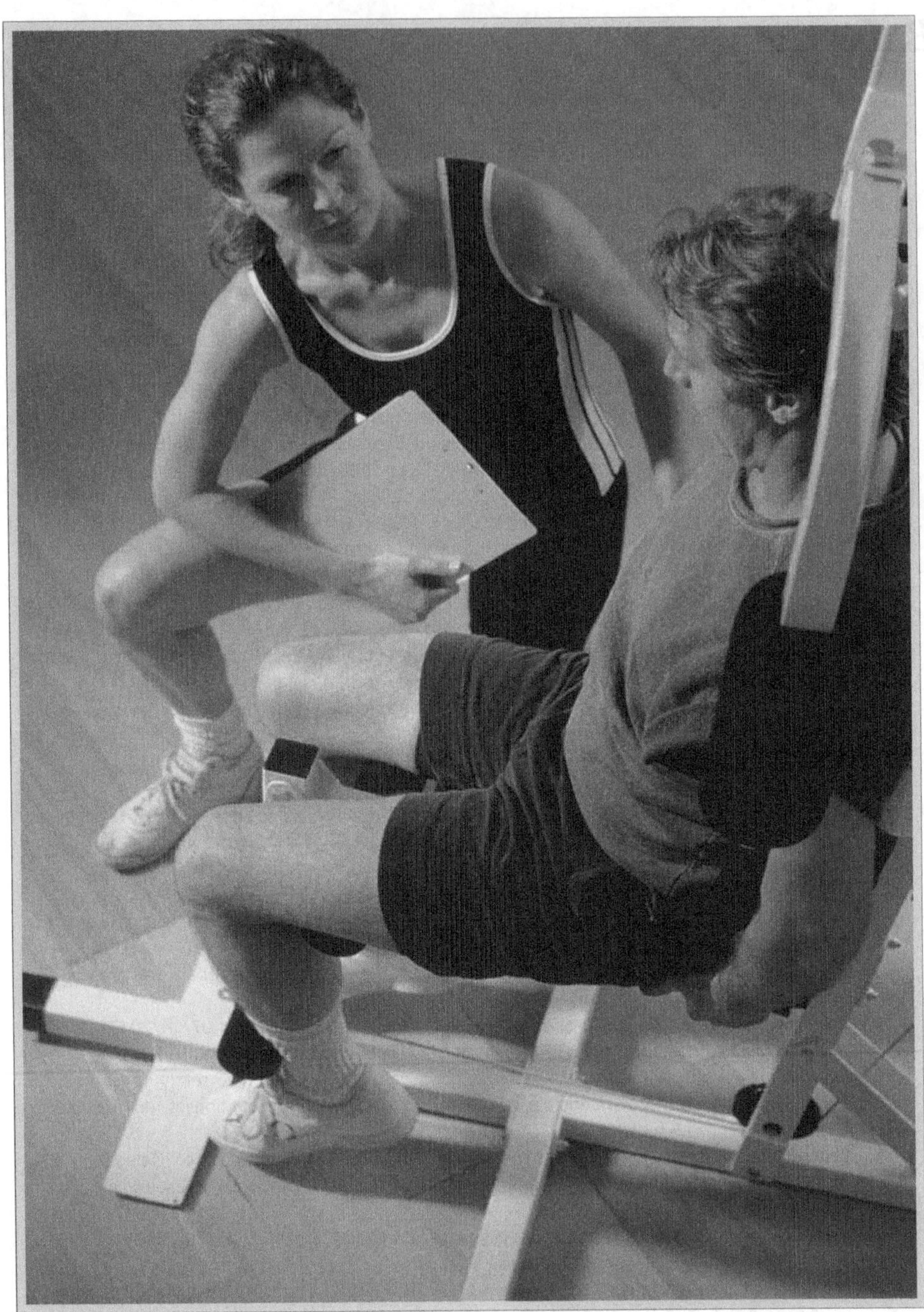

Chapter 12 - Implementing Nutrition Programs

This chapter will focus on details of how to implement a nutrition program in conjunction with a fitness/wellness program. Discussion will focus on the process of working with clients including the steps involved in implementation of an individual nutrition program; a group program; a child and teen program; a program for seniors, athletes, and vegetarians.

Objectives

After reading and studying this chapter, you should be able to:

1. Describe body composition measurements, evaluate caloric needs and list types of food intake documentation methods.
2. Discuss the components involved in the implementation of an individual nutrition program.
3. Explain the components involved in developing a group nutrition program.
4. Describe the components of a nutrition program for children and teens.
5. Discuss the components involved in developing nutrition programs for seniors, athletes, and vegetarians.
6. Explain the process by which you would deal with an obese individual.

Introduction

The challenge facing professionals today is the idea held by the public that a "quick fix" exists when it comes to health. We are bombarded with new products daily that promise to make us healthier, thinner, and more attractive. As professionals, we embark on the daunting task of convincing the "gullible" public that there is no such thing as a quick fix. Just as you can't plant a seedling in March and expect fruit in April, the public needs to understand that it's impossible to obtain fitness and wellness overnight. We need to renew the belief that moderation along with small, slow lifestyle changes are the ingredients necessary to promote health and fitness. The changes must be ones that the public can live with without feeling deprived. For example, going from whole milk to 2% milk is a much easier transition than trying to go from whole milk to skim milk. As professionals dedicated to teaching healthy lifestyles, we need to develop patience and not try to bring individuals to our level of fitness overnight.

While exercise is not a major component of this textbook, it is assumed that the reader is familiar with exercise prescription and recommendations. Building muscle and burning fat must include aerobic exercise, muscle strengthening exercise (assuming flexibility as well), and proper nutrition to fuel the body. The statement "a calorie is a calorie, etc." may be true in dieting but not in body composition change. In muscle building and fat burning, it's not only calories, but the type of calories and when those calories are eaten (in conjunction with exercise). The information contained in this chapter will produce muscle building and fat burning only if the program includes aerobic exercise, muscle strengthening exercise, proper eating, and control of catabolic factors (see Chapter 5 for more information on catabolic factors).

The following program outlines are suggestions. There are many possible variations, and we will focus our attention on one option in each category. Before attempting to implement any of the suggested programs in this chapter, be sure that you have studied previous chapters in this textbook. It is assumed that you understand the biochemistry of the energy nutrients, energy production, supplements, nutrition research, and the prerequisites involved before implementing a program.

Information in this chapter should not be used to alter a medically prescribed regimen or as a form of self treatment. Implementing any of the programs in this chapter requires working directly with a qualified, licensed professional and/or using materials developed by qualified, licensed professionals.

NOTE: As a professional, it is important to be practicing within the scope of practice and standard of professional care based on education, training, credentialing, and experience.

This is especially true with special populations and higher risk clients. This includes, but not limited to, individuals with medical conditions, pregnant women and neonates, children under the age of 2, geriatric patients, and psychiatric disorders.

Body Composition Measures

There is much confusion surrounding why measuring body composition rather than scale weight is a better way to gauge success in health and weight management. In Chapter 13, we will discuss how the scale does not indicate "size" or health. For example, two objects such as a softball and a beach ball can weigh the same but are clearly different sizes. There are several ways to measure size and health status including Body Mass Index, percent body fat, and waist to hip ratio. Body mass index is a way to judge weight in relation to height. Waist circumference and body mass index (BMI) are indirect methods to assess body composition. Percent body fat, a more direct method, can be determined in several ways. The goal of weight loss is loss of stored body fat. The most popular tool for measuring fat loss is scale weight. However, traditional scales are unable to differentiate between fat, muscle, bone or body fluid, which makes up our total body weight. If an individual has only a small amount of weight to lose, the scale may not change significantly as lean muscle mass increases and body fat decreases.

Body Mass Index

BMI, calculated from height and weight measurements, is a useful tool to measure overweight and obesity. It is an indirect, approximate estimate of body fat and an indicator of disease risk (1). The higher the BMI, the higher the risk for certain diseases such as heart disease, high blood pressure, type 2 diabetes, gallstones, breathing problems, and certain cancers (2). BMI has several limitations (2):

- It may overestimate body fat in athletes and others who have a muscular build.
- It may underestimate body fat in older persons and others who have lost muscle.

Body Mass Index Norms	
Emaciated	Less than 15
Severely Underweight	15.0 to 16.9
Underweight	17.0 to 18.9
Normal Weight	19.0 to 24.9
Overweight	25.0 to 29.9
Obese	30.0 to 39.9
Severely Obese	40.0 or more

The BMI calculation provides a figure that is sometimes difficult to interpret; but, nonetheless, important as a predictor of disease. Body Mass Index is determined by the following equation:

Body Mass Index Calculation
weight ÷ 2.2 (height (inches) x .0254)2
Example: weight is 220 pounds and height is 6 feet 4 inches step 1 - 220 ÷ 2.2 = 100 step 2 - 76 inches x .0254 = 1.93 step 3 - 1.93 x 1.93 = 3.72 step 4 - 100 ÷ 3.72 = 26.88 *Body Mass Index is 26.88 and is considered overweight*

A Body Mass Index calculator is available on line at http://fnic.nal.usda.gov/fnic/interactiveDRI/ (47,48).

Waist-to-Hip Ratio

Waist-to-hip ratio (WHR) is another index associated with disease risk (1). Measuring waist circumference helps screen for possible health risks associated with overweight and obesity (2). An increased risk of heart disease and type 2 diabetes exists in individuals with more body fat around the waist rather than the hips. A person who is not overweight but has considerable amounts of fat stored around the waist will have a greater risk for developing one of these diseases. This risk goes up with a waist size that is greater than 35 inches for women or greater than 40 inches for men (2). The waist is measured at the narrowest point, and the hips are measured at the widest point. The waist measurement is then divided by the hip measurement and the ratio determines risk. Increased risk is indicated if a female has a ratio above .8 and above .9 for a male.

Waist-to-Hip Ratio Calculation
A man has a waist of 39 inches, and a hip measurement of 40 inches. Step 1: 39 ÷ 40 = .98
This man is at increased risk for the chronic diseases mentioned above.

Percent Body Fat

There is no single ideal percentage of body fat for everyone. Levels of body fat are epidemiologically dependent on gender and age (8). Different authorities have developed different recommendations for ideal body fat percentages. The table below from the American Council on Exercise shows how average percentages differ according to specified groups and categories (9):

Description	**Women**	**Men**
Essential Fat	10-13%	2-5%
Athletes	14-20%	6-13%
Fitness	21-24%	14-17%
Average	25-31%	18-24%
Obese	32% +	25% +

Essential fat is the level below which physical and physiological health would be negatively affected. Controversy exists as to whether a particular body fat percentage is better for one's health. The leanest athletes typically compete at levels of about 6–13% for men or 14–20% for women (9).

Percentage of body fat is strongly associated with the risk of several chronic diseases, but accurate measurements are difficult (5). Too little body fat is linked to problems with healthy functioning in both men and women and can lead to problems with reproduction in women, as well as amenorrhea. Too much body fat increases the risk of many diseases, including type 2 diabetes, high blood pressure, stroke, heart disease, and certain cancers (4,5).

Percent body fat can be measured by a variety of methods such as Bioelectric Impedance Analysis, calipers, hydrostatic/underwater weighing, air displacement (Body Pod), and dual energy x-ray absorptiometry (DEXA Scan). Bioelectrical Impedance Analysis (BIA) is a relatively simple, quick, and non-invasive technique to measure body composition (3). It measures body fat accurately in controlled clinical conditions, but its performance in the field is inconsistent. Dehghan M, et al. concluded that BIA measurements validated for specific ethnic groups can accurately measure body fat in these populations, but not in others and suggest that for large epidemiological studies with diverse populations BIA may not be the appropriate choice for body composition measurement (3).

Calipers measure the subcutaneous fat underneath the skin (6). The amount of fat under the skin is correlated to total body fat using a "standard measure". There is also a margin of error associated with this method. While not totally accurate, this method offers precision, i.e., consecutive readings over months can be consistent. Peterson, et al. determined the accuracy of percent body fat estimates from seven different bioelectrical impedance analysis (BIA) models and a seven site skin fold formula (SKF) compared with air displacement. Skin fold measures were found to be the most reliable field method of estimating body composition but require more training than BIA (7).

Caloric Requirements

As mentioned before, building lean muscle tissue requires proper nutrition to fuel the body. The following tables summarize the caloric recommendations for the macronutrients (31,32):

Recommendations (40,41)	Grams/Day	Percentage of Daily Calories
Carbohydrates	130 grams for men and women	45% to 65%
Sugar	NA	Less than or equal to 10%
Total Fats	NA	20 % to 35%
Saturated and Trans Fat	NA	Limit saturated fats, keep trans fat intake as low as possible
Proteins	.8 grams to 1.8 grams	15 to 20%

Fiber Recommendations	Men (g/day)	Women (g/day)
Adults under 50 years old	38	25
Adults over 50 years old	30	21

Carbohydrates

Adults should get 45 percent to 65 percent of their daily calories from carbohydrates (31,32). Acceptable ranges for children are similar. The Recommended Dietary Allowances express recommendations in terms of grams per day - 130 grams per day for both men and women. Consensus in the field of sports nutrition has departed from calculating carbohydrate requirements as a percentage to expressing requirements as grams per kilogram (g/kg) body weight (BW) (34) while still maintaining a range of 45% to 65% of total caloric needs. The table below reiterates the recommendations by the AND, ACSM, and IOC for athletes.

AND, ACSM Carbohydrate Recommendations (33)	IOC Carbohydrate Recommendations (34)
6 to 10 g/kg BW/day.	3 to 5 g/kg BW/day, low intensity/skill-based activities;
	5 to 7 g/kg BW/day, moderate/high intensity (1 hour/day)
	6 to 10 g/kg BW/day, moderate/high intensity (1- 3 hours per day)
	4 to 7 g/kg BW/day for strength athletes
	8 to 12 g/kg BW/day, extreme commitment (4 to 5 hours per day).

Refined and added sugar intake should be kept as low as possible with a maximum of 10% of total caloric intake.

Fats

The acceptable macronutrient range for fat intake is 20 to 35% of energy (31). The fat requirements for sedentary individuals and athletes are similar but slightly higher for athletes. Intake should not decrease below 20% of total energy intake because intake of dietary fat is important for the absorption of fat-soluble vitamins and essential fatty acids (33). Intake of saturated fats should be limited and trans fat intake should be kept as low as possible (33).

Proteins

Much debate still exists concerning protein requirements. As discussed in Chapter 5, according to the recommended dietary allowance (RDA), the general protein requirement for a sedentary person is 0.8 g/kg BW/day (33,36,37). This requirement appears to suffice for general fitness and can be slightly elevated to 1.0 g/kg BW/day (36).

Dietary protein requirements are elevated with strength, speed, or endurance training (35,36). The AND and ACSM recommend daily protein requirements for strength and endurance athletes of 1.2-1.7 g/kg BW/day The IOC protein guidelines for athletes are 1.3-1.8 g/kg BW/day and 1.6-1.7 g/kg BW/day for strength-training athletes (38). Hence, the range of protein varies from .8 g/kg BW/day to 1.8 g/kg BW/day.

Estimated Energy Requirements (EER)

For reasons already discussed, we will be applying the EER calculation to estimate total energy requirements for adults. The Dietary Reference Intakes (DRI) (31) and the Dietary Guidelines (39) provide energy recommendations for men and women who are slightly active to very active. Estimated Energy Requirement (EER) is the average dietary energy intake that is predicted to maintain energy balance in healthy, normal weight individuals of a defined age, gender, weight, height, and level of physical activity consistent with good health. In children and pregnant and lactating women, the EER includes the needs associated with growth or secretion of milk at rates consistent with good health (40,41). The following table lists the EER calculations for men and women 19 years and older (weight in kilograms and height in meters).

Men 19 Years and Older
EER = [662 – (9.53 x Age)] + PA X [(15.91 x Weight) + (539.6 x Height)]
Women 19 Years and Older
EER = [354 – (6.91 x Age)] + PA X [(9.36 x Weight) + (726 x Height)]

The following table lists the physical activity (PA) factor.

Men > 19 Years (1)	Women > 19 Years	Physical Activity
Sedentary: 1.0	Sedentary: 1.0	Daily living activities
Low Active: 1.11	Low Active: 1.12	Plus 30-60 min. moderate activity
Active: 1.25	Active: 1.27	Plus >60 min. moderate activity
Very Active: 1.48	Very Active: 1.45	Plus >60 min. moderate activity and 60 min. vigorous activity or 120 min. moderate activity

Body Fat Adjusted Estimated Energy Requirements (EER)

The BMR component of EER does not take into account body composition, which includes the percentages of muscle and fat in the body. Muscle burns many more calories, while fat cells utilize much less. Leaner bodies need more calories than bodies that are less lean. Hence, a person with an above average amount of muscle will have a higher BMR than calculated and therefore a higher EER; and a person with a below average amount of muscle will have a lower BMR than calculated and therefore a lower EER (39,40). The "ideal" lean body mass is based on the ideal body fat percentage of 15% for men and 22% for women. These "factors" will be included in the final total energy expenditure calculation.

Males - Body Fat Adjusted EER
Adjusted Percent = 100% - (Actual % Body Fat – Average % Body Fat)
Body Fat Adjusted EER = EER X Adjusted percent
Example: Male that is 29 years old; 6'1" tall; weighs 190 pounds; activity level is low-active; body fat is 28% EER = 3019 calories Adjusted Percent = 100 – (28%-15%) = 87% or .87 Body Fat Adjusted EER = 3019 x .87 =2627

Females - Body Fat Adjusted EER
Adjusted Percent = 100% - (Actual % Body Fat – Average % Body Fat)
Body Fat Adjusted EER = EER X Adjusted percent
Example: Female that is 33 years old; 5'4" tall; weighs 127 pounds; activity level is low-active; body fat is 26% EER = 2057 Adjusted Percent = 100% – (26%-22%) = 96% or .96 Body Fat Adjusted EER = 2057 x .96 = 1975

See case studies at the end of this chapter for examples of how these calculations are used when when implementing a nutrition program.

Lifestyle Journal

It is important to obtain accurate lifestyle and nutrition information from clients. In this discussion the term "clients" will refer to the public at large including patients, students, etc. As discussed in detail in Chapter 11, it is illegal in most states for a non-licensed professional to complete a diet analysis for clients unless working directly with and under the guidance of a licensed professional. Wellness/fitness professionals may however legally request information about lifestyle and eating patterns. There are several ways to document eating patterns.

A diet history is created when someone recalls what they ate in the past; this method is not very accurate since it is easy for people to forget or omit certain items.

Food frequency is determined by providing a person a list of foods and asking the person how often the particular food is eaten. This form of food intake is typically used when conducting research. Individuals are asked questions such as how often do you eat strawberries in season: daily weekly, monthly, or never. As you can see, this method is not very accurate, but in research, if you see a statistically significant difference in responses, then you know you have a difference.

A diet record is a record of what is eaten throughout the day. This method requires that the client recall foods eaten previously and is not as accurate as a food log.

A Food log or a food diary consists of a person writing down everything eaten on a daily basis. You should be aware that not all persons will be completely honest. It is vital to educate the client on the importance of providing accurate information. Explain that you are trying to help this person make healthy lifestyle changes; you can't help if you are not provided with an accurate picture of the person's present lifestyle. A food log should contain the types of foods eaten, quantities eaten, time of day, mood and other factors such as participation in exercise. These last points will be especially important when trying to identify patterns of eating that must be altered. The food log also allows the fitness/wellness professional to help coach a client to incorporate practical, small changes. For success, food preferences must be incorporated into the clients menu planning. The fitness/wellness professional should make it clear that the purpose of keeping a lifestyle journal is for educational purposes and to help guide the client to come up with appropriate lifestyle changes.

Food Chart

The following food chart is an aid in estimating portion sizes. Be sure to reiterate that these estimates are not to be viewed as "what should be eaten." Estimates of portion sizes include: ½ cup of cut up fruit or grapes is the size of a light bulb; one pancake is the size of a CD, 1 cup of salad (packed) is the size of a baseball; 1 cup of pasta, rice or potatoes is the size of a fist; 1 oz. of cubed cheese is the size of 4 small dice; 1 medium fruit is the size of a tennis ball; 1 teaspoon of oil is the size of a quarter; 3 oz. of meat or fish cooked is the size of a deck of cards; ¼ cup raisins is the size of a large egg; 1 medium potato is the size of a computer mouse; 1 slice of bread is (slightly larger) than an audio cassette; and 1 oz. nuts is the size of 2 shot glasses.

In the next section, we will discuss steps involved in implementing a nutrition program for adults that have no medical conditions as defined in Chapter 11. We will then discuss implementation of group programs, children and teen programs, programs for athletes, older adults, and vegetarians. As a reminder exercise must be a component of all programs; building muscle and burning fat must include aerobic exercise, muscle strengthening exercise (assuming flexibility as well), and proper nutrition to fuel the body.

You Are What You Eat . . .
Are Your Portion Sizes Too Much?

Living a healthy lifestyle involves making the right choices about food, exercise and other daily activities. Americans are waging a war against an epidemic of obesity, partly due to eating too much food. Over half of the adults in the United States are overweight or obese—and today, obesity in children is rapidly becoming a major health crisis. Heart disease, type 2 diabetes and some types of cancers are just a few of the health risks associated with being overweight. Choosing healthier foods in the right proportion and exercising regularly can make a difference in your quality of life. Here are some easy ways to help you understand serving sizes.

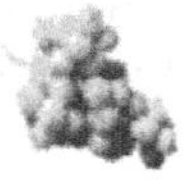
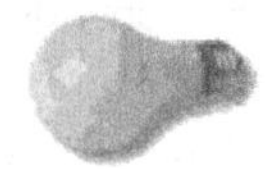

1/2 cup of grapes = light bulb

SERVING SIZE SAME SIZE AS

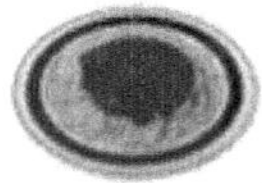
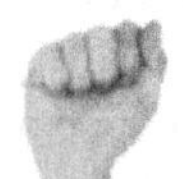

1 cup of pasta, rice or potatoes = fist

SERVING SIZE SAME SIZE AS

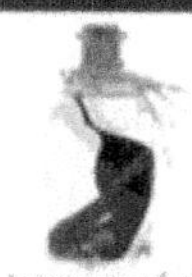
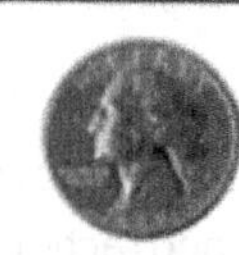

1 teaspoon of oil or mayo = quarter

SERVING SIZE SAME SIZE AS

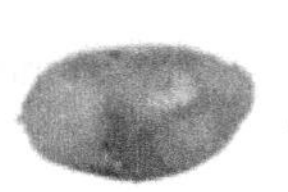
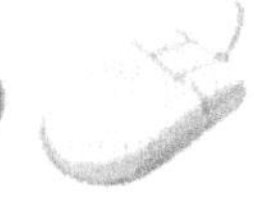

1 medium potato = computer mouse

SERVING SIZE SAME SIZE AS

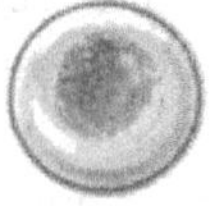
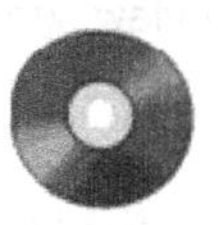

1 pancake = compact disc

SERVING SIZE SAME SIZE AS

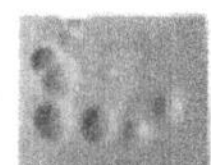
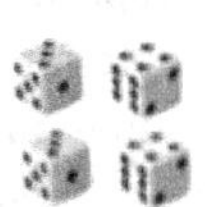

1 oz. of cubed cheese = 4 dice

SERVING SIZE SAME SIZE AS

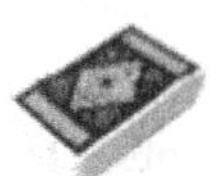

3 oz. of cooked meat, fish, or poultry = deck of cards

SERVING SIZE SAME SIZE AS

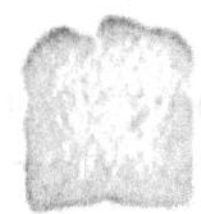
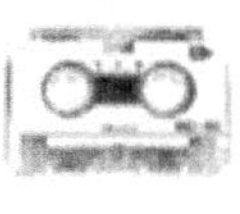

1 slice of bread = audiocassette

SERVING SIZE SAME SIZE AS

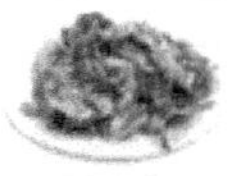
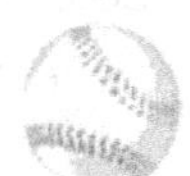

1 cup of green salad = baseball

SERVING SIZE SAME SIZE AS

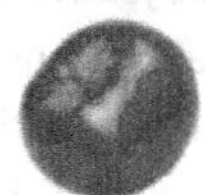
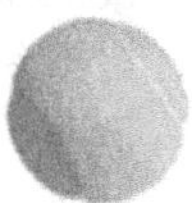

1 medium fruit = tennis ball

SERVING SIZE SAME SIZE AS

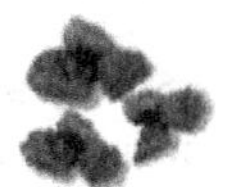

1/4 cup of raisins = large egg

SERVING SIZE SAME SIZE AS

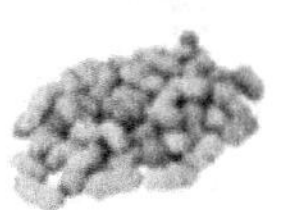
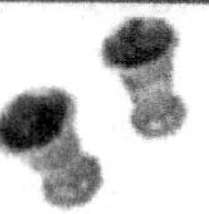

1 oz. nuts = 2 shot glasses full

Individual Program

The following information summarizes the steps involved in the implementation of an individual nutrition program.

- Interview. This step includes determining the "Stage of Readiness to Change"; describing and selling your program; receiving payment; instructions for first appointment and setting a date for the first appointment
- First appointment. This step includes signing agreements (if not signed during the interview); completing a client profile; assisting the client in setting goals and objectives; completing body composition measurements; instructing the client on how to keep a lifestyle journal; and providing the client with a hand out (educational sheet); meeting wrap up and date for next appointment.
- Before next appointment. Determine body composition measures, estimated energy requirements (EER), and appropriate menu plan.
- Second appointment. Review goals and objectives; provide EER and body composition results; using coaching skills, assist the client in setting one or two goals; provide a hand out (educational sheet) and menu plan; wrap up the meeting; and set a date for the next appointment.
- Third appointment. Review goals and objectives and lifestyle journal; set new goals and objectives, if appropriate; provide a hand out (educational sheet); wrap up the meeting; and set a date for the next appointment.
- Follow up sessions. Follow same outline as in the third appointment.
- Ending a program. Determine when the client is ready to move on.

Interview

The first step in instituting a nutrition program is to set up a preliminary interview (15 minutes) with all potential clients. This can be done in person or over the phone. The goal as a coach is to work with clients in the preparation and action phases, support clients in maintenance, and help clients through any times of relapse. This interview is designed to determine the client's stage of change.

The section on coaching described methods to determine the client's stage of change. In review, one way to test the "Stage of Readiness to Change" is by questioning. Examples of questions include:

1. How can I help you?
2. What do you hope to accomplish in working with me/this program?
3. On a scale of 1 to 10, how confident are you in your ability to make positive lifestyle changes?
4. What will changing do for you; what will happen if you don't change?

Trying to work with individuals in the precontemplative stage will only cause frustration and can actually induce failure on the part of the client. It's important to understand that some individuals are not ready to make lifestyle changes. As much as we wish we could "save everyone", we cannot. The role of the fitness/wellness professional during the interview is to identify which individuals are ready and which are NOT ready to make lifestyle changes.

Watch for excuses! Potential clients in the precontemplation stage do not take responsibility but rather provide lots of excuses concerning their lack of success. If you "hear the blame game," this potential client is not a good candidate. You can feel comfortable saying to this person, "I hear you are frustrated with your situation, but unless you can take the responsibility for your current choices and situation, I can't help you. Can you tell me what you can do to change your current situation to make it better for your health?" Then let the person think about it. If the person comes up with some solid answers that reveal the desire for personal change then there is a glimmer of hope. It is also important to recognize with individuals that are not ready to change that sometimes they are simply looking for someone else to blame for their inability to live a healthier lifestyle. In working with a client that is not ready to change, he or she may likely attempt to blame you as the coach for their lack of success.

If a potential client is in the precontemplation stage, the next course of action is to explain that your program may not be the best program for him/her. If this individual is thinking about making changes or is ready to make changes, the interview then becomes your chance to convince him/her that nutrition is a large component to success in body composition change.

It is important to note here that many individuals believe they know what to eat. They are convinced that they are not successful because they do not have the willpower to follow through. However, the truth of the matter is most individuals do not know what to eat. Quizzing the individual on his or her knowledge of nutrition will quickly make the individual aware that he/she does not understand how to fuel the body properly to optimize muscle building and fat burning. The following questions are helpful in understanding how much the person does or does not know about the basics of body composition change and the importance of nutrition:

1. Can you list several dietary sources of protein?
2. Do you know what types of fat in the diet are stored as fat in fat cells?
3. Can you list several food sources of essential fats?
4. Do you know what the consequences are of not consuming enough carbohydrates on a daily basis?
5. Do you know how many servings of fruits and vegetables should be consumed

every day?

6. Do you know how much water you should drink daily?

The next component of the interview is to describe your services in detail. What can the client expect from you, and what will his/her responsibilities be? You will want to provide details concerning your program, such as the cost of the program, the length of the program, services you will provide, etc.

It's important to note that many individuals in the fitness/wellness profession do not perceive themselves as sales people; but in a very real sense they are. They are selling the most valuable commodity there is in life - health.

Once the individual signs up for your program, the rest of the interview consists of receiving payment, having the new client sign a legal agreement, a responsibility clause, and discussing preparations for the first appointment.

Receiving payment is absolutely essential. Payment must be received before the first appointment and it is also important to have a cancellation policy. A belief has been fostered that requesting payment somehow diminishes "dedication" to the profession. This is absolutely false. There are several important reasons to never work for "free." First, a financial commitment on the part of the client produces accountability. Second, if fitness professionals do not charge (and charge a substantial amount) for their services, they will not be perceived as professional. It is a known fact in business that the higher the cost for a product/service the greater the perceived value. To be perceived as an expert, fitness professionals must charge industry rates. It is also important to have a cancellation policy.

If a fitness professional has a hard time asking for money, the process can be scripted. An example of such a script might consist of the following: "Great - I believe we will work well together. So how would you like to pay for the program? We accept credit cards, cash, and check." If a potential client says he/she does not have the money, the script may continue: "Oh darn, that's too bad. I do believe this program would be a great fit for you. As soon as you do have the money, let me know, and we will set up an appointment." Or you can go through the questioning process and point out that it may not be a matter of finances, but a matter of priorities. In either case, professionals need to write their own "script".

By the end of the interview (or before the first appointment), you should have obtained a clearance form to exercise, a physician's approval if necessary, and a legal agreement. The client must also sign a "responsibility" agreement. At this point in the interview, the client should be aware that responsibility for success rests with him/her. This must be emphasized and clearly stated at the beginning of the program. The client should read the agreement out loud then sign the agreement. The fitness/wellness professional must then sign the agreement, as well. Keep in mind that as the fitness/wellness professional you are not responsible for success or failure. Responsibility rests with the client.

The final component of the interview is to provide the client with details concerning what to expect during the first appointment: completion of a comprehensive client profile sheet; assistance in goal setting; completion of baseline body composition measurements and instruction on how to complete a lifestyle journal. You'll want to describe the body composition measures that will be done, reasons for taking the measurements, and details of how to dress, etc. Lastly, be sure to set the outline and time expectation of the first and following appointments. It is very easy for a client to bombard you with questions and monopolize your time. As a professional, you likely have a schedule to keep, and it is much easier to stick to the schedule when upfront about the expectations with the client.

First Appointment

If not completed during the initial interview the client must sign a clearance form to exercise, a physician's approval if necessary, a legal agreement, and a responsibility agreement. At this point in the interview, the client should be aware that responsibility for success rests with him/her. This must be emphasized and clearly stated at the beginning of the program. If not already done, the client should read the agreement out loud then sign the agreement. The fitness/wellness professional must then sign the agreement as well.

Responsibility Agreement

Welcome to ____. The next ________weeks are crucial to ensuring your success in lifelong weight management. Please make this program your top priority. Many obstacles to your success will undoubtedly crop up in the next few weeks. Don't let these obstacles stand in your way. Be aware that you will probably go through several psychological stages during your program. We will ask you to determine what causes you to overeat and/or what prevents you from exercising. In some cases, eating issues are a cover up for other more deep rooted problems. During your program you must continuously ask yourself if the changes you are making are lifestyle changes - changes you can live with the rest of your life without feeling deprived or stressed. If these changes are difficult and "unpleasant", then we must "talk". We will work with you to make this program the "beginning of the rest of your life". We will also be asking you to periodically keep a food log of everything you eat. A food log can actually decrease your obsession with food. Remember, the only way we can help you is if we have all the facts. We are here to educate, motivate, and support you, not to judge you.

We, the staff of ____________ are at your disposal to help ease you into lifestyle transitions. However, you must do all the work. Therefore, we ask that you read the agreement below carefully, and sign only if you are in complete agreement:

I ________________________ agree to follow the exercise program as prescribed in our sessions; I ________________________ also agree to make changes in my eating patterns as agreed upon.

The next step after signing and completing the agreements is to collect pertinent data on the client which can be classified into the following categories: demographics, personal history, physical activity history, weight history, eating patterns/eating issues, stress levels, goals, and objectives.

Demographics refers to information such as name, address, telephone number, etc. Personal history refers to information such as age, gender, height, weight, smoking history, body composition, and other lifestyle variables. Information concerning weight history is included in the personal history section and is valuable in providing information concerning large weight fluctuations and any possible eating disorders. Clients with large weight fluctuations – also known as yo-yo dieters— will have a much harder time with body composition change. Yo-yo dieting leads to loss of muscle mass and the addition of fat stores. These individuals have low metabolism. It's best not to make comments on any of the information the client provides you at this time. Ask questions, yes, but don't give opinions or make judgments. Remember, weight history is a delicate issue for most people. Let your clients answer honestly in a non-judgmental atmosphere. You will approach each "red flag" in a very supportive manner in future appointments.

As previously discussed, stress is catabolic, and in order to maintain health, stress must be controlled. Hence, it is critical to obtain information concerning the client's perceived stress levels. On a scale of 1 to 10, with 10 being high, ask the client what his/her stress levels are at home and at work. Stress levels 7 or above indicate a possible catabolic response is occurring in the body. While we are not experts on stress reduction, we can provide clients details concerning health implications associated with high stress levels.

A physical activity or exercise questionnaire should provide all the information necessary to prescribe a safe and effective exercise program. It should provide detailed information concerning past exercise, any injuries due to exercise, and current exercise habits.

Medical and disease history refers to questions concerning past and present health issues. There are many forms and variations of health history questionnaires. The most commonly used form is known as the Par-Q. Refer to your exercise manuals for a copy of a health history questionnaire, or combine the best features of a few forms to create your own. Also see "Client Profile" in the case studies at the end of this chapter.

Another important component of a client's profile deals with dietary history which addresses eating patterns and food issues. It is important to learn whether your client eats when depressed or stressed; this can be indicative of an emotional eating pattern. If a client admits that he/she eats when depressed, you can advise him/her to keep track of this in the journal, and you will discuss possible solutions. Another critical component is addressing whether or not the individual believes he or she has, or has ever had, an eating disorder. If a possible eating disorder is present, you must refer this individual to your licensed dietitian and a mental health profession specializing in eating disorders. If you suspect that the client may have needs that exceed your scope, an easy question to ask is "are you open to meeting with someone who has more experience or expertise in this area?" If so, "I have someone I can refer you to. His/ her name is ...."

Once the client profile is complete, the next step is to assist the client in setting several goals and objectives that can be accomplished in a prescribed time period. It is important to set realistic goals utilizing coaching skills. Be sure to review the section in Chapter 11 on setting effective goals and objectives. Once several goals and objectives have been agreed upon they can be listed in the client profile. You will also want to indicate the client's "Stage of Readiness to Change" on the client profile sheet.

In order to obtain an accurate picture of your client's disease risk, you will want to perform the three body composition measures previously discussed (BMI, waist to hip ratio, percent body fat) during your first appointment, and document the results on the client profile sheet. You may choose NOT to provide all three results to the client, but they are nonetheless important for your records. You'll want to explain to the client at this time what it is you will be doing with the information that has been collected. You can also reveal that you will be doing your own homework before the next session. Using the body composition numbers and the client's profile sheet, you will be determining estimated energy requirements (EER). You will return to the second appointment armed with a pre-approved menu plan for someone in your client's particular caloric range as determined by the estimated energy requirements.

You will want to provide the client with a lifestyle journal and provide instructions on how to complete the journal. You can reiterate that you are BOTH highly invested in your client's success, and that while you understand that keeping a journal can be a time consuming and daunting task, it is a valuable tool in promoting success. Explain that you will use the information from the journal in establishing future goals and objectives.

If time allows, you may want to include a one day food recall (documented in the client profile) to obtain an initial "picture" of the client's eating patterns. Depending on the discussion during this meeting, you will want to provide the client with an educational sheet. For example, if the client indicates that he/she is highly "stressed," you will want to give him/her an educational sheet on how to decrease stress. You can wrap up the session by setting up a date for the next appointment.

Before the Next Appointment

With the information you collected in the first session, you'll want to enter the body composition results on the "DRI results sheet" (see case studies). Using the online calculator at http://fnic.nal.usda.gov/fnic/interactiveDRI/, you will want to enter the client's information and either print the results from the website or enter the results using your own documents. Take a few minutes to review the client's profile sheet, body composition results, and the estimated energy requirements and make some notes regarding issues you think might deserve discussion. You will also want to choose an appropriate and corresponding caloric menu plan.

Second Appointment

At the beginning of the second appointment, you will want to collect the client's lifestyle journal and give it a quick look. Did the client exercise? Did the client write down what he/she ate? Ask the client how the process was for him/her, and if he/she has any specific questions about keeping a journal. Are there a few small issues you see right away from the journal that deserve mention?

If you did your homework, you will be armed with the client's body composition measures, EER, and the appropriate, corresponding menu plan. Take some time to go over these results, and perhaps draw on the lifestyle journal. Compare and contrast the menu plan with the lifestyle journal. Typically, clients are surprised at the estimated energy requirements. Any discussion here is good, as it gets the client thinking about making changes. Remember not to make value judgments; just listen and state facts.

Discuss previous goals set in the first appointment. Was the client able to complete the goals and objectives that were set? If not, use coaching skills to discuss what happened. This is a crucial point. When you begin coaching nutrition clients, their actions must be their choice, not yours! You can make recommendations, of course, but no goal will be achieved unless it is the client's chosen goal. You'll need to use your fitness knowledge and give your client an honest appraisal of achievable goals. Remember in this session ask questions: "Would you like more information on that topic? How could we make that goal more achievable? What are some action steps you could make to attain that goal? How realistic to think this goal is to achieve in this time frame?"

Are the chosen goals too far out of reach for the chosen time frame? Remember, it's better to start small and set long term, larger goals as the client moves through the program. The client will not need to keep a lifestyle journal, but you might explain the benefits of continuing to keep a journal. It's a good idea to explain that this process is time intensive but provides a means of ensuring success.

Wrap up the meeting by providing the client with an educational sheet, and set up a time for the next appointment.

Third Appointment

In the third appointment, you will want to continue the process of reviewing the lifestyle journal (if completed), and discuss previous goals and objectives. Ask the client about his/her SMART goals at this time, and help make sure they meet all the requirements. If they don't meet the criteria, assist the client to include the missing components. Above all, make sure the goals are realistic. Even if you want your client to stop drinking a 6-pack of beer a night, if he/she says, "I guess I could drink light beer instead this week," go with it! The client is changing and will change at a pace that is right for him/her. You made a recommendation to, "Look at alcohol content because it contributes to empty calories." The client grasped the severity of that comment and chose the goal.

Always conclude a session with the following: a fresh set of SMART goals to be achieved before the the next appointment; an educational sheet on a relevant topic; and set a date for the next appointment.

Follow-up Appointments

Each session from here on out will include a discussion of the goals set at the previous appointment and how the client fared. You can introduce other topics that you feel the client might be ready to tackle, and you can use the approved educational handouts. Your main goal with each session is to ensure that the client understands that he/she is making progress every week and that lifestyle change is a SLOW process. You'll have to use every ounce of compassion and every bit of knowledge to help the client understand that he/she can't lose 6 sizes in 4 weeks. Always focus on the positive changes the client is making, and reflect on how far he/she has come already just by signing up for a program such as yours.

Note that the first 3 sessions include a lot of background work. It's very important to spend those first 3 sessions really getting into the nitty gritty of a client's history, specific measurements, and goals, so that your program will be built on a strong foundation. You've got to spend those first 3 sessions really figuring out what that client has come to you for and how your work together can help change his/her life. The rest of your sessions from then on can be "more relaxed".

Ending a Program

Once your client is satisfied with his/her own efficacy in regard to lifestyle change, begins to set SMART goals, and understands the steps needed to continue, it's your job to ask if the client is ready to move on without your help. If the client no longer needs your guidance and is ready to go it alone, you've done your job! Ask the client for feedback about the program. Giving clients a pre-written questionnaire is always a great idea. Use open-ended questions, such as "What parts of your program did you find the most helpful?" and "Was there anything you had hoped to learn during your program that you did not get to explore? If so, what?" This way, the client provides invaluable help as you fine-tune your programs and services.

Group Program

Group programs offer an added benefit of interaction with other individuals with similar goals. This can be seen from the success of groups such as Weight Watchers. Fitness professionals can build on this concept by providing an exercise prescription and more detailed nutrition information. It is important to structure a group program that includes a "curriculum" with learning objectives. A curriculum ensures that participants will complete the program with a new level of acquired information.

Informational Meeting

An informational meeting is an excellent way to get the word out about your group program. You will want to advertise the program in such a way as to "provide something for free" such as a "lecture on why dieting doesn't work"! Groups should be formed with common goals. For example, everyone in the group does the cooking, or grocery shopping, or wants to lose weight, etc. Once your chosen group is established, the group program should include discussion of goals and objectives, exercise regimen, and how to keep a food log.

Be sure to have your advertising materials, business card, and a sign up sheet ready at the beginning of the informational meeting. Begin the meeting by introducing yourself (see Keys to A Successful Class on the next page) and describing the program. Include the date and time of the weekly sessions and clearly specify the commitments required of participants: attend all meetings, commit to an exercise program, keep a lifestyle journal, etc. Explain that the program requires a commitment "to change" on their part. Be sure to explain that all attendees will receive a follow up phone call. This is a critical component. All attendees must be contacted. For those individuals not chosen explain the reason for their non-acceptance (class is filled, not willing to exercise, not willing to remove problem foods from the home). Also critical is to offer non-chosen attendees other options. This may include a discounted membership to an exercise facility; possibly a one-on-one program; discounted personal training session; or a referral to a sports dietitian, etc.

Design a ten minute presentation on why diets don't work (Chapter 13). Provide details on why dieting doesn't work and has never worked (see section on diets). Display a hard ball and beach ball, and explain that both balls weigh the same.

Allow time for questions and answers. Don't worry if you don't know all the answers. Let participants know that you work directly with a qualified/licensed professional that can answer questions (through you).

It's impossible to address each participant's individual concerns during a group program, so it works best to choose a topic based on participant interest or need. Successful programs can include as many meetings as needed for participants to become successful in making lifestyle changes. A simple solution to help stay on track when in a group setting is to create a "parking lot". On a white board or flip chart, keep a list of topics or questions that come up but are too off topic and steer away from your planned curriculum. You can state that you will come back to these items if there is time, or you will discuss after the class is over.

Group meetings should contain similar topics as individual programs. In a pilot program completed by Lifestyle Management Associates, the group program consisted of 8 sessions. At the end of the 8 week program, participants were invited to return in 4 weeks for a free body composition analysis. During these follow up appointments participants were offered options for continued support: individual consultations, another group program, weekly meetings, etc. The program was very successful in that all participants indicated that they had learned everything they needed to know about a healthy eating program centered on food preferences.

Keys to a Successful Class

Below are some keys to implementing a successful class include:

1. Create a non-threatening environment. It takes courage to attend an informational meeting. Many individuals, if not most, have failed many times at weight management. Be sure your meetings are situated in a non-threatening environment. Having a meeting in the middle of a workout area, with lots of "fit" people in skimpy outfits is very threatening to overweight and inactive people.
2. Take Charge. Help make individuals comfortable by introducing yourself. Humor is always a great way to make people feel comfortable. Be sure your comments are humorous to everyone. Ask questions. People like to talk about themselves. Keep the questions light (so what do you do; do you live close by; are you a member here, etc.). Be sure not to allow any one individual to

monopolize the conversation.

3. Positive Attitude. One of the greatest assets you can bring to the group is a positive attitude. Always maximize the positive, and "eliminate the negative".
4. Welcome each participant. It is important to be sure that you specifically welcome everyone to the informational meeting. Let them know that you appreciate their taking time from their busy schedules to attend. Have each individual introduce themselves. This is also a great time to ask light questions.
5. Remember names. People always feel special when someone remembers their name. As people introduce themselves, jot down notes to help you remember their names. Along with remembering names, it is also important to jot down something that the person has said about themselves. This is also a great way to remember names.
6. Working with individuals. Even though you are facilitating a group program, the program is made up of individuals with very different reasons for attending and very different needs.
7. Learn to listen. We so often feel like we have to do all the talking. After all, we're the teachers. But listening is even more important. Through careful listening, you can learn and understand each person's needs.
8. Show empathy. Empathy is defined as "understanding of another's feelings." While you may not have the same experiences as participants, there is always "commonality" of experiences. Dr. Pentz describes that as an obese child she could empathize with anyone that is overweight or obese. While she never had an eating disorder, she can empathize about poor body image, etc. This will also help build rapport.
9. Remember to coach. Your role in this program is that of educator and coach. Coaching is a co- creative partnership between a qualified coach and a willing client that supports the client through desired life changes. In other words, you don't tell people what needs to be changed, you assist them in discovering what needs to be changed. See section on coaching for further details.
10. Recruit volunteers. Group programs provide a great opportunity to ask for volunteers to help with future programs.

Follow Up

Upon completion of the program, it is important to provide follow up options for participants. Participants can be invited back for a follow up body composition analysis. Follow up options can include: one-on-one consultations; another group program; weekly meeting with other program graduates; personal training; etc.

Child and Teen Program

For the first time in history, children will have shorter and less healthy lives than their parents, and all fitness/wellness professionals are strongly encouraged to include children and teens in their programs. Before listing the steps involved in implementing a nutrition program with children and teens, we will discuss: obesity rates and associated conditions; the definition of overweight and obesity; how to determine caloric needs for children; recommended number and size of servings of the 5 food groups; and the AASDN star-associated food rating system.

Childhood Obesity Rates and Associated Conditions

Globally, an estimated 43 million preschool children (under age 5) were overweight or obese in 2010, a 60 percent increase since 1990 (20). The problem affects countries rich and poor and by sheer numbers places the greatest burden on the poorest. Of the world's 43 million overweight and obese preschoolers, 35 million live in developing countries. By 2020, if the current epidemic continues unabated, 9 percent of all preschoolers will be overweight or obese—nearly 60 million children (20).

Obesity increases a child's risk of numerous health problems and can create emotional and social issues. Obese children are also more likely to be obese as adults, increasing their risk of serious health problems such as heart disease and stroke (21-26).

Some health problems are much more likely to affect obese children than non-obese children such as (21-26):

- Asthma, especially severe asthma
- Diabetes, type 2
- High blood pressure
- High cholesterol
- Heart failure
- Liver problems ("fatty liver")
- Bone and joint problems in the lower body
- Growth abnormalities
- Emotional and social problems
- Breathing problems such as sleep apnea
- Rashes or fungal infections of the skin, acne

Diabetes is one of the most common chronic diseases in children and adolescents affecting about 151,000 people below the age of 20 years (27).

Obesity and the form of diabetes linked to it (Type 2) are taking an even worse toll on America's children than medical experts had realized (27). A new study indicates that the disease progresses more rapidly in children than in adults and is harder to treat. "It's frightening how severe this disease is in children," said Dr. David M. Nathan, an author of the study (27). Why the disease is so hard to control in children and teenagers is not known. The researchers said that rapid growth and the intense hormonal changes at puberty might play a role (27). Clearly, today's younger generation faces serious health consequences due to obesity.

Defining Childhood Obesity

As with adults, Body Mass Index (BMI) is a number calculated from a child's weight and height and is a reliable indicator of body fatness for most children and teens. It does not measure body fat directly, but research has shown that it correlates to measures of body fat. Additionally, BMI is an inexpensive and easy-to-perform method of screening for weight categories that may lead to health problems (28).

After BMI is calculated for children and teens, the BMI number is plotted on the CDC BMI-for-age growth charts (for either girls or boys) to obtain a percentile ranking. Percentiles are the most commonly used indicator to assess the size and growth patterns of individual children in the United States (29). The percentile indicates the relative position of the child's BMI number among children of the same gender and age.

The BMI-for-age percentile is used to interpret the BMI number because BMI is both age- and gender-specific for children and teens. These criteria are different from those used to interpret BMI for adults — which do not take into account age or gender. Age and gender are considered for children and teens for two reasons:

- The amount of body fat changes with age. (BMI for children and teens is often referred to as BMI-for-age.)
- The amount of body fat differs between girls and boys. The CDC BMI-for-age growth charts for girls and boys take into account these differences and allow translation of a BMI number into a percentile for a child's or teen's gender and age.

BMI-for-age weight status categories and the corresponding percentiles are shown in the following table (29).

Weight Status Category	Percentile Range
Underweight	Less than the 5th percentile
Healthy weight	5th percentile to less than the 85th percentile

Weight Status Category	Percentile Range
Overweight	85th to less than the 95th percentile
Obese	Equal to or greater than the 95th percentile

Child and Teen Caloric Needs

Caloric requirements for children vary according to the rate at which they burn calories, gender, and age. Average calorie needs increase as a child ages, with peak number of calories between 2,200 and 3,000 daily calories during adolescence. The "Merck Manuals" (also known as *The Merck Manual of Diagnosis and Therapy)* list nutritional needs for infants and children using a formula of calories per pound of body weight (42).

Babies and Toddlers

The "Merck Manuals" suggested required daily calories formula for an infant equals 50 to 55 calories per pound (kcal/lb) up to 6 months of age and then drops to 45 kcal/lb at one years old (42). One year olds generally need about 850 calories each day. During infancy and into the toddler years, around age 3, calorie requirements are the same for boys and girls (42). Children between the ages of 1 and 3 consume roughly 1,300 calories daily (42). Please note, working with toddlers under 2 years old is beyond the scope of practice for all AASDN Nutrition Specialists.

4 to 8 Years Old

Starting as early as 4 years old, children's caloric requirements may differ according to their gender (43). Boys typically require a higher calorie intake than girls, as reported by the National Heart, Lung and Blood Institute (NHLBI), but each child's needs vary according to activity level (43). The NHBLI estimates that 4 to 8 year-old boys require between 1,400 and 2,000 daily calories while girls need approximately 200 calories less than boys for each developmental stage and activity level (43).

The NHLBI defines "active" as performing the equivalent of walking at least three miles a day, at a rate of 3 to 4 miles per hour (43). At this age, "active" may include running around at recess, participating in physical education at a high effort level. Sedentary is classified as being involved in "day to day" activities, such as eating, going to school and going through a typical daily schedule with not a lot of extra activity.

9 to 13 Years Old

The "tween" age, between 9 and 13, is a time for growing and approaching puberty. Children in this age group continue to require large numbers of calories to support their growth and sustain their body weight. The NHLBI recommendations for caloric intake for 9 to 13 year-old boys are between 1,800 to 2,600 calories, with more active boys requiring more calories (43). Girls in this age group generally need to consume 1,600 to 2,000 daily calories.

Teenagers

The USDA Dietary Guidelines for Americans show that children hit their peak in terms of caloric requirements in their teen years between the ages of 14 and 18 years old (44). Children in this age group are typically active with sports and approach their full height. Boys who are more sedentary may only need to consume 2,200 to 2,400. Girls with a less active lifestyle typically require 1,800 to 2,000 calories daily. Boys that function at a high activity level during their teen years usually require between 2,800 and 3,200 calories daily, with girls close behind in the 2,400 calorie range. The "Merck Manuals" uses a formulation of 20 kcal/lb when determining caloric requirements for middle teens, around 15 years of age (42).

Serving Sizes

Below is a list of recommended serving sizes from the 5 food groups taken from ChooseMyPlate.gov.

Grains
1 slice bread, waffle or pancake (1 ounce equivalent)
½ cup cooked oatmeal (1 ounce equivalent)
½ bagel, hamburger bun, or English muffin (1 ounce equivalent)
½ cup cooked rice, pasta or cereal (1 ounce equivalent)
1 cup ready to eat cereal (1 ounce equivalent)
Vegetables
¾ cup (6 fluid ounces) 100% vegetable juice
1 cup raw, leafy vegetables or salad
½ cup cooked or canned vegetables
Fruits
1 medium apple, orange or banana
½ cup fruit (canned, cooked or raw)
½ cup (4 fluid ounces) 100% fruit juice
¼ cup dried fruit (raisins, apricots or prunes)
Milk
1 cup milk or yogurt
2 ounces processed cheese (American)
1 ½ ounces natural cheese (cheddar)
Meat and Beans

1 tablespoon of peanut butter counts as 1 ounce
¼ cup nuts or 20-24 almonds
1 medium size egg
2-3 ounces of poultry, meat or fish (2-3 servings)
¼ cup of beans

The following table lists the number of servings per day based on age for each of the 5 groups (reprinted from ChooseMyPlate.gov).

	Servings /Day	**One Serving 1- 3 years**	**One Serving 4-5 years**	**One Serving 6-12 years**	**One Serving 12 years - adults**
Grains	5 or less	½ slice or ¼cup	½ slice or 1/3 cup	1 slice or ½ cup	1 slice or ½ cup
Vegetables	3 to 5	¼ cup	1/3 cup	½ cup	½ cup
Fruits	2 to 4	¼ cup	1/3 cup	½ cup	½ cup
Dairy	2 to 3	½ cup	¾ cup	1 cup	1 cup
Meat/Bean/Nuts	2 to 3	1 oz or ¼ cup	1 ½ oz or 1/3 cup	2 oz or ½ cup	2 to 3 oz or ½ cup

Calories	**1000**	**1200**	**1400**	**1600**	**1800**	**2000**
Grains	3 oz eq	4 oz eq	5 oz eq	5 oz eq	6 oz eq	6 oz eq
Vegetables	1 cup	1 ½ cups	1 ½ cups	2 cups	2 ½ cups	2 ½ cups
Fruits	1 cup	1 cup	1 ½ cups	1 ½ cups	1 ½ cups	2 cups
Dairy	2 cups	2 cups	2 cups	3 cups	3 cups	3 cups
Meat/Bean/Nuts	2 oz eq	3 oz eq	4 oz eq	5 oz eq	5 oz eq	5 ½ oz eq

Calories	**2200**	**2400**	**2600**	**2800**	**3000**	**3200**
Grains	7 oz eq	8 oz eq	9 oz eq	10 oz eq	10 oz eq	10 oz eq
Vegetables	3 cups	3 cups	3 ½ cups	3 ½ cups	4 cups	4 cups
Fruits	2 cups	2 cups	2 cups	2 ½ cups	2 ½ cups	2 ½ cups
Dairy	3 cups	3 cups	3 cups	3 cups	3 cups	3 cups
Meat/Bean/Nuts	6 oz eq	6 ½ oz eq	6 ½ oz eq	7 oz eq	7 oz eq	7 oz eq

Motivating Children–AASDN Star Associated Food Rating System

In January of 2012, for the first time in 15 years, the USDA issued new guidelines for school lunches (45). These new guidelines increase offerings of fruits, vegetables and whole grain-rich foods. AASDN supports these efforts through development of colorful, interactive tools aimed at educating, inspiring, and motivating children to make healthy eating choices.

The star-associated food rating system developed by AASDN is implemented through the use of placemats. The *AASDN Placemats*™ incorporate a "star" associated food rating system on the front side of the placemats. Foods are rated according to their nutritional value: 5 stars (Gold) – best choices, 4 stars (Green) - good choices, 3 stars (Blue) – OK choices, 2 stars (Red) – less healthy choices, and 0 stars (Grey) – avoid these choices. The first placemat developed was the "Shoot for 20 Stars Day" placemat. On November 2nd 2012, almost 3000 children across the country participated in our first "Shoot for 20 Stars Day" utilizing this placemat. This first Initiative produced data indicating that the participating children consumed more fruits, vegetables, and whole grains as a direct response to the AASDN Placemat. The exciting results of the 2012 NSLAI Initiative led to the creation of a collaborative research project with The University of South Florida. The purpose of the project is to determine the impact of the AASDN placemat on the fruit and vegetable intake of 2nd grade school age children.

AASDN has developed three colorful, laminated, star-associated food tracking placemats to meet the needs of all educational settings. These laminated, reusable interactive placemats allow children to use enclosed washable markers to color in stars and reward themselves for good decision making!

Steps Involved in Implementing a Child and Teen Program

Step 1 – Stage or Readiness to Change.

As with adults, the first step in instituting a nutrition program is to set up a preliminary interview (15 minutes). It is especially important to ascertain as to whether or not the child/teen is "invested" in making changes. Often times it is a parent, teacher or coach that is invested in wanting the child to make changes and not the child. Just as with adults, working with children that are in the precontemplative stage will not produce success. Also, working with children may, at times, require a working relationship with the parent or guardian. The goals of the child may not be the same as the goals of the parent or guardian.

Step 2 – BMI

The CDC and the American Academy of Pediatrics (AAP) recommend the use of BMI to screen for overweight and obesity in children beginning at 2 years old (29). Below are the steps involved in determining BMI for children and teens:

1. Before calculating BMI, obtain accurate height and weight measurements.
2. Calculate the BMI and percentile using the Child and Teen BMI Calculator at http://apps.nccd.cdc.gov/dnpabmi/.
3. Find the weight status category for the calculated BMI-for-age percentile as shown in the following table. These categories are based on expert committee recommendations (29). See the following chart.

Weight Status Category	Percentile Range
Underweight	Less than the 5th percentile
Healthy weight	5th percentile to less than the 85th percentile
Overweight	85th to less than the 95th percentile
Obese	Equal to or greater than the 95th percentile

See the following example of how some sample BMI numbers would be interpreted for a 10 year old boy (30).

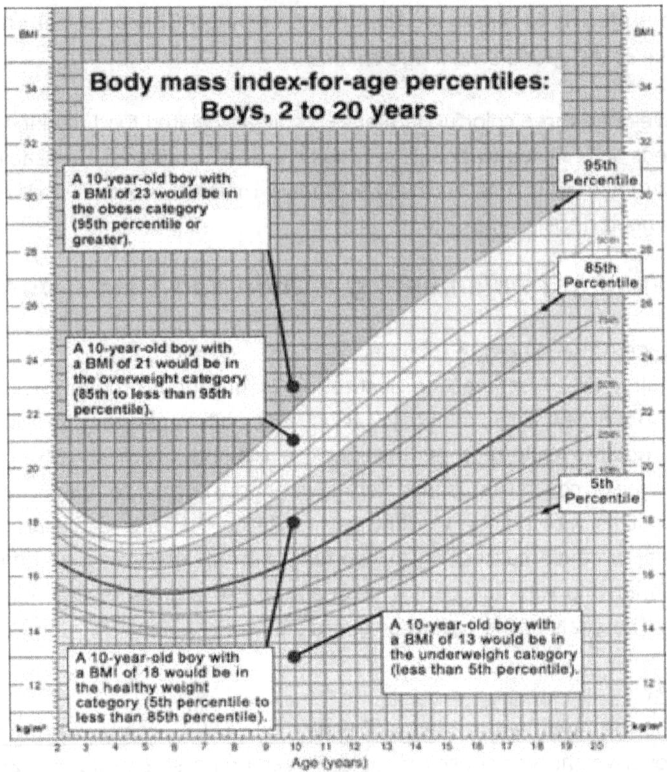

<u>Step 3 - Caloric Needs</u>

The Institute of Medicine utilizes information taken from the IOM Dietary Reference Intakes report (2002) in determining caloric needs for children. This method utilizes "Reference size," as determined by IOM. Reference size is based on median height and weight for children ages up to age 18 years of age (following table).

Gender	Age (years)	Sedentary [b]	Moderately Active [c]	Active [d]
Child	2-3	1,000	1,000-1,400	1,000-1,400
Female	4-8 9-13 14-18	1,200 1,600 1,800	1,400-1,600 1,600-2,000 2,000	1,400-1,800 1,800-2,200 2,400
Male	4-8 9-13 14-18	1,400 1,800 2,200	1,400-1,600 1,800-2,200 2,400-2,800	1,600-2,000 2,000-2,600 2,800-3,200

a These levels are based on Estimated Energy Requirements (EER) from the Institute of Medicine Dietary Reference Intakes macronutrients report, 2002, calculated by gender, age, and activity level for reference-sized individuals. "Reference size," as determined by IOM, is based on median height and weight for ages up to age 18 years of age.

[b] Sedentary means a lifestyle that includes the light physical activity associated with typical day-to-day life.

[c] Moderately active means a lifestyle that includes physical activity equivalent to walking about 1.5 to 3 miles per day at 3 to 4 miles per hour, in addition to the light physical activity associated with day-to-day life

d Active means a lifestyle that includes physical activity equivalent to walking more than 3 miles per day at 3 to 4 miles per hour, in addition to the light physical activity associated with typical day-to-day life.

Step 4 - AASDN Meal Plans

AASDN has developed several meal plans for each of the caloric categories listed in the table above. These meal plans illustrate portion sizes and meal and snack breakdown; and these plans also incorporate the AASDN star associated food rating system.

1000 calorie menu plans	1200 calorie menu plans	1400 calorie menu plans
1600 calorie menu plans	1800 calorie menu plans	2000 calorie menu plans
2200 calorie menu plans	2400 calorie menu plans	2600 calorie menu plans
2800 calorie menu plans	3000 calorie menu plans	3200 calorie menu plans

1. Determine the appropriate caloric meal plan from the table in step 3.
2. Print the appropriate meal plans.
3. Become familiar with the pattern and portion sizes included in the meal plan and begin with small changes. The changes must be palatable to the child. Small changes may include choosing lower fat dairy products and increasing small amounts of fruits and vegetables that the child likes; and limited processed foods.
4. AASDN laminated placemats are a colorful, fun, and interactive way to motivate children and teens and reward themselves for good decision making! Visit http://aasdnschoollunchinitiative.blogspot.com/p/placemats.html for details.

These meal plans can be accessed free of charge at http://www.aasdn.org/childrens-menu-plans/. See the Appendix for samples of meal plans and AASDN placemats.

Obese Population

The simplistic definition of obesity is excess body fat that accumulates when people take in more food energy than they expend. Many factors are involved in this simplistic definition. Obesity has many interrelated causes and is not simply a matter of what one eats. Obesity is a combination of behavioral, psychological, biological, genetic, metabolic, and dietary components. It is important to recognize that it cannot be assumed that because someone is obese that he/she simply eats too much. While it is likely at one point the individual consumed too many calories, it is important to meet the client where they are in the present and build on their current lifestyle. The client may currently be on a very low calorie diet. This again goes back to coaching. With the disastrous effects of fad dieting (physical and psychological), it may be difficult to facilitate a paradigm shift away from dieting. This can be true with any client not just a client that is obese.

For adults, overweight and obesity ranges are determined by using body mass index (BMI) (49). BMI is used because, for most people, it correlates with their amount of body fat.

- An adult who has a BMI between 25 and 29.9 is considered overweight.
- An adult who has a BMI of 30 or higher is considered obese.

See the table below for an example of how BMI correlates to a person who is 5' 9" inches tall.

Height	Weight Range	BMI	Considered
5' 9"	124 lbs or less	Below 18.5	Underweight
	125 lbs to 168 lbs	18.5 to 24.9	Healthy weight
	169 lbs to 202 lbs	25.0 to 29.9	Overweight
	203 lbs or more	30 or higher	Obese

It is important to remember that although BMI correlates with the amount of body fat, BMI does not directly measure body fat. As a result, some people, such as athletes, may have a BMI that identifies them as overweight even though they do not have excess body fat.

The steps in working with obese clients are similar to working with non-obese populations. Your exercise program should contain all the components of a program designed for obese persons as recommended by the American College of Sports Medicine.

Aging Population

When you see an older, frail woman, do you automatically think "little old lady" and assume that she is slow, incompetent, or senile? This is a form of prejudice called ageism (14). Ageism is stereotyping and discriminating against individuals or groups because of their age. It is a set of beliefs, attitudes, norms, and values used to justify age based prejudice, discrimination, and subordination (14). The term was coined in 1969 by Robert Neil Butler to describe discrimination against seniors, and patterned on sexism and racism (15). Butler defined ageism as a combination of three connected elements. Among them were prejudicial attitudes towards older people, old age, and the aging process; discriminatory practices against older people; and institutional practices and policies that perpetuate stereotypes about older people (16). Our language and our humor toward the aging reflect this prejudice in terms such as over the hill, fuddy-duddy, little old lady, old hag, old coot, dirty old man. Our own individual ageist attitudes can be identified and eliminated through continuous exposure to and working with older adults.

There is no denying it. We are all aging daily. We look in the mirror and wonder who is the aging person looking back at us. For most of us, the aging process is unwanted and dreaded. Our only option is to age as gracefully as possible. While we have very little control over the outward signs of aging, we do have tremendous control over the physiological aspects of aging. In essence, everything we do either contributes to or prevents aging, and many of the choices that prevent aging are easy and simple to incorporate.

Aging is one of those vague terms that we use constantly but can't define with precision. We can point to friends and relatives who are old, but a specific definition eludes us. We are born; we grow from childhood to adulthood; and then we grow old. An English gerontologist defined aging as an increased liability to die (11).

Researchers at Tufts University have focused on a more positive definition of aging. They resurrected a concept that the medical research community has used for years. The term "biomarkers" is used to refer to biological markers of aging (12). Researchers at Tufts have narrowed the definition to include only the physiological functions that can be altered for the better by changes in a person's lifestyle (12).

Biologically, as people age, they become more diverse than the younger population; i.e., younger people are much more similar physiologically than are older persons (12). Some eighty year olds look more like thirty year olds when measuring physiological parameters; similarly, some twenty five year olds physiologically look more like fifty year olds. People age at a similar rate until they reach their late twenties or mid thirties (11). Then, between the ages of 28 and 36, most individuals reach a transition point from growing to aging. As people age chronologically, variability among individuals becomes great; so much so that averages become meaningless. Certain functions, such as mental activity and IQ, in some individuals show almost no decline and even improve from chronological age 35 to 75.

A common belief that aging is mostly inherited is unfounded (12). Genetics accounts for less than 30 percent of all aging effects and becomes less important as a person ages so that by the age of eighty, lifestyle choices account for almost 100% of a person's overall health and longevity. Even if sedentary individuals begin at 50 years old to implement exercise and healthy eating, they can regain 90 percent of the health benefits of their younger counterparts by age 70.

Up until the mid-1980's, it was assumed that muscle loss (sarcopenia) was age related and inevitable (12). However, in the mid-1980's, Walter Frontera, completed research at Tufts University that revised the way we look at exercise (13). Dr. Frontera investigated the effects of resistance training in sixty and seventy old males (13). They performed exercises at 80 percent of their one repetition maximum. In just twelve weeks, muscle hypertrophy increased 10 to 12 percent, and muscle strength increased 100 to 175%. The amount of hypertrophy was as much as was expected in young people doing the same amount of exercise (13). Hence, many of the factors once associated with aging are now known to be due to inactivity (fat gain, muscle loss, diabetes, heart disease, etc.). Strength training can prevent sarcopenia. It can also improve balance, help prevent osteoporosis, and lessen arthritis pain through stronger muscles which can ease the strain.

The challenges facing this diverse group of older adults who span more than five decades are also varied. As individuals approach their seventies and eighties, many of the challenges they face are actually a reversal of the challenges they faced in their younger years.

The 50 to 70 Year Old Adult

The 50 to 70 year old must still face the battle of added weight gain and increased risk of chronic diseases associated with weight gain (diabetes, heart disease, hypertension, etc.). Also many adults in this age range are still working and face similar challenges of a hectic, stressful lifestyle as their younger counterparts (12). No matter what physical limitations exist, everyone must exercise to remain physiologically young. Exercise is the closest thing we do have to a "magic pill". As previously mentioned, physiological variability in this group is great, and heart rate varies widely among individuals. In determining exercise intensity, the BORG scale is recommended. The goal using the BORG scale is to reach an intensity of 15/16 on the original scale, or 7 on the new scale (46). If the older person has any trace of heart disease a cardiovascular event may occur. The problem is seriously compounded if the older person sits or lies down immediately, takes a hot shower or plunges into a hot tub or steam room. These situations should be avoided for at least 45 minutes to an hour.

A resistance training program for this population should concentrate on a minimum of exercises encompassing all large muscle groups. The participants in the above cited research performed 5 exercises to failure. It is not necessary to add several exercises per muscle group for this population. Maintaining flexibility is critical for this age group if they are to maintain their activities of daily living (12).

The Over 70 Year Old Adult

Many adults over 70 are faced with very different challenges than their younger counterparts. If exercise has been lacking, this group is typified by decreased muscle mass (sarcopenia) and increased body fat (12). Rather than facing obesity, they face decreased caloric intake associated with sarcopenia and are therefore at increased risk for nutritional deficiencies (12). Nutritional status surveys have indeed shown a marked increase in risk of malnutrition and sub-clinical deficiencies in this group. Dietary quality becomes difficult to ensure since overall energy intake becomes so low.

If successful aging is to continue in this age group, cardiovascular exercise is a must. In addition to the aerobic benefits, cardiovascular exercise increases appetite, which in turn can help ward off nutritional deficiencies typically seen in this group. Precautions for this group are similar to that for the 50 to 70 year old adult. However, this group is typified by more limitations to exercise and exercise, prescription may have to be modified. Tufts University guidelines emphasize the use of the BORG scale for this population, as well, and recommend a 10 minute warm up and cool down (12).

Resistance training also becomes more critical in this group if successfully aging is to occur. Not only is it possible for individuals over 70 to increase muscle mass, but all individuals, even centurions, can build muscle. In 1990, Dr. Maria Fiatarone published her research in which men and women in their eighties and nineties increased muscle strength by 175% and muscle hypertrophy by 10% in 8 weeks (17). Resistance training can prevent sarcopenia and hence prevent the nutritional deficiencies associated with it (17).

MyPlate for Older Adults

Working with the aging population follows the same steps as with younger adults except that caloric needs decline with age due to a decrease in metabolism and physical activity. Nutrition scientists at the Jean Mayer USDA Human Nutrition Research Center on Aging (USDA HNRCA) at Tufts University have developed the MyPlate for Older Adults, which corresponds with the federal government's MyPlate symbol (18). Nutritional requirements for some nutrients increases for this population, and the MyPlate for Older Adults provides examples of high density foods - foods that contain high levels of vitamins and minerals.

MyPlate for Older Adults

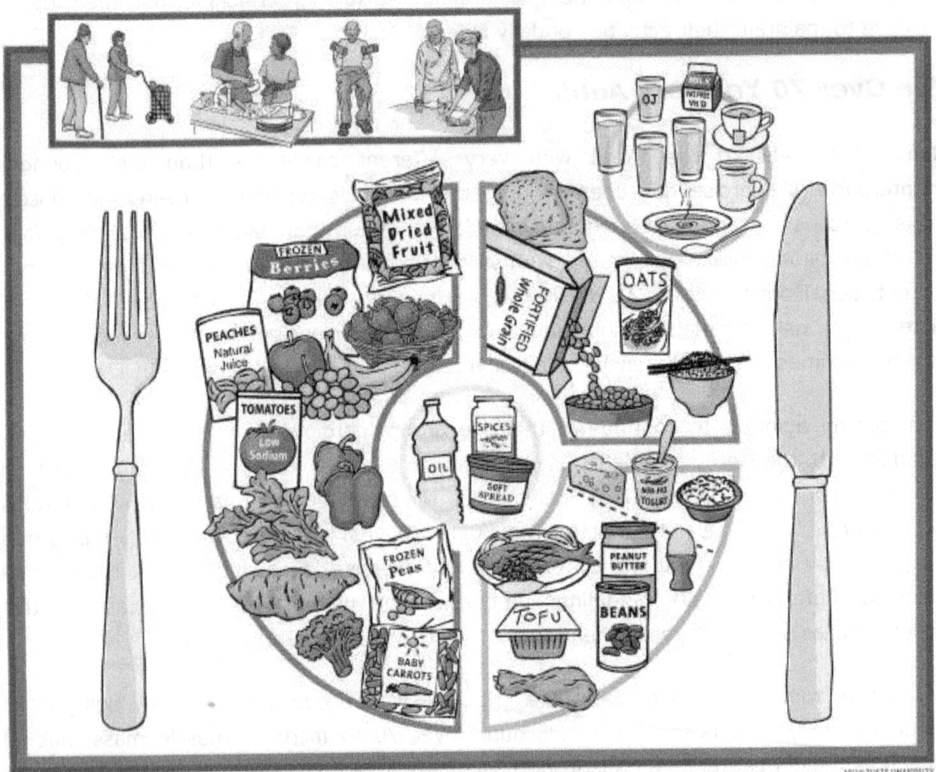

Reprinted with permission from Betsy Hayes, Tufts University (18).

The drawing features different forms of vegetables and fruits that are convenient, affordable, and readily available. Unique components include icons for regular physical activity and emphasis on adequate fluid intake, both of particular concern for older adults (18).

The following foods, fluids, and physical activities are represented on My Plate for Older Adults:

- Bright-colored vegetables such as carrots and broccoli.
- Deep-colored fruit such as berries and peaches.
- Whole, enriched, and fortified grains and cereals such as brown rice and 100% whole wheat bread.
- Low- and non-fat dairy products such as yogurt and low-lactose milk.
- Dry beans and nuts, fish, poultry, lean meat, and eggs.
- Liquid vegetable oils, soft spreads low in saturated and *trans* fat, and spices to replace salt.
- Fluids such as water and fat-free milk.
- Physical activity such as walking, resistance training, and light cleaning.

MyPlate for Older Adults promotes regular physical activity with icons depicting common activities that include daily errands and household chores. Although some of those chores do not take the place of more formalized exercise routines involving cardiovascular exercises, those included serve to remind older adults that there is a variety of options for regular physical activity.

Athletic Population

Working with athletes is very similar to working with other populations. Special considerations include the amounts of carbohydrates, water, fats, proteins, vitamins, and minerals. Please review Chapter 5 for recommendations by the Academy of Nutrition and Dietetics (AND), the American College of Sports Medicine (ACSM), and the International Olympic Committee (IOC).

Vegetarian Population

Working with vegetarians follows the same steps as working with other adults. Lactovegetarians omit meats, eggs, fish, and poultry but include dairy products. Lacto-ovo-vegetarians include milk products and eggs but exclude meat, poultry, fish and seafood. Vegans exclude all animal products including meat, poultry, fish, eggs, and dairy products (19).

Vegetarians can easily obtain large quantities of most nutrients with only a few possible exceptions. By choosing whole, unprocessed grains; vegetables; beans, legumes, and lentils, vegetarians can obtain all necessary protein needs.

Research on the health benefits of vegetarian diets is complex since this population differs in other respects, as well. Vegetarians are typically active, use little alcohol, and refrain from smoking. Available research does point to health benefits of vegetarian diets. In general, vegetarians maintain a lower and healthier body weight than non-vegetarians (19). Vegetarians tend to have lower blood pressure and lower rates of hypertension than non-vegetarians, and the incidence of heart disease is much lower. Vegetarians have a significantly lower rate of cancer than the general population (19).

It is recommended that vegetarians also pay attention to iron intake. The absorption of iron in plant foods is enhanced by vitamin C (chili has iron in the beans and the tomatoes have lots of vitamin C); hence, vegetarians are not any more likely to be iron deficient than the general public (19). As long as they eat a variety of whole foods, a plant based diet provides all needed iron.

Zinc is similar to iron in that meat provides the richest sources of iron, in the standard American diet and plant sources are not as well absorbed. Also, high intake of soy interferes with zinc absorption. Vegetarians are advised to include lots of whole grains, nuts, and legumes in their daily food plan(19).

Vitamin B12 is found in animal products hence vegetarians must rely on fortified sources or supplements to obtain this vitamin. Without adequate amounts of B12 nerve damage can occur (19).

Summary

The challenge facing professionals today is the idea that a "quick fix" exists when it comes to health. We are bombarded with new products daily that promise to make us healthier, thinner, sexier, etc. As professionals, we embark on the daunting task of convincing the "gullible" public that there is no such thing as a quick fix. Just as you can't plant a seedling in March and expect fruit in April, the public needs to understand that you can't obtain fitness and wellness overnight. We need to renew the belief that moderation along with small, slow lifestyle changes are the ingredients necessary to promote health and fitness. The changes must be ones that the public can live with without feeling deprived. For example, going from whole milk to 2% milk is a much easier transition that trying to go from whole milk to skim milk. As professionals,dedicated to teaching healthy lifestyles, we need to develop patience and not try to bring individuals to our level of fitness overnight.

There is much confusion surrounding why measuring body composition rather than scale weight is a better way to gauge success in health and weight management. In Chapter 13, we will discuss how the scale does not indicate "size" or health. For example, two objects such as a softball and a beach ball can weigh the same but are clearly different sizes. There are several ways to measure size and health status including Body Mass Index, percent body fat, and waist to hip ratio. Body mass index is a way to judge weight in relation to height. Waist circumference and body mass index (BMI) are indirect methods to assess body composition. Percent body fat, a more direct method, can be determined in several ways.

The goal of weight loss is loss of stored body fat. The most popular tool for measuring fat loss is scale weight. However, traditional scales are unable to differentiate between fat, muscle, bone or body fluid, which makes up our total body weight. If an individual has only a small amount of weight to lose, the scale may not change significantly as lean muscle mass increases and body fat decreases.

Adults should get 45 percent to 65 percent of their daily calories from carbohydrates. Acceptable ranges for children are similar. The Recommended Dietary Allowances express recommendations in terms of grams per day - 130 grams per day for both men and women. Sugar intake should be kept as low as possible with a maximum of 10% of total caloric intake. The acceptable macronutrient range for fat intake is 20 to 35% of energy. The fat requirements for sedentary individuals and athletes are similar but slightly higher for athletes. Intake should not decrease below 20% of total energy intake because the intake of fat is important for the absorption of fat-soluble vitamins and essential fatty acids. Saturated fat and trans fat should be kept as low as possible. Much debate still exists concerning protein requirements. Dietary protein requirements are elevated with strength, speed or endurance training. The AND and ACSM recommend daily protein requirements for strength and endurance athletes of 1.2-1.7 g/kg BW/day t. The IOC protein guidelines for athletes are 1.3-1.8 g/kg BW/day and 1.6-1.7 g/kg BW/day for strength-training athletes (38). Hence the range of protein varies from .8 g/kg BW/day to 1.8 g/kg BW/day.

The Dietary Reference Intakes (DRI) (31) and the Dietary Guidelines provide energy recommendations for men and women who are slightly active to very active. The Dietary Reference Intakes (DRIs) define the daily requirement for energy as the Estimated Energy Requirement (EER). Estimated Energy Requirement (EER) is the average dietary energy intake that is predicted to maintain energy balance in healthy, normal weight individuals of a defined age, gender, weight, height, and level of physical activity consistent with good health. In children and pregnant and lactating women, the EER includes the needs associated with growth or secretion of milk at rates consistent with good health.

It is important to obtain accurate lifestyle and nutrition information from potential clients. In our discussion clients will refer to the public at large including patients, students, etc. It is illegal in most states for a non-licensed professional to complete a diet analysis for clients unless working directly and under the guidance of a licensed professional. Wellness/fitness professionals may however legally request information about lifestyle and eating patterns. There are several ways to document eating patterns.

The steps involved in the implementation of an individual nutrition program include: an interview; a first appointment; EER and body composition analysis before next appointment; the second appointment; the third appointment; follow up sessions; and details concerning ending a program. Group programs offer an added benefit of interaction with other individuals with similar goals. This can be seen from the success of groups such as Weight Watchers. Fitness professionals can build on this concept by providing exercise prescription and more detailed nutrition information at each meeting. It is important to structure a group program that includes a "curriculum." A curriculum ensures that participants will complete the program with a new level of acquired information.

For the first time in history, children will have shorter and less healthy lives than their parents, and all fitness/wellness professionals are strongly encouraged to include children and teens in their programs. Globally, an estimated 43 million preschool children (under age 5) were overweight or obese in 2010, a 60 percent increase since 1990 (20). The problem affects countries rich and poor, and by sheer numbers, places the greatest burden on the poorest. Of the world's 43 million overweight and obese preschoolers, 35 million live in developing countries.

Obesity increases a child's risk of numerous health problems and can create emotional and social issues. Obese children are also more likely to be obese as adults, increasing their risk of serious health problems such as heart disease and stroke. Diabetes is one of the most common chronic diseases in children and adolescents affecting about 151,000 people below the age of 20 years. As with adults, Body Mass Index (BMI) is a number calculated from a child's weight and height and is a reliable indicator of body fatness for most children and teens. It does not measure body fat directly, but research has shown that it correlates to measures of body fat. Additionally, BMI is an inexpensive and easy-to-perform method of screening for weight categories that may lead to health problems.

Caloric requirements for children vary according to the rate at which they burn calories, their body type, and their age. Caloric requirements for children are largely based on a certain number of calories in relation to a child's body weight. Average calorie needs increase as a child ages, with peak number of calories between 2,200 and 3,000 daily calories during adolescence. The "Merck Manuals" (also known as *The Merck Manual of Diagnosis and Therapy)* lists nutritional needs for infants and children using a formula of calories per pound of body weight.

The steps involved in implementing a youth program include: an interview to determine the stage of readiness to change of the child; BMI calculation; determination of caloric needs based on age, gender, and activity level; choosing the corresponding, appropriate menu plan.

Working with the aging population follows the same steps as with younger adults except that calorie needs decline with age due to a slow-down in metabolism and physical activity. Nutrition scientists at the Jean Mayer USDA Human Nutrition Research Center on Aging (USDA HNRCA) at Tufts University have developed the MyPlate for Older Adults which corresponds with the federal government's MyPlate symbol. Nutritional requirements remain the same, and in some cases, increases. MyPlate for Older Adults provides examples of foods that contain high levels of vitamins and minerals and are consistent with the federal government's 2010 Dietary Guidelines for Americans.

Working with athletes is very similar to working with other populations. Special considerations include the amounts of carbohydrates, water, fats, proteins, vitamins and minerals. Please review Chapter 5 for recommendations by the Academy of Nutrition and Dietetics, the American College of Sports Medicine ACSM), and the International Olympic Committee (IOC).

Working with vegetarians follows the same steps as working with adults. Vegetarians can easily obtain large quantities of most nutrients with only a few possible exceptions. By choosing a whole food, plant based diet with minimal processed foods, vegetarians can obtain all adequate nutrients. One possible exception is vitamin B12. Vitamin B12 is found in animal products hence vegetarians must rely on fortified sources or supplements to obtain this vitamin. Without adequate amounts of B12 nerve damage can occur.

Chapter 12 - Sample Test

1. For each case study (following pages), read the Client Profile which includes background information; personal, medical, exercise information; disease and dietary history; and a one day food recall; and provide the following information:
    i. Identify the "Stage of Readiness to Change". Is this client someone you can help? Explain your answer.
    ii. Do the stated goals and objectives follow the SMART. Rule? Explain your answer.
    iii. Read the client profile and identify any "red flags" that might indicate a reason for collaborating with a licensed professional. Explain your answer.
    iv. Identify body composition results and activity level. Why was this activity level chosen?
    v. Determine the estimated energy requirements (EER), and calculate the body fat adjusted EER (if applicable).
    vi. How did you determine the recommended daily caloric intake?
    vii. How was the body fat adjusted daily caloric intake determined?
    viii. Read the one day food recall. Approximately how many calories is the person ingesting?
    ix. Discuss the caloric differences between the one day food recall and the recommended daily caloric intake. Does this individual have to increase or decrease calories? How much of a caloric change would you recommend?
    x. Identify key coaching opportunities / keeping in mind lifestyle changes.
    xi. Using your expertise and coaching skills explain how you would present the results and assist the person in setting goals and objectives.

Case Studies

Case Study 1 – Sally Stressed

Name	Sally Stressed	Date	07/05/13

Background

Sally is a 28 year old single nurse who has always been overweight. During high school and college she was "big" but she gained more weight after a relationship of several years ended. She has been working with a trainer for 6months and has managed to lose 20 pounds but she has plateaued at 200 pounds. She is 5'10" tall. She strength trains 3 times a week with her trainer and does a cardio workout three times a week for 30 minutes. Sally has decided to seek your help with a nutrition program.

Signed Agreements

Legal Agreement	Yes	Responsibility Agreement	Yes	Par-Q or equivalent	Yes

Demographic Information

Street Address	555 Glenn Drive
City/Town	West Palm Beach
State/Zip Code	FL 33419
Telephone	555.555.5555
Emergency Contact	
Emergency Phone	

Personal History

Age	28	Blood Type	A positive	Smoker	No
Date of Birth	01/15/85	Wt at Heaviest	228	Ever Smoked	No
Gender	Female	Wt at Lightest	180	Date Quit	NA
Height	5'10"	BMI	28.7	Occupation	Nurse
Weight	200 lbs	Waist/Hip	0.95	Stress Level	6
		% Body Fat	43.00%	Activity Level	Low-Active

Physical Activity

Describe Exercise Program	Weight training 3x/week, cardio 3x/week for 30 minutes
For How Long	Working with trainer for 6 months
Limitations to Exercise	None

Comments	

Medical History

Seeing a physician for any reason?	No
Taking any medications? If so list under comments.	No
Taking any over-the-counter medications? If so list under comments.	No
Taking any supplements? If so list under comments.	No
Comments:	

Disease History*

Does the client have any health related issues?	No
Does the client have any known diseases?	No
Disease Risk:	
Is the client a male over the age of 45 or female over the age of 55?	No
Has a parent or sibling experienced a heart attack before the age of 65?	No
Does the client have high blood pressure, diabetes, high cholesterol?	No
Does the client have any known allergies? If so describe under comments.	No
Does the client have any known eating disorders	No
Comments	
* If the client has any medical issues, diseases, indicators of disease risk or allergies you must receive written permission from a licensed professional before working with this client.	

Dietary History

What is the client's largest meal?	Dinner
Does the client snack during the day?	Yes
If yes, what types of snacks?	Fruit, Candy, Cookies
Does the client eat after dinner?	Yes
If so, what types of snacks?	Fruit, Candy, Cookies
What size does the client consider his/her meals to be?	Medium
Does the client eat when stressed?	Yes
Does the client eat when depressed?	Yes

Does the client feel he/she has or ever had an eating disorder?	No
Comments	

One Day Food Recall

	Breakfast	Snack	Lunch	Snack	Dinner	Snack
Day 1	Coffee with cream, 1 cup Cheerios, 1 cup non-fat milk water	Medium banana, 16 almonds, water	Protein drink	Raisins, water	Baked potato, broccoli (1 cup), salad with ½ cup dressing, 3 oz turkey. glass of wine (6 oz)	Cheese and crackers, Diet Soda
Calories						
					Total Calories	

Stage of Readiness to Change/ SMART Goals

Stage of Readiness to Change	
Goals:	
S	
M	
A	
R	
T	
Comments	

Case Study 2 - Stacy Teen

Name	Stacy Teen	Date	07/20/13

Background

Two parents come to you for help with their daughter - Stacy who is 16 years old. She is a great high school basketball player, and they have dreams of her getting a basketball scholarship. The daughter is obese, and the parents want you to help her lose weight. However, after speaking privately with the Stacy, you find out that she hates basketball, and she doesn't think she's fat! Upon further investigation, you discover that she does not want to disappoint her father so she agrees to work with you.

Signed Agreements

Legal Agreement	Yes	Responsibility Agreement	Yes	Par-Q or equivalent	Yes

Demographic Information

Street Address	222 Teen Drive
City/Town	Boston
State/Zip Code	MA, 02132
Telephone	555.555.5555
Emergency Contact	
Emergency Phone	

Personal History

Age	16	Blood Type	B positive	Smoker	No
Date of Birth	01/20/97	Wt at Heaviest	260	Ever Smoked	No
Gender	Female	Wt at Lightest	150	Date Quit	NA
Height	6'2"	BMI	33.4	Occupation	Student
Weight	260 lbs	Waist/Hip	0.95	Stress Level	7
		% Body Fat	39.00%	Activity Level	Active

Physical Activity

Describe Exercise Program	No weight training, basketball almost every day
For How Long	Two years
Limitations to Exercise	None
Comments	Stacy says she doesn't like basketball, and her coach is always screaming at her. While talking to you she begins to cry.

Medical History

Seeing a physician for any reason?	No
Taking any medications? If so list under comments.	No
Taking any over-the-counter medications? If so list under comments.	No
Taking any supplements? If so list under comments.	No
Comments:	

Disease History*

Does the client have any health related issues?	No
Does the client have any known diseases?	No
Disease Risk:	
Is the client a male over the age of 45 or female over the age of 55?	No
Has a parent or sibling experienced a heart attack before the age of 65?	No
Does the client have high blood pressure, diabetes, high cholesterol?	No
Does the client have any known allergies? If so describe under comments.	No
Does the client have any known eating disorders	No
Comments	
* If the client has any medical issues, diseases, indicators of disease risk or allergies you must receive written permission from a licensed professional before working with this client.	

Dietary History

What is the client largest meal?	Dinner
Does the client snack during the day?	Yes
If yes, what types of snacks?	Fruit, Candy, Cookies
Does the client eat after dinner?	Yes
If so, what types of snacks?	Fruit, Candy, Cookies
What size does the client consider his/her meals to be?	Medium
Does the client eat when stressed?	Yes
Does the client eat when depressed?	Yes

Does the client feel he/she has or ever had an eating disorder?	No
Comments	

One Day Food Recall

	Breakfast	Snack	Lunch	Snack	Dinner	Snack
Day 1	No breakfast	ice cream sandwich	2 slices of pizza, 24 oz coke,	Snickers candy bar orange slices at practice water	Macaroni and cheese, 2 cokes	2 Snickers bars (Mon and Dad don't know)
Calories						
					Total Calories	

Stage of Readiness to Change/ SMART Goals

Stage of Readiness to Change	
Goals:	
S	
M	
A	
R	
T	
Comments	

Case Study 3 – Randy Runner

Name	Randy Runner	Date	08/01/13

Background

Randy is a 20 year old collegiate cross country athlete. Randy is going into his third year on the team and is getting pressure to improve on his times. As a result, his coach strongly advised him to meet with you to improve his eating habits. While somewhat reluctant, he recognizes he could make better choices when it comes to nutrition and mentioned he wants to learn more about what to eat after practice. The team is currently doing two-a-day practices with a 5:45 am and 3:30 pm practice. Randy rarely eats breakfast, usually consumes a large lunch, and eats snack food throughout the evening.

Signed Agreements

Legal Agreement	Yes	Responsibility Agreement	Yes	Par-Q or equivalent	Yes

Demographic Information

Street Address	13 Elm Street
City/Town	Kalamazoo
State/Zip Code	MI 49006
Telephone	555.555.5555
Emergency Contact	
Emergency Phone	

Personal History

Age	20	Blood Type		Smoker	No
Date of Birth	07/24/93	Wt at Heaviest	152	Ever Smoked	No
Gender	Male	Wt at Lightest	138	Date Quit	NA
Height	5' 8"	BMI	22	Occupation	Student
Weight	145 lbs	Waist/Hip	0.93	Stress Level	6
		% Body Fat	8.20%	Activity Level	High

Physical Activity

Describe Exercise Program	Two-a-day practices includes running and light weight training.
For How Long	3+ years
Limitations to Exercise	None
Comments	

Medical History

Seeing a physician for any reason?	No
Taking any medications? If so list under comments.	No
Taking any over-the-counter medications? If so list under comments.	No
Taking any supplements? If so list under comments.	No
Comments:	

Disease History*

Does the client have any health related issues?	No
Does the client have any known diseases?	No
Disease Risk:	
Is the client a male over the age of 45 or female over the age of 55?	No
Has a parent or sibling experienced a heart attack before the age of 65?	No
Does the client have high blood pressure, diabetes, high cholesterol?	No
Does the client have any known allergies? If so describe under comments.	No
Does the client have any known eating disorders	No
Comments	
* If the client has any medical issues, diseases, indicators of disease risk or allergies you must receive written permission from a licensed professional before working with this client.	

Dietary History

What is the client's largest meal?	Lunch
Does the client snack during the day?	Yes
If yes, what types of snacks?	Chips, energy bars, sports drinks
Does the client eat after dinner?	Yes
If so, what types of snacks?	Chips
What size does the client consider his/her meals to be?	Medium
Does the client eat when stressed?	No
Does the client eat when depressed?	No

Does the client feel he/she has or ever had an eating disorder?	No
Comments	

One Day Food Recall

	Breakfast	Snack	Lunch	Snack	Dinner	Snack
Day 1	Skip	Energy bar	Pasta, red sauce, juice, garlic bread, cookie	16.9 oz. Gatorade,	Two slices of pizza, six buffalo wings	Chips
Calories		250	Large serving	110		200
					Total Calories	

Stage of Readiness to Change/ SMART Goals

Stage of Readiness to Change	
Goals	
S	
M	
A	
R	
T	
Comments	

References

1. American Heart Association. Frequently asked questions about BMI. (accessed 07/16/2013). http://www.heart.org/HEARTORG/GettingHealthy/WeightManagement/BodyMassIndex/Frequently-Asked-Questions-about-BMI_UCM_307892_Article.jsp.
2. National Heart, Lung, and Blood Institute. Assessing your weight and health risk. (accessed 07/13/2013). http://www.nhlbi.nih.gov/health/public/heart/ obesity/lose_wt/risk.htm.
3. Dehghan M. Merchant AT. (2008). Is bioelectrical impedance accurate for use in large epidemiological studies? Nutrition Journal. 7:26 doi:10.1186/1475-2891-7-26.
4. Shape Up American. Body fat and health risk. (accessed 07/13/2013). http://www.shapeup.org/bfl/risk1.html.
5. Kim JY. Han SH. Yang BM.Implication of high-body-fat percentage on cardiometabolic risk in middle-aged, healthy, normal-weight adults. *Obesity (Silver Spring).* 2012 Aug 28. doi: 10.1002/oby.20020.
6. Nieman D. (1991). Ftness and Sports Medicine. Bull Publishing: Palo Alto, Ca.
7. Peterson J, et al. (2011). Accuracy of consumer grade bioelectrical impedance analysis devices compared with air displacement plethysmography. nt J Exerc Sci 4(3): 176-184.
8. Jackson, AS; Stanforth, PR; Gagnon, J; Rankinen, T; Leon, AS; Rao, DC; Skinner, JS; Bouchard, C et al. (2002). "True". *International Journal of Obesity* 26 (6): 789–96.
9. ACE (2009) What are the guidelines for percentage of body fat loss? American Council on Exercise (ACE). Ask the Expert Blog. December 2, 2009.
10. Friedl, KE. Moore RJ. Martinez-Lopez LE. Vogel JA. Askew EW. Marchitelli LJ. Hoyt RW. Gordon CC (1994). "Lower limit of body fat in healthy active men.". *J Appl Physiol.* 77(2):933-40.
11. Comfort, A. The biology of senescence, 3rd ed. NY: Elsever, 1979.
12. Evans, W, IH Rosenberg. *Biomarkers.* NY: Simon & Schuster, 1991.
13. Fronter W, et al. (1991). A cross-sectional study of muscle strength and mass in 45-78 year old men and women. J Appl. Physiol. 71)2):664-650.
14. Kirkpatrick, George R.; Katsiaficas, George N.; Kirkpatrick, Robert George; Mary Lou Emery (1987). Introduction to critical sociology. Ardent Media. p. 261. ISBN 978-0-8290-1595-9. Retrieved 28 January 2011.
15. Kramarae, C. and Spender, D. (2000) *Routledge International Encyclopedia of Women: Global Women's Issues and Knowledge.* Routledge. p. 29.
16. Wilkinson J and Ferraro K, Thirty Years of Ageism Research. In Nelson T (ed). Ageism: Stereotyping and Prejudice Against Older Persons. Massachusetts Institute of Technology, 2002.
17. Fiatarone, MA, et al. High intensity strength training in nonagenarians: Effects on skeletal muscle, *Journal of the American Medical Association,* 263:3029-3034, 1990.
18. Hayes, B. My Plate for Older adults. Tufts University Faculty and Research. (accessed 07/17/2013). http://nutrition.tufts.edu/research/myplate-older-adults. Reprinted with permission Betsy Hayes, Tufts University.
19. P.K.Newby, K.L. Tucker, et al. Rish of overweight and obesity among semivegetarian, lactoveg- etarian, and vegan women. Amer J of Clinical Nutrition. 81: 1267-1274. 2005.
20. de Onis M. Blossner M. Borghi E. (2010). Global prevalence and trends of overweight and obesity among preschool children. *Am J Clin Nutr.* 92:1257-64.
21. Daniels SR, Arnett DK, Eckel RH, et al. Overweight in children and adolescents: pathophysiology, consequences, prevention, and treatment. *Circulation* 2005;111;1999–2002.
22. Office of the Surgeon General. (2010). The Surgeon General's Vision for a Healthy and Fit Nation. Rockville, MD, U.S. Department of Health and Human Services.
23. Freedman DS, Zuguo M, Srinivasan SR, Berenson GS, Dietz WH. (2007). Cardiovascular risk

factors and excess adiposity among overweight children and adolescents: the Bogalusa Heart Study. *Journal of Pediatrics.* 150(1):12–17.

24. Li C, Ford ES, Zhao G, Mokdad AH. (2009). Prevalence of pre-diabetes and its association with clustering of cardiometabolic risk factors and hyperinsulinemia among US adolescents: NHANES 2005–2006. *Diabetes Care.* 32:342–347.
25. CDC. National diabetes fact sheet: national estimates and general information on diabetes and prediabetes in the United States. (2011)Atlanta, GA: U.S. Department of Health and Human Services.
26. Dietz WH. (2004). Overweight in childhood and adolescence. *New England Journal of Medicine.* 350:855-857.
27. Nathan D. (2012). Obesity-linked diabetes in children resists treatment. New Eng Journal Med. 17:1557-1650.
28. Centers for Disease Control and Prevention. Basics about childhood obesity. (accessed 07/17/2013). http://www.cdc.gov/obesity/childhood/basics.html.
29. Centers for Disease Control and Prevention. What is a percentile? (accessed 07/17/2013). http://www.cdc.gov/growthcharts/growthchart_faq.htm.
30. Centers for Disease Control and Prevention. How is BMI calculated and interpreted for children and teens? (accessed 07/18/2013). http://www.cdc.gov/healthyweight/assessing /bmi/childrens_BMI/about_childrens_BMI.html.
31. Otten J. Hellwig J. Meyers L, ed. (2006). *Dietary Reference Intakes: The Essential Guide to Nutrient Requirements.* Washington (DC): The National Academies Press.
32. Institute of Medicine. (2005). *Dietary Reference Intakes for Energy, Carbohydrate, Fiber, Fat, Fatty Acids, Cholesterol, Protein, and Amino Acids.* Washington (DC): The National Academies Press.
33. Rodriquez NR. DiMarco NM. Langley S. (2009). Position of the American Dietetic Association, Dietitians of Canada, and the American College of Sports Medicine: Nutrition and athletic performance. *J Am Diet Assoc.* 109(3):509-527 [homepage on the Internet]. c2012. Available from: http://journals.lww.com/acsm-msse/Fulltext/2009/03000/ Nutrition_and_Athletic_Performance.27.aspxPrev Chronic Dis. 2006 October; 3(4): A129. Published online 2006 September 15. PMCID: PMC1784117.
34. International Olympic Committee (IOC) consensus statement on sports nutrition 2010. J Sports Sci. 2011;29(SI):S3-S4.
35. Kreider RB. Wilborn CD. Taylor L, et al. (2010). ISSN exercise and sport nutrition review: research and recommendations. *Int J Soc Sports Nutr.* 7:7 [homepage on the Internet]. c2012. Available from: http://www.biomedcentral.com/content/pdf/1550-2783-7-7.pdf.
36. Phillips SM. Van Loon LJC. (2011). Dietary protein for athletes: from requirements to optimum adaptation. *J Sport Sci.* 29 Suppl 1):S29-S38.
37. Nutrition Information Centre, Stellenbosch University.(2003). Dietary reference intakes. Washington: The National Academies Press; 2003.
38. Slater G. Phillips SM. (2011). Nutrition guidelines for strength sports: sprinting, weightlifting, throwing events, and bodybuilding. *J Sports Sci.* 29(S1):S67-S77.
39. GlobalRPH. Insittute of Medicine – EER Requirements. EER online calculators: http://www.globalrph.com/estimated_energy_requirement.htm. (Accessed 06/08/2013).
40. Gerrior S. WenYen J. Basiotis P. (2006). An Easy Approach to Calculating Estimated Energy Requirements. Prev Chronic Dis. 2006 October; 3(4): A129. http://www.ncbi.nlm.nih. gov/pmc/articles/PMC1784117/.
41. Dietary Reference Intakes For Energy, Carbohydrate, Fiber, Fat, Fatty Acids,Cholesterol, Protein,and Amino Acids, Institute of Medicine of the National Academies, 2002 and 2005, The National Academy Press. Washington, DC 20001.
42. Colson, ER, et al (Full review/revision 2010). The Merck Manual for Health Care Professionals. Nutrition in Infants. Modified 2012. http://www.merckmanuals.com/professional/

pediatrics/approach_to_the_care_of_normal_infants_and_children/nutrition_in_infants.html#v1076437.

43. US Department of Health & Human Services. National Heart, Lung, and Blood Institute. Balance Food and Activity. Updated Feb. 13, 2013. (accessed 07/21/2013). http://www.nhlbi.nih.gov/ health/public/heart/obesity/wecan/healthy-weight-basics/balance.htm.
44. United States Department of Health and Human Services and United States Department of Agriculture. (2005). *Dietary Guidelines for Americans*. Washington (DC): US Government Printing Office. (http://www.health.gov/dietaryguidelines/dga2005/report/HTML/D3_Disccalories.htm).
45. USDA Food and Nutrition Service. Nutrition Standards for School Meals. Healthy Hunger-Free Kids Act. (accessed 07/21/2013). Modified 07/10/2013. http://www.fns.usda.gov/cnd/governance/legislation/nutritionstandards.htm.
46. Centers for Disease Control and Prevention. Physical Activity. Perceived Exertion (Borg Rating of Perceived Exertion Scale). Last updated March 2011. (accessed 07/22/2013). http://www.cdc.gov/physicalactivity/everyone/measuring/exertion.html.
47. Centers for Disease Control and Prevention. Healthy Weight – it's not a diet, it's a lifestyle. Adult Body Mass Index calculator. Revised May 4, 2011. (accessed 07/22/2013). http://www.cdc.gov/healthyweight/assessing/bmi/adult_bmi/english_bmi_calculator/bmi_calculator.html.
48. Centers for Disease Control and Prevention. Healthy Weight – it's not a diet, it's a lifestyle. BMI Percentile Calculator for Child and Teen. Revised May 4, 2011. (accessed 07/22/2013).
49. Centers for Disease Control and Prevention. Overweight and Obesity. Defining Overweight and Obesity. Updated April 12, 2012. (accessed 07/23/2013). http://www.cdc.gov/obesity/adult/defining.html.
50. Sunset Vegetarian Cooking. Ed, of Sunset Books and Sunset Magazine. (1991). Lane Publishing Company.

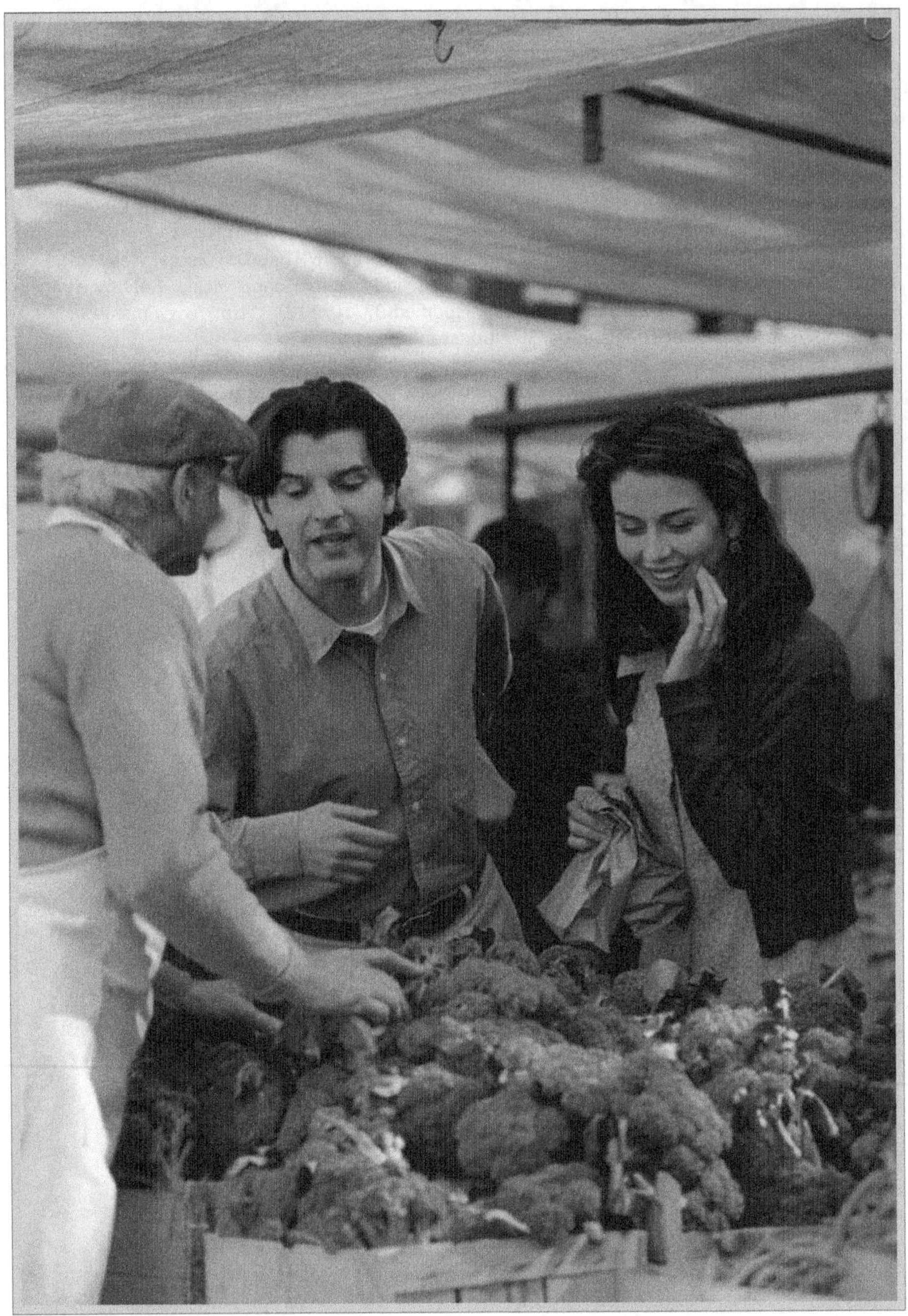

Chapter 13 - Promoting Success

This chapter focuses on factors involved in promoting success in health and life long weight management. Topics include many of the pitfalls associated with dieting; ambiguous and misleading labeling regulations; pitfalls of eating out; and other sabotaging effects such as friendly saboteurs, holidays, meeting, etc. We will conclude with a discussion on practices that are necessary to begin and maintaining a successful, life-altering nutrition business.

Objectives

After reading and studying this chapter, you should be able to:

1. Describe the history of dieting and debunk some of the latest fad diets.
2. Explain why dieting doesn't work in long term weight management.
3. Provide details concerning labeling regulations by the FDA and USDA.
4. Discuss unregulated terms and non governmental logos.
5. Provide details concerning healthy choices when eating out.
6. Describe the components necessary to build a successful nutrition business.

Introduction

Success in maintaining life long health requires acquiring important skills. This chapter will focus on some of the pitfalls that sabotage people from being more successful.

An entire section is dedicated to diets. We are a nation addicted to dieting even though diets don't work and they have never worked. So why are we still addicted to a process that simply doesn't work? The history of dieting sheds light on how we became a nation addicted!

This chapter will then look at labeling laws. Many well intentioned clients, athletes, and patients are making what they believe to be healthy choices but are instead being sabotaged by inconsistencies and often ambiguous labeling regulations. "Whole grain" doesn't mean whole grain; "93% lean ground beef" isn't 93% lean by calories; and the definition of "free-range" is far from what you may envision.

Next, the discussion will focus on eating out. Most people are totally unaware of what they are eating when they eat out. Other sabotaging practices will also be discussed including eating too many calories in the evening, dealing with problem foods in the home, deprivation of favorite foods, eating too fast, shopping when hungry, not planning, eating by the numbers, friendly saboteurs, and stress eating.

The final section will look at components necessary to build a successful, life altering nutrition business.

Diet – A Four Letter Word

The diet industry is now a $20 billion industry with 100 million dieters (1,2). Despite all our "diet foods" we are still getting fatter. Despite all the money spent yearly on dieting, more than one-third of adults are obese (3). Obesity has now been classified as a disease by the American Medical Association (4) and has reached epidemic proportions.

History of Dieting

Dieting has been around for thousands of years, although not in any structured way like we see all around us today. It wasn't very common until the 1800's simply because only the rich and well to do were overweight (5). As time progressed, many more people became wealthy and thus had much greater access to the same foods as the wealthy; eating and drinking too much became a sign of affluence (5).

But strangely enough it wasn't entirely the health or wealth factors that started the diet craze; it was the war against sin (5,6)! Yes, the immorality of excess from gluttony would cause a more sinful world according to the American Presbyterian minister Sylvester Graham. After being ordained in 1826, Pastor Graham began to preach the ills of physical, moral, and spiritual health which he believed could be remedied by a basic vegetarian diet (5,6). He also encouraged such behavior as; sleeping on hard and unyielding mattresses, the opening of bedroom windows (whatever the weather), regular cold showers, brisk hearty exercise, clothing to include only loose garments, learning about the benefits of drinking pure water, and of course chastity (5,6). This temperance movement by Pastor Graham in the city of Philadelphia was not very popular among certain groups, and he was referred to as 'Dr. Sawdust' by opponents; his followers became known as the "Grahamites." The word spread, and thousands began to attend his lectures. Pastor Graham, also the originator of graham flour and the flat bread known as graham crackers, stated that the vitality, strength and all-round health of his followers proved that vegetarianism was the "way." He also tirelessly campaigned against all alcohol, coffee, tea, and tobacco as stimulants (5,6).

In the 1850's in England, a man called William Banting was seriously obese (7,8,9). This poor man was so fat that he supposedly could not tie his own shoes, and it is said that he had to go downstairs backwards. Advice from doctors concerning exercise, steam baths, temporary starvation, and chemical purges did little to reduce his weight. One medical practitioner had suggested that he might find the answer by not eating any more than a minimum of sugars and starches (5,7,8,9). William Banting followed this advice, and lost fifty pounds in a year. He was so excited at his success that he wrote a book, titled: "Letter on Corpulence Addressed to the Public," that was published in 1862 (5,9). Hence, not only was the world's first diet book was born but the first low carbohydrate diet was also born.

William Banting's obesity had been cured but the British Medical Association (BMA) immediately attacked this approach because Banting was not a scientist. BMA claimed that Banting's book had no scientific value and would not work for others (9,10). The public however was impressed, and people all over the English speaking world read Banting's book and lost weight. It proved so popular, that it was translated into other languages and spread to other countries (5,9,10).

Around the end of the nineteenth century, William Ewart Gladstone, the four time British Prime Minister, had apparently advised that a person should always masticate (chew) thirty-two times before swallowing (5,11). Why thirty-two? Thirty-two is the same number as the total of teeth in the mouth. He claimed that this lead to a decrease in appetite and subsequent weight loss (5,11).

Horace Fletcher, nicknamed the "Chew-Chew Man" and the "Great Masticator", took the enthusiasm for chewing to much greater heights. He believed that chewing should continue until the food becomes a liquid in the mouth; and any food that does not become liquid (like fiber) should not be chewed in the first place. Leaving fiber out of a diet leads to constipation, as those caught up in the frenzy discovered. But Fletcher, who lost over sixty pounds, persisted that he was right and a small price to pay (5).

Dr. John Kellogg thought that the advice from Fletcher to avoid fiber was so "very wrong" that he founded a cereal company - Kellogg - because he wanted to make sure Americans were getting plenty of fiber in their diets (5).

Medical historian and author of Calories and Corset: A History of Dieting over 2,000 years, Louise Foxcroft reports that in the early 1900s the tapeworm diet started to be advertised. Rumors and reports of tapeworm use during the early 20th century in jockeys, celebrities and models litter the web (87). More recently, the "Tapeworm Diet" made it on the "Tyra Banks Show" in 2009. Fortunately, the "experts" on the show demonstrated and discussed the serious sides effects of ingesting parasites in general, much less for weight loss. Unfortunately, while illegal in the US, there are still sites that sell tapeworms online for dieting purposes and sadly there is apparently a market for them (88).

In 1918, Wilbur Atwater, a chemist, developed the theory that thermal energy was given off by foodstuffs (calories) when burned. Lulu Hunt Peters, a Californian doctor, then introduced the concept of counting calories to aid in weight loss. In her bestselling book *Diet and Health with a Key to the Calories,* she stated that calories were the scientific way of looking at weight loss, and her work is still influential today (12). She also showed that a lot of money could be made by anyone coming up with new ideas to help overweight people. More and more people were becoming overweight, and the public's obsession with fat was off to a running start (5).

Diet books hit bookshelves with variations of this same idea along with new ideas, such as all that matters is combinations of foods that are consumed at the same time. The first of these was William Hay, who recommended that proteins, starches, and sugars be eaten separately to avoid putting on excess fat (13). He also advised that having an enema each and every day was a key to proper health (13). Other authors took the same unscientific, unproven theory and altered it slightly, claiming that some food could change properties of other foods, if digested together. This same theory is still being proclaimed by many today (5). See below for more examples.

Diets, More Diets, and More Diets

And people are still eating more, weighing more, and dieting more. There have been far too many diet books published to document them all, but below is a timeline that includes a few notable points in dieting history (5):

- 1930's - The Hollywood Diet (soon to be better known as the Grapefruit Diet) is introduced. Seaweeds such as kelp and bladder wrack are promoted as the food of choice to end weight problems (14).
- 'Diet Guru' Victor Lindlahr, regularly broadcasts on the nation's radios to spread news of `reverse calorie foods' (15,16). This is a catabolic system of weight loss he states where some foods use up more calories to be digested, than they give out to the body; like celery and apples.
- 1940's and 1950's - "Ideal Weight" charts are invented by matching a weight with gender, height, and frame (17).
- Diet pills are introduced that are based on Amphetamine derivatives. It is soon realized that they are dangerous (18).
- 1960's - A woman named Jean Nidetch and friends hold a meeting in her apartment to share support and advice on dieting; and thus began Weight Watchers (19).
- Dr. Atkins releases his plan for weight loss: a high protein, high fat, and low carbohydrate diet which causes a storm of controversy that still rages today (20).
- The Pritikin Diet Program with low fat and high fiber is introduced for those with heart problems but is quickly taken up by others for weight loss (21).
- The eating disorder anorexia nervosa is described for the first time by psychiatrists, as many continual dieters are becoming underweight (22).
- A new diet drug called fenfluramine is introduced which makes the brain think the stomach is full (23).
- Dr. Robert Linn invents a protein drink called Prolinn, which is made up of slaughterhouse byproducts like crushed horns and hooves and hides, which are treated with artificial flavorings and enzymes. In his book, *the Last Chance Diet,* he urges people to completely omit food and break "the fast" only by the use of his protein drink. Somewhere around 3 million people used his "supplement" (24).
- The book entitled Fit for Life is written by Harvey and Marilyn Diamond. In it are claims that the human body has changing physiological needs for certain foodstuffs depending on the time of the day (25).
- 1980's - The Beverly Hills Diet becomes the latest dieting craze. It holds that only fruit should be eaten for the first ten days of the plan (26).
- An anti-diabetes system called The Glycemic Index is developed by Dr. David Jenkins and a team of scientists at the University of Toronto (27). To help simplify

the problems suffered by diabetics, this index charts how quickly a range of diverse foodstuffs affects blood sugar levels. This research is also often misappropriated by authors of fad diets to back up their weight loss claims.

- TV personality Oprah Winfrey loses almost 70 pounds on a liquid diet (5).
- Health writer Susan Powter advises her female readers to diet less and exercise more (28).
- The diet pills containing fenfluramine and the related dexfenfluramine are withdrawn by their manufacturers as the FDA reports on them being a cause of heart valve disease (29).
- 2000's - Some researchers claim that for the first time in recorded human history, the number of underfed people in the world has been equaled by those overweight (89).

How to Write Your Own Diet Book

Bonnie Liebman, in "How to Write a Diet Book", provides details on how to create a diet book (30). "After all," she says, "You've been eating all your life haven't you? Don't worry about having any expertise or degree (30)!"

In Step 1, Bonnie says to name your book after a trendy place (South Beach, Beverly Hills, Scarsdale, etc.). Next, make up a diet that will banish unwanted fat forever. It doesn't matter what it is, people will believe it. Then, personalize it by tailoring it to the masses (Eat Right 4 Your Type, Carbohydrate Addict's Diet, The Zone, etc.). Zero in on a body part (Abs Diet, Cellulite Breakthrough, The Butt Book, etc.) Single out a food that currently isn't in vogue (Grapefruit Diet, Cabbage Soup Diet) and single out a nutrient (low carb, low-fat, etc.) (30).

In Step 2, tell people they won't be hungry on your diet; people on your diet will lose weight even when all other diets failed; tell people they will not only lose weight, but they will have more energy, be healthier and will show no signs of aging. Also, tell people that they don't have to give up their favorite foods, don't have to count calories, will lose weight fast, and will detox their body. Be sure to tell people that your diet is backed by scientific research, and to boost sales, tell people that the scientific community has completely ignored your research.

Step 3 - Keep it complicated (or simple). For people who don't like to read, fill chapters with foods to avoid, recipes, blank pages that people can write on, and lots of charts listing fiber, calories, etc. For science lovers, deluge people with scientific evidence, especially if it has been ignored. Use scientific names (lipoprotein lipase, cortisol, leptin, etc.), and be sure to explain how your diet will prevent diseases. Be sure to have at least 50 references and a list of supplements to take. You can even create your own supplements.

Step 4 - Think outside the box. Go beyond what's been done. "You can think of it as a creative writing course," says Bonnie (30).

And on and on we go. As a last word on this topic, Bonnie states that Winnie the Pooh, that well loved bear, once asked how long it took to get thin. The answer, it appears, is still not fully available!

AASDN "Spoof" on Diets

Maybe it'll take me 8 weeks!
Beer and Prune Diet
You can look like this in six weeks!

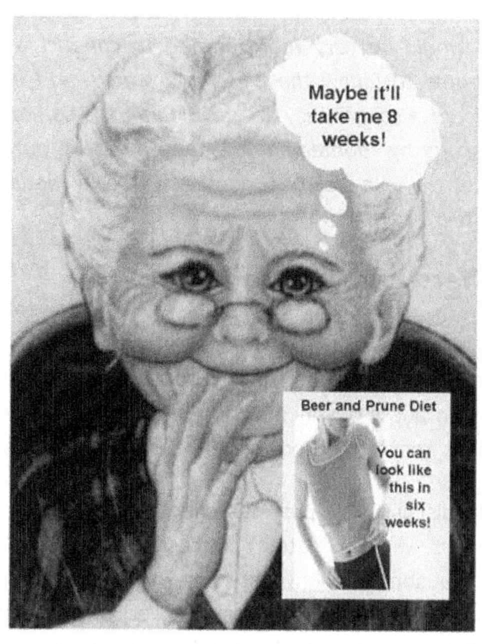

Using the steps above, Dr. Jane Pentz and colleagues at AASDN have developed the *Boston Beer and Prune Diet.* Scientific evidence convincingly shows that people can lose up to 15 to 25 pounds in six weeks. Participants stated that they had more energy and were not hungry while following the *new AASDN fat burning diet*. Dr. Pentz explains that compounds in beer, regardless of the type, contain over 560 aromatic compounds (78) that not only contribute to the overall aroma of beer but several compounds also have appetite suppressant properties (78). Compounds such as ethyl acetate, isoamyl acetate, and linalool, not only provide flavorful aroma found in beer but are also known to reduce appetite. Prunes are dried plums, fruits of Prunus domestica L., cultivated and propagated since ancient times. Certain dried prunes are produced from cultivar d'Agen (79). Prunes cultivated from cultivar d'Agen have "cleansing properties" specific to this type of cultivated prune (78). The combination of the compounds ethyl acetate, isoamyl acetate, and linalool, in combination with the cleansing properties of d'Agen cultivated prunes, has been shown increase weight loss in all participants. All individuals following the diet also lost body fat, particularly around the waist.

The diet calls for one 8 ounce glass of warm beer at breakfast with 2 d'Agen prunes. Lunch consists of another 8 ounce glass of warm beer with 4 d'Agen prunes. Why warm beer?

The appetite suppressant properties of ethyl acetate, isoamyl acetate, and linalool are enhanced when the beer is at room temperature. Dinner consists of vegetables, 4 ounces of meat or fish, another glass or warm been, and 4 d'Agen prunes. All participants in the study stated that they felt full and were not hungry. For more details and success stories visit www.BostonBeerPruneDiet.com.

Note: Anyone astute enough to look up the references listed above will see that beer does indeed have over 560 aromatic compounds, but the research has nothing to do with weight loss; and most (if not all) prunes are cultivated from d'Agen. No references are made to actual studies on the diet itself.

It would be very ***inexpensive*** *to conduct a research project on this diet by asking 10 people to follow the diet for 2 weeks and extrapolate the weight loss for 6 weeks. It would also be easy to do BMI and waist to hip ratio on each person and "fudge" the results by "tightening" the tape measure during measurements. People following such a diet will lose weight! Could it be due to the low caloric nature of the diet and the laxative effect of prunes?*

Diets and Muscle Loss

Dieting doesn't work for many reasons, but first and foremost, low calorie diets utilize lean muscle as an energy source—hence, fat burning machinery is lost. The scale goes down but is destined to go right back up. When the weight is gained back, it's all fat. The only known method of permanent weight loss is exercise and healthy eating (31).

As discussed in previous chapters and worth reiterating here, fasting (twelve to sixteen hours without eating) forces the body to switch to a wasting metabolism; i.e., exhausting carbohydrate reserves and drawing on vital protein tissues. In the first few days of a fast or a low calorie diet, body protein provides about 90 percent of the needed glucose (31). If body proteins were to continue to be utilized at this rate, death would ensue within weeks (31). However, as the low calorie diet or fast continues, the body finds a way to use fat by-products (ketones) as a fuel source for some cells, such as muscle cells. Other cells, such as brain cells and nervous system cells, require glucose; hence body protein continues to be degraded. This is a dangerous process since ketones can cause a metabolic disorder known as acidosis. In acidosis, changes in pH occur, and large perturbations in pH can eventually cause death. Fasting reduces energy output, and the body conserves both its fat and lean tissue. As the lean organ tissues shrink, they perform less metabolic work and so demand less energy (31,32).

Consider the following example. The beach ball and baseball in this picture weigh the same. Hence, weight provides no information about size - only weight. Most Americans use the scale as a measure of determining size and health status. However, body composition is the appropriate measure to determine size.

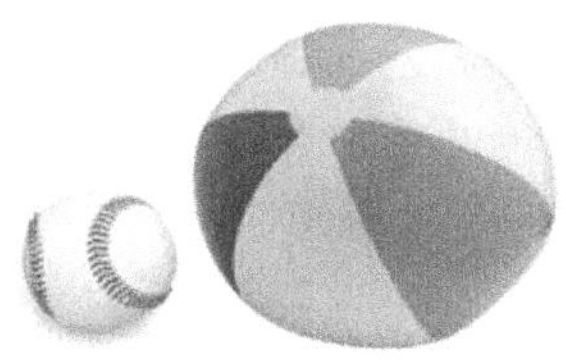

Consider another example. Mike is a 55-year-old executive trying desperately to win the battle of the bulge. He steps on the scale every morning to monitor his weight. At six foot, two inches and 200 pounds, he doesn't look "obese," but Mike is frustrated. He eats less (by skipping lunch) and exercises more in order to keep his weight from creeping up, and he now buys clothes a size larger. He is always tired and hungry, and often cranky. To add to Mike's frustration, his twin brother who also weighs 200 pounds, is obviously leaner looking, wears clothes several sizes smaller than Mike and eats much more than Mike does.

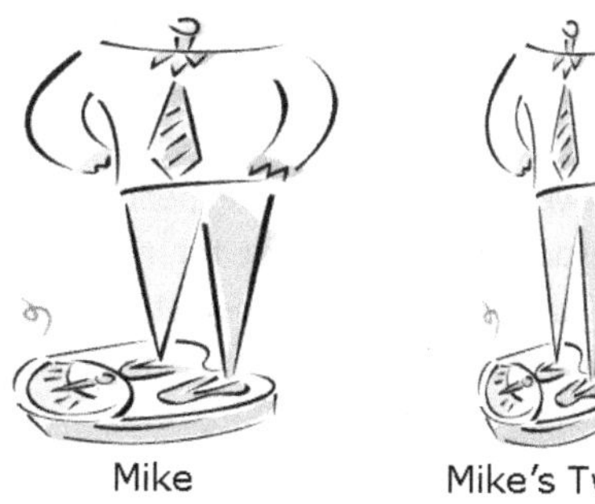

The scale is deceiving Mike. The scale only measures his total mass - 200 pounds. The question the scale answers for Mike is, "How much do I weigh?" It cannot answer the more important question, "How much of those 200 pounds is calorie-burning muscle versus metabolically inactive fat?" Therefore, the scale provides an unreliable "picture" of Mike's true condition. Mike, like millions of Americans, believes his body is burning fat when he does not eat, but the truth of the matter is that by following his low-calorie regimen, he is actually losing muscle at a rate equal to or greater than his loss of fat.

To end this vicious cycle of eating less and increasing his body fat, Mike must fuel his muscles with adequate amounts of calories and carbohydrates every day. He must be sure to limit saturated fat in his diet and incorporate adequate amounts of protein. As discussed in the previous chapter, small, slow lifestyle changes are key to success in body composition change.

Eating Enough and On Time

Changing body composition (building muscle and utilizing fat stores for energy) requires fueling the body not dieting (31,32,33). ACSM Health & Fitness Journal provides an in-depth discussion of the necessity to fuel the body in exercise, and the consequences associated with inadequate caloric intake (33). When healthy people exercise during a time of severe energy deprivation, the potential benefits of exercise can be lost (33). Also, energy inadequacies may be the reason that people turn to performance enhancing ergogenic aids. They can be fooled into thinking that ergogenic aids are conferring benefits when, in reality, they are simply filling an energy or nutrient void that could be more effectively met by eating sufficient energy with a healthy distribution of nutrients (33).

Again, dieting forces the resting metabolic rate to make adjustments. These and other factors influence a person's total energy requirement. Energy balance requires an appropriate adjustment on the consumption side of the energy equation, i.e., decreased metabolic rate must be accompanied by decreased caloric intake, or weight gain will occur (33). On the other hand, overeating does not result in an equivalent increase in resting energy expenditure. Studies support the notion that energy restrictive diets often fail because they induce a lower resting energy expenditure that ultimately impedes weight loss (33). While this is particularly a problem for people who are disposed to gaining weight, it is also likely to be a problem in others because the reduction in resting energy expenditure is greater than would be expected by the weight loss from inadequate energy intake.

Adaptations that occur from energy imbalance have been known for some time. For example, it's been shown that runners clearly expend more energy than non-runners, yet they can maintain weight despite energy intakes equivalent to that of the non-runners. In one study, the runners ran approximately 54 kilometers per week but maintained weight on an energy intake that was calculated to be about 645 calories below the predicted energy requirement (33).

There is evidence that muscle mass may actually be reduced when caloric needs are not met (33). This may be associated with the long accepted idea that carbohydrates have a protein-sparing effect; that is, proteins are used as a source of energy when there is inadequate carbohydrate energy (31). A low energy intake (likely to be low in carbohydrates) would require that protein be used as a fuel rather than be spared for anabolic (muscle building) purposes (31). A low carbohydrate diet should be a red flag for exercisers who are trying to improve conditioning and muscle hypertrophy. It would be hard to imagine anything more counterproductive than utilizing the very tissue you're trying to improve because of an insufficient level of appropriate energy from carbohydrates (31).

A person may consume sufficient energy to satisfy the general daily need for energy but if these energy providing foods are consumed at the wrong time or are not the right type, the energy requirement may not be satisfied (33). A person who has an estimated daily energy requirement of 2,000 kilocalories can expect clearly different outcomes if the required energy is consumed in one meal at the end of the day or broken up into several meals spread throughout the day (33). Since exercise produces an insulin response, more glucose and amino acids enter cells after exercising. The determinant of how soon after exercise to eat depends on how long it takes for the individual to cool down so that blood flow can be diverted from working muscles to the gastrointestinal tract for absorption of nutrients.

The person who misses breakfast and lunch is likely to experience low blood sugar(31). It is common among elite athletes to complete an early morning exercise session before any source of energy is consumed (33). People commonly exercise in an energy-deficient state because the assumption is (albeit an incorrect one) that the body will run without fuel or will easily burn undesirable fat for fuel. Not true!

In addition to the reductions in energy expenditure during caloric restriction, other acute compensator changes occur, such as a reduction in levels of leptin and cholecystokinin (CCK) and increases in ghrelin and appetite, which all promote weight regain (90-94). Leptin and ghrelin are two hormones that have a major influence on energy balance (95). Leptin's roles are to mediate long term energy balance and to suppress food intake. The role of ghrelin, a fast acting hormone, is meal initiation. CCK is a peptide that plays numerous roles in appetite control and body weight regulation throughout the GI tract and CNS, with physiological effects on gallbladder contraction, pancreatic and gastric acid secretion, slowing emptying, and suppression of energy intake (96). While short-term weight-loss can be achieved through dietary/caloric restriction, the majority of people gain back the weight they lost due to adaptions in hormonal changes which can last up to 12 months after the caloric restriction (97). The hormonal and peptide changes that occur during caloric restriction dieting further support that dieting does not work. The key to sustainable healthy weight management is eating the right amounts of the right foods at the right time.

Labeling Regulations

Many well-intentioned clients, athletes, and patients are making what they believe to be healthy choices at the grocery store and in restaurants, but they are instead being sabotaged by inconsistencies and often ambiguous labeling regulations. Deciphering food labels and health claims has become an exercise in understanding legal rhetoric. "Whole grain" doesn't mean whole grain; "93% lean ground beef" isn't 93% lean by calories; and the definition of "free-range" is far from what you may envision. The goal of this section is **NOT** to have individuals throw away their can of Pam spray, or to totally eliminate beef from their diets. To be healthy, individuals need to know how much they should eat, and how much of each nutrient they should eat. The goal is to educate them on how to make healthier more informed choices. It can be viewed similar to maintaining a "budget", i.e. a calorie budget. Understanding labeling regulations can help protect individuals from fraudulently being "cheated" out of their hard earned calories.

The Food and Drug Administration (FDA) is responsible for regulating most food products, while the United States Department of Agriculture (USDA) is responsible for regulating dairy, meat, and poultry products (36,37). Each organization developed labeling requirements that are unique to their respective products and requirements. The National Labeling and Education Act (NLEA) passed by Congress in 1990 required mandatory nutrition labeling to appear on most packaged foods regulated by the FDA (34). The NLEA pertains only to those labels of food products regulated by FDA, which has labeling authority over the majority of foods. However, meat and poultry product labels are under the authority of Food Safety and Inspection Service (FSIS) in the USDA, and alcoholic beverage product labels are under the authority of the Alcohol and Tobacco Tax and Trade Bureau of the Department of the Treasury, formerly the Bureau of Alcohol, Tobacco and Firearms (37). No regulations have been passed requiring the USDA to make meat labels comparable to the packaged food labels. This makes it very difficult for consumers to compare products. Prepackaged pizza with meat topping falls under USDA rules while cheese pizza is labeled according to FDA rules (35).

FDA Regulations (Most Food Products)

To reiterate The National Labeling and Education Act (NLEA) passed by Congress in 1990 required mandatory nutrition labeling to appear on most packaged foods regulated by the FDA (35).

Whole Grain

There are several factors in determining the content of whole grain in various products.

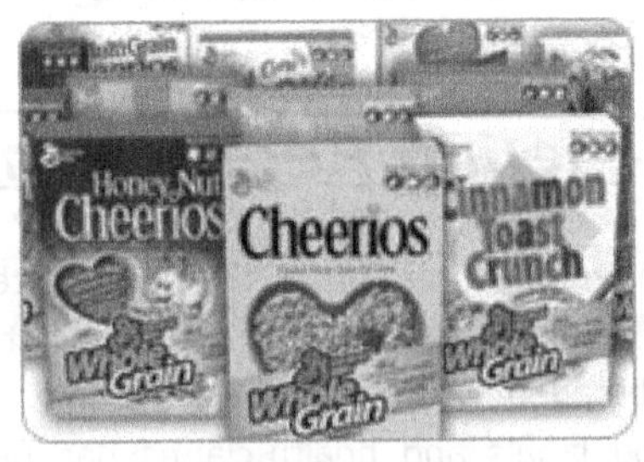

- The definition "made with whole grain" does not specify an amount of whole grain the product must contain (31,32,36). Hence, the product can have "some" amount of whole grain or almost no whole grain.
- "Made with whole grain" means a product may contain either a little or a lot of

whole grain- a specified amount is not required.

- "An excellent source of whole grain" means a product must contain at least 16 grams per serving or approximately nearly half of what most serving sizes are (30 to 55 grams).
- "A good source of whole grain" means there can be as little as 8 grams per serving. Is this truly a good source when the product may be less than 50% whole grain?
- "Multigrain" is a mixture of grains that can be mostly refined with minimal nutritional value.

General Mills claims their whole grain cereals are "made with whole grains." So how do the newer cereals stack up against their older counterparts? By comparing older ingredient labels with the new ones, it is clear the only thing that changed is the label. You can Visit www.wholegrainscouncil.org for more information about whole grains and where to find them in foods (80).

Fat Free/Calorie Free

Are products that claim to be calorie and fat-free truly free of calories and fat? Not exactly (31,32,36,38)!

- If a serving size contains less than 5 calories, per serving it can be called "calorie free."
- If a serving size contains 1/2 gram of fat, or less the product can be called "non-fat."
- The nutrition label on a can of Pam fat free cooking spray reads: serving size 1/3 second, calories 0, calories from fat 0. A side panel compares the fat in the Pam spray to the fat in butter. In a one second spray, Pam has 7 calories while a tablespoon of butter has 104 calories. A low fat alternative to be sure, but 7 calories per second does not mean calorie free. The can contains 702 (1/3 second) servings, in other words, 234 seconds; hence, the can contains 1638 calories (234 seconds x 7calories/second). The labeling law states that if the serving size contains 1/2 gram of fat or less it can be called non fat, and if the serving size contains less than 5 calories per serving, it can be called calorie free. So the 1/3 second serving size fulfills the legal requirements.
- Promise Ultra Fat-Free is 100% fat.
- This same regulation holds true for "trans-fats." Many new products are not truly free of trans-fats.

USDA Regulations

The USDA labeling regulations allow meat, poultry, and dairy products to label fat content by volume or weight rather than by calories as with the FDA labeling regulations (31,32,36,38,39).

Meat

A label of ground beef can legally state that it is 85% lean but that doesn't mean that the product is 15% fat by calories. The 85% lean, refers to fat content by weight (not by calories). Beef that is 85% lean can be 45 to 50% fat by calories. Hence, by legal definition:

- 93% lean ground beef (7% fat by weight) is actually 45% fat by calories.
- 97% lean pre-packaged meat is actually 18% fat by calories.

Dairy

The dairy industry is also regulated by the USDA and falls under the same category as meat and poultry products (31,38,39):

- Milk labeled 1% fat is 18% fat by calories.
- Milk labeled 2% fat is 36% fat by calories.
- Whole milk is almost 50% fat by calories. By definition, the FDA's guideline of low-fat is "a product containing three grams of fat or less ". Therefore, under the USDA labeling guidelines, milk labeled 2% (containing 5 grams of fat) could make the low-fat claim. However, in 1998 the FDA disallowed the use of low-fat for 2% milk. The term that is now used to replace low-fat is reduced- fat.

Organic

The USDA is responsible for managing the National Organic Program implemented in October 2002 (40). Organic is a labeling term that indicates: "the food or other agricultural product has been produced through approved methods that integrate cultural, biological, and mechanical practices that foster cycling of resources, promote ecological balance, and conserve biodiversity" (41). Synthetic fertilizers, sewage sludge, irradiation, and genetic engineering may not be used. By definition, organic farming avoids the use of most artificial inputs, such as synthetic pesticides and fertilizers. Also banned are the use of animal byproducts, antibiotics, and sewage sludge, among other practices (41).

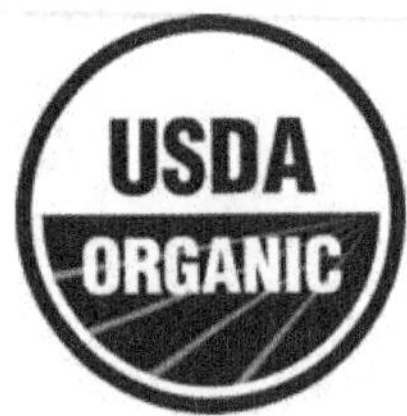

Organic certification agencies inspect and verify that organic farmers, ranchers, distributors, processors, and traders are complying with the USDA organic regulations. In order to sell, label, or represent their products as organic, operations must follow all of the specifications set out by the USDA organic regulations (31,32). Items labeled "certified organic" must pass a clearly defined certificating process by federal agents. Items labeled "certified organic" can not be genetically modified or irradiated; produce cannot be farmed with most synthetic pesticides or fertilizers; organic dairy, poultry, meat, and eggs are produced without growth hormones and antibiotics (40,41).

Any food product (except fish) using the word "organic" must be certified by an official USDA accredited organization. Definitions include (31,32):

- Foods made with 100 percent organic ingredients may claim "100% organic" and use the organic seal.
- "Organic" must contain at least 95% organically produced ingredients.
- A "made with organic" label means a product must contain at least 70% organic ingredients.
- Products that contain fewer than 70% organic ingredients cannot bear the USDA Organic seal or display the word "organic" on the front of the package. They may list them on the side panel but cannot make any claims on the front.
- Farms and handling operations that sell less than $5000 a year are exempt from certification and can label their products organic but can not use the USDA Organic seal.
- Grocery stores or restaurants do not have to be certified.
- Consumers can determine which fruits and vegetables are organic by reading the product code on produce stickers. Codes for conventionally grown produce are 4 digits; codes for organic produce are five digits; and codes for genetically modified produce are also five digits but begin with an 8 (31).

Since 1997, organic sales have more than quintupled with $18.9 billion in sales in 2007 (98). Because of the consumer demand for organic products, challenges with the organic regulatory program emerged. As a result, the 2008 Farm Act provided many provisions to help domestic producers meet the challenges of organic agriculture and meet the demand of the consumer (98).

National Organic Program (NOP) was audited in 2010, and the results were not favorable for consumers who place their trust in the logo. Here is a brief summary of the findings (99):

1. National Organic Program needs to improve its enforcement of organic operations that violate regulations. Prior to this report, NOP officials had not developed written policies for violators. As a result, months and years went by on the five

organic operations that were caught marketing non organic food products.

2. Processing of program complaints needed more timely action. Accordingly to the report, NOP did not resolve 19 of 41 program complaints in a timely matter.
3. NOP did not properly approve and manage the California State Organic Program. California was allowed to operate without required compliance and enforcement since 2004.
4. NOP did not incorporate periodic residue testing of organic products into its regulations. None of the five certifying agents the audit visited conducted periodic testing.
5. Evaluations of NOP's accreditation process were not performed annually.
6. Need for a more effective process for identifying inconsistent operating practices and clarify program requirements. The auditors visited four agents and 20 of their certified organic operations and found that all four agents were enforcing different requirements.
7. NOP oversight of foreign certifying agents needs significant improvement. NOP failed to complete required on site reviews at 5 of 44 foreign certifying agents.

It is not yet clear whether all or some of the recommendation from the report for the NOP have been implemented. However, it is clear that there are major issues with the oversight of the NOP.

Expect to pay 50-100% more for organic foods because it is more labor intensive, and without the help of pesticides, the yield is not always as large (43). You can keep costs down by shopping sale items, comparing prices, buying locally grown products at farmers' markets, or joining a co-op. Large grocery store chains are now offering organic foods which will help to keep prices down (43). Organic dollars should be spent primarily on produce (43). Fruits and vegetables are conventionally treated with pesticides, and fertilizers to enhance growth and prevent infestation and are most likely to contain residues (43).

The Environmental Working Group (EWG), a DC based nonprofit group, recommends going organic on what they call the "dirty dozen" which includes: peaches, apples, sweet bell peppers, celery, strawberries, cherries, imported grapes, spinach, lettuce, potatoes, blueberries, kale (44). The group also lists produce with the least or no pesticide residues which includes: cabbage, kiwi, sweet peas, asparagus, mango, pineapple, corn, avocado, onions, eggplant, cantaloupe, honeydew melon, watermelon, grapefruit, sweet potatoes (44). In 2011, some scientist challenged the EWG's claim of the dirty dozen stating that the commodity list are at negligible levels of pesticides and the methods used by EWG were insufficient (100).

Despite the concept that organic foods are healthier because of the lack of pesticides and fertilizers used, the evidence does not support these claims. Two large scale systematic reviews of the literature conclude that there is a lack of evidence that organic foods are significantly more nutritious, and there are nutrition related health effects from consuming organically produced food (191,102).

While the benefits of human consumption are still up for debate, there are some environmental benefits, such as reduced nutrient pollution, carbon sequestration, reduced pesticides residues in water, and enhanced biodiversity (103).

The USDA has not developed organic certification standards for seafood. Wild or farmed fish can be labeled "organic" despite the presence of mercury, PCBs, and other contaminants.

At this point, there isn't a right or wrong choice when deciding to consume organic or not. The decision boils down to what do you as the consumer believe is best for your health and well-being. The reality for many Americans is that enough fruits and vegetables and lean proteins aren't consumed in the first place; organic or not is a second, third, or fourth thought for most.

Health Claims

Unlike nutrition information, health messages on labels were strictly forbidden until 1987 (45). Since 1987, some scientifically based health statements have been permitted on labels subject to FDA approval (45). Health messages such as "Diets low in sodium may reduce the risk of high blood pressure," meant that the FDA had examined scientific evidence and reached the conclusion that there was a clear link between diet and health. Food manufacturers wanted to be allowed to inform consumers about possible benefits based on less than clear and convincing evidence (45,46). Food manufactures took their fight to court and the court ruled in their favor. The FDA must now allow claims that are **not** backed by convincing scientific evidence. There are now several "grades" of health claims that manufacturers can use. See the following table (45,46).

Grade	Level of Confidence	Required Disclaimer
Grade A	High: Significant scientific agreement	Does not require a disclaimer.
Grade B	Moderate: Evidence is supportive but not conclusive	Disclaimer: "Although there is scientific evidence supporting this claim, the evidence is not conclusive"
Grade C	Low: Evidence is limited and not conclusive	Disclaimer: "Some scientific evidence suggests (health claim). However, FDA has determined that this evidence is limited and not conclusive."
Grade D	Very Low: Little scientific evidence supporting this claim.	Disclaimer: "Very limited and preliminary scientific evidence research suggests (health claim). FDA concludes that there is little scientific evidence supporting this claim."

Structure-Function Claims

Unlike health claims, which require food manufacturers to collect scientific evidence and petition the FDA, structure-function claims can be made without any FDA approval (45,46). Manufacturers can add claims such as "improves bone health" or improves "cholesterol health" without any proof. However, manufacturers can not mention a disease or symptom. So claiming that a product "improves cholesterol levels" is illegal, but claiming that the product improves "cholesterol health" is legal. One can see how the public can be misled into believing product claims when no evidence exists.

Label Terms

The following is a summary of information that must be provided on labels (36) Basic packaging information must include: the common name of the product; the name and address of the manufacturer, packer or distributor; the net contents; the ingredient list; the serving size and number of servings; the quantities of specified nutrients and constituents.

Ingredient List:

1. The FDA requires that all ingredients be listed in descending order of predominance by weight and to state on the label that they have done so.
2. When more than one sweetener is used, manufacturers must put them all together under the term "sweeteners" and list them in order of predominance. So if the label specifies sweeteners as the second ingredient then the total of sweeteners is the second largest component of the product.
3. Manufacturers are also required to list the specific fats and oils they have used. They can no longer use the terms and/or clause (soybeans and/or coconut).

4. Manufacturers must now also list all additives.

Serving Size:

1. Labels must identify the size of a serving and the number of servings.
2. The standard serving size for beverages is 8 ounces.
3. Any package that contains less than 2 servings is considered a single serving item and the label must reflect the contents of the entire package.

Nutrition Information:

1. The label must show the quantities of certain nutrients, total calories, and calories from fat.
2. The label must indicate grams from total fat, saturated fat, cholesterol, and sodium.
3. The label must indicate total grams of carbohydrate, sugars, fiber, and protein.
4. Labels must present nutrient content information as compared with the percentage of recommended intakes: vitamin A, vitamin C, iron, calcium.

General Terms:

- Free. Nutritionally trivial and unlikely to have a physiological consequence; synonyms include without, no, and zero.
- High. 20% or more of the Daily Value for a given nutrient per serving.
- Less. At least 25% less of a given nutrient than the comparison food. Synonyms include fewer and reduced.
- Light or lite. Any use of the term, other than as defined below, must specify what it is referring to (for example, light in color, or light in texture).
- Low. An amount that would allow frequent consumption of a food without exceeding the dietary guidelines. A food that is naturally low in a nutrient may make such a claim but only as it applies to similar foods (for example, "fresh cauliflower, a low sodium food"); synonyms include little, few, low source of.
- More. At least 10% more of a given nutrient than the comparison food; synonyms include "added".
- Good source of. Product provides between 10 and 19% of the Daily Value for a given nutrient per serving.

Cholesterol Terms:

- Foods containing more than 13 g total fat per serving or per 50 g must indicate those contents immediately after a cholesterol claim. All cholesterol claims are prohibited when the food contains more than 2 grams saturated fat/serving.

- Cholesterol-free. Less than 2 mg cholesterol per serving and 2 grams or less saturated fat per serving.
- Low in cholesterol. 20 mg or less per serving and 2 grams or less of saturated fat per serving.
- Less cholesterol. 25% or less cholesterol than the comparison food (reflecting a reduction of fat at least 20 mg per serving) and 2 grams or less saturated fat per serving.

Energy Terms:

- Kilocalorie-free. Fewer than 5 kcal per serving.
- Light. One-third fewer kilocalories than the comparison food.
- Low kilocalorie. Less than 40 kcal per serving.

Fat Terms:

- Extra lean. Less than 5 grams of fat, 2 g of saturated fat, and 95 mg of cholesterol per serving and per 100 grams of food.
- Fat-free. Less than 0.5 grams of fat per serving (and no added fat or oil).
- Lean. Less than 10 grams fat, 4 g saturated fat, and 95 mg cholesterol per serving/per 100 grams of food.
- Less fat. 25% or less fat than the comparison food.
- Less saturated fat. 25% or less saturated fat than the comparison food.
- Low fat. 3 grams or less fat per serving.
- Low saturated fat. 1 gram or less saturated fat per serving.
- Percent fat-free. May be used only if the product meets the definition of low fat or fat free and must reflect the amount of fat in 100 grams.
- Light. 50% or less of the fat than in the comparison food (for example, 50% less fat than our regular cookies).

Fiber Terms

- High fiber. 20% or more of the Daily Value for fiber.
- High-fiber claim. Can be made on a food that contains more than 3 grams of fiber per serving and per 100 grams; must also declare total fiber.

Sodium Terms

- Sodium-free and salt-free. Less than 5 mg of sodium per serving.
- Low sodium. Less than 140 mg per serving.
- Light. A low kilocalorie, low-fat food with a 50% reduction in sodium.
- Light in sodium. No more than 50% of the sodium in the comparison food.
- Very low sodium. Less than 35 mg per serving.
- Sodium-free. Less than 0.5 grams per serving.

Voluntary Labeling

Labeling regulations that are voluntary include livestock products, such as meat and eggs. Animal raising claims must be truthful and not misleading. USDA's Food Safety Inspection Service verifies the truthfulness of these claims (31,32,36):

- *Free-range*. This label indicates that the flock was provided shelter in a building, room, or area with unlimited access to food, fresh water, and continuous access to the outdoors during their production cycle. The outdoor area may or may not be fenced and/or covered with netting-like material. This label is regulated by the USDA.
- *Cage-free*. This label indicates that the flock was able to freely roam a building, room, or enclosed area with unlimited access to food and fresh water during their production cycle.
- *Natural*. As required by USDA, meat, poultry, and egg products labeled as "natural" must be minimally processed and contain no artificial ingredients. However, the natural label does not include any standards regarding farm practices and only applies to processing of meat and egg products. There are no standards or regulations for the labeling of natural food products if they do not contain meat or eggs.
- *Grass-fed*. Grass-fed animals receive a majority of their nutrients from grass throughout their life, while organic animals' pasture diet may be supplemented with grain. Also USDA regulated, the grass-fed label does not limit the use of antibiotics, hormones, or pesticides. Meat products may be labeled as grass-fed organic.
- *Pasture-raised*. Due to the number of variables involved in pasture-raised agricultural systems, the USDA has not developed a federal definition for pasture-raised products.
- *Humane*. Multiple labeling programs make claims that animals were treated humanely during the production cycle, but the verification of these claims varies widely. These labeling programs are not regulated under a single USDA definition.
- *No added hormones*. A similar claim includes "Raised without Hormones." Federal regulations have never permitted hormones or steroids in poultry, pork, or goat.
- *Gluten-free*. The U.S. Food and Drug Administration published a regulation defining the term "gluten-free" for voluntary food labeling on August 2, 2013 (104). The FDA was directed to issue the new regulation by the Food Allergen Labeling and Consumer Protection Act (FALCPA), which directed the FDA to set guidelines for the use of the term "gluten-free" (104). It requires that, in order to use the term "gluten-free" on its label, a food must meet all of the requirements of the definition, including that the food must contain less than 20 parts per million of gluten. The rule also requires foods with the claims "no gluten," "free of

gluten," and "without gluten" to meet the definition for "gluten-free" (104). Food manufacturers have one year to bring their labels into compliance with the new requirements. Adherence to a gluten-free diet is key in treating celiac disease, and the FDA's new 'gluten-free' definition will help people with this condition make food choices that will help them to manage their health. The term "gluten" refers to proteins that occur naturally in wheat, rye, barley, and cross-bred hybrids of these grains. In people with celiac disease, foods that contain gluten trigger production of antibodies that attack and damage the lining of the small intestine. Such damage limits the ability of celiac disease patients to absorb nutrients and puts them at risk of other very serious health problems, including nutritional deficiencies, osteoporosis, growth retardation, infertility, miscarriages, short stature, and intestinal cancers.

Unregulated Terms

The FDA does not evaluate or regulate terms placed on labels outside of the nutrition facts panel (31,32,36).

Net Carbs

The term "net carbs" does not have a legal definition and is not used by the FDA or the American Diabetes Association (47).

The term "net carbs" came about when companies were seeking a way to market their products as being low in carbohydrates. Some food companies created the term "net carbs" and defined it as the total grams of carbohydrate minus the grams of sugar alcohols, fiber, and glycerin.

Nutrition Facts

Serving Size: 1 Bar (60g)
Servings Per Container: 1

Amount Per Serving	
Calories 220	**Calories from Fat 80**
	% Daily Value*
Total Fat 9g	14%
Saturated Fat 6g	30%
Trans Fat 0g	
Cholesterol 0mg	0%
Sodium 120mg	5%
Total Carbohydrate 27g	9%
Dietary Fiber 11g	44%
Sugar 1g	
Sugar Alcohol 4g	
Protein 17g	34%

• Vitamin A 25%	• Vitamin C 25%
• Calcium 35%	• Iron 10%
• Vitamin E 15%	• Vitamin K 15%
• Thiamin 15%	• Riboflavin 15%
• Niacin 15%	• Vitamin B6 15%
• Folate 15%	• Vitamin B12 15%
• Biotin 25%	• Magnesium 15%
• Phosphorus 10%	• Pantothenic Acid 15%
• Zinc 15%	• Selenium 15%
• Chromium 10%	

*Percent Daily Values are based on a 2,000 calorie diet. Your daily values may be higher or lower depending on your calorie needs:

	Calories	2,000	2,500
Total Fat	Less Than	65g	80g
Sat Fat	Less Than	20g	25g
Cholesterol	Less Than	300mg	300mg
Sodium	Less Than	2400mg	2400mg
Total Carbohydrate		300g	375g
Dietary Fiber		25g	30g
Protein		50g	65g

The FDA requires that the total carbohydrate count is listed on a nutrition label and must include the full amount of grams from sugar alcohols and fiber (31,32,36). However, these carbs have less impact on blood glucose than others because they are only partially converted to glucose or not at all (47). This equation is not entirely accurate because some of the sugar alcohols and fiber are absorbed by the body. In fact, about half of the grams of sugar alcohols are metabolized to glucose (47).

Consumers should ignore the net carb definition and read the nutrition facts and ingredients list for more information. Diabetics on intensive insulin management who must manage their diabetes with carb-to-insulin ratios should understand (47):

1. If the product's sugar alcohol content is greater than 5 grams, subtract half the grams of sugar alcohols from the total carbohydrates and count this as the "available carbohydrate" for insulin adjustment purposes. However, if erythritol is the only sugar alcohol listed, subtract all of the grams of sugar alcohol.
2. Total fiber in foods comprises many different types of natural fiber and manufactured ingredients. If insoluble fiber is listed on the nutrition facts panel under "Total Carbohydrate," subtract all of the insoluble fiber from the total carbohydrates and from the total fiber grams. If the fiber quantity is still greater than 5 grams, subtract half the grams of dietary fiber from the total carbohydrates, and use the result as the available carbs for insulin adjustment purposes.

Food Production / Commodities

Current agricultural policies are another contributing factor to the poor health of Americans (48-51). Government payments are skewed towards overproduction of commodity foods containing mostly processed, high calorie foods (48). Cheap commodities allow retailers and restaurants (and schools) to sell their products at a low cost (58,63,64). Not only are these commodities cheap, but farmers are also subsidized by the government which makes them lucrative crops to grow (63,64).

Commodity programs, or Title I of the U.S. Farm Bill, is the main federal mechanism for influencing American agriculture (49). The 2008 Farm Bill was to expire in 2012, but a temporary extension was granted until the end of 2013 at which time Congress must produce a final bill to be signed into law (53,54). The American farm policy is effectively driving the production and propagation of cheap sugars and oils that lead to widespread availablilty in the food supply, which many believe is contributing to the "growing" nation. Although subsidies provide a necessary safety net to farmers, existing support programs continue to create strong economic incentives to overproduce a select number of crops at the expense of American health (48).

The U.S. food market provides 3900 calories per capita each day, or twice the average person's caloric requirement (55). Between 1970 and 2000, the consumption of added fats per person increased by 38% and that of sugars increased by 20% (4). The consumption of high-fructose corn syrup (HFCS) increased more than 1000% between 1970 and 1990, which today accounts for more than 40% of caloric sweeteners added to food and beverages (56). The situation is exacerbated because these foods provide extremely cheap caloric options (57) and most consumers place more importance on cost when purchasing food (58,59,60).

The business of food is the most ubiquitous and powerful industry in the world (48). It is dominated by influential stakeholders, interest groups, and public health organizations have had little influence in the process. Because of the scale and complexity of the obesity epidemic, any one intervention cannot reasonably be expected to reverse obesity trends in the immediate future (48). Although policy reform is only one of the many fronts to combat obesity, a revision of agricultural priorities is crucial (48). Public health interventions will remain limited in their impact until they can influence decisions that are made at every level of the American food chain, from growers to consumers (48).

Eating Out

Eating out can produce panic in individuals embarking on new lifestyle changes. Individuals need to be educated in making healthy choices when eating out. Yes, people can eat out and still maintain healthy habits, but, it's not easy; it can be a very confusing, difficult task.

America has been called a "fast food nation," and for good reason (65,66). Everyday, one out of four Americans eats fast food (65,66). Most do it for the convenience as well as cost; fast food restaurants are often the cheapest option. Unfortunately, they are not the most nutritious option. Generally, fast food meals are higher in calories, sodium, and fat, and are often lacking in important vitamins and minerals (31,32). Restaurant dining poses similar challenges. Restaurant meals also tend to include too much fat, salt, or sugar, and portions are almost always larger than normal.

The good news is that many fast food and dining restaurants are adding healthier menu options. It is now possible to eat a fairly nutritious meal on the go.

Hints On Eating Out

Eating at a restaurant does not have to sabotage a healthy lifestyle plan. Using smart-eating strategies when eating out can eliminate many calories and reduce sodium and fat intake (81).

Have a plan.
Eat a light dinner if you ate a big lunch that day, or r if you know ahead of time that you're going to a restaurant, cut back on calories during other meals that day.

Menu terms.

Knowing menu terms and cooking basics makes ordering easier, especially if you need to control calories or fat. Look for foods that are steamed, broiled, baked, or grilled, and limit fried and sautéed items or foods described as "crispy," "rich" or "au gratin."

Choosing a Restaurant.

Think ahead. Consider meal options at different restaurants and look for places with a wide range of menu items. Check online menus if available for menu and nutrition information.

Ordering.

Balance your meal by including foods from all the different food groups: meat, dairy, fruits, vegetables, and grains. Look for freshly made entrée salads that give you "balance in a bowl." For example, entrée salads with chicken, hard boiled eggs, or seafood provide protein along with fiber and vitamins. If you are counting calories, use a low-fat dressing, or skip some of the extras like croutons. For sandwich toppings, go with low-fat options like lettuce, tomato, and onion; use condiments like ketchup, mustard or relish, or low-fat dressings. Round out your meal by ordering healthy side dishes, such as a side salad with low-fat dressing, baked potato, or fruit. Boost the nutritional value of your baked potato by topping it with vegetables, salsa, or chili.

Substitute

Ask for a side salad with low-fat dressing to replace fries in a combination meal. Many restaurants honor requests so don't be afraid to be assertive, ask menu questions and make special requests to meet your nutritional needs. Many restaurants serve huge portions, sometimes enough for two or three people. Order menu items that contain fewer calories, and eat a smaller portion. Bring leftovers home for another meal, or order an appetizer in place of an entrée and add a small salad. Order sauce and dressing on the side. By asking for sauces and dressings on the side, you can control the amount that you eat. Often, you can use less than is normally used and still enjoy the same taste.

Eating

Eat slowly. It takes about 20 minutes for your brain to get the message from your stomach that you are no longer hungry. Fast eaters often are over-eaters, while slow eaters tend to eat less and are still satisfied. Avoid buffets. All-you-can-eat buffets promote overeating. If the temptation isn't in front of you, you are less likely to overindulge. Stick to the light menu, and make careful menu selections. Many restaurants indicate healthy choices on their menus, and most sit-down places will modify menu items on your request.

Knowing how food is prepared can be a good indication of whether it will work with your diet or ruin it. Main courses which have been baked, broiled, roasted, poached or steamed will be more healthy than anything fried. Salads with plenty of fresh fruits and vegetables and lighter dressings will be better than salads with croutons, cheeses, meats, and heavy dressings.

When choosing a soup, keep in mind that cream-based soups are higher in fat and calories than most other soups. Soup can serve as a great appetizer to a meal, or as an entree. Most soups are low in calories and will fill you up so you eat less. When ordering grilled fish or vegetables, ask that the food either be grilled without butter or oil or prepared "light," with little oil or butter. When ordering pasta dishes, look for tomato-based sauces rather than cream-based sauces. Tomato-based sauces are much lower in fat and calories. In addition, the tomato sauce (or marinara sauce) can count as a vegetable! Drink water, seltzer, or unsweetened tea or coffee instead of regular soda or alcoholic beverages. This will save a lot of calories each day.

<u>Share</u>

Sharing entrees, appetizers, and desserts with dining partners is a great idea. It allows you to sample something that you really want to have while also helping you avoid the temptation to overindulge. If you are sharing with a friend or your partner, your portion size is automatically reduced and there is less available to eat. It is still important to make good menu choices, but sharing might make dessert (or something else indulgent) more of an option.

<u>Eating Out with Kids</u>

Choose a restaurant that caters to children and has a healthy children's menu that includes smaller portion sizes and meals designed to provide ample nourishment for smaller bodies. For kids' meals, opt for milk as a beverage and fruit for dessert. Order plain foods with sauce on the side. Substitute healthier "sides" in place of fries, like carrots or apple slices. Choose two or three suitable menu items, then let your child pick one. Let kids order their familiar favorites when they eat out. For new foods, offer a bite or two from your order.

Calcium is important at all ages, but especially for growing bones. To get adequate calcium, drink low-fat or fat-free plain or chocolate milk or add a slice of cheese to sandwiches. Choose dairy-based treats like yogurt, a smoothie or frozen dairy dessert. Non-dairy options include calcium fortified juices and almond, soy or rice milks. Also selecting dark green, leafy vegetables (broccoli, kale, collards) and beans on a regular basis can increase calcium consumption.

Restaurants may be intimidating to people trying to stick to a healthy diet, but with preparation and confidence, you can enjoy your restaurant meal without abandoning healthy eating.

The big picture.

Think of eating out in the context of your whole diet. If it is a special occasion or a fun social occasion and you know you want to order your favorite meal at a nice restaurant, cut back on your earlier meals that day. Moderation is always key, but planning ahead can help you relax and enjoy your dining out experience without sacrificing good nutrition or diet control.

Other Sabotaging Practices

Portion Distortion

Advertisers and food distributors have truly distorted our view of serving sizes. How many times have you seen supersize, all you can eat, double or even triple burgers, big foot pizza, or 16 ounce sirloin? The average portion sizes for nearly every category of food have increased since the late 1970s both at home and at restaurants (82,83). Many popular foods and beverages are now manufactured in sizes up to five times larger than when they were introduced (84). Portions for many of these foods now exceed federal recommended standards by as much as eight times (84)! Years ago a meal at a fast food restaurant might consist of a 4-ounce hamburger, 3-ounce serving of French fries, and a 10-ounce soda; compare that to the 7.6-ounce burger, 7-ounce serving of fries, and 32-ounce drink you might order today. Eating out in restaurants has also taught consumers to adopt the supersize mentality at home. So how do we help clients deal with portion sizes? The food chart presented in Chapter 12 is a very useful tool in helping clients understand how much they are eating.

Eating Too Many Calories in the Evening

Dieters who eat their main meal earlier in the day lose significantly more weight than those who eat later in the day even when caloric intake is similar (85). Someone consuming 1000 calories at night and not eating during the day will not be successful in weight management. Muscle will be utilized during the day for energy and the body will store many of the 1000 calories eaten at night as fat. Changing eating patterns is a very difficult obstacle to overcome. As already discussed, many people with stressful, harried lifestyles associate eating in the evening with "unwinding" and "taking care of themselves." These individuals will need to find other alternatives to "fill in the gap." This is where a fun list is helpful. A fun list can help individuals replace the eating with a more positive activity. The client/student is asked to make a fun list consisting of at least five things that he or she enjoys. This fun list should be displayed in an area where it is readily seen (as on the refrigerator). When the problematic period approaches, the client then picks one of the fun activities instead of eating. While this sounds easy, in most cases it is not. Some persons may have a hard time coming up with a fun list and then have tremendous difficulty implementing it. However, it's well worth the effort because it works.

Problem Foods in the Home

Temptation needs to be minimized, especially for beginners. Problem foods need to be removed from the home temporarily, if not permanently. Help your clients reach the understanding that this in no way means they are "failures" but is simply a part of human nature.

Deprivation of Favorite Foods

Deprivation produces binge-eating. Favorite foods can be eaten in moderation. Moderation is the key! Goals need to be set as to the timing of these favorite foods, i.e., "I'll have a piece of chocolate cake next weekend." To reiterate, these favorite foods should not be kept in the home but should be bought in one serving sizes or eaten out.

Shopping When Hungry

Never shop when hungry. Hungry people make lousy choices. The temptation is too great—no one should ever go food shopping when hungry. Have a healthy snack first, then attempt "entering the candy store without buying candy".

Not Planning

Not planning is surely one of the biggest obstacles to overcome. For persons to be successful in long term weight management, planning must become part of their lifestyle. Planning does not take extra time—it requires thinking ahead of time. If healthy choices are not available, the hungry individual will undoubtedly make "lousy choices." This doesn't mean that the only choices are carrots and celery (rabbit food). Good choices can include yogurt, bagels, cereals, pretzels, fruits, milk, etc.

Eating by The Numbers

Prescribing a computerized list of foods that should be eaten does not produce success. Telling someone that they must eat cottage cheese every day when they hate cottage cheese will lead to failure. What will produce long term success is incorporating the individual's food preferences with changes centered on those preferences. For example, if your client loves cream cheese on his/her bagel for breakfast, switching to low fat cream cheese is an acceptable alternative. Eventually, switching to nonfat cream cheese may also be an acceptable alternative. However, telling your client that cream cheese is a bad food and never to be eaten again may produce immediate results but eventually will produce failure. Remember, no one can sacrifice forever. Also, it is important to work with clients/students to help come up with acceptable alternatives. If the same client as above hates low fat cream cheese, another alternative may be to put jelly on the bagel 6 out of 7 days, and on the seventh day, indulge in the "real" thing.

<u>Friendly Saboteurs</u>

Saboteurs are essentially people who target behaviors for their own purposes. They offer food when it is not wanted, advice whether it is wise or not, and commentary not generally designed to facilitate attainment of goals. Saboteurs come in so many forms that it is often difficult to spot them until after the fact. Some mean well but produce harm through their ignorance, others are deliberately trying to sabotage, and yet others are simply selfish. The only commonality is that regardless of their motives, saboteurs try to alter behavior from what should be done to what they want done. There are several steps in gaining the upper hand over people's efforts to control. The first is to really convince individuals that they have the right to say no. The second is to identify the principal saboteurs; they are not always obvious. The next step is to master strategies to produce assertiveness in your clients.

<u>Stress Eating</u>

Have you ever had this experience? You come home from a long day feeling tired, down, and lonely. The day has been super-stressful, and you have no one to greet you at the door. You look in the refrigerator for something to eat; you really do not feel like cooking dinner for yourself, so you have a snack of cheese and crackers. You have more cheese and crackers and decide that this was dinner. Then, since you have eaten a lousy dinner, dessert would fit right in. You open the freezer and have a few bites of ice cream. After thinking about your day and how you feel, you continue eating the ice cream until it's all gone. This type of stress eating is very common. Strategies to deal with stress eating at night can include a fun list, healthy snacks available, etc.

Another strategy is to "never be hungry". Hungry, starving people make unhealthy choices. Here are some helpful hints and strategies: always be sure to eat breakfast; eat every 3 to 4 hours during the day; carry emergency food in the car or at the office; eat a snack before reaching home; on the drive home plan dinner.

Sometimes the thought of cooking dinner at the end of a long day is just overwhelming. This is an area where planning is key. Individuals should try to plan meals in advance of this "critical time period". If they are too tired to cook, options need to be determined. For example, cottage cheese and fruit with a baked potato and salsa fulfills all of the nutritional requirements of a healthy meal (may not be a great sounding combination) and requires very little effort. Frozen vegetables added to broth-based soup with a slice of whole grain bread will also fulfill the requirements for a healthy meal. Of course, there is always the option of eating out, but beware; this is a time when it is easy to give in to all the temptations (I deserve it). If opting to eat out rules, the restaurant should be familiar and the choice made before entering the restaurant.

<u>Traveling</u>
Learning to eat healthy when traveling requires fortitude. Making healthy choices when traveling is a process of "trial and error". Carrying healthy snacks may be the only alternative. Another pitfall is those "social" alcoholic drinks.

<u>Meetings</u>
Many people feel compelled to eat at business meetings, while others eat because of boredom. Teach your clients to try to eat a healthy snack before meetings and to have water available to drink. If possible, they should bring their own healthy snacks. After the meeting, they should go back to their healthy eating program.

<u>Holidays/Being a Guest</u>
The problem with holidays is not one holiday but many holidays and the days surrounding them. For some clients, holidays are terrifying; some people worry about holidays months ahead of time. They are afraid to say no to any food that their host presents (they do not want to be rude). This can be a very huge stumbling block for some clients. They will be dealing with psychological factors that have been ingrained for many years. The key to helping these clients is to emphasize the importance of becoming assertive enough to be able to say no (see the section on friendly saboteurs). Other strategies include filling up on vegetables and taking smaller portions of high fat alternatives— just enough to be polite. Offering to bring a low fat alternative can also be very helpful.

Building a Successful Nutrition Business

Whether you work for yourself or another company, implementing a nutrition component requires an understanding of entrepreneurial skills. Starting a new business - the Business of Nutrition - can be a daunting task.

In 2010, there were 27.9 million small businesses in the U.S. and over three-quarters of these small businesses had no employees (86). Every year, over a million people in this country start a business (68). Statistics indicate that over 40 percent of these businesses will fail by the end of the first year. Within five years, that number rises to more than 80% (68).

To be included in the 20% of businesses that succeed well beyond five years, you will need not only passion and fortitude, but you will need to understand business "disciplines." You will need to become a "juggler" combining the roles of boss, employee and technician.

This section will focus on helping you get started. However, to be successful you will need to go beyond the information presented in this textbook. There are many great books about owning and running your own business. Beyond books, there are courses available. The Small Business Administration - http://www.sba.gov/ - offers free online programs and information.

EMyth

What is the EMyth? The "EMyth," or Entrepreneurial Myth, is the flawed assumption that people who are an expert at a certain technical skill will therefore be successful running a business of the same kind (69):

In Michael Gerber's first book, The EMyth Revisited, he describes many common mistakes small business owners make (68). "It's a common misconception that because someone understands the nuts-and-bolts of technical work, they will similarly understand how a business providing that sort of product or service should function." From the EMyth point of view, small business owners struggle to achieve success because they are working *in* their business when they need to be working *on* their business (68).

The exciting process, developed by Michael Gerber, ensures that building a successful business does not depend on "luck" or "magic." A successful business follows the "Business Development Process." Its foundation includes three integrated activities:

i nnovation, quantification, and orchestration (68).

The difference between creativity and innovation is the difference between thinking about getting things done and actually getting them done. Creativity thinks up new things; innovation does new things. Innovation is the signature of a bold, imaginative hand (68).

In Michael Gerber's second book, The EMyth Mastery, he describes the "Seven Essential Disciplines for Building a World Class Company (67). In great detail, Michael defines the qualities required to build a successful business.

The exciting take-home point is running a successful business requires following predetermined "rules." Success does not depend on "chance". Each one of us can be successful in business if we follow the rules. Not following the rules can be a "recipe" for disaster.

Before Getting Started

Before getting started, it is critical to weigh the pros and cons of being an entrepreneur. Prepare for crazy-long hours, including weekends, and a work load that's also taxing for an entrepreneur's family. Many spouses/partners don't understand this and may not be able to tolerate it. Aside from these considerations, here's what the experts say are the required attributes to be a successful entrepreneur (68).

It's Not Just the Money

Two of the USA's most famous entrepreneurs — Bill Gates at Microsoft and Warren Buffett at Berkshire Hathaway — are also the two richest Americans. They were driven to create great companies not just huge fortunes (68). Indeed, Gates and Buffett have combined their riches to create a $60 billion philanthropic powerhouse in the Bill & Melinda Gates Foundation (72). "Entrepreneurs" are much more interested in wealth rather than riches (68). Riches are piles of money but wealth is broader encompassing less-tangible rewards such as respect and independence. So as a would-be entrepreneur you need to examine how you expect to be rewarded. If the compensation is just cash then the practice of entrepreneurship will not be very rewarding (68)."

Passion

When something is important to you, you not only know it in your heart but in your brain. You infect others with your passion which makes them believe in you (68). You don't just think you've built a better business — you feel it in your gut, and you know the world will be much better when you can get your idea to market. Passion must be the driving force to withstand the downside of owning your own business, ie., the workload and long hours.

Risk-taking

Business success isn't guaranteed. Would-be entrepreneurs must be calculated risk-takers. The thought of failing can't slow your steps as things get tougher. True entrepreneurs strive to control risk while still thriving on it (68).

Strong Ethics

Start-ups depend heavily on strong ethics. In a hyper-competitive economy, any whiff of dishonesty can deep-six a new enterprise. Penn State University's Anthony Warren, who advises venture capitalists, says honesty and trustworthiness are high on the list of attributes he looks for when he considers recommending a venture to potential investors (73). "Who wants to be in business with someone you can't trust," says Warren, director of the school's Farrell Center for Corporate Innovation and Entrepreneurship (73). The founders of Google, Sergey Brin and Larry Page, famously created a "don't be evil" mantra when they took Google public (73).

Tech Ease

Feeling comfortable with technology is crucial because computers, software, and other gadgets are key to launching a successful business in the service sector (72). Start-up costs have decreased since the prices for powerful computers and software have fallen. These lower prices came as the internet allows entrepreneurs to tap global markets. Setting up a small office with a laptop, fax machine, cellphone, etc. can cost as little as $5,000 (72). Add a professional-looking website for $500 or so, and you can compete with bigger, more established companies. But you can't take advantage of those lower costs if you aren't comfortable using popular word-processing, database, spreadsheet, and presentation programs (72).

Tenacity

Sometimes the best business ideas fail to take hold — not because there isn't demand but because the start-up was under-capitalized, or the entrepreneur lacked management know-how. (72). A nobody entrepreneur who started a variety store in Arkansas in 1945 eventually lost the business when his landlord wouldn't renew his lease, but he didn't give up. "I've never been one to dwell on reverses," Sam Walton recalled in his autobiography, "and I didn't do so then (72)." The company he fought to start, WalMart, is now the USA's biggest private employer with more than 1.3 million workers (72).

Pros and Cons

Benefits of having your own business are numerous. As a consultant, you are your own boss. You decide how much to charge and you decide when you want to work and when you want to play. You don't have a boss telling you what to do and when to do it. You decide where to work, whether it's in a health setting, a corporate setting, club setting, physical therapy setting, or your own facility. You negotiate percentages when consulting with health facilities. Another reason to work as an independent consultant is the tax benefits. As a business owner, you get to deduct expenses, in some circumstances travel (when it is related to your work), home office space and more.

One of the biggest problems associated with owning your own business is "you are your own boss." Now it's your job to accumulate income, pay bills, find new business, etc. For some, the benefits far outweigh any negatives. For others, the "uncertainty" and lack of "guaranteed" income are terrifying. Before you begin a journey as an entrepreneur, be sure you are in the former category not the latter.

Steps to Starting a Business

New businesses face many challenges from planning, to regulations, to opening a bank account, and creating a web site. Regardless of where you are in the process, the following preparatory steps are required for success in implementing a new business (70).

1. Write a business plan and form goals and objectives for your new company. A successful start to any business requires a detailed outline of what you plan to accomplish. Whether you use your own savings or obtain loans, starting a business requires money. The loan process can take months to complete, so start early. Lenders often request a completed business plan prior to approval of funding. Forming a corporation or LLC can protect owners' personal assets from business debts. Additionally, incorporating can provide credibility and tax benefits (71).
2. Identify a location for the business and establish a business address. Businesses must maintain an address where legal documents can be received (70,71).
3. Will your corporation or LLC do business under a name other than its legal name filed with the Secretary of State? If so, it must file a DBA (Doing Business As) name (70,71).
4. Businesses file names on a per-state basis, so other companies may be using the same or a similar name in other states. Conducting a trademark search ensures your unique company name isn't already in use (74).
5. Obtain a Federal Employer Identification Number (EIN) (71). Incorporated

businesses and companies that hire employees must obtain an EIN. Most state, county, and local governments require businesses to obtain licensing before they begin to operate (70).

6. Incorporating or forming an LLC does not provide a company with business insurance. Most companies obtain general business insurance from an insurance provider. Corporations and LLCs that hire employees also typically obtain unemployment and workers compensation insurance (70).
7. Establish a web presence (70). Not having an effective website eliminates opportunities for new customers and more profit.
8. To protect personal assets, businesses must maintain separate business and personal accounts and records. Establish a separate business bank account so that your personal assets are not co-mingled with business funds (70).
9. Establish proper accounting procedures and follow government rules. Operating a small business means satisfying ongoing government and legal requirements to maintain the company's good standing. Identify where to get help. Smart business owners know where and when to seek advice from other sources (70) Such as the Small Business Administration (http://www.sba.gov/).

After all these steps have been taken, you're still not quite ready to get started. There are several more steps before "opening day" (68).

Your Unique Perspective

Your business must reflect "you." What is it that makes you unique? What is it that draws you to this profession? Success rests on your ability to differentiate your services from others. Your personal reasons are what will make your business different and successful. After answering these questions you are ready to go on to the next step.

Choosing a Client Base

In Chapter 10, we discussed identifying clients that are ready to make lifestyle changes. It must be reiterated again if an individual is in the "precontemplative" stage, no changes will be made. This type of individual will "blame" you for their inability to live a healthier lifestyle. In working with a client that is not ready to change, he or she may likely attempt to blame you as the coach for their lack of success. You will simply be frustrating yourself and setting your business up for failure. There is no quicker way to destroy a business than this type of "bad" publicity.

Choosing your client base means deciding on which "type" of client you would like to work with (75). To answer this question, begin scripting an answer to what it is you do. Have you ever met someone who asked you what you do? How did you answer? Many entrepreneurs don't know how to answer this simple question. Often people respond with their job title or general profession. "I'm a personal trainer" or "I'm a nutrition coach." For example, let's say you bumped into someone you hadn't seen in several years. You ask them, "What do you do?" They respond, "I'm a teacher." Well that's nice, but it doesn't tell you very much. Now say they responded with, "I enrich young minds and inspire children to follow their passion." This statement provides a much better understanding of "what this person does." An appropriate answer for a fitness/wellness professional might begin with: "I help people pursue their health and wellness goals." This response does not answer what **you** do! What unique group do you serve (75)? You can generate even more interest by leading off with a question before using the introduction you just developed. After you're asked, "What do you do?" try something simple like, "You know how lots of people are trying to lose weight? Well what I do is help (your target population) to adjust their lifestyle to pursue their goals." Another example might be, "You know how there is all kinds of confusion about the healthiest way to eat? Well, what I do is help (your target population) to sift through the information and develop an individual healthy eating plan." These examples are referred to as "scripting". Scripting may seem artificial at first, but as you get more comfortable with your personal script, it will come across natural. Scripting clarifies thoughts and produces confidence (75).

After answering the question "What do you do" you now have a clearer idea of the group that you want to work with. You now have an individual introduction that inspires you and gets you excited to meet new people.

Developing a Pricing Scheme

Before deciding on pricing options, research other "diet" programs in your community. It's important to price your program relative to other programs in your area. One mistake many fitness professionals make is to price a nutrition program relative to personal training programs. The public pays much more for nutrition/diet programs than personal training. There is also hidden preparation time that must be included in your pricing scheme. A suggested pricing scheme is to multiply personal training rates in your area by 1.25 to 1.5. For example, if training rates average $50 an hour you should charge $62.50 to $75 per hour for nutrition services.

Attracting Business - Sales

Thoughts determine actions, and actions determine results (75). So the first step to attracting new business is "positive" thinking. How do you feel when you think of selling or promoting your business? Your confidence attracts confident clients. If you appear uncomfortable or uneasy about your services, you will attract uncomfortable and uneasy clients.

Many nutrition professionals mention all kinds of negative emotions when it comes to sales, marketing, and public relations. It's important to feel comfortable with promoting your services. Although you may not have any formal training in attracting business, it has more to do with your attitude than your aptitude on the subject. You want to display a confidence in the quality of your services and inspire the belief that you can truly help your clients; this may never be spoken, but you will emanate a level of confidence that your clients can feel. This confidence will motivate and inspire them to work harder and believe in their abilities to succeed when working with you (75).

Making the Sale

In order to stay in business and remain competitive in the field, you must earn money. Money is not the only driving force behind what you do, but it is absolutely necessary to stay in business. Your main goal is to help people achieve their goals, to stretch themselves, and to be better than they ever thought they could be (75); but without income, you won't be able to stay in business and help them achieve their goals.

The truth is selling is positive, and in order to be successful selling your services, you need to believe it's great to sell! What both you and your client are really looking for is a positive relationship. Knowing that you are looking for a relationship and not just a sale can help you to relax and enjoy talking to new and potential clients. Sure, a one time sale is okay, but in order to build a strong nutrition business, you need to attract repeat and long-term customers who will refer more business in your direction. Nutrition is an intimate business, and it typically takes several sessions to get results. You'll be learning a lot about your client and you will want to develop a strong relationship during the promotion and sale.

Most people in health care professions enjoy people. Talking to people typically comes natural. However, if you feel like you're trying to "sell" then you may feel uncomfortable and appear less confident. You also may seem stiff and tend to lack the passion that most clients are seeking. So forget about "selling" and simply get to know the person. Ask questions, develop rapport, and enjoy the process. Remember, you are providing a service that they should be desperate to receive. You have the solutions to their questions.

Although many people think "closing" a sale is complex, if you've effectively used questions to attract your client to your services, the close is relatively easy. Here are several examples of effective closing statements (75):

- "The nutrition coaching seems to appeal to you. When would you like to get started?"
- "It sounds like you are ready to make an investment in your health. When is a good time for your first appointment?"
- "You look eager to get started. The next step is for us to set-up an initial 1-hour appointment. Do you prefer mornings or afternoons?"
- "If I can fit you in my schedule this week, would you like to get started?"
- "If it's okay with you, I'll grab my schedule book so we can get you started right away."

In the ideal world, everyone would say "yes" and sign-up right then. However, there are two other things to consider. One is that you may feel your services don't meet the client's needs. In which case an easy way to check is, "Based on what you're telling me this may not be for you, what do you think?" This is an easy way to let the client out of an uncomfortable situation and leave the door open for future business opportunities.

The second thing that may happen is the client has some objection. You should immediately go back to asking questions. Have the client explain their objection in more detail and remember to never disagree – this is a sure way to lose a new client. Before providing an alternative solution, you need to know more about the objections. Here are some potential questions used to further discuss the objection:

- "Obviously you have a good reason for saying that. May I ask what it is?"
- "I understand how you feel. Others have felt the same way when I have spoken to them, but after our initial appointment, they found this was the perfect solution for them. What do you think?" (this particular style is often referred to as a "feel, felt, found statement")
- "Let me see if I understand your concerns, (restate what they said) you're worried that you won't be able to follow the plan."

Happy clients are more than willing to provide a testimonial (75). Testimonials are a great way for prospective clients to learn about how others have benefited from your services. After spending so much time attracting a new client, it's important to continue the relationship even after the coaching sessions are complete. One of the best ways to gain new business is through results and referrals. If your clients get results, others will see this and ask them about it. Most people are thrilled to send more business your way if you helped them achieve their goals. Referrals do not always come that easily though. Sometimes you have to ask for them. This may be as simple as asking a question at the end of a session: "Do you know anyone else who could benefit from my services?" It can also be beneficial to ask for referrals at the end of the initial sale, "Can you give me the names of three people who are in a similar situation?" I would even encourage you to ask for referrals from people who choose not to work with you. Try, "Who do you know who could benefit from the services we've just discussed?"

Provide present clients with brochures, your website, etc. Provide present clients with incentives for referrals (discount on sessions, etc.). Other trainers that are not providing nutrition services can benefit by referring clients to you for your nutrition program. You can provide incentives to the trainers for such referrals. Ask all of your clients for permission to contact their doctors and periodically provide the physicians with the clients progress (fax a one page summary monthly). This is a great way for physicians to become familiar with seeing your name and will connect your name with patient improvement. Once you have one physician referring clients to you, send letters to other physicians letting them know that one of their colleagues is referring patients. Before you know it, you will have other physicians referring patients (75).

Other ways to obtain referrals include letters, emails, and newsletters. Thank you cards, special offers, etc, all provide opportunities to gain qualified referrals.

Professional

If you want people to believe in you and your services, they have to see you as a professional. There are many aspects to being professional. One of the basics is dressing professionally and appropriately for the services you're offering. If you're trying to close a sale for a nutrition presentation at a local gym, a suit may be overdressed, while shorts and a tank top are probably too casual (unless you're Richard Simmons). It's important to know your audience and dress appropriately.

Certainly your attitude and speech are critical to a professional demeanor. Carry yourself confidently, and avoid sarcasm and arrogance. Be careful with the types of humor you use. There's also danger in being over confident and almost coming across as arrogant. The best way to open with a new client is to compliment them or something they own. Let's say you are meeting a potential new client in her office to discuss your nutrition services. When you enter the room, find a nice picture or piece of art, say something positive, and ask a simple question: "That's a beautiful picture, where did you find it?" If the new client is coming to you, compliment him on his decision to improve his health. Make sure your compliment is sincere and something you really believe to be admirable or positive. Once again, follow with a question. For example, if I walked into your office to learn more about your services, you might say, "How did you hear about me? (or) What have you heard about my services?" This will get the meeting off to a great start, as the potential client immediately feels you are interested in him/her.

Research Your Competition

Research your competition. It's important to know what's available in your area that's competing for the same business. Some of the obvious services are Weight Watchers, fad diets, internet based programs, and the latest "best selling" book. Compare what you are offering to what's available. Look at all of the benefits of what you provide. Some examples might include individual attention, personal training, availability, experience, flexibility, and investment. It's important not to bad mouth your competition – the focus is what you offer that is unique to you – not what they don't offer.

As part of your research, look into why some people are choosing other services. Are they offering something unique that you might want to add to your service or product line? Investigate the pricing structure. Typically clients are looking for the best "deal" not necessarily the lowest price. What makes your service a better deal to the client? Don't try to be all things to all people. Remember what you are offering, and stay true to your vision.

It's important not to make promises you can't keep or offer services that you are not positioned to provide at a high standard of quality. This shows in your speech and in the energy you bring to the initial meeting. If you have positioned yourself to provide a service that you are not prepared to offer, it shows, and the client will recognize the discomfort.

Another aspect of knowing your competition is that sometimes you are actually better off referring clients to your competition. This might sound like a poor business tactic, but it is actually a sound business tool. If a client asks about a group setting and your services are based on one-on-one nutrition coaching, you're better off referring this client to a another program. In the long run you're both going to be more successful. The client will respect you for providing an option that is more appropriate.

Marketing

Marketing is the wide range of activities involved in making sure that you're continuing to meet the needs of your customers and getting value in return. Marketing is usually focused on one product or service (77). Thus, a marketing plan for one product might be very different than for another product. Marketing activities include "inbound marketing," such as market research to find out what groups of potential customers exist, what their needs are, which of those needs you can meet, how you should meet them, etc. Inbound marketing also includes analyzing the competition, positioning your new product or service (finding your market niche), and pricing your products and services. "Outbound marketing" includes promoting a product through continued advertising, promotions, public relations, and sales (77).

If you are like the majority of small business owners, your marketing budget is limited. The most effective way to market a small business is to create a well rounded program that combines sales activities with your marketing tactics. Your sales activities will not only decrease your out-of-pocket marketing expense, but it also adds the value of interacting with your prospective customers and clients. This interaction will provide you with research that is priceless (77).

Does having a limited marketing budget mean you can't run with the big companies? Absolutely not! It just means you have to think a little more creatively. Consider launching your marketing campaign by doing one of the following (77):

- Call your vendors or associates, and ask them to participate with you in co-op advertising.
- Take some time to send your existing customers' referrals and buying incentives.
- Have you thought about introducing yourself to the media? Free publicity has the potential to boost your business. By doing this , you position yourself as an expert in your field.
- Invite people into your place of business by piggybacking onto an event. Is there a "race" coming to town? Are you willing to help? It could mean free publicity.

- When you do spend money on marketing, do not forget to create a way to track those marketing efforts. You can do this by coding your ads, using multiple toll-free telephone numbers, and asking prospects where they heard about you. This enables you to notice when a marketing tactic stops working. You can then quickly replace it with a better choice or method.
- By being diligent in your marketing and creating an easy strategy, such as holding yourself accountable to contact ten customers or potential customers daily five days a week, you will see your business grow at an exceptional rate. The great thing is it will not take a large marketing budget to make it happen.

Advertising Materials

Most small businesses budget more for print advertising than any other type. Print ads include postcards, brochures, ads in journals and magazines, and sales support materials. Print ads should always include a headline, a subhead, a visual and an action statement.

Want Your Carbs Back?
✓Tired of crazy diets?
✓Want to lose the fat and keep it off?
✓Want to learn more?
Come to our informational meeting on March 10 at 7 pm. Refreshments and snacks will be served!
Contact Jane at 555.555.5555

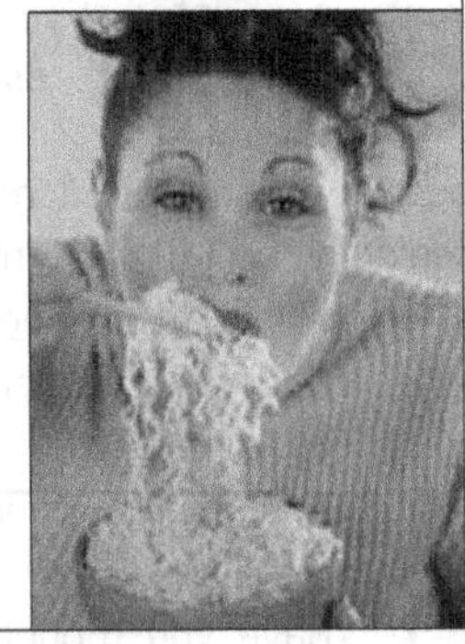

The headline is the most important aspect of any print materials (78). This ad filled an entire room with standing room only and provided many great leads.

Seventy to eighty percent of sales are decided on the headline alone. Your headline must attract the reader to want to continue reading. A visual is optional but pictures catch people's eye. You, of course, want to include your logo and contact information. A second crucial component (second to the headline) is an action statement. You want the reader to be moved to perform an action. The action may be to visit your website, call you, or send you an email. Action statements include, but are not limited to, providing something for free. Pay attention to ads you see that attract your attention. What attracted you? Were you moved to perform an action? A word of caution! Some ads attract a particular portion of the population, and the same ad can upset another segment of the population, which is why it is equally important to test your ad. Send it to friends, family, and acquaintances, and ask for their opinions. You'll be amazed at how much you can learn from people's first impressions (78).

TV combines visual and verbal exposure in real-time. We all have our favorite TV ads. What is it that makes some ads memorable and others we "want to forget"? TV differs by combining action, audio and video. You can also demonstrate a product feature through TV advertising. The visual and verbal modes reinforce each other. TV advertising is also great for evoking emotions. A good ad generates the right emotion for the product. So when you think TV advertising, think emotion. Which TV venues work best for your ad? What programs provide the best audience for your services and/or products? Radio is similar to television advertising. Listeners see through "imagination." Sound can be used to provoke images in the mind of the listener. A car screeching, a child crying, a phone ringing all invoke images. These images can be used in a similar manner as a television ad (78).

Should you develop your own website? The answer is ABSOLUTELY! Hosting a website is inexpensive and a great way for your clients to learn about you and your services without the expense of color brochures, etc. Some internet providers offer a free site. Many of the same rules used in print advertising apply to websites. We've all been on websites that we find frustrating and websites we can navigate easily. Visit many, many websites and pattern your website after the ones you like. Just as with print ad, your website should reflect you (78).

Purchasing tables at special events and trade shows can become an expensive venture. Often, however, you can barter for a free table by providing a lecture or volunteering to help. Preparing for these shows is also crucial. Determine the demographics of your audience in advance. Ask for names of other presenters. If you know any presenters personally, contact them, and let them know that you will be available to discuss your programs. Ask the event organizers if there are any avenues for you to advertise. Be sure to have marketing materials on hand. Before the event let everyone you know that you will be there. Have lots of brochures and business cards on hand. It is also a great idea to have a "giveaway" for people who will provide you with contact information (75).

Take advantage of free advertising by writing articles for local newspapers, local clubs, local churches, and other local organizations (75). Provide free lectures. At the end of the lecture provide details about your program; be sure to have business cards and brochures. Free lectures entice people to come listen to you discuss a "hot topic."

Attend meetings for local organizations and clubs. If you are a runner attend a local race. If you are interested in working with new moms, attend a local mother's group, etc. Volunteering for your favorite organization is also a great way to get people to know "what you do" (78).

Summary

The diet industry is now a $20 billion industry with a 100 million dieters (1,2). Despite all our "diet foods" we are still getting fatter. Despite all of the money spent yearly on dieting, more than one-third of adults are obese. Obesity has now been classified as a disease and is reaching epidemic proportions.

Dieting has been around for thousands of years, although not in any structured way like we see all around us today. It wasn't very common until the 1800's simply because people who were overweight were not very common; only the rich and well to-do were overweight so being fat was not a problem for most Americans. As time progressed, many more people became wealthy and thus had much greater access to the same foods as the wealthy. Eating and drinking too much became a sign of affluence, but strangely enough, it wasn't entirely the health factors of being overweight that started the diet craze; it was the war against sin! The American Presbyterian minister Sylvester Graham began to preach the ills of physical, moral, and spiritual health could all be remedied by a basic vegetarian diet. Pastor Graham, also the originator of graham flour and the flat bread known as graham crackers, stated that the vitality, strength, and health of his followers proved that vegetarianism was the "way." He tirelessly campaigned against all alcohol, coffee, tea, and tobacco as stimulants.

In the 1850's England, a man called William Banting was seriously obese. One medical practitioner had suggested that he might find the answer by not eating any more than a minimum of sugars and starches. Banting lost fifty pounds in a year. He was so excited at his success that he wrote a book, and hence, the world's first diet book was born; and the first low carbohydrate diet was also born. Around the end of the nineteenth century, William Ewart Gladstone, the four time British Prime Minister, had apparently advised that a person should always masticate (chew) thirty two times before swallowing. Horace Fletcher, nicknamed the "Chew-Chew Man" and the "Great Masticator", took the enthusiasm for chewing to much greater heights. He believed that chewing should continue until the food becomes a liquid in the mouth; and any food that does not (like fiber) should not be chewed in the first place. Leaving fiber out of a diet leads to constipation as those caught up in the frenzy discovered. Dr. John Kellogg thought that the advice from Fletcher to avoid fiber was so wrong that he founded his famous cereal company - Kellogg; he wanted to make sure Americans were getting plenty of fiber in their diets (5).

Lulu Hunt Peters, a Californian doctor, introduced the concept of counting calories to aid in weight loss. In her bestseller book *Diet and Health with a Key to the Calories* she stated that calories were the scientific way of looking at things. Diet books hit bookshelves with variations of a new idea that all that matters is what combinations of foods are consumed at the same time. This same theory is still being proclaimed by many today.

Bonnie Liebman, in "How to Write a Diet Book," provides details on how to create a diet book. "After all," she says, "You've been eating all your life haven't you? Don't worry about having any expertise or degree." Bonnie says to name your book after a trendy place; tell people they won't be hungry on your diet; for science lovers, deluge people with scientific evidence, especially if it has been ignored.

Dieting doesn't work for many reasons, but first and foremost low calorie diets utilize lean muscle as an energy source—hence fat burning machinery is lost. The scale goes down but is destined to go right back up. When the weight is gained back, it's all fat. The only known method of permanent weight loss is exercise and healthy eating. Changing body composition (building muscle and utilizing fat stores for energy) requires fueling the body, not dieting. ACSM Health & Fitness Journal provides an in-depth discussion of the necessity to fuel the body in exercise, and the consequences associated with inadequate caloric intake.

Many well-intentioned clients, athletes, and patients are making what they believe to be healthy choices at the grocery store and in restaurants, but they are instead being sabotaged by inconsistencies and often ambiguous labeling regulations. Deciphering food labels and health claims has become an exercise in understanding legal rhetoric. "Whole grain" doesn't mean whole grain; "93% lean ground beef" isn't 93% lean by calories; and the definition of "free-range" is far from what you may envision.

The Food and Drug Administration (FDA) is responsible for regulating most food products, while the United States Department of Agriculture (USDA) is responsible for regulating meat and poultry products. Each organization developed labeling requirements that are unique to their respective products and requirements. The National Labeling and Education Act (NLEA) passed by Congress in 1990 required mandatory nutrition labeling to appear on most packaged foods regulated by the FDA . The NLEA pertains only to those labels of food products regulated by FDA, which has label authority over the majority of foods. However, meat and poultry product labels are under the authority of Food Safety and Inspection Service (FSIS) in the USDA. No regulations have been passed requiring the USDA to make meat labels comparable to the packaged food labels. This makes it very difficult for consumers to compare products. Prepackaged pizza with meat topping falls under USDA rules, while cheese pizza is labeled according to FDA rules.

The USDA is responsible for managing the National Organic Program implemented in October 2002. Organic is a labeling term that indicates that: "the food or other agricultural product has been produced through approved methods that integrate cultural, biological, and mechanical practices that foster cycling of resources, promote ecological balance, and conserve biodiversity." Synthetic fertilizers, sewage sludge, irradiation, and genetic engineering may not be used. By definition, organic farming avoids the use of most artificial inputs, such as synthetic pesticides and fertilizers. Also banned are the use of animal byproducts, antibiotics and sewage sludge, among other practices.

The FDA does not evaluate or regulate terms placed on labels outside of the nutrition facts panel. The term "net carbs" came about when companies were seeking a way to market their products as being low in carbohydrates. The FDA requires that the total carbohydrate count is listed on a nutrition label and must include the full amount of grams from sugar alcohols and fiber. Some food companies created the term "net carbs" and defined it as the total grams of carbohydrate minus the grams of sugar alcohols, fiber, and glycerin. This equation is not entirely accurate because some of the sugar alcohols and fiber are absorbed by the body. In fact, about half of the grams of sugar alcohols are metabolized to glucose.

Eating out can produce panic in individuals embarking on new lifestyle changes. Individuals need to be educated in making healthy choices when eating out. Yes, people can eat out and still maintain healthy habits, but it's not easy; it can be a very confusing, difficult task. Eating at a restaurant does not have to sabotage a healthy lifestyle plan. Using smart-eating strategies when eating out can eliminate many calories and reduce sodium and fat intake. Other sabotaging practices include: portion distortion; eating too many calories in the evening; having problem foods in the home; deprivation of favorite foods; shopping when hungry; not planning; friendly saboteurs; stress eating; traveling; holidays, etc.

Whether you work for yourself or another company, implementing a nutrition component requires an understanding of entrepreneurial skills. Starting a new business - the Business of Nutrition - can be a daunting task. A successful business follows the "Business Development Process" and includes three integrated activities: innovation, quantification, and orchestration.

Chapter 13 – Sample Test

1. Describe the history of dieting and why diets don't work.
2. Provide details on how to write your own diet book.
3. Does a label stating 85% lean indicate that the contents are 15% fat by calories? Explain your answer.
4. Discuss the levels of "health claims" that manufacturers can use.
5. Describe the differences between the USDA labeling guidelines and the FDA guidelines.
6. Discuss ways of choosing healthier choices when eating out.
7. What would you say to a client who tells you that he or she does not have time to eat?
8. What are friendly saboteurs?
9. What does EMyth refer to? Provide details of the "Business Development Process."
10. What are the pros and cons of running your own business?
11. Describe the details of choosing a client base.

References

1. Reisner, R. (2008). The diet industry: A Big Fat Lie. *Bloomberg Business Week.* (accessed 07/24/2013). http://abcnews.go.com/Health/100-million-dieters-20-billion-weight-loss-industry/story?id=16297197#.T-pLJhxAhvZ. /archives/2008/03/the_diet_industry_a_big_fat_lie.html.
2. ABC News Staff. 100 Million Dieters, $20 Billion: The Weight-loss industry by the numbers. (2012). *ABC News.* (accessed 07/24/2013). http://abcnews.go.com/Health/100-million-dieters-20-billion-weight-loss-industry/story?id=16297197.
3. Centers for Disease Control and Prevention. (2012). Adult obesity facts: Obesity is common, serious and costly. (accessed 07/24/2013). http://www.cdc.gov/ obesity/data/adult.html.
4. Moyer, C. (2013). Delegates declare obesity as a disease. AMA Annual Meeting. (accessed 07/24/2013). http://www.amednews.com/assets/PDF/prhd0701.pdf.
5. Martel J. (2008). The history of dieting – our love of food. TheHistoryOf.net. (accessed 07/24/2013). http://www.thehistoryof.net/the-history-of-dieting.html.
6. International Vegetarian Union. USA: 19th Century Sylvester Graham (1795-1851. (accessed 07/24/2013). In: *Burrows, Edwin G. and Mike Wallace, _Gotham: A History of New York City to 1898_; New York and Oxford: Oxford University Press, 1999. http://www.ivu.org/ history/usa19/graham.html*
7. Every day in history. Penguin Pocket On This Day. (2006) Penguin Reference Library. Penguin Publishing (Division of Simon & Shuster): England. http://books.google.com/books/about /Penguin_ Pocket_On_This_Day.html?id=5FgUAAAACAAJ.
8. *Harrison. R.* William Banting Biography". Oxford Dictionary of National Biography. (accessed 07/24/2013). http://dx.doi.org/10.1093/ref:odnb/1320.
9. Groves, PhD, Barry (2002). "WILLIAM BANTING: The Father of the Low-Carbohydrate Diet". Second Opinions. (accessed 07/24/2013). http://www.second-opinions.co.uk/ banting.html#.Ue_tYG1jn5k.
10. Biography of Banting. (1948). Br Med J. 1:1084.3. http://www.bmj.com/content/1/4561/ 1084.3.
11. Halliday S. (2011). Amazing & Extraordinary facts – Great Britain. William Gladstone. F & W Media Inc: Cincinnati, OH.
12. Peters L. (1918). *Diet and Health: With Key to the Calories.* Reilly and Lee: Baltimore, MD.
13. Hay, William Howard. *Health via Food.* Sun-Diet Health Service, 1929. Public domain material, Soil and Health Library. (accessed 07/24/2013). http://www.soilandhealth.org / 02/0201hyglibcat/020165.hay.pdf.
14. Dunford RE. (2002). *The Grapefruit and Apple Cider Vinegar Combo Diet.* The Magni Company: McKinney, TX.
15. Buxton, Frank; Bill Owen (1972). *The big broadcast, 1920-1950.* Viking Press. p. 250.
16. Levenstein, Harvey A. (2003). *Paradox of plenty: a social history of eating in modern America, Part 12.* University of California Press. p.11.
17. Applebaum, M. The myth of the ideal weight.http://www.drapplebaum.com/fitness %20rants/the%20myth%20of%20the%20ideal%20weight.htm. (accessed 07/24/2013).
18. Rasmussen, N. (2008). America's first amphetamine epidemic 1929-1971. Am J Public Health. 98(6):974-985. http://www.ncbi.nlm.nih.gov/pmc/articles/PMC2377281/.
19. Weight Watchers. Philosophy who we are. (accessed 07/24/2013). https://www.weight watchers.com/about/his/history.aspx.
20. Atkins R. (1979). Dr. Atkins' Diet Revolution. D. McKay Co: England: London.
21. Pritikin N. (1984). The Pritikin program for diet and exercise. Bantam Publishing: NY, NY.
22. Bruch H. (1978). The golden cage: The enigma of anorexia nervosa. Harvard University Press: Cambridge, MA.

23. Weintraub M, et al. (1984). "A double-blind clinical trial in weight control. Use of fenfluramine and phentermine alone and in combination". *Archives of Internal Medicine* 144 (6): 1143–1148.
24. Linn R. (1977). The last chance diet-When everything else has failed: Dr. Linn's protein-sparing fast program. Lyle Stuart Publisher. NJ: Fort Lee.
25. Davidson T. (2007). Fit for Life diet. In Jacqueline L. Longe. *The Gale Encyclopedia of Diets: A Guide to Health and Nutrition*. Thomson Gale. MI: Farmington Hills. P 383–385.
26. Mazel J. (1981). *Beverly Hills Diet*. Sidgwick & Jackson Ltd. England: London.
27. Jenkins D, et al. (1981). Glycemic index of foods: a physiological basis for carbohydrate exchange. Am J Clin Nutr. 34(3). 362-366. http://ajcn.nutrition.org/content/34/3/362.long.
28. Powter S. Stop the Insanity. (1993). Gallery Books. IL: Chicago.
29. U.S. Food and Drug Administration (1997). FDA announces withdrawal fenfluramine and dexfenfluramine. P97-32. (accessed 07/24/2013). http://www.fda.gov/Drugs/DrugSafety/PostmarketDrugSafetyInformationforPatientsandProviders/ucm179871.htm.
30. Liebman, B. *How to Write A diet Book*. Nutrition Action Healthletter. July/August 2006. (accessed 07/24/2013). http://media.sethroberts.net/reviews/2006-07-01_How_to_write_a_diet_book.pdf.
31. Whitney, E & Rolfes S. (2013). *Understanding Nutrition,13th ed.* Belmont,CA:Wadsworth, Cengage Learnin (48-61, 234-237, 640-641).
32. Ross, C (Shils) et al. (2012). *Modern Nutrition in Health & Disease, 11th ed.* Philadelphia PA: Lipincott Wilillians & Wilikins (1480-1501).
33. Bernardot D and Thompson W. (1999). *E*nergy from food for Physical Activity, Enough and on Time. *ACSM's Health & Fitness Journal.* July/August 1999.
34. Meadows M. (2006). U.S. Food and Drug Administration. A Century of ensuring safe foods and cosmetics. *FDA Consumer Magazine.* Updated 2009. (accessed 07/24/2013). http://www.fda.gov/AboutFDA/WhatWeDo/History/FOrgsHistory/CFSAN/ucm083863.htm.
35. NLEA. Public Law 101-585. Nov 8, 1990.
36. U.S. Food and Drug Administration Center for Food Safety & Applied Nutrition. A food labeling guide. May, 1997. (accessed 07/24/2013) http://www.fda.gov/Food/Guidance Regulation/GuidanceDocumentsRegulatoryInformation/DietarySupplements/ucm2006823.htm
37. Wartella, E, et al. (2010). Examination of front-of-package nutrition rating systems and symbols: Phase 1 Report. The National Academy Press. (Chapter 2 – History of Nutrition labeling). http://www.nap.edu/catalog.php?record_id=12957.
38. U.S. Food and Drug Administration. FDA video – don't let your food take you by surprise. Read the Label. (accessed 07/26/2013). http://www.accessdata.fda.gov/scripts/video/food.cfm?yid=rIeNUV6LtxA.
39. Liebman, B. (1997). Where's the ground beef labeling?. Nutrition Action Health Letter. (accessed 07/26/2013). http://www.cspinet.net/nah/junebeef.htm.
40. USDA. Organic Certification. National Organic Program. Last modified 11/15/2011. (accessed 07/26/2013). http://www.usda.gov/wps/portal/usda/usdahome?navid=ORGANIC_CERTIFICATIO.
41. USDA National Organic Program. Consumer Information. Updated 10/17/2012. (accessed 07/26/2013). http://www.ams.usda.gov/AMSv1.0/ams.fetchTemplate Data.dotemplate=TemplateC&navID=ConsumerInfoLinkNOPOrganicSeal&rightNav1=ConsumerInfoLinkNOPOrganicSeal&topNav=&leftNav=NationalOrganicProgram&page=NOPConsumers&resultType=&acct=nopgeninf.o
42. Smith-Spangler C. Brandeau ML. Hunter GE. Bavinger JC. Pearson M. Eschbach PJ. Sundaram V. Liu H. Schirmer P. Stave C. Olkin I. Bravata DM (2012). "Are organic foods safer or healthier than conventional alternatives?: a systematic review.". *Annals of Internal Medicine* 157 (5): 348–366.

43. Zelman, K. Organic foods – are they worth the price tag. *United Healthcare: Organic Foods.* (accessed 07/26/2013). http://www.uhc.com/source4women/health_wellness_tools_resources/nutrition/organic_foods.htm.
44. Environmental Working Group. (2013). Shoppers guide to pesticides in produce. (accessed 07/26/2013). http://static.ewg.org/reports/2013/foodnews2013/ docs/pdf/2013 EWGPesticideGuide.pdf.
45. U.S. Food and Drug Administration. Label Claims. Types of claims: definitions, guidance, regulatory information, and permitted claims. Updated 05/17/2013. (accessed 07/26/2013). http://www.fda.gov/Food/IngredientsPackagingLabeling/ LabelingNutrition/ucm2006873.htm.
46. U.S. Food and Drug Administration. (2003). Claims that can be made for conventional foods and dietary supplements. Updated 06/07/2013. (accessed 07/26/2013). http://www.fda.gov/Food/IngredientsPackagingLabeling/ LabelingNutrition/ucm111447.htm.
47. Wheeler, M. (2010). What are net carbs? Diabetes Forecast. The Healthy Living Magazine.
48. Franck, et al. (2013). Agricultural subsidies and the American obesity epidemic. Am J of Preventive Medicine. Vol 45 Issue 3.
49. Story M. Kaphingst KM. Robinson-O'Brien R. Glanz K. (2008). Creating healthy food and eating environments: policy and environmental approaches. *Annu Rev Public Health*. 29:253–72
50. Story M. Hamm MW. Wallinga D. (2009). Food systems and public health: linkages to achieve healthier diets and healthier communities. *J Hunger Environ Nutr.* 4:219–24.
51. Jackson RJ, et al. (2009). Agriculture policy is health policy. J Hunger Environ Nutr. 4:393–408.
52. Weber JA, Becker N. (2006). Framing the farm bill. J Am Diet Assoc. 106: 1354–7.
53. Stalled farm bill is pushed for its savings (2012). *New York Times.* www.nytimes.com/ 2012/12/06/us/politics/stalled-farm-bill-could-help-with-deficit-reduction. Html.
54. U.S. Congress issues short-term farm bill extension. International Centre for Trade and Sustainable Development. *Bridges Weekly Trade News Digest.* 17(1). ictsd.org/i/news/bridgesweekly/152578.
55. Ludwig DS. Nestle M. (2008). Can the food industry play a constructive role in the obesity epidemic? *JAMA.* 300:1808–11.
56. Bray GA. Nielsen SJ. Popkin BM. (2004). Consumption of high-fructose corn syrup in beverages may play a role in the epidemic of obesity. *Am J Clin Nutr.* 79:537–43.
57. Ruhm CJ. (2012). Understanding overeating and obesity. *J Health Econ.* 31:781–96.
58. Tillotson J. (2004). America's obesity: conflicting public policies, industrial economic development, and unintended human consequences. *Annu Rev Nutr.* 24:617–43.
59. Horrigan L. Lawrence RS. Walker P. (2002). How sustainable agriculture can address the environmental and human health harms of industrial agriculture. *Environ Health Perspect.* 110:445–56.
60. Morris MN. Misra S. Sibary S. (2008). Global fattening: designing effective approaches to reducing obesity. *J Am Acad Bus.* 12:249–55.
61. Novak NL, Brownell KD. (2011). Obesity: a public health approach. *Psychiatry Clin North Am.* 34:895–909.
62. Wallinga D. (2010). Agricultural policy and childhood obesity: a food systems and public health commentary. *Health Aff (*Millwood). 29:405–10.
63. Fields S. (2004). The fat of the land: do agricultural subsidies foster poor health? *Environ Health Perspect.* 112:A820–A823.
64. Miner J. (2006). Market incentives could bring U.S. agriculture and nutrition policies into accord. *Cal Ag.* 60:8–13.
65. Schlosser, Eric (2001). *Fast Food Nation.* New York: Houghton Mifflin Co.
66. Schlosser, Eric (2001). The bitter truth about fast food. *The Guardian.* (accessed 07/26/2013). http://www.guardian.co.uk/books/2001/apr/07/features.weekend.

67. Gerber, M. E-Myth Mastery. Harper Collins, USA, 2005.
68. Gerber, M. EMyth Revisited, Harper Collins, USA, 2002.
69. Emyth – Our story. http://www.e-myth.com/pub/htdocs/about
70. Ten step to starting a business. The Company Corporaton. (accessed (07/26/2013). https://www.incorporate.com/completing_startup_tasks.html.
71. Internal Revenue Service. Checklist for starting a business (accessed 07/26/2013) http://www.irs.gov/businesses/small/article/0,,id=98810,00.html.
72. Gates B. Gates M. Bill & Melinda Gates Foundation. Letter from Bill and Melinda Gates. (accessed 07/26/2013). http://www.gatesfoundation.org/Who-We-Are/General-Information/Letter-from-Bill-and-Melinda-Gates.
73. Hopkins J. (2006). Starting a business: What it takes. (accessed 07/26/2013). http://usatoday30.usatoday.com/money/smallbusiness/2006-07-30-starting-your-business_x.htm
74. U.S. Patent and Trademark Office. Trademark electronic search system (TESS). (accessed 07/26/2013). http://tmsearch.uspto.gov/bin/gate.exe?f=tess&state=4803:3h6z8r.1.1.
75. Pentz J. Salgueiro G. (2006). The Business of Nutrition 1 – Attracting New Business. LMA Publishing: Boston, MA.
76. Small Business Administration. Starting a small business. (accessed 07/26/2013). http://www.sba.gov/smallbusinessplanner/index.html.
77. Chapman L. All about marketing. Management Help. (accessed 07/26/2013). http://managementhelp.org/marketing/index.htm.
78. Chemir Evans Analytical Group. Winter 2008 Newsletter. What's in your holiday brew. Accessed 07/26/2013). http://www.chemir.com/chemistry-of-beer.html.
79. Stacewica-Sapuntzakis M, et al. (2001). Chemical compositon and potential health effects of prunes: A functional food? Crit Rev Food Sci Nutr. 41(4):251-86.
80. Whole Grains Council. (accessed 07/26/2013). http://wholegrainscouncil.org/.
81. Spark People. 85 tips and strategies for dining out. (accessed 07/26/2013). http://www.sparkpeople.com/resource/nutrition_articles.asp?id=544.
82. Zelman K. (2003). Avoid portion distortion. *WebMd Weight Loss Clinic.* Updated 2005. (accessed 07/26/2013). http://www.webmd.com/diet/features/avoid-portion-distortion.
83. Rolls B. Morris E. Roe LS. (2002). Portion size of food effects energy intake in normal-weight and overweight men and women. *Am J Clin Nutr.* Vol. 76 no. 6 1207-1213.
84. Young LR. Nestle M. (2003). Expanding portion sizes in the US marketplace: implications for nutrition counseling. *J Am Diet Assoc.* 103(2):231-4.
85. Garaulet M, et al. (2013). Timing of food intake predicts weight loss effectiveness. Int J of Obesity. 37: 604-611. http://www.nature.com/ijo/journal/v37/n4/full/ijo2012229a.html.
86. SBA Office of Advocacy. (2010). Frequently asked questions: How many small businesses are there. (accessed 07/26/2013). http://www.sba.gov/sites/default/files/FAQ_Sept_2012.pdf.
87. Winterman D. (2013). History's weirdest fad diets. BBC News Magazine. http://www.bbc.co.uk/news/magazine-20695743.
88. Khan A. (2009). Tyra Banks and the tapeworm diet. Los Angeles Times. (accessed 08/04/2013.) http://latimesblogs.latimes.com/booster_shots/2009/12/tyra-banks-show-tapeworm-diet.html.
89. Gardner G. Halweil. (2000). Escaping hunger, escaping excess. Worldwatch Institute. (accessed 08/04/2013).http://www.worldwatch.org/node/488.
90. Sumithran, P. et. al. (2011). Long-term persistence of hormonal adaptations to weight loss. N Engl J Med 365:1597.604.
91. Leibel RL, Hirsch J. (1984). Diminished energy requirements in reduced-obese patients. Metabolism 33:164-70.
92. Geldszus R, Mayr B, Horn R, Geisthovel F, von zur Mühlen A, Brabant G. (1996). Serum leptin and weight reduction in female obesity. Eur J Endocrinol 135: 659-62.

93. Chearskul S, Delbridge E, Shulkes A, Proietto J, Kriketos A. (2008). Effect of weight loss and ketosis on postprandial cholecystokinin and free fatty acid concentrations. Am J Clin Nutr 87:1238-46.
94. Cummings DE, Weigle DS, Frayo S, et al. (2006). Plasma ghrelin levels after diet-inducedweight loss or gastric bypass surgery. N Engl J Med 346:1623-30.
95. Klok MD. et. al. (2007). The role of leptin and ghrelin in regulation of food intake and body weight in humans: a review. Obes Rev 8(1): 21-34.
96. Little TJ. Et. al. (2005). Role of cholecystokinin in appetite control and body weight regulation. Obes Rev. 6(4):294-306.
97. Sumithran P. et. al. (2011). Long-term persistence of hormonal adaptations to weight loss. *N Engl J Med* 365:1597.604.
98. Greene C. et. al. (2009). Emerging issues in the US organic industry. US Department of Agriculture.
99. Harden GH. (2010). Oversight of the national organic program. Office of Inspector General. http://www.usda.gov/oig/webdocs/01601-03-HY.pdf.
100. Winter CK & Katz JM. (2011). Dietary exposure to pesticide residues from commodities alleged to contain the highest contamination levels. *J of Toxicology* 1-7.
101. Dangour AD. et. al. (2010). Nutrition-related health effects of orgainic food: a systemic review. *Am J Clin Nutr.* 1-8.
102. Spangler CS. Et al. (2012). Are organic foods safer or healthier than conventional alternatives? *Annals of Internal Medicine* 157:348-366.
103. Greene C. et. al. (2009). Emerging issues in the US organic industry. US Department of Agriculture. http://www.ers.usda.gov/publications/eib-economic-information-bulletin/eib55.aspx.
104. U.S. Food and Drug Administration. FDA News Release. FDA defines "gluten-free" for food labeling. (2013). (accessed 08/05/2013). http://www.fda.gov/NewsEvents/Newsroom/PressAnnouncements/UCM363474.htm.

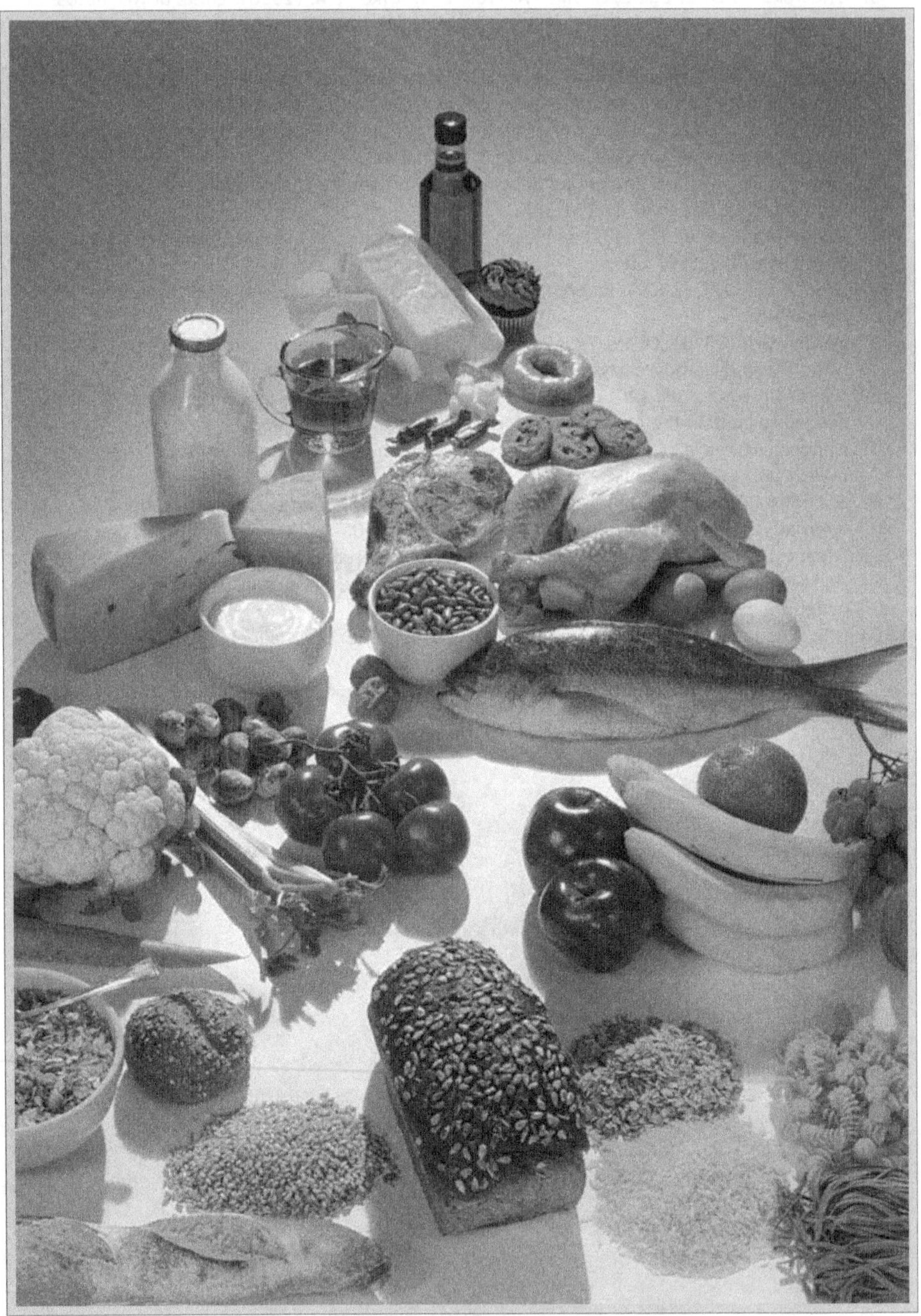

Appendix

Glossary....476

Equations / Requirements....492

Legal and Responsibility Agreement....496

AASDN Children's Meal Plans....498

AASDN Star-Associated Food Rating Placemats....500

Index....502

Glossary

A

absorption: the uptake of nutrients by the cells of the small intestine for transport into either the blood or the lymph.

Acceptable Daily Intake (ADI): the estimated amount of a sweetener that individuals can safely consume each day over the course of a lifetime without adverse effects.

acetyl CoA (ass-eh-teel, or ah-SEET-il, coh-AY): a 2-carbon compound (acetate, or acetic acid) to which a molecule of CoA is attached.

acidosis (assi-DOE-sis): above-normal acidity in the blood and body fluids.

additives: substances not normally consumed as foods but added to food either intentionally or by accident.

Adequate Intake (AI): the average daily amount of a nutrient that appears sufficient to maintain a specified criterion; a value used as a guide for nutrient intake when an RDA cannot be determined.

adipose (ADD-ih-poce) **tissue:** the body's fat tissue; consists of masses of triglyceride-storing cells.

adrenal glands: glands adjacent to, and just above, each kidney.

alcohol: a class of organic compounds containing hydroxyl (OH) groups.

alcohol dehydrogenase (dee-high-DROJ-eh-nayz)**:** an enzyme active in the stomach and the liver that converts ethanol to acetaldehyde.

amino (a-MEEN-oh)**:** building blocks of proteins. Each contains an amino group, an acid group, a hydrogen atom, and a distinctive side group, all attached to a central carbon atom.

amino acid pool: the supply of amino acids derived from either food proteins or body proteins that collect in cells and circulating blood and stand ready to be incorporated in proteins and other compounds or used for energy.

ammonia: a compound with the chemical formula NH3, produced during the deamination of amino acids.

anabolic steroids: drugs related to the male sex hormone, testosterone, that stimulate the development of lean body mass.

anabolism (an-AB-o-lism)**:** reactions in which small molecules are put together to build larger ones. Anabolic reactions require energy.

anaerobic (AN-air-ROE-bic)**:** not requiring oxygen.

anemia (ah_NEE-me-ah)**:** literally, "too little blood". Anemia is any condition in which too few red blood cells are present, or the red blood cells are immature (and therefore large) or too small or contain too little hemoglobin to carry the normal amount of oxygen to the tissues. Anemia is not a disease itself but can be a symptom of many different disease conditions, including many nutrient deficiencies, bleeding, excessive red blood cell destruction, and defective red blood cell formation.

anorexia (an-oh-RECK-see-ah) **nervosa:** an eating disorder characterized by a refusal to maintain a minimally normal body weight and a distortion in perception of body shape and weight.

antioxidants: in the body, substances that significantly decrease the adverse effects of free radicals on normal physiological functions.

arachidonic (a-RACK-ih-DON-ic) **acid:** an omega-6 polyunsaturated fatty acid with 20 carbons and four double bonds; present in small amounts in meat and other animal products and synthesized in the body from linoleic acid.

arteries: vessels that carry blood from the heart to the tissues.

artificial sweeteners: sugar substitutes that provide negligible, in any, energy sometimes called *nonnutritive sweeteners.*

ascorbic acid: one of the two active forms of vitamin C. Many people refer to C by this name.

aspartame (ah-SPAR-tame or ASS-par-tame)**:** an artificial sweetener composed of two amino acids (phenylalanine and aspartic acid); approved for use in both the United States and Canada.

atherosclerosis (ATH-er-oh-scler-OH-sis)**:** a type of artery disease characterized by plaques (accumulations of lipid-containing material) on the inner walls of the arteries.

ATP or **adenosine** (ah-DEN-oh-seen) **triphosphate** (try-FOS-fate): a common high-energy compound composed of a purine (adenine), a sugar (ribose), and theree phosphate groups.

B

basal metabolic rate (BMR): the rate of energy use for metabolism under specified conditions: after a 12-hour fast and restful sleep, without any physical activity or emotional excitement, and in a comfortable setting. It is usually expressed as kcalories per kilogram body weight per hour.

bile: an emulsifier that prepares fats and oils for digestion; an exocrine secretion made by the liver, stored in the gallbladder, and released into the small intestine when needed.

body composition: the proportion of muscle, bone, fat, and other tissue that make up a person's total body weight.

body mass index (BMI): an index of a person's weight in relation to height determined by dividing the weight (in kilograms) by the square of height (in meters).

bolus (Boh-lus)**:** a portion; with respect to food, the amount swallowed at one time.

bomb calorimeter (KAL-oh-RIM-eh-ter)**:** an instrument that measures the heat energy released when foods are burned, thus providing an estimate of the potential energy (kcalories) of the foods.

branched-chain amino acids: the essential amino acids leucine isolecine, and valine, which are present in large amounts in skeletal muscle tissue; falsely promoted as fuel for exercising muscles.

bulimia (byoo-LEEM-ee-ah) **nervosa:** an eating disorder characterized by repeated episodes of binge eating usually followed by self-induced vomiting, misuse of laxatives or diuretics, fasting, or excessive exercise.

C

caffeine: a natural stimulant found in many common foods and beverages, including coffee, tea, and chocolate; may enhance endurance by stimulating fatty acid release. High doses cause headaches, trembling rapid heart rate, and other undesirable side effects.

Calories: units by which energy is measured. Food energy is measured in kilocalories (1000 calories equal 1 kilocalorie), abbreviated kcalories or kcal. One kcalorie is the amount of heat necessary to raise the temperature of 1 kilogram (kg) of water 1°. The scientific use of the term kcalorie is the same as the popular use of the term calorie.

carbohydrate loading: a regimen of moderate exercise followed by the consumption of a high-carbohydrate diet that enables muscles to store glycogen beyond their normal capacities; also called *glycogen loading* or *glycogen super compensation.*

cardiovascular disease (CVD): a general term for all diseases of the heart and blood vessels. Atherosclerosis is the main cause of CVD. When the arteries that carry blood to the heart muscle become blocked, the heart suffers damage known as coronary heart disease (CHD).

carnitine (CAR-neh-teen)**:** a nonessential, nonprotein amino acid made in the body from lysine that helps transport fatty acids across the mitochondrial membranes. As a supplement, carnitine supposedly "burns" fat and spares glycogen during endurance events, but in reality it does neither.

carotenoids (kah-ROT-eh-noyds)**:** pigments commonly found in plants and animals, some of which have vitamin A activity. The carotenoid with the greatest vitamin A activity is beta-carotene.

catabolism (ca-TAB-o-lism)**:** reactions in which large molecules are broken down to smaller ones. Catabolic reactions release energy.

celiac disease: an intestinal disorder in which the inability to absorb the protein portion of gluten results in an immune response that damages intestinal cells; also called *celiac sprue* or *gluten-sensitive enteropathy.*

cell differentiation (DIF-er-EN-she-AY-shun)**:** the process by which immature cells develop specific functions different from those of the original that are characteristic of their mature cell type.

cell membrane: the thin layer of tissue that surrounds the cell and encloses its contents; made primarily of lipid and protein.

chylomicrons (kye-lo-MY-cronz)**:** the class of lipoproteins that transport lipids from the intestinal cells to the rest of the body.

cis: on the near side of; refers to a chemical configuration in which the hydrogen atoms are located on the same side of a double bond.

CoA (Coh-AY)**:** coenzyme A; the coenzyme derived from the B vitamin pantothenic acid and central to energy metabolism.

coenzymes: complex organic molecules that work with enzymes to facilitate the enzymes' activity. Many coenzymes have B vitamins as part of their structures.

complementary proteins: two or more dietary proteins whose amino acid assortments complement each other in such a way that the essential amino acids missing from one are supplied by the other .

conditionally essential amino acid: an amino acid that is normally nonessential, but must be supplied by the diet in special circumstances when the need for it exceeds the body's ability to produce it.

CP, or **creatine phosphate:** a high-energy compound in muscle cells that acts as a reservoir of energy that can maintain a steady supply of ATP. CP provides the energy for short bursts of activity; also called *phosphocreatine.*

C-reactive protein (CRP): a protein released during the acute phase of infection or inflammation that enhances immunity by promoting phagocytosis and activating platelets. Its presence may be used to assess a person's risk of an impending heart attack or stroke.

creatine: (KREE-ah-tin): a nitrogen-containing compound that combines with phosphate to form the high-energy compound creatine phosphate (or phosphocreatine) in muscles.

D

daily values (DV): reference values developed by the FDZ specifically for use on food labels.

dehydration: the condition in which body water output exceeds water input. Symptoms include thirst, dry skin and mucous membranes, rapid heartbeat, low blood pressure, and weakness.

diabetes (DYE-uh-BEET-eez)**:** chronic disorders of carbohydrate metabolism, usually characterized by hyperglycemia resulting from insufficient or ineffective insulin; clinically called diabetes mellitus (MELL-ih-tus or MELL-eye-tus).

Dietary Reference Intakes (DRI): a set on nutrient intake values for healthy people in the United States and Canada. These values are used for planning and assessing diets and include: Estimated Average Requirements (EAR), Recommended Dietary Allowance (RDA), Adequate Intakes (AI), and Tolerable Upper Intake Levels (UL).

dietary supplement: any pill, capsule, tablet, liquid, or powder that contains vitamins, minerals, herbs, or amino acids; intended to increase dietary intake of these substances.

disordered eating: eating behaviors that are neither normal nor healthy, including restrained eating, fasting, binge eating, and purging.

diverticulitis (DYE-ver-tic-you-LYE-tis): infected or inflamed diverticula.

diverticulosis (DYE-ver-tic-you-LOH-sis)**:** the condition of having diverticula.

double-blind experiment: an experiment in which neither the subjects nor the researchers know which subjects are members of the experimental group and which are serving as control subjects, until after the experiment is over.

E

Eating disorders: disturbances in eating behavior that feopardize a person's physical or psychological health

edema (eh-DEEM-uh)**:** the swelling of body tissue caused by excessive amounts of fluid in the interstitial spaces; seen in protein deficiency (among other conditions).

eicosanoids (eye-COSS-uh-noyds)**:** derivatives of 20-carbon fatty acids; biologically active compounds that help to regulate blood pressure, blood clotting, and other body functions. They include prostaglandins (PROS-tah-GLAND-ins), thromboxanes, throm-BOX-ains), and leukrotrienes (LOO-ko-TRY-eens).

epinephrine (EP-ih-NEFF-rin)**:** a hormone of the adrenal gland that modulates the stress response; formerly called adrenaline. When administered by injection, epinephrine counteracts anaphylactic shock by opening the airways and maintaining heartbeat and blood pressure.

epithelial tissue: the layer of the body that servers as a selective barrier between the body's interior and environment. Examples are the cornea of the eyes, the skin, the respiratory lining of the lungs, and the lining of the digestive tract.

ergogenic (ER-goJEN-ick) **aids:** substance or techniques used in an attempt to enhance physical performance.

esophangus (ee-SOF-ahgus)**:** the food pipe; the conduit from the mouth to the stomach.

essential amino acids: amino acids that the body cannot synthesis to meet physiological needs.

essential fatty acids: fatty acids that the body cannot synthesize in amounts sufficient to meet physiological needs.

essential nutrients: nutrients a person must obtain from food because the body cannot synthesize them in amounts sufficient to meet physiological needs; also called indispensable nutrients. About 40 nutrients are currently known to be essential for human beings.

Estimated Average Requirement (EAR): the average daily amount of a nutrient that will maintain a specific biochemical or physiological function in half the healthy people of a given age and gender group.

Estimated Energy Requirement (EER): the average dietary energy intake that maintains energy balance and good health in a person of a given age, gender, weight, height, and level of physical activity.

F

fatty acid: an organic compound composed of a carbon chain with hydrogens attached and an acid group (COOH) at one end and a methyl group (CH3)at the other end.

flavonoids (FLAV-von-oyds)**:** yellows pigments in foods; phytochemicals that may exert physiological effects on the body.

food intolerances: adverse reactions to foods that do not involve the immune system.

food-borne illness: illness transmitted to human beings through food and water, caused by either an infectious agent (food-borne infection) or a poisonous substance (food intoxication); commonly known as food poisoning.

G

gallbladder: the organ that stores and concentrates bile. When it receives the signal that fat is present in the duodenum, the gallbladder contracts and squirts bile through the bile duct into the duodenum.

gastric juice: the digestive secretion of the gastric glands of the stomach.

Gastroesophageal reflux disease (GERD): a condition characterized by the backflow of stomach acid into the esophagus two or more times a week.

generally recognized as safe (GRAS): food additives that have long been in use and are believed to be safe. First established by the FDA in 1958, the GRAS list is subject to revision as new facts become known.

H

HDL (high-density lipoprotein): the type of lipoprotein that transports cholesterol back to the liver from the cells; composed primarily of protein.

heartburn: a burning sensation tin the chest area caused by backflow of stomach acid into the esophagus; medically known as gastroesophageal reflux.

hemochromatosis (HE-moh-KRO-ma-toe-sis)**:** a genetically determined failure to prevent absorption of unneeded dietary iron that is characterized by iron overload and tissue damage.

hemoglobin (HE-moh-GLO-bin)**:** the oxygen-carrying protein of the red blood cells that transports oxygen from the lungs to tissues throughout the body; hemoglobin accounts for 80 percent of the body's iron.

hepatic vein: the vein that collects blood from the liver and returns it to the heart.

high-fructose corn syrup (HFCS): a syrup made from cornstarch that has been treated with an enzyme that converts some of the glucose to the sweeter fructose; made especially for use in processed foods and beverages, where it is the predominant sweetener.

homeostasis (HOME-ee-oh-STAY-sis): the maintenance of constant internal conditions (such as blood chemistry, temperature, and blood pressure)by the body's control systems. A homeostatic system is constantly reacting to external forces to maintain limits set by the body's needs.

hormones: chemical messengers. Hormones are secreted by a variety of glands in response to altered conditions in the body. Each hormone travels to one or more specific target tissues or organs, where it elicits a specific response to maintain homeostasis.

I

immune system: the body's natural defense against foreign materials that have penetrated the skin or mucous membranes.

indispensable amino acids: essential amino acids.

inflammation: an immunological response to cellular injury characterized by an increase in white blood cells.

insoluble fibers: nonstarch polysaccharides that do not dissolve in water. Examples include the tough, fibrous structures found in the strings of celery and skins of corn kernels.

insulin (IN-suh-lin)**:** a hormone secreted by special cells in the pancreas in response to (among other things) elevated blood glucose concentrations. Insulin controls the transport of glucose from the bloodstream into the muscle and fat cells.

intracellular fluid: fluid within the cells, usually high in potassium and phosphate. Intracellular fluid accounts for approximately two thirds of the body's water.

irritable bowel syndrome: an intestinal disorder of unknown cause. Symptoms include abdominal discomfort and cramping, diarrhea, constipation, or alternating diarrhea and constipation.

J

joule: a measure of work energy; the amount of energy expended when 1 kilogram is moved 1 meter by a force of 1 newton.

K

kcalorie: a unit by which energy is measured. One kcalorie is the amount of heat necessary to raise the temperature of 1 kilogram (kg) of water 1° C. The scientific use of the term kcalorie is the same as the popular use of the term calorie.

ketone (KEE-tone) **bodies:** compounds produced during the incomplete breakdown of fat when glucose is not available in the cells.

ketosis (kee-TOE-sis)**:** an undesirably high concentration of ketone bodies in the blood and urine.

Kreb's cycle: named after the scientist who elucidated this biochemistry, a series of metabolic reactions that break down molecules of acetyl CoA to carbon dioxide and hydrogen atoms; also called the citric acid cycle or the TCA cycle.

L

lacto-ovo-vegetarians: people who include milk, milk products, and eggs, but exclude meat, poultry, and seafood from their diets.

lactose (LAK-tose)**:** a disaccharide composed of glucose and galactose; commonly known as milk sugar.

lactovegetarians: people who include milk and milk products, but exclude meat, poultry, seafood, and eggs from their diet.

LDL (low-density lipoprotein): the type of lipoprotein derived from very-low-density lipoproteins (VLDL) as triglycerides are removed and broken down; composed primarily of cholesterol.

lignans: phytochemicals present in flaxseed that are converted to phytosterols by intestinal bacteria and are under study as possible anticancer agents.

limiting amino acid: the essentials amino acid found in the shortest supply relative to the amounts needed for protein synthesis in the body. Four amino acids are most likely to be limiting: lysine, methionine, threonine, and tryptophan.

lipids: a family of compounds that includes triglycerides, phospholipids, and sterols. Lipies are characterized by their insolubility in water.

lipoprotein lipase (LPL): an enzyme that hydrolyzes triglycerides passing by in the bloodstream and directs their parts into the cells, where they can be metabolized for energy or reassembled for storage.

lipoproteins (LIP-oh-PRO-teenz)**:** cluster of lipids associated with proteins that serve as transport vehicles for lipids in the lymph and blood.

M

macronutrients: carbohydrate, fat and protein; the nutrients the body requires in relatively large amounts (many grams daily)

macrophages (MAK-roe-fay-jez)**:** large phagocytic cells that serve as scavengers of the blood, cleaning it of old or abnormal cells, cellular debris, and antigens.

metabolic syndrome: a combination of risk factors – insulin resistance, hypertension , abnormal blood lipids, and abdominal obesity – that greatly increase a person's risk of developing coronary heart disease; also called Syndrome X, insulin resistance syndrome, or dysmetabolic syndrome.

metabolism: the sum total of all the chemical reations that go in living cells. Energy metabolism includes all the reactions by which the body obtains and expends the energy from food.

micelles (MY-cells)**:** tiny spherical complexes of emulsified fat that arise during digestion; most contain bile salts and the products of lipid digestion, including fatty acids, monoglycerides, and cholesterol.

Microgram (μg RAE): micrograms retinol activity equivalents; a measure of vitamin A activity.

micronutrients: vitamins and minerals; the nutrients the body requires in relatively small amounts (milligrams or micrograms daily).

microvilli (MY-cro-VILL-ee or MY-cro-VILL-eye)**:** tiny, hair like projections on each cell of very villus that can trap nutrient particles and transport them into the cells; singular microvillus.

N

neurotransmitters: chemicals that are released at the end of a nerve cell when a nerve impulse arrives there. They diffuse across the gap to the next cell and alter the membrane of that second cell to either inhibit or excite it.

niacin equivalents (NE): the amount of niacin present in food, including the niacin that can theoretically be made from its precursor, tryptophan.

nitrogen balance: the amount of nitrogen consumed (N in) as compared with the amount of nitrogen excreted (N out) in a given period of time.

nonessential amino acids: amino acids that the body can synthesize.

nonheme iron: the iron in foods that is not bound to proteins; found in both plant-derived and animal-derived foods.

nonnutritive sweeteners: sweeteners that yield no energy (or insignificant energy in the case of aspartame).

nutrients: chemical substances obtained from food and used in the body to provide energy, structural materials, and regulating agents to support growth, maintenance, and repair of the body's tissues. Nutrients may also reduce the risks of some diseases.

Nutrition: the science of food and the nutrients and other substances they contain, and of their actions within the body (including ingestion, digestion, absorption, transport, metabolism, and excretion). A broader definition includes the social, economic, cultural, and psychological implications of food and eating.

O

obese: overweight with adverse health effects; BMI 30 or more.

oils: lipids that are liquid at room temperature (77° F or 25° C).

omega-3 fatty acid: a polyunsaturated fatty acid in which the closest double bond to the methyl (CH3)end of the carbon chain is three carbons away.

omega-6 fatty acid: a polyunsaturated fatty acid in which the closest double bond t the methyl (CH3) end of the carbon chain is six carbons away.

organic: in chemistry, a substance or molecule containing carbon-carbon bonds or carbon-hydrogen bonds. This definition exclude coal, diamonds, and a few carbon-containing compounds that contain only a single carbon and no hydrogen, such as carbon dioxide (CO2), calcium carbonate (CaCO3), magnesium carbonate (MGCO3), and sodium cyanide (NaCN).

organic: on food labels, that at least 95 percent of the product's ingredients have been grown and processed according to USDA regulations defining the use of fertilizers, herbicides, insecticides, fungicides, preservatives, and other chemical ingredients.

P

pancreas: a gland that secretes digestive enzymes and juices into the duodenum. (The pancreas also secretes hormones into the blood that help to maintain glucose homeostasis.)

peer review: a process in which a panel of scientists rigorously evaluates a research study to assure that the scientific method was followed.

pesticides: chemicals used to control insects, weeds, fungi, and other pests on plants, vegetables, fruits, and animals. Used broadly, the term includes herbicides (to kill weeds), and fungicides (to kill fungi).

pH: the unit of measure expressing a substance's acidity or alkalinity. The lower the pH, the higher the H+ ion concentration and stronger the acid. A pH above 7is alkaline, or base (a solution in which OH- ions predominate).

pharmacological effect: the body's response to a large dose of nutrient (levels commonly available only from supplements) that overwhelms some body system and acts like a drug.

phosphocreatine (PC): a high-energy compound in muscle cells that acts as a reservoir of energy that can maintain a steady supply of ATP and provides the energy for short bursts of activity; also called creatine phosphate (CP).

R

Recommended Dietary Allowance (RDA): the average daily amount of a nutrient considered adequate to meet the known nutrient needs of practically all healthy people; a goal for dietary intake by individuals.

resistant starches: starches that escape digestion and absorption in the small intestine of healthy people.

resting metabolic rate (RMR): similar to the basal metabolic rate (BMR), a measure of the energy use of a person at rest in a comfortable setting, but with less stringent criteria for recent food intake and physical activity. Consequently, the RMR is slightly higher than the BMR.

S

sarcopenia (SAR-koh-PEE-nee-ah)**:** loss of skeletal muscle mass, strength, and quality.

sickle-cell anemia: a hereditary from of anemia characterized by abnormal sickle – or crescent – shaped red blood cells. Sickled cells interfere with oxygen transport and blood flow. Symptoms are precipitated by dehydration and insufficient oxygen (as may occur at high altitudes) and include hemolytic anemia (red blood cells burst), fever, and severe pain in the joints and abdomen.

small intestine: a 10 foot length of small-diameter intestine that is the major site of digestion of food and absorption of nutrients. Its segments are the duodenum, jejunum, and ileum.

soluble fibers: nonstarch polysaccharides that dissolve in water to form a gel. An example is pectin from fruit, which is used thicken jellies.

sphincter (SHINK-ter)**:** a circular muscle surrounding, and able to close, a body opening. Sphincters are found at specific points along the GI tract and regulate the flow of food particles.

stroke: an event in wich the blood flow t a part of the brain is cut off; also called cerebrovascular accident (CVA).

sugar alcohols: sugar like compounds that can be derived from fruits or commercially produced from dextrose; also called polyols. Sugar alcohols are absorbed more slowly than other sugars and metabolized differently in the human body; they are not readily utilized by ordinary mouth bacteria. Examples are maltitol, mannitol, sorbitol, xylitol, isomalt, and lactitol.

T

TCA cycle or tricarboxylic (try-car-box-ILL-ick)**:** acid cycle: a series of metabolic reactions that break down molecules of acetyl CoA to carbon dioxide and hydrogen atoms; also called the citric acid cycle of the Kreb's cycle after the biochemist who elucidated its reactions.

thermic effect of food (TEF): an estimation of the energy required to process food (digest, absorb, transport, metabolize, and store ingested nutrients); also called the specific dynamic effect (SDE) of food or the specific dynamic activity (SDA) of food. The sum of the TEF and any increase in the metabolic rate due to overeating is known as diet-induced thermogenesis (DIT).

Tolerable Upper Intake Level (UL): the maximum daily amount of a nutrient that appears safe for most healthy and beyond which there is an increased risk of adverse health effects.

type 1 diabetes: the less common type of diabetes in which the pancreas produces little to no insulin. Type 1 diabetes usually results from autoimmune destruction of pancreatic beta cells.

type 2 diabetes: the more common type of diabetes in which the cells fail to respond to insulin. Type 2 diabetes usually accompanies obesity and results from insulin resistance coupled with insufficient insulin secretion.

U

unsaturated fatty acid: a fatty acid that lacks hydrogen atoms and has at least one double bond between carbons (includes monounsaturated and polyunsaturated fatty acids). An unsaturated fat is composed of triglycerides in which most of the fatty acids are unsaturated.

V

Vegans (VEE-gans)**:** people who exclude all animal-derived foods (including meat, poultry, fish, eggs, and milk and milk products) from their diets; also called pure vegetarians, strict vegetarians, or total vegetarians.

vegetarians: a general term used to describe people who exclude meat, poultry, fish, or other animal-derived foods from their diets.

Veins (VANES)**:** vessels that carry blood to the heart.

villi (VILL-ee, VILL-eye)**:** fingerlike projections from the folds of small intestine; singular villus.

vitamins: organic, essential nutrients required in small amounts by the body for health. Vitamins regulate body processes that support growth and maintain life.

W

whole grain: a grain that maintains the same relative proportions of starchy endosperm, germ, and bran as the original (all but the husk); not refined.

Equations / Requirements

Volume

1 cup = 1/2 pint = 8 fluid ounces = 237 milliliters
4 cups = 1 quart = 32 fluid ounces = 0.946 liter
4 quarts = 1 gallon = 128 fluid ounces = 3.785 liters
1 milliliter = .03 ounces
2 tablespoons = 1 fluid ounce = 30 milliliters
16 tablespoons = 1 cup = 237 milliliters
3 teaspoons = 1 tablespoon = 15 milliliters
4 cups = 1 quart
1 gallon = 3.79 liters

Weight

one ounce = 28.35 grams 3 1/2 ounces = 100 grams
1 pound = 16 ounces = 453.6 grams
1 kilogram = 1000 grams = 2.2 pounds
1 gram = 100 micrograms

Length

1 inch = 2.54 centimeters
1 foot = 30.48 centimeters
1 meter = 39.37 inches

Waist-to-Hip Ratio Calculation
A man has a waist of 39 inches, and a hip measurement of 40 inches. Step 1: 39 ÷ 40 = .98
This man is at increased risk for the chronic diseases mentioned above.

Body Mass Index

Body Mass Index Calculation
weight ÷ 2.2 (height (inches) x .0254)2
Example: weight is 220 pounds and height is 6 feet 4 inches step 1 - 220 ÷ 2.2 = 100 step 2 - 76 inches x .0254 = 1.93 step 3 - 1.93 x 1.93 = 3.72 step 4 - 100 ÷ 3.72 = 26.88 *Body Mass Index is 26.88 and is considered obese*

Body Mass Index Norms	
Emaciated	Less than 15
Severely Underweight	15.0 to 16.9
Underweight	17.0 to 18.9
Normal Weight	19.0 to 24.9
Overweight	25.0 to 29.9
Obese	30.0 to 39.9
Severely Obese	40.0 or more

EER -Adults

Men 19 Years and Older
EER = [662 – (9.53 x Age)] + PA X [(15.91 x Weight) + (539.6 x Height)]
Women 19 Years and Older
EER = [354 – (6.91 x Age)] + PA X [(9.36 x Weight) + (726 x Height)]

Body Fat Adjusted EER

Males - Body Fat Adjusted EER
Adjusted Percent = 100% - (Actual % Body Fat – Average % Body Fat)
Body Fat Adjusted EER = EER X Adjusted percent
Example: Male that is 29 years old; 6'1" tall; weighs 190 pounds; activity level is low-active; body fat is 28% EER = 3019 calories Adjusted Percent = 100 – (28%-15%) = 87% or .87 Body Fat Adjusted EER = 3019 x .87 =2627

Females - Body Fat Adjusted EER
Adjusted Percent = 100% - (Actual % Body Fat – Average % Body Fat)
Body Fat Adjusted EER = EER X Adjusted percent
Example: Female that is 33 years old; 5'4" tall; weighs 127 pounds; activity level is low-active; body fat is 26% EER = 2057 Adjusted Percent = 100% – (26%-22%) = 96% or .96 Body Fat Adjusted EER = 2057 x .96 = 1975

EER Activity Coefficients

Men > 19 Years (1)	Women > 19 Years	Physical Activity
Sedentary: 1.0	Sedentary: 1.0	Daily living activities
Low Active: 1.11	Low Active: 1.12	Plus 30-60 min. moderate activity
Active: 1.25	Active: 1.27	Plus >60 min. moderate activity
Very Active: 1.48	Very Active: 1.45	Plus >60 min. moderate activity and 60 min. vigorous activity or 120 min. moderate activity

Percent Body Fat Norms

Description	Women	Men
Essential Fat	10-13%	2-5%
Athletes	14-20%	6-13%
Fitness	21-24%	14-17%
Average	25-31%	18-24%
Obese	32% +	25% +

Caloric Requirements

Recommendations	Grams/Day	Percentage of Daily Calories
Carbohydrates	130 grams for men and women	45% to 65%
Sugar	NA	≤ 10.00%
Fats	NA	20 % to 35%
Proteins	.8 grams to 1.8 grams	15 to 20%

Fiber Recommendations	Men (g/day)	Women (g/day)
Adults under 50 years old	38	25

Fiber Recommendations	Men (g/day)	Women (g/day)
Adults over 50 years old	30	21

Dietary Reference Intakes – Child and Teen Caloric Needs)

Gender	Age (years)	Sedentary [b]	Moderately Active [c]	Active [d]
Child	2-3	1,000	1,000-1,400	1,000-1,400
Female	4-8 9-13 14-18	1,200 1,600 1,800	1,400-1,600 1,600-2,000 2,000	1,400-1,800 1,800-2,200 2,400
Male	4-8 9-13 14-18	1,400 1,800 2,200	1,400-1,600 1,800-2,200 2,400-2,800	1,600-2,000 2,000-2,600 2,800-3,200

Child and Teen Weight Status Categories

Weight Status Category	Percentile Range
Underweight	Less than the 5th percentile
Healthy weight	5th percentile to less than the 85th percentile
Overweight	85th to less than the 95th percentile
Obese	Equal to or greater than the 95th percentile

Responsibility Agreement

Welcome to ____. The next ________weeks are crucial to ensuring your success in lifelong weight management. Please make this program your top priority. Many obstacles to your success will undoubtedly crop up in the next few weeks. Don't let these obstacles stand in your way. Be aware that you will probably go through several psychological stages during your program. We will ask you to determine what causes you to overeat and/or what prevents you from exercising. In some cases, eating issues are a cover up for other more deep rooted problems. During your program you must continuously ask yourself if the changes you are making are lifestyle changes - changes you can live with the rest of your life without feeling deprived or stressed. If these changes are difficult and "unpleasant", then we must "talk". We will work with you to make this program the "beginning of the rest of your life". We will also be asking you to periodically keep a food log of everything you eat. A food log can actually decrease your obsession with food. Remember, the only way we can help you is if we have all the facts. We are your educators, motivators, and your confidants - not your judges.

We, the staff of ____________ are at your disposal to help ease you into lifestyle transitions. However, you must do all the work. Therefore, we ask that you read the agreement below carefully, and sign only if you are in complete agreement:

I ________________________ agree to follow the exercise program as prescribed in our sessions; I ________________________ also agree to make changes in my eating patterns as agreed upon.

Legal Waiver

I am aware that exercise can be physically stressful and in certain instances can even be harmful and result in death; I am also aware that unknown incidences can arise from changing eating patterns. I am aware that anyone who smokes; has ever had elevated blood pressure; is over 45 (men) or 55 (women) years of age; presently does not exercise; has ever had cardiac (heart) problems; is overweight; has diabetes; has a family history of cardiovascular problems; is susceptible to or has ever had orthopedic problems; or is pregnant; is more at risk while exercising and changing eating patterns. I understand that I should consult with my personal physician before I begin or continue any such program. I also understand it is recommended that I have a physician identify any limitations on my exercise or eating patterns that I may have if any of these conditions exist. I understand that my participation in the **Nutrition Specialist Program** through AASDN, which includes exercise, meal planning, and nutrition education – developed by qualified licensed dietitians/nutritionists - is voluntary and at my own risk. I hereby release AASDN; affiliates, subsidiaries and parent companies; any of its or their respective officers, directors, agents or employees from and agree to hold any and all of the released individuals or entities harmless against, any claims or liability arising out of my participation in any of the programs and facilities. I further agree not to sue or make any claim of any nature whatsoever relating to or arising out of my participation in any of the Nutrition Specialist programs, or use of facilities in any court, agency, or other forum or proceeding against any individual or entity whom I have released and agreed to hold harmless in the preceding sentence.

I have read this form and fully understand the above waiver, release, and assumption of risk. I have had the opportunity to ask questions. I understand that I have given up substantial rights by signing this waiver, release, and assumption of risk and I sign it voluntarily. I have sufficient information to give my informed consent to participate in the referenced program and its facilities. I also understand that group classes may be audio/video taped for educational purposes only.

Signature ____________________________

Witness ___________________________ Date ____________________

The information obtained in this program is designed to optimize safety and foster attainment of personal goals. All information will be kept strictly confidential and will only be available to Nutrition Specialist personnel, and the program dietitian, unless otherwise authorized in writing by you.

1000 Calorie Menu Plan - 1

Breakfast
½ cup cooked oatmeal
1 Tbsp nuts and 1 Tbsp raisins (added to cereal)
8 oz fat free or 1% milk
½ cup fruit (strawberries, blueberries, peaches, apples)

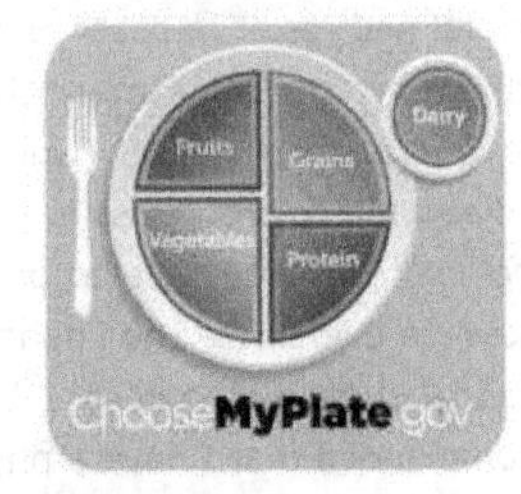

Snack
1 oz whole wheat cracker
1/4 cup cubed vegetable

Lunch
Sandwich - ½ slice whole wheat bread (½ oz) and 2 slices turkey or chicken breast (1 oz)
½ tsp light mayonnaise and lettuce
½ cup cubed vegetable
4 oz fat free milk

Snack
½ cup cottage cheese (1% low fat)
½ cup fruit

Dinner
½ cup cooked brown rice or ½ cup cubed sweet potato
1 oz grilled chicken, or turkey or fish
½ cup green salad and 1 tsp extra virgin olive oil and 1 tsp vinegar

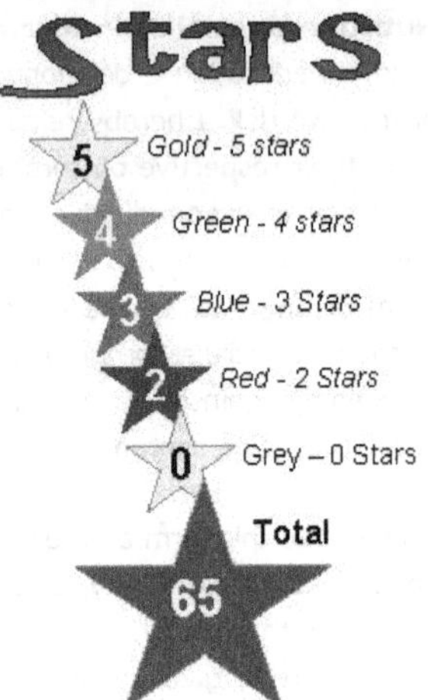

Total Daily Stars

60 Stars or more – Great
45 - 59 Stars – Good
44 Stars or less – Not so good!

Calorie Breakdown: 1015 to 1035 Kcal

Food Group	Amount	Stars
Vegetable	1 cup	10 Stars
Fruit	1 cup	10 Stars
Grains	3 ounces	15 Stars
Milk/Dairy	2 cups	15 Stars
Meat/Bean	3 ounces	15 Stars*

* Protein in the dairy products increase protein to equal 15 stars.

1000 Calorie Menu Plan - 2

Breakfast
1 cup whole grain cereal (Cheerios, Chex, Great Grains, Kashi, Life, Mini Wheats)
1 Tbsp raisins (added to cereal)
8 oz fat free or 1% milk
½ cup fruit (strawberries, blueberries, peaches, apples)

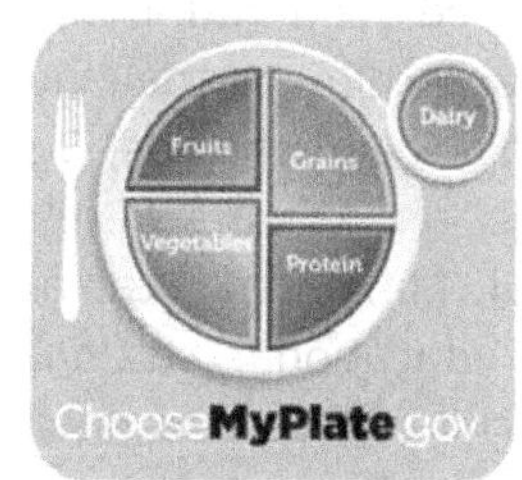

Snack
1 oz whole wheat cracker
1/4 cup cubed vegetable

Lunch
Sandwich - ½ slice whole wheat bread (½ oz) and 1 Tbsp all natural peanut butter
½ cup cubed vegetable
4 oz fat free milk

Snack
½ cup cottage cheese (1% low fat)
½ cup fruit

Dinner
½ cup cooked brown rice or ½ cup cubed sweet potato
1½ oz grilled chicken, or turkey or fish
½ cup green salad and 1 tsp extra virgin olive oil and 1 tsp vinegar

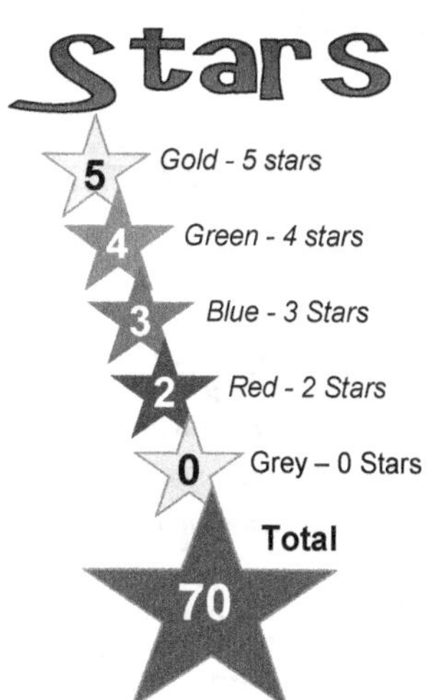

Total Daily Stars

60 Stars or more – Great
45 - 59 Stars – Good
44 Stars or less – Not so good!

Calorie Breakdown: 1050 to 1070 Kcal

Food Group	Amount	Stars
Vegetable	1 cup	10 Stars
Fruit	$1\frac{1}{2}$ cups	15 Stars
Grains	3 ounces	15 Stars
Milk/Dairy	$1\frac{1}{2}$ cups	15 Stars
Meat/Bean	$2\frac{1}{2}$ ounces	15 Stars*

* Protein in the dairy products increase protein to equal 15 stars.

* Meal plans (1000-00 calories) available online at http://www.aasdn.org/obesitypart4.htm

AASDN Placemats

The AASDN star-associated food rating system is implemented utilizing colorful and interactive placemats. The *AASDN Placemats™* incorporate a "star" associated food rating system on the front side of the placemats. Foods are rated according to their nutritional value: 5 stars (Gold) - best choices, 4 stars (Green) - good choices, 3 stars (Blue) - Ok choices, 2 stars (Red) - less healthy choices, and 0 stars (Grey) - avoid these choices. AASDN has developed three colorful, laminated, star-associated food tracking placemats to meet the needs of all educational settings. These laminated, reusable, interactive placemats allow children to use enclosed washable markers to color in stars and reward themselves for good decision making! Visit www.aasdn.org (click on NSLAI) for more details.

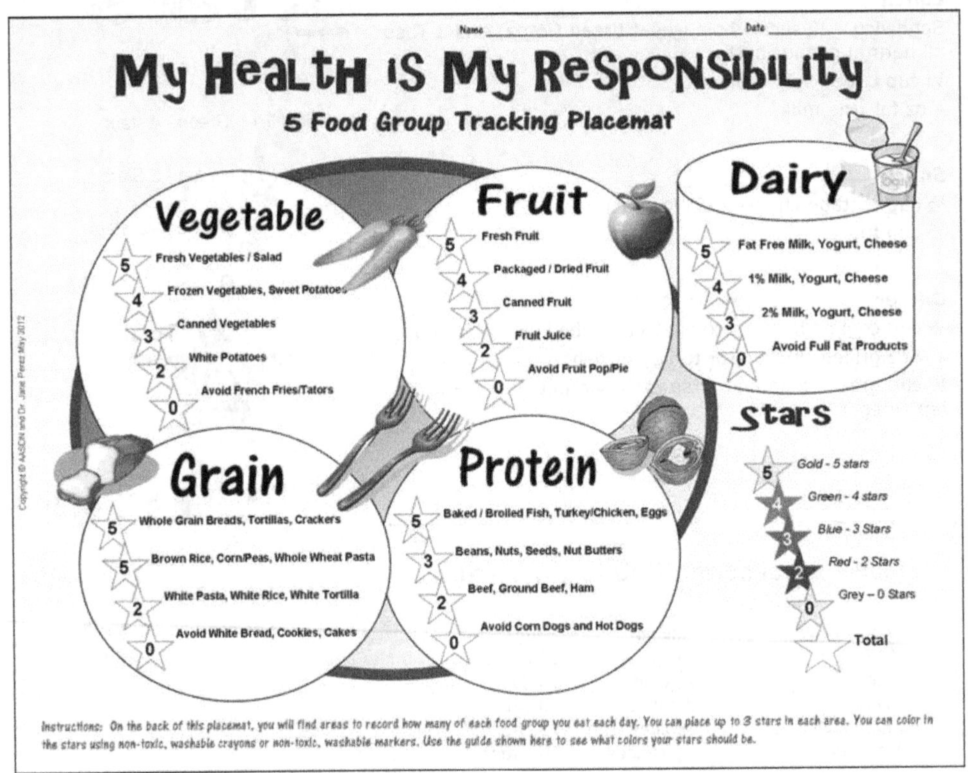

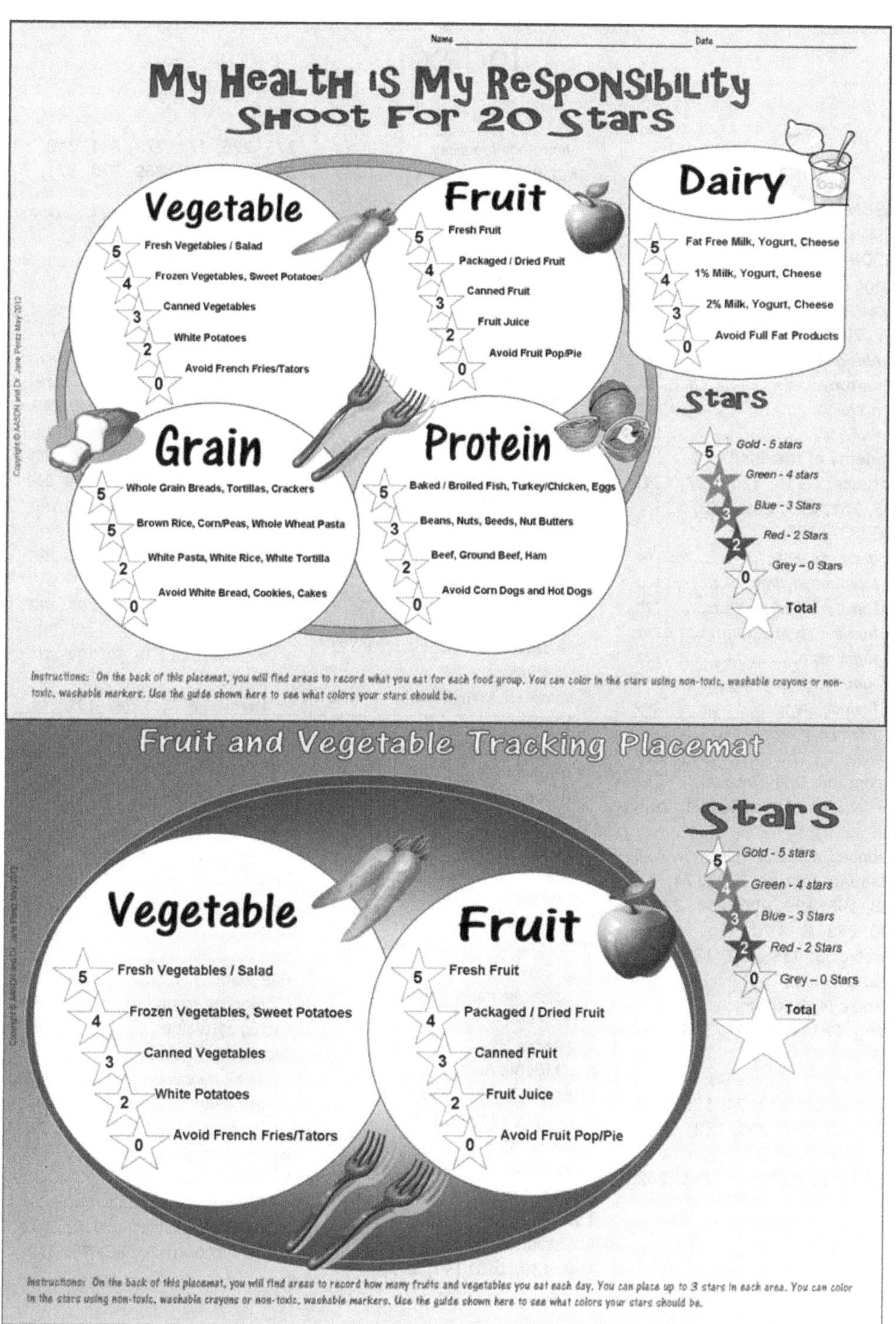

Name
Date
My Health is My Responsibility
Shoot For 20 Stars
Vegetable
5 Fresh Vegetables / Salad
4 Frozen Vegetables, Sweet Potatoes
3 Canned Vegetables
2 White Potatoes
0 Avoid French Fries/Tators
Fruit
5 Fresh Fruit
4 Packaged / Dried Fruit
3 Canned Fruit
2 Fruit Juice
0 Avoid Fruit Pop/Pie
Dairy
5 Fat Free Milk, Yogurt, Cheese
4 1% Milk, Yogurt, Cheese
3 2% Milk, Yogurt, Cheese
0 Avoid Full Fat Products
Grain
5 Whole Grain Breads, Tortillas, Crackers
5 Brown Rice, Corn/Peas, Whole Wheat Pasta
2 White Pasta, White Rice, White Tortilla
0 Avoid White Bread, Cookies, Cakes
Protein
5 Baked / Broiled Fish, Turkey/Chicken, Eggs
3 Beans, Nuts, Seeds, Nut Butters
2 Beef, Ground Beef, Ham
0 Avoid Corn Dogs and Hot Dogs
Stars
5 Gold - 5 stars
4 Green - 4 stars
3 Blue - 3 Stars
2 Red - 2 Stars
0 Grey – 0 Stars
Total
Instructions: On the back of this placemat, you will find areas to record what you eat for each food group. You can color in the stars using non-toxic, washable crayons or non-toxic, washable markers. Use the guide shown here to see what colors your stars should be.
Fruit and Vegetable Tracking Placemat
Stars
5 Gold - 5 stars
4 Green - 4 stars
3 Blue - 3 Stars
2 Red - 2 Stars
0 Grey – 0 Stars
Total
Vegetable
5 Fresh Vegetables / Salad
4 Frozen Vegetables, Sweet Potatoes
3 Canned Vegetables
2 White Potatoes
0 Avoid French Fries/Tators
Fruit
5 Fresh Fruit
4 Packaged / Dried Fruit
3 Canned Fruit
2 Fruit Juice
0 Avoid Fruit Pop/Pie
Instructions: On the back of this placemat, you will find areas to record how many fruits and vegetables you eat each day. You can place up to 3 stars in each area. You can color in the stars using non-toxic, washable crayons or non-toxic, washable markers. Use the guide shown here to see what colors your stars should be.

Index

A

AASDN Placemat..............393
AASDN Scope of Practice....341
AASDN Star Associated Food Rating System.................392
Absorption......7, 9, 12, 13, 27, 179, 203, 204, 206, 210, 211
Absorption Rate....................41
Carbohydrates......................36
microvilli...............................7
Proteins.............................101
Academy of Nutrition and Dietetics....115, 120, 127, 131, 135, 261, 272, 289, 323, 326, 336, 337, 405
Basal Metabolic Rate...........134
Low-Carbohydrate Diet.........120
Low-Carbohydrate Diets........120
Nutrient Timing...................131
Nutrients............................127
Nutritive Sweeteners.............54
Position Stand.....................289
Vitamins - Minerals.............272
Acai........................272, 279
Acceptable Daily Intake........52
Acetyl CoA. 118, 119, 201, 202, 216
Acidosis..........................428
Adequate Intake 17, 28, 74, 97, 128, 198, 199, 206, 214, 228, 230, 238
Aerobic. .3, 118, 122, 139, 169, 172, 366, 399
Aerobic Metabolism...........118
Aging. 170, 171, 397, 398, 399, 405
Alanine................98, 99, 102
Alcohol......123, 124, 126, 157, 158, 166, 172, 208, 232
Calories..............................50
Alternative Medicine. .261, 262, 263, 279
Alternative Medicine...............
Dietary Supplements............263
Mind-Body Practices............264
NCCAM..............................261
Supplements......................265
American College of Sports Medicine....115, 127, 131, 145, 168, 186, 272, 289, 396, 401, 405
Fats..................................129
Fluid.................................133
Micronutrients.............131, 133
Nutrient Timing...................131
Protein...............................129
Amino Acid Score.............104
Amino Acids....8, 9, 12, 13, 39, 40, 93, 95, 96, 97, 100, 101
Alanine................................98
BCAA...................................99
Deamination..........................97
Essential Amino Acids.12, 96, 97, 98, 101, 107, 108
Glucogenic..................100, 123
Glutamine............................98
Ketogenic Amino Acids..........100
Nitrogen..............................99
Nonessential Amino Acids.......98
Transamination.....................97
Transport Systems........101, 102
Ammonia..........8, 97, 98, 274
Anabolic. .9, 12, 121, 123, 227, 274, 275
Anhydrous..........................8
Antibodies.................95, 442
Antioxidants......133, 200, 213, 218, 290
Supplementation...141, 290, 296
Vitamin C...........................200
Vitamin E...........................213
Arachidonic Acid...........76, 85
Artery 7, 78, 86, 158, 159, 164, 169, 170, 171, 182, 183
Ascorbic Acid............205, 324
Aspartame............51, 52, 318
Atherosclerosis....45, 157, 158, 159, 163, 164, 170, 171
Athletes.....122, 127, 128, 129, 130, 139, 140, 141, 273, 274, 275, 276, 277, 278, 284, 290, 291, 325, 367, 369, 370, 371, 401
ATP....116, 118, 119, 121, 122, 236, 251, 276

B

B Vitamins...........................
B Vitamins Toxicity..............199
Biotin.....18, 197, 199, 200, 202, 230
Folate.......18, 50, 200, 203, 205
Niacin.......18, 96, 197, 199, 200
Pantothenic Acid....18, 197, 199, 200, 201
Riboflavin.......18, 133, 141, 197, 198, 199, 200
Thiamin....18, 50, 197, 198, 199, 200, 201
Vitamin B12.....18, 50, 199, 203, 204, 406
Vitamin B6.....18, 162, 197, 199, 200, 204
Water Soluble Vitamins...50, 199 203
Basal Metabolic Rate.....16, 39, 134, 136
BMR............115, 135, 137, 372
Beriberi...................199, 201
Beta-Carotene...........206, 207
Bias........................308, 310
Bile..................................6
Bile Acids.................6, 81, 82
Bioelectric Impedance........369
Biological Value................104
Biotin.................................
Biotin Deficiency.................202
Biotin Roles........................202
Biotin Toxicity.....................202
Bitter Orange...................279
Blood.................................
Platelets................................8
Blood Brain Barrier............102
Blood Clotting..77, 85, 86, 213,

218, 230, 242
Blood Pressure. .22, 44, 46, 77, 120, 124, 157, 164, 165, 166, 167, 168, 169, 170, 180, 235, 237, 275, 280, 388, 402
Cardiovascular.....................157
Essential Fatty Acids..............77
High Fiber Diet......................46
Insulin Resistance..................44
Stress................................124
Body Composition Measures.....
Body Mass Index..................367
Percent Body Fat.................368
Waist-to-Hip Ratio................368
..368
Body Fat....40, 41, 69, 84, 131, 135, 137, 367, 368, 372, 389, 396, 403
Body Mass Index..................367
Equations............................135
Essential Fat........................369
Ideal Body Fat.....................141
Waist-to-Hip Ratio................368
..368
Body Fat Adjusted Estimated Energy Requirements.........372
Botanical.................270, 271
Brain...50, 102, 159, 169, 171, 208, 244, 246, 274, 445
Building a Successful Nutrition Business..............................
Advertising..........................462
Attracting Business - Sales....457
Before Getting Started..........452
Choosing a Client Base.........455
Developing a Pricing Scheme.456
EMyth................................451
It's Not Just the Money.........452
Marketing...........................461
Passion..............................452
Professional........................459
Pros and Cons.....................454
Research Your Competition...460
Risk-taking..........................453
Steps to Starting a Business..454
Strong Ethics......................453
Tech Ease...........................453
Tenacity.............................453
Your Unique Perspective.......455
................................456, 457

C

C-Reactive Protein......163, 164
Caffeine......14, 122, 124, 161, 178, 179, 212, 232, 277, 280, 281, 290
Calciferol.........................209
Calcium13, 133, 164, 165, 176, 214, 230, 231
Absorption............231, 232, 234
Calcium Absorption210, 231, 232
Calcium Deficiency...............233
Calcium Malabsorption..........176
Calcium Roles......................233
Calcium Toxicity...................233
Calories....3, 4, 10, 11, 14, 16, 18, 20, 22, 25, 34, 37, 52, 54, 68, 127, 128
Body Fat Adjusted Estimated Energy Requirements...........372
Body Fat Adjustment............137
Physical Activity...................136
Cancer....24, 40, 46, 172, 173, 184, 207, 281, 288, 402
Breast Cancer..............173, 174
Cancer and Physical Activity..173
Colon.................................179
Colon Cancer.......................173
Endometrial Cancer 174
Lung Cancer.................171, 174
Prostate......................174, 275
Vegetarians.........................402
Vitamin E...........................213
Carbohydrate............2, 6, 7, 9
Absorption............35, 36, 37, 46
Calories.......................128, 135
Carbohydrate - Complex.........10
Carbohydrate - Protein Sparing 97
Carbohydrate - Simple...........10
Digestion...................33, 35, 50
Disaccharide.........................34
Fiber...................................46
Gluconeogenesis...................39
Glucose...............................38
Glucose 37
Glucose Time Curve..............38
Glycemic Index.....................41
Glycemic Load.......................43
Glycogen.............................36
Insulin Resistance..................44
Low-Carbohydrate Diets........120
Metabolic Syndrome...............45
Monosaccharide.....................34
Monosaccharides...................36
Oligosaccharide.....................34
Polysaccharide.......................34
Recommended Intake............47
..35
Carbon Chain................69, 81
Cardiovascular Disease......124, 165, 168, 171, 182, 183, 185, 186, 201, 237, 251
Coronary Heart Disease........157
Heart Disease......................157
Homocysteine......................162
Physical Activity...................165
Stress................................124
Case Studies....................408
Catabolic. 9, 98, 122, 123, 124, 126, 139, 227, 366, 381
Catabolic Factors...................
Age...................................123
Alcohol..............................126
Alcohol 123
Caffeine.............................124
Fasting and Starvation..........123
Gender..............................123
Genetics.............................122
Illness...............................124
Inadequate Rest..................127
Nutrition............................123
Stress................................124
Celiac Disease..................175
Cells...................................
Animal Cells............................1
Brain..........27, 38, 40, 274, 428
Cytoplasm.............................2
Cytosol.................................2
Digestive Tract........................5
Epithelial Cells.........................3
Eukaryotic..............................2
Fat Cells................................1
Membrane..............................2
Mitochondria...........................3
Muscle Cells............................1
Nerve Cells.............................1
Nucleus.................................2
Plant Cells..............................1
Prokaryotic.............................2

Red Blood Cells........................1
Cellulose..................2, 10, 34
Certification.....................344
Childhood Obesity......388, 389
Chloride....17, 19, 28, 228, 230
Chloride Deficiency...............235
Chloride Roles.....................234
Chloride Toxicity..................235
Cholesterol.....11, 20, 35, 44, 45, 80, 81, 83, 158, 159, 160, 161
Cholesterol Lowering Medication 158, 160
Choline.............................70
Chromium. 17, 19, 28, 239, 248
Chromium Deficiency............248
Chromium Roles..................248
Chromium Toxicity...............248
Glucose-Tolerance Factor......248
Chronic Kidney Disease......179
Chylomicron...........82, 83, 87
Circulatory System...............7
Coaching Skills.................345
Coenzyme..116, 118, 119, 200, 201, 202, 203, 204
Coenzyme A......118, 200, 201, 202, 216
Collagen......95, 158, 200, 206, 246, 252
Complementary Alternative Medicine.........................262
Conflict of Interest............308
Federal Conflict-of-Interest Regulations 312
Intangible...........................309
Tangible.............................311
ConsumerLab.com............283
Copper...19, 28, 239, 243, 246
Absorption..........................246
Copper Absorption...............246
Copper Deficiency................246
Copper Roles.......................246
Copper Toxicity............246, 247
Coronary Calcium Scan......164
Coronary Heart Disease......73, 157, 159, 164
Creatine..................275, 276
Cretinism..................239, 244
Critical Analysis of Research 315
Questions to be Answered.....320
Reputable Resources............326
Study Design.......................315
Crohn's Disease. 175, 176, 177, 178, 185
Cytoplasm......2, 101, 109, 116
Cytosol........16, 116, 118, 119

D

Daily Values.......................17
Dash-Sodium Diet.............167
Deamination......................97
Dehydration...40, 41, 133, 151, 228, 229, 235, 273, 287
DHA...........................74, 75
DIAAS............................105
Diabetes............151, 154, 156
Diabetes and Physical Activity156
Gestational Diabetes............153
Hypoglycemia.......127, 156, 185
Preventing Diabetes.............154
Type 1 Diabetes...................151
Type 2 Diabetes...................152
..152
Diet.........................120, 422
AASDN "Spoof" on Diets.......427
Diets and Muscle Loss...........428
Diets, More Diets, and More Diets 425
Eating Enough and On Time. .429
History of Dieting.................422
How to Write Your Own Diet Book..................................426
Diet Record......................373
Dietary Fiber....43, 46, 58, 443
Dietary Guidelines...19, 21, 23, 24, 28, 391
Dietary Reference Intakes...17, 28, 135, 136, 137
Digestion.....4, 6, 27, 116, 198, 271
Bile.......................................6
Digestive Juices..................4, 6
Digestive Tract........................4
Esophagus.............................5
Liver......................................6
Stomach.................................5
Digestive..............................
Glands....................................6
Digestive System.........4, 7, 47
Disaccharide...........10, 34, 35
Dispensable Amino Acids........8
DNA......2, 200, 203, 204, 213, 217, 242, 245, 251, 252
Docosahexaenoic Acid..........74
Double Bonds....71, 72, 73, 74, 84, 85
Duodenum..........................7

E

Eating Disorders.........381, 409
Eating Out.......................444
Eicosanoids..................76, 85
Eicosapentaenoic Acid..........74
Electrolytes. 132, 133, 234, 292
Electron Transport Chain..........
Mitochondria......................119
EMyth.....................451, 452
Endocrine.............................
Glands.................................3
Endocrine System................3
Endogenous....82, 83, 87, 236, 290
Energy....................115, 116
Adenosine Triphosphate (ATP) 118
Electron Transport Chain.......118
Energy Production................116
Energy Utilization.................119
Mitochondria.......................119
Nutrient Timing....................131
Phosphocreatine..................118
Tricarboxylic acid (TCA)........118
Energy Drinks.....125, 278, 290
Energy Expenditure...115, 127, 134, 135, 136, 372
Energy Utilization.............119
Age....................................123
Diet....................................119
Exercise Duration.................122
Exercise Intensity................121
Fitness Level.......................122
Gender...............................123
Genetics.............................122
Low-Carbohydrate Diets........119
Muscle Mass........................122
Nutrition.............................123
Rest...................................121
Enzymes...6, 7, 11, 35, 80, 81,

86, 95, 96, 99, 100, 101, 116, 201, 203, 204, 205, 206, 232, 233, 236, 242, 246, 247, 425
Ephedra..........................280
Epinephrine........16, 37, 38, 96
Epithelial Cells......3, 36, 82, 87
Ergogenic Aids.......................
Amino Acids........................274
Anabolic Steroids.................274
Caffeine..............................277
Carbohydrates/Proteins........273
Creatine..............................275
Energy Bars........................278
Energy Drinks......................278
Water.................................273
Weight Loss Supplements.....279
.......................................273
Esophagus......4, 5, 49, 50, 59, 178, 185
Essential..............................
Amino Acids.....................97, 98
Essential Fatty Acids 67, 69, 74, 76, 77, 78, 82, 85, 129, 371
Essential Nutrients.........9, 102
Carbohydrate........10, 27, 33, 34
Carbohydrates.........................9
Lipids...................................68
Estimated Average Requirements........17, 28, 198
Estimated Energy Requirements (EER). 135, 136, 137, 372, 376, 382, 383
Exercise. 14, 46, 118, 121, 122, 126, 129, 130, 131, 132, 133
Exogenous.....82, 87, 152, 236

F

FAD.........................200, 201
Fad Diets...........421, 426, 460
Fasting and Starvation.......123
Fat Cells.....1, 3, 4, 36, 83, 372
Fat Soluble Vitamins......12, 13, 206
Vitamin A.......18, 197, 199, 206, 207, 208
Vitamin D. 18, 81, 133, 206, 209, 210, 211, 212, 290
Vitamin E...18, 69, 78, 206, 213, 218
Vitamin K..............18, 207, 214
................................209, 213
Fatty Acids.............58, 69, 70
Essential Fatty Acids. .67, 69, 74, 76, 77, 78, 82, 129, 371
Polyunsaturated Fatty Acids...20, 74, 82
Saturated Fatty Acids............71
FDA......52, 53, 54, 55, 56, 86, 126, 176, 215, 262, 265, 266, 267, 268, 269, 270, 273, 280, 281, 284, 286, 323, 426, 432, 434, 437, 438, 441, 442
Ferritin...............96, 240, 242
Fiber. 2, 11, 18, 34, 35, 41, 46, 47, 128, 161, 178, 370, 440, 442, 443, 467
Fiber...................................
Cancer....................46, 53, 157
Cellulose.................................2
Dietary Fiber.........................58
Dietary Fibers........................46
Fiber Content of Foods...........47
High Fiber Diet.....................46
Irritable Bowel Syndrome......178
Recommended Intake...........47
Fish Oil...........................272
Fluoride. 17, 74, 228, 238, 239, 431, 432
Folate....18, 50, 176, 200, 203, 204, 205, 296
Folate - Deficiency...............203
Folate - Roles......................203
Folate Toxicity.....................203
Food Chart.......................374
Food Frequency................373
Food Log.........................373
Food Production / Commodities 443
Free Radicals..............13, 213

G

Galactose....................10, 34
Gallbladder..........6, 8, 81, 431
Gastrointestinal Disorders...175
Gastrointestinal Reflux Disease (GERD)......175, 178, 179, 185
Gastrointestinal Tract. 176, 184, 199, 201, 203, 214, 217, 431
Gestational Diabetes..151, 152, 153
Glands......................5, 6, 37
Glucagon..........................16
Gluconeogenesis..........39, 100
Glucose.....4, 8, 10, 15, 34, 36, 37, 38, 39, 40, 41, 42, 45, 50, 97, 99, 100, 118, 119, 121, 123, 124, 151, 156, 165, 171, 230, 248
Gluconeogenesis..................100
Glucose Intolerance........45, 127
Glucose-Alanine Cycle............98
Glucose-Tolerance Factor......248
Glycolysis...........................118
Hypoglycemia..............127, 156
Gluten-Free. 175, 176, 441, 442
Glycemic Index..41, 42, 43, 44, 140
Glycerol. 39, 69, 80, 81, 82, 83, 116, 124
Glycogen. 8, 10, 11, 16, 34, 36, 37, 38, 39, 40, 120, 122, 123, 132, 133, 229
Glycolysis. .116, 118, 119, 122, 138
Cytosol...............................118
Pyruvate.............................118
GRAS 52, 53, 54, 55, 59, 78, 86
Green Tea.......................281

H

HDL...45, 73, 82, 83, 159, 160, 161, 172, 182, 238
Healthy Eating Plate..24, 25, 26
Heart Disease....24, 44, 45, 55, 73, 78, 150, 151, 157, 159, 160, 161, 162, 163, 164, 170, 171, 242, 243, 272, 367, 368, 369, 388, 398, 402
Heme.................96, 204, 240
Hemochromatosis.......241, 242
Hemoglobin...95, 96, 107, 201, 217, 239, 240, 251
Herbal 270, 271, 278, 280, 281, 343
High Fructose Corn Syrup....33, 50, 55
High-Sensitivity C-Reactive

Protein....163
Homeostasis....14
Homocysteine....162
Hormones....15
Epinephrine....16, 38, 96
Glucagon....16, 37, 38, 41
Growth Hormone....95, 435
Insulin. 15, 38, 40, 58, 152, 156, 185, 242, 248, 443
Thyroid....16, 95, 239, 243, 244, 245, 252
....37
Hydration....14, 123, 133, 278
Hydrogenation....12, 73
Hyperglycemia....163, 248
Hypertension....165
Blood Pressure....165, 166, 167, 168, 169, 170
Hypertrophy....119, 122, 123, 124, 127, 130, 131, 139, 140, 398
Hypoglycemia....127

I

Immune System 11, 12, 46, 50, 69, 76, 77, 78, 98, 124, 151, 152, 208, 210, 218, 231, 237, 242, 251
Implementing Nutrition Programs....
Aging Population....397
Body Composition Measures..367
Case Studies....408
Certification....344
Child and Teen Program....388
Choosing a Licensed Professional 344
Coaching Skills....345
Estimated Energy Requirements (EER)....371
Group Program....385
Individual Program....376
Legal Considerations....336
Lifestyle Journal....373
MyPlate for Older Adults....400
Obese Population....396
Percent Body Fat....368
Prerequisites....335
Program Materials....344
Promoting Success....421
Scope of Practice....341
State Licensure Laws....339
Waist-to-Hip Ratio....368
....368, 373
Indispensable Amino Acids. .97, 103, 105, 107, 110
Inflammation...46, 77, 85, 163, 175, 176, 177, 183, 184, 199, 201, 292
Inorganic....13, 14, 228, 245, 248, 252
Insulin....15, 37, 38
Insulin Resistance....44, 45
International Olympic Committee. 115, 127, 131, 272, 277, 289, 290, 401, 405, 418
Iodine....19, 228, 239, 243
Iodine Deficiency....244
Iodine Roles....244
Iodine Toxicity....244
Iron....13, 18, 96, 133
Absorption....240
Iron Deficiency....208, 211
Iron-Deficiency Anemia....175
Irritable Bowel Syndrome (IBS) 175, 178
Isoleucine 97, 98, 99, 100, 102, 202

K

Keshan Disease....239, 245
Ketoacidosis....41, 152
Ketogenic Diet....40, 100
Ketones....8, 40, 120, 428
Ketosis....39, 40, 41, 122
Kidney Disease....179
Phosphorus....181, 236
Potassium....180
Sodium....180
....180
Kilocalorie....116, 431, 440

L

L-Carnitine....162
Labeling....
Fat Free/Calorie Free 433
FDA Regulations....432
Food Production / Commodities 443
General Terms....439
Gluten-Free....441
Health Claims....437
Ingredient List....438
Label Terms....438
Net Carbs....442
Nutrition Information....439
Organic....434
Structure-Function Claims....438
Unregulated Terms....442
USDA Regulations....434
Voluntary Labeling....441
....433
Lactose....10, 34, 178
Lactose Intolerance....176, 232
Large Intestine...4, 35, 46, 177
LDL. 73, 83, 159, 161, 162, 171
Lean Body Mass. 134, 137, 141, 290, 372
Lecithin....70
Leucine..98, 99, 100, 102, 130, 140
Lifestyle Journal....373
Limiting Amino Acid...103, 104, 109
Linoleic Acid....74, 75
Linolenic Acid....74, 75
Lipids 9, 46, 49, 67, 68, 82, 96, 201, 217, 237
Absorption....67, 68, 81, 82, 371
Alcohol..8, 10, 15, 21, 49, 50, 69
Calories....68
Digestion....67, 81, 86
....49
Lipoprotein....8, 9, 82, 83, 87, 158, 159, 160, 163, 165, 198
Liver...6, 8, 16, 34, 35, 36, 37, 38, 39, 50, 81, 82
Low-Carbohydrate Diets....
Diets....120
lymphatic system....7, 8, 9
Lysine....97, 98, 100, 102, 103, 104

M

Macronutrients....1, 9, 41, 128,

370
Carbohydrate 2, 9, 10, 27, 33, 34
Lipids............................11, 68
Magnesium....13, 19, 166, 228, 230, 231, 251
Magnesium...........................
Magnesium Deficiency..........238
Magnesium Roles.................237
Magnesium Toxicity.............238
Major Minerals......................
Calcium..13, 164, 165, 214, 230, 231
Chloride.....17, 19, 28, 228, 230, 234
Magnesium......13, 19, 166, 228, 230, 231, 237, 251
Phosphorus......13, 19, 180, 181, 236, 251
Potassium. 13, 18, 180, 230, 234
Sodium 13, 18, 20, 81, 166, 167, 230, 232, 234, 440
Sulfur................9, 13, 230, 236
.......................................180
Malabsorption....175, 176, 199, 213, 237
Manganese.....19, 28, 239, 252
Manganese Deficiency..........247
Manganese Roles.................247
Manganese Toxicity..............247
Marketing........................461
Mediterranean Diet 167
Menadione.......................215
Mercury............................78
Metabolic Syndrome44, 46, 184
Metabolism..3, 4, 9, 15, 16, 35, 50, 82, 83, 87, 97, 100
Methionine...98, 102, 162, 204, 236, 245, 250
Micronutrients. 9, 13, 131, 133, 197, 290
Microvilli.............................7
Mind-Body Practices...........264
Minerals 7, 8, 9, 10, 13, 18, 35, 47, 59, 228, 230, 238, 263, 265, 267, 272, 400, 405
Mitochondria...3, 4, 16, 70, 98, 116, 118, 119
Molecule...3, 4, 7, 8, 9, 13, 14, 36, 50, 69, 71, 72, 80, 94, 95, 96, 101, 102, 116, 119, 200
Molybdenum....17, 19, 28, 239, 249
Molybdenum Deficiency........249
Molybdenum Roles...............248
Molybdenum Toxicity............249
Monosaccharide. 10, 34, 35, 36, 43
Monounsaturated 12, 20, 70, 71
Multivitamin......131, 265, 286, 287, 288, 289, 290
Muscle Mass......123, 134, 135, 139, 274, 399, 430
My Plate for Older Adults....401
Myoglobin.....95, 107, 239, 240

N

NAD.........................200, 202
NCCAM......261, 262, 263, 265, 279, 280, 294, 295
NCCAM Classifications............
Dietary Supplements............263
Mind and Body Approaches...281
Mind-Body Practices.............264
Supplements.......................265
Neotame......................51, 52
Nervous System...................3
Net Carbs........................442
Net Protein Utilization........105
Neurotransmitters. 96, 200, 201
Niacin....18, 96, 197, 199, 200, 202
Niacin Deficiency..................202
Niacin Roles........................202
Niacin Toxicity.....................202
Nicotinamide.............202, 217
Nicotinic Acid.............202, 217
Nitrogen.....................99, 100
Nonessential.........................
Amino Acids..........................98
Nonnutritive Sweeteners..........
Acesulfame Potassium............51
Aspartame............................51
Neotame...............................51
Saccharin.............................51
Stevia.............................51, 53
Sucralose.............................51
Norepinephrine.............37, 38
NSF International.......283, 284
Nucleic Acid......9, 99, 236, 251
Nucleotide......................9, 36
Nucleus..............................2
Nutrient. .2, 3, 4, 6, 7, 8, 9, 10, 13, 14, 16, 17, 18, 19, 20, 35, 41, 47, 70, 80, 102, 116, 119, 127
Nutrient Timing.....................
Carbohydrates.....................131
Fluid..................................133
Micronutrients.....................133
Proteins..............................132
Nutrition and Disease.........149
Atherosclerosis....................158
Cancer................................172
Cancer and Physical Activity..173
Cardiovascular Disease.........157
Cardiovascular Disease and Physical Activity...................165
Celiac Disease.....................175
Cholesterol..........................159
Chronic Kidney Disease.........179
Coronary Calcium Scan.........164
Crohn's Disease...................176
Dash Diet............................166
Dash-Sodium Diet................167
Diabetes.............................151
Diabetes and Physical Activity156
Diagnosing Diabetes.............153
Gastrointestinal Reflux Disease 178
Gestational Diabetes............153
GI Disorders and Physical Activity...............................179
High-Sensitivity C-Reactive Protein...............................163
Hypertension.......................165
Hypertension and Physical Activity...............................168
Irritable Bowel Syndrome......178
L-Carnitine..........................162
Mediterranean Diet 167
Preventing Diabetes.............154
Stroke................................169
Stroke and Physical Activity...172
Type 1 Diabetes...................151
Type 2 Diabetes...................152
Ulcerative Colitis..................178
................................152, 156
Nutrition Research.............307
Bias...................................308

Conflict of Interest...............308
Federal Regulations 312
Intangible Conflicts 309
Managing Conflicts of Interest 314
Scientists Behaving Badly.....312
Tangible Conflicts.................311
The Bayh-Dole Act 311
..310
Nutritive Sweeteners..............
High Fructose Corn Syrup.......55
Natural Sweeteners................52
Sugar Alcohols.................52, 54

O

Obesity....44, 45, 55, 152, 157, 171, 172, 184, 326, 367, 368, 388, 389, 393, 396, 399, 405, 422, 444
Office of Dietary Supplements (ODS)............................266
Oil...21, 25, 68, 69, 70, 71, 73, 75, 78
Omega-3 Fatty Acids74, 77, 78, 80, 168, 272
Organelles......................2, 69
Organic. 2, 3, 9, 13, 43, 49, 80, 94, 198, 248, 434, 435, 436, 437, 441, 467
Osteomalacia.....206, 207, 210, 211, 212
Osteoporosis40, 175, 176, 206, 208, 212, 233, 246, 398
Oxidation. 3, 97, 119, 130, 133, 239, 246
Oxygen. 2, 7, 9, 34, 49, 74, 78, 96, 118, 119, 121, 122, 170, 171, 198, 217, 239, 241

P

Pancreas. 6, 15, 16, 37, 38, 44, 45, 58, 151, 152, 242, 252, 276
Pantothenic Acid. .18, 197, 199, 200, 201
Pantothenic Acid Deficiency...202
Pantothenic Acid Roles..........201
Pantothenic Acid Toxicity......202
PCB.................................79
PDCAAS....................105, 140
Peer Review..............320, 321
Pellagra...................199, 202
Peptide Bond......................94
PER................................105
Peristalsis...........................5
Pernicious Anemia.............199
pH...................................15
Phosphocreatine 118, 121, 139, 276
Phospholipids.8, 11, 68, 69, 70, 72, 80, 231, 236
Phosphorus. . .13, 19, 180, 181, 236, 251
Phosphorus - Roles..............236
Phosphorus Deficiency..........237
Phosphorus Toxicity.............237
Photosynthesis.....................2
Phylloquinone...................214
Phytate.............236, 240, 242
Placebo.....207, 274, 275, 276, 319, 321
Platelets......8, 76, 77, 85, 159, 242, 252
PLP.........................204, 217
Polypeptide........................94
Polysaccharide.....9, 34, 35, 36
Polyunsaturated. 12, 20, 70, 71, 74, 76, 82
Portal Vein..........................8
Portion Size. 43, 154, 374, 395, 446, 447
Position Stands................289
Potassium.....13, 18, 180, 230, 234
Potassium Deficiency............235
Potassium Roles...................234
Potassium Toxicity........235, 236
Promoting Success...........421
Building a Successful Nutrition Business............................451
Deprivation of Favorite Foods 448
Diet - A Four Letter Word.....422
Diets and Muscle Loss...........428
Eating Enough and On Time. .429
Eating Out..........................444
Eating Too Many Calories in the Evening.............................447
FDA Regulations..................432
Friendly Saboteurs...............449
Labeling Regulations............431
Not Planning.......................448
Portion Distortion................447
Problem Foods in the Home...448
Stress Eating.......................449
USDA Regulations................434
................................433, 450
Prostaglandins....76, 77, 85, 86
Protein Quality...........102, 103
Amino Acid Score................104
Biological Value..................104
DIAAS...............................105
Essential Amino Acids...........102
Net Protein Utilization...........105
PDCAAS.............................105
Protein Efficiency Ratio 105
................................103, 104
Proteins...............................
Absorption........93, 99, 101, 103
Digestion. 93, 100, 101, 108, 109
Pyridoxal..........................204
pyridoxamine....................204
Pyridoxine........................204
Pyruvate......98, 100, 118, 119, 202

R

Recommended Dietary Allowances. 1, 17, 27, 128, 198, 370
Red Blood Cells. . .1, 8, 70, 151, 203, 213, 217, 240, 241
Requirements........................
Calories..............................370
Carbohydrate......................128
Carbohydrates.....................370
Fats..................................371
Fluids................................131
Lipids................................129
Proteins.......................129, 371
...............................131, 371
Resistance Training....123, 127, 132, 134, 169, 276, 398, 399, 401
Responsibility Agreement....380
Resting Metabolic Rate (RMR) 134

Retinoic Acid....................207
Retinol.............206, 207, 208
Riboflavin....18, 133, 141, 197, 198, 199, 200
Riboflavin (B2) Deficiency.....201
Riboflavin (B2) Roles...........201
Riboflavin (B2) Toxicity.........201
Riboflavin Roles..................200
Rickets 175, 206, 210, 211, 212
RNA.......2, 8, 9, 217, 236, 251

S

Saccharin................51, 52, 53
Saliva..........................35, 81
Salivary Glands...............6, 35
Sarcopenia................398, 399
Saturated Fatty Acids....12, 20, 71, 72
Scientific Method..............308
Scurvy.............200, 205, 206
Selenium......19, 228, 239, 245
Kashin-Beck Disease............245
Selenium Deficiency............245
Selenium Roles...................245
Selenium Toxicity................245
Serotonin..................96, 204
Sibutramine.....................281
Skeletal Muscle 3, 98, 100, 122, 123, 124, 126, 229, 238, 246, 274, 276
Small Intestine..4, 6, 7, 35, 46, 49, 59, 81, 82, 101, 175, 204, 228, 240, 251, 442
SMART Rule......................355
Smooth Muscle.....................3
Sodium....18, 20, 81, 101, 166, 167, 230, 232, 234, 437, 440
Sodium Deficiency...............235
Sodium Toxicity...................235
Soluble Fiber.................46, 47
Sorbitol................52, 54, 178
Soy Protein. 103, 105, 109, 130
Sphincter.....................5, 178
Sports Drinks.....273, 290, 415
Stages of Readiness to Change 348
Starch.........10, 11, 34, 35, 43
State Licensure Laws.........339
Steroids......80, 270, 273, 274, 275, 286
High Blood Pressure............275
Sterol....................11, 68, 80
Stevia....................51, 52, 53
Stomach 4, 5, 6, 35, 46, 49, 50, 81, 86, 100, 124, 204, 213, 230, 278, 280, 281, 445
Stress....16, 38, 122, 123, 124, 139, 158, 353, 380, 381, 408, 422
Stress Eating....................449
Stroke. 46, 150, 151, 153, 158, 159, 161, 162, 163, 165, 168, 169, 170, 171, 172, 280, 281, 369, 388
Study Design....................315
Sucralose.....................51, 52
Sugar Alcohol 52, 54, 442, 443, 467
Sulfur.......9, 13, 200, 230, 236
Sulfur Deficiencies...............236
Sulfur Roles........................236
Sulfur Toxicities..................236
Supplement Categories..........
Botanicals..........................270
Ergogenic Aids.....................273
Vitamins - Minerals.............272
Supplements....................265
Claims..............................268
ConsumerLab.com...............283
Definitions/Regulations.........267
Is It Effective.......................286
Is It Required......................287
Is It Safe...........................285
Multivitamin 287
NSF..................................283
Office of Dietary Supplements 266
Position Stand....................289
Safety...............................270
Side Effects........................287
Standardization...................269
Supplement Categories.........270
Supplement Label................268
USP..................................284
Verification Programs...........283
...............................282, 283
Sweeteners.......................51
Nonnutritive Sweeteners...51, 52
Nonnutritive Sweeteners 51
Nutritive Sweeteners...51, 52, 54

T

TCA.................116, 118, 119
TEE...............................136
Testosterone..80, 81, 123, 126, 274, 275
Tetrahydrofolate (THF) 203, 217
Thermic Effect of Food.......135
Calories............................135
Thiamin. 18, 50, 198, 199, 200, 201
Thiamin Roles....................201
Thiamin Deficiency........200, 201
Thiamin Toxicity...........200, 201
Thiamin Pyrophosphate (TPP) 201, 216
Thyroid..........16, 95, 243, 252
Tolerable Upper Intake Level (UL).......17, 28, 199, 235, 238
Trace Minerals.......................
Chromium....13, 17, 19, 28, 239, 248
Copper 13, 19, 28, 239, 243, 246
Fluoride.............................239
Iodine.......13, 19, 228, 239, 243
Iron...........13, 18, 96, 133, 238
Manganese. 13, 17, 19, 239, 247, 252
Molybdenum 17, 19, 28, 239, 249
Selenium...13, 19, 228, 239, 245
Zinc 19, 133, 208, 238, 239, 242, 243, 288
.......................................247
Trans Fatty Acid.................72
Transamination...................13
transport....................7, 9, 33
Triglyceride. 11, 41, 69, 83, 160
Tryptophan..................96, 98
Tyrosine.........96, 98, 100, 102

U

U.S. Pharmacopeia.....284, 285
Ulcerative Colitis 175, 177, 178, 185
Unsaturated Fatty Acid. .71, 72, 74

USDA. .19, 21, 23, 24, 28, 166, 214, 218, 288, 326, 391, 392, 400, 432, 434, 435, 437, 441, 466, 467

V

Vascular System..................7
Vegetarian...21, 103, 109, 133, 141, 168, 184, 205, 401
Calcium............................133
Iron...........................133, 141
Riboflavin...........................133
Vitamin B12.................133, 205
Vitamin D...........................133
Zinc.......................13, 133, 402
Vein.................7, 8, 157, 182
Vitamin A....18, 197, 206, 207, 286
Vitamin A Deficiency.............208
Vitamin A Roles...................208
Vitamin A Toxicity.........208, 286
Vitamin B12...18, 50, 133, 199, 203, 204, 406
Vitamin B12 Deficiency.........204
Vitamin B12 Roles................204
Vitamin B12 Toxicity.............204
Vitamin B6...18, 162, 197, 199, 200, 204
Vitamin B6 - Toxicity 204
Vitamin B6 Deficiency...........204
Vitamin B6 Roles..................204
Vitamin C....13, 161, 199, 200, 205, 241, 246, 402
Vitamin C - Deficiency..........206
Vitamin C - Toxicity.............206
Vitamin C Deficiency............206
Vitamin C Roles..................205
Vitamin C Toxicity................206
Vitamins - Water Soluble........13
Vitamin D......18, 81, 133, 176, 206, 209, 210, 211, 212, 290
Vitamin D Roles..................210
Vitamin D Deficiency............211
Vitamin D Toxicity 211
Vitamin E 18, 78, 206, 213, 218
Vitamin E Deficiency............213
Vitamin E Roles....................213
Vitamin E Toxicity................213
Vitamin K...........18, 207, 214
Menaquinone.......................214
Phylloquinone......................214
Vitamin K Deficiency.............214
Vitamin K Roles...................214
Vitamin K Toxicity................214
Vitamins..............................
B Vitamins13, 50, 198, 199, 200, 216, 217, 237, 251

W

Waist-to-hip Ratio.....171, 367, 368, 408
Water. .9, 10, 14, 25, 131, 227, 228, 229, 273
Water Soluble Vitamins...........
B Vitamins.13, 50, 199, 200, 202
Vitamin C 18, 161, 199, 200, 205
Weight Loss Supplements........
Acai...................................279
Bitter Orange.......................279
Ephedra.............................280
Green Tea...........................281
Sibutramine.........................281
.......................................279
Wheat......42, 43, 48, 106, 247
whole grain..............432, 433

Z

Zinc......13, 19, 133, 208, 238, 239, 242, 288
Absorption..................242, 243
Athletic Population..............401
Vegetarian Population...........401
Zinc Absorption....................402
Zinc Deficiency....................242
Zinc Roles...........................242
Zinc Toxicity........................242
.......................................401

CPSIA information can be obtained at www.ICGtesting.com
Printed in the USA
LVOW02*2353110315

430087LV00003B/7/P